HOST RESPONSE TO BIOMATERIALS

HOST RESPONSE TO BIOMATERIALS

THE IMPACT OF HOST RESPONSE ON BIOMATERIAL SELECTION

Edited by

STEPHEN F. BADYLAK

Department of Surgery, McGowan Institute for
Regenerative Medicine, University of Pittsburgh, PA, USA

AMSTERDAM • BOSTON • HEIDELBERG • LONDON
NEW YORK • OXFORD • PARIS • SAN DIEGO
SAN FRANCISCO • SINGAPORE • SYDNEY • TOKYO

Academic Press is an imprint of Elsevier

Academic Press is an imprint of Elsevier
125, London Wall, EC2Y 5AS
525 B Street, Suite 1800, San Diego, CA 92101-4495, USA
225 Wyman Street, Waltham, MA 02451, USA
The Boulevard, Langford Lane, Kidlington, Oxford OX5 1GB, UK

Notices
Knowledge and best practice in this field are constantly changing. As new research and experience broaden our understanding, changes in research methods, professional practices, or medical treatment may become necessary.

Practitioners and researchers must always rely on their own experience and knowledge in evaluating and using any information, methods, compounds, or experiments described herein. In using such information or methods they should be mindful of their own safety and the safety of others, including parties for whom they have a professional responsibility.

To the fullest extent of the law, neither the Publisher nor the authors, contributors, or editors, assume any liability for any injury and/or damage to persons or property as a matter of products liability, negligence or otherwise, or from any use or operation of any methods, products, instructions, or ideas contained in the material herein.

ISBN: 978-0-12-800196-7

British Library Cataloguing-in-Publication Data
A catalogue record for this book is available from the British Library

Library of Congress Cataloging-in-Publication Data
A catalog record for this book is available from the Library of Congress

For information on all Academic Press publications
visit our website at http://store.elsevier.com/

Typeset by MPS Limited, Chennai, India
www.adi-mps.com

Printed and bound in the United States

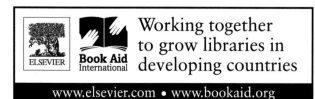

CONTENTS

LIST OF CONTRIBUTORS

Steven D. Abramowitch
Department of Bioengineering, University of Pittsburgh, Pittsburgh, PA, USA; Magee-Womens Research Institute, University of Pittsburgh, Pittsburgh, PA, USA

James Anderson
Department of Pathology and Biomedical Engineering, Case Western Reserve University, Cleveland, OH, USA

Mahender N. Avula
Department of Bioengineering, University of Utah, UT, USA; Research and Development, Catheter Connections, Inc., Salt Lake City, UT, USA

Stephen F. Badylak
Department of Surgery, University of Pittsburgh, Pittsburgh, PA, USA; McGowan Institute for Regenerative Medicine, University of Pittsburgh, Pittsburgh, PA, USA

David W. Baker
Bioengineering Department, University of Texas at Arlington, Arlington, TX, USA

William R. Barone
Department of Bioengineering, University of Pittsburgh, Pittsburgh, PA, USA

Bryan N. Brown
Department of Bioengineering, McGowan Institute for Regenerative Medicine, University of Pittsburgh, Pittsburgh, PA, USA

Stephanie Cramer
Department of Biomedical Engineering, Case Western Reserve University, Cleveland, OH, USA

Jonathan M. Fishman
Honorary Clinical Lecturer University College London, UCL Institute of Child Health, London, UK

Maria Rosaria Galdiero
Division of Clinical Immunology and Allergy, University of Naples Federico II, Naples, Italy; Humanitas Clinical and Research Hospital, Rozzano, Milan, Italy

Uri Galili
Department of Surgery, University of Massachusetts Medical School, Worcester, MA, USA

Stuart Goodman
Department of Orthopaedic Surgery, Stanford University, Stanford, CA, USA; Department of Bioengineering, Stanford University, Stanford, CA, USA

David W. Grainger
Department of Bioengineering, University of Utah, UT, USA; Research and Development, Catheter Connections, Inc., Salt Lake City, UT, USA; Department of Pharmaceutics and Pharmaceutical Chemistry; Early Development Analytics Department, Alcon Laboratories, Inc., Norcross, GA, USA

Kim Jones
Department of Chemical Engineering and School of Biomedical Engineering, McMaster University, Hamilton, ON, Canada

Benjamin G. Keselowsky
J. Crayton Pruitt Family Department of Biomedical Engineering, University of Florida, Gainesville, FL, USA

Themis R. Kyriakides
Department of Biomedical Engineering, Yale University, New Haven, CT, USA

Jamal S. Lewis
J. Crayton Pruitt Family Department of Biomedical Engineering, University of Florida, Gainesville, FL, USA

Tzu–Hua Lin
Department of Orthopaedic Surgery, Stanford University, Stanford, CA, USA

Ricardo Londono
McGowan Institute for Regenerative Medicine, University of Pittsburgh, Pittsburgh, PA, USA; School of Medicine, University of Pittsburgh, Pittsburgh, PA, USA

Samuel T. Lopresti
Department of Bioengineering, McGowan Institute for Regenerative Medicine, University of Pittsburgh, Pittsburgh, PA, USA

Alberto Mantovani
Humanitas University, Rozzano, Milan, Italy; Humanitas Clinical and Research Hospital, Rozzano, Milan, Italy

Pamela A. Moalli
Magee-Womens Research Institute, University of Pittsburgh, Pittsburgh, PA, USA

Jukka Pajarinen
Department of Orthopaedic Surgery, Stanford University, Stanford, CA, USA

Archana N. Rao
Department of Pharmaceutics and Pharmaceutical Chemistry; Early Development Analytics Department, Alcon Laboratories, Inc., Norcross, GA, USA

Buddy D. Ratner
Department of Bioengineering, University of Washington, Seattle, WA, USA

Taishi Sato
Department of Orthopaedic Surgery, Stanford University, Stanford, CA, USA

Liping Tang
Bioengineering Department, University of Texas at Arlington, Arlington, TX, USA

Katherine Wiles
Department of Surgery, UCL Institute of Child Health, London, UK

Kathryn J. Wood
Transplantation Research Immunology Group, Nuffield Department of Surgical Sciences, University of Oxford John Radcliffe Hospital Headley Way, Headington, Oxford, UK

Zhenyu Yao
Department of Orthopaedic Surgery, Stanford University, Stanford, CA, USA

Jun Zhou
Bioengineering Department, University of Texas at Arlington, Arlington, TX, USA

FOREWORD

The evolution and emergence of new biomaterials, medical devices, and prostheses is continuously marked by disruptive technology and innovation; however, success or failure in the clinical setting is ultimately dependent upon the host response following *in vivo* placement. Therefore, an understanding of the host response to biomaterials is both timely and necessary. This text provides an understanding of our current knowledge of the host response and identifies areas of ongoing research that will play a significant role in not only our further understanding of the response to biomaterials but also provide design criteria for new biomaterials. The respective chapters in this text target specific types of responses, but overall the text provides a basis for current and future understanding of the following: factors that promote implant success; rates, patterns, and mechanisms of implant failure; effects of patient and medical device factors on performance; the determination of dynamics, temporal variations, and mechanisms of tissue–material interactions; future design criteria for medical devices; and the determination of the adequacy and appropriateness of animal models.

Many factors may play a role in the failure or success of medical devices, e.g., blood/material interactions or mechanical property mismatch, but the host response will continue to be the most significant factor in determining downstream clinical efficacy.

While many implant failures can be characterized as implant- or material-dependent or clinically or biologically dependent, many modes and mechanisms of failure are dependent on both implant and biological factors. This text focuses on biological factors in the context of the host responses and provides not only an understanding of our current knowledge of this response but also relevant information for the safety (biocompatibility), efficacy (function), and the future design and development of next generation biomaterials, medical devices, and prostheses.

Dr. James Anderson
Department of Pathology and Biomedical Engineering,
Case Western Reserve University, Cleveland, OH, USA

PREFACE

This textbook is intended to be a resource and guide for biomaterial scientists, tissue engineers, biomedical engineering instructors and students, and importantly, for clinicians and surgeons with an interest in understanding the factors that influence the host (patient) response to biomaterials. There are many textbooks and journals that describe and characterize the physical, mechanical, and material properties of biomaterials, and great effort is expended in customizing the properties of biomaterials for specific clinical applications. Although these characteristics are certainly important, they are typically relevant only at the time of implantation since the host begins an immediate and relentless response to the presence of any foreign material. The integrity of these biomaterial properties at 6 months, 1 year, 10 years and beyond will ultimately determine clinical success. The host response to the biomaterials following implantation is clearly the driving factor in determining eventual success (or failure).

The host response is dependent upon a combination of factors including surgical technique, biomaterial properties, host factors, and an understanding of the innate and acquired immune systems when designing biomaterials. This textbook provides the perspective of experts within each of these disciplines. Exposure to different viewpoints regarding host response is important, and attempts have been made to identify where differences in opinion exist. The chapter by David Grainger describes the effects of age-related factors upon the host response. The concept of biocompatibility is addressed in Chapters 2 and 3 by Drs. James Anderson and Buddy Ratner, respectively, but is also discussed in numerous other chapters since it is such a fundamental concept and in some ways synonymous with the host response. The role of dendritic cells, the innate immune system, and the acquired immune system are covered by Drs. Keselowsky, Mantovani, and Wood, respectively. The surgical perspective of the clinical disciplines within orthopedics and urogynecologic surgery is provided by Drs. Goodman and Moalli in Chapters 12 and 13, respectively. Drs. Kyriakides and Tang discuss the important concepts of protein deposition on the surface of biomaterials and methods for evaluating various aspects of the host response.

This textbook is certainly not exhaustive since the breadth of disciplines involved in the host response is great. However, it is hoped that the contents of this book provide a useful guide and stimulate further investigation and discussion of the host response to biomaterials.

Stephen F. Badylak
Department of Surgery, McGowan Institute for Regenerative Medicine,
University of Pittsburgh, PA, USA

ACKNOWLEDGMENTS

I would like to acknowledge several individuals for their assistance in making this textbook a reality.

First, my wife Sherry for her patience and understanding of the time commitment in completing this work.

Second, a big thank you to Allyson LaCovey for her organizational skills and editing assistance.

And finally, the students and faculty of the McGowan Institute for their support and willingness to answer endless questions, provide images and artwork, and give unbiased feedback from start to finish.

CHAPTER 1

Factors Which Affect the Host Response to Biomaterials

Ricardo Londono[1,2] and Stephen F. Badylak[1,3]
[1]McGowan Institute for Regenerative Medicine, University of Pittsburgh, Pittsburgh, PA, USA
[2]School of Medicine, University of Pittsburgh, Pittsburgh, PA, USA
[3]Department of Surgery, University of Pittsburgh, Pittsburgh, PA, USA

Contents

INTRODUCTION

The ability of a biomaterial to perform its intended *in vivo* function is dependent on many factors including its composition, mechanical and material properties, surface topography and molecular landscape, ability to resist infection, and proper surgical placement, among others. However, the ultimate determinant of success or failure is the host response to the biomaterial.

The host response begins immediately upon implantation and consists of both the response to the inevitable iatrogenic tissue injury during device placement and the response to the material itself. In most cases, the implantation-induced component resolves quickly as part of the normal wound healing process. However, the response to the material will last for the length of time the material is present in the host. Materials which elicit a persistent proinflammatory response are likely to be associated with abundant fibrous connective tissue deposition and the downstream consequences of the effector molecules secreted by recruited inflammatory cells. Materials which

Host Response to Biomaterials.
DOI: http://dx.doi.org/10.1016/B978-0-12-800196-7.00001-3

Table 1.1 Host-related and biomaterial-related factors which affect the host response and chapters in which they are discussed
Factors that affect the host response to biomaterials

Biomaterial-related factors	Chapters	Host-related factors	Chapters
Composition (material)	2, 3	Age	11
Degradability	3	Anatomic location	12, 13, 14
Mechanical properties		Previous interventions	14
Sterility		Comorbidities	
Antigenicity	4, 5, 8, 10	Immune response	2, 6, 7, 8, 9
Active ingredients (drugs)		Medications	

either rapidly degrade or reach a steady state of tolerance with adjacent host tissue (see Chapter 3) are typically associated with minimal scarring, a quiescent population of resident inflammatory cells, and tissue types appropriate for the anatomic location.

The host response to an implanted material includes factors that relate to the biomaterial itself and factors that relate to the host (Table 1.1). Biomaterial-related factors have been the focus of studies for many years. Such factors include the base composition of the material (e.g., polypropylene versus polytetrafluoroethylene versus extracellular matrix), surface texture, surface ligand landscape, degradability, and device design parameters such as pore and fiber size, among others. Host-related factors, on the other hand, have been underappreciated as a determinant of the response. These factors include age, nutritional status, body mass index, comorbidities such as diabetes, previous interventions at the treatment site, and medications being taken by the patient, among others. No biomaterial is inert and the interplay between material and host-related factors should be considered in the design and manufacture of all biomaterials.

BIOMATERIAL–HOST INTERACTION

Although the physical and mechanical properties of a material at the time of implantation are important for obvious reasons, these properties are equally important at 1 month, 1 year, 5 years, and beyond, especially for those materials intended to remain *in situ* for the life span of the patient. The host response can degrade, destroy, encapsulate, or otherwise alter the composition of the biomaterial over time resulting in changes to the form and mechanical properties of the material itself (Figure 1.1) (Badylak, 2014). Hence, it is not the degree to which the physical characteristics of the material resemble the targeted anatomic location before implantation that determines the performance of a biomaterial, but rather the host response over time.

The host response is initiated with the activation of the innate immune system as a result of cell and tissue damage during biomaterial implantation (see Chapters 2, 3, 4). Upon contact with the host tissues, the surface of the biomaterial is coated with blood and plasma proteins through a process known as the Vroman effect (Slack et al., 1987).

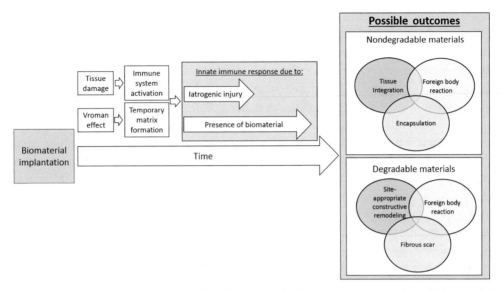

Figure 1.1 *Host response to biomaterial implantation.* The host response to implanted biomaterials depends upon many factors. Although the initial stages of the biomaterial–host interaction are shared among all materials and include tissue damage during implantation and protein adsorption to the surface of the material, the host response quickly transitions into complex phases that depend directly upon the type of material being implanted and other factors. These phases involve cellular and molecular components of the innate immune system and the wound healing response, and will ultimately determine the clinical outcome (i.e., encapsulation vs. scar formation vs. constructive remodeling).

Depending on the type of biomaterial and surface topography (i.e., type I collagen vs. polytetrafluoroethylene vs. titanium), the type and amount of adsorbed molecules will vary, and consequently, so will the composition and arrangement of the interface molecules that exist between the host tissues and the implant.

As a result of the Vroman effect, host cells typically do not interact directly with the surface of the biomaterial but rather with the adsorbed protein layer. This protein layer—sometimes in conjunction with clot formation during hemostasis—forms a temporary matrix that bridges and mediates the interaction between the host tissues and the biomaterial. With degradable materials (e.g., non-cross-linked biologic scaffolds, poly(lactic-co-glycolic acid), polyglactin), this temporary matrix serves as a bridge that facilitates cellular access and promotes infiltration toward or into the material. With nondegradable biomaterials (e.g., permanent titanium alloy implants, polypropylene), the adsorbed protein layer serves as an interface that provides sites for cell attachment and mediates the interaction between the host and the implanted construct.

Within minutes of implantation, the cellular response becomes predominated by neutrophils at the host–biomaterial interface. The neutrophil response peaks within 48–72 h after implantation and is the hallmark of the acute innate immune response. In addition to eliminating pathogens that may be present at the treatment site, neutrophils play important roles in the immune response such as establishment of signaling gradients that attract and activate other components of the innate immune system (Wang and Arase, 2014), initiation of granulation tissue formation, and in the case of degradable biomaterials, secretion of enzymes such as collagenases and serine proteases (Nauseef and Borregaard, 2014) that initiate the process of biomaterial degradation and remodeling of the treatment site (Londono and Badylak, 2014).

As a result of signaling gradients established by neutrophils, the innate immune response transitions to a macrophage dominant infiltrate that slowly replaces the accumulated neutrophils at the host–biomaterial interface. The type and magnitude of the macrophage response will depend primarily on the material and host factors identified in Table 1.1. Degradable biologic materials placed in anatomic locations within healthy, vascularized tissue can degrade within weeks (Carey et al., 2014; Record et al., 2001) and promote a pro-remodeling M2 macrophage-associated response that leads to functional, site-appropriate tissue deposition (Badylak et al., 2011; Sicari et al., 2014). Alternatively, certain types of synthetic biomaterials can promote pro-inflammatory processes that will lead to the foreign body reaction, scar tissue formation, and chronic inflammatory processes associated with an M1 macrophage phenotype (Anderson et al., 2008; Klinge et al., 1999; Leber et al., 1998). Permanent, nondegradable biomaterials, such as metallic plates or screws, typically lead to a foreign body reaction as a result of "frustrated phagocytosis" and can promote inflammation, seroma formation, and eventually encapsulation. The degree to which each type of response is deemed acceptable will depend upon the type and specific performance expectations of the biomaterial in each given anatomic location (e.g., temporary orthopedic support vs. functional organ replacement vs. tissue fillers in reconstructive applications).

HOST FACTORS

Host factors that affect the biomaterial–host interaction are typically underappreciated, and as a result, have not been thoroughly evaluated in the context of patient outcomes. As stated previously, the initial host response to implanted biomaterials is primarily orchestrated by plasma proteins and the innate immune system. As such, any factors or underlying conditions that may affect these variables will inevitably alter the biomaterial–host interaction.

AGE

The aging process affects every organ system and associated functions including immunocompetence. In fact, immunosenescence is thought to be one of the major predisposing factors to increased incidence of infection in older individuals (Hazeldine and Lord, 2014). Some of the most important age-related changes in the cellular component of the innate immune system are summarized in Table 1.2.

The cellular component of the innate immune system and its role in responding to the presence of foreign materials is closely examined in Chapters 2, 3, and 6. Although absolute numbers of neutrophils and macrophages are not typically affected by aging, important functional changes including the ability to mobilize, establish chemical gradients, and phagocytize pathogens and foreign elements are usually observed with advanced age. These changes can affect the process of biomaterial-associated tissue repair by affecting material degradation, cell migration and proliferation, angiogenesis, neo-matrix deposition, and tissue remodeling.

In addition to affecting the immune system, the aging process alters adult stem cell function and behavior (Ludke et al., 2014; Oh et al., 2014). Stem cells are necessary for homeostasis and the wound healing response. These precursor cells maintain organ function and are necessary for tissue repair. In turn, therapeutic approaches that rely on

Table 1.2 Age-related changes of innate immunity

Effect of age in cellular component of innate immunity

Cell type	Changes in composition	Changes in function	References
Monocytes/ macrophages	No change in absolute number	Decreased phagocytosis	Hearps et al. (2012), McLachlan et al. (1995)
	No change in circulating frequency	Decreased ROS production	Nguyen et al. (2005), Qian et al. (2012)
	Increased percentage of CD14+ 16++ nonclassical monocytes	Increased TNF-α production via TLR-4	Seidler et al. (2010), van Duin et al. (2007)
	Reduced percentage of CD14+ 16− classical monocytes	Decreased IL-6 and TNF-α production via TLR1/2	
Neutrophils	No change in circulating numbers	Reduced chemotaxis *in vitro*	Born et al. (1995), Butcher et al. (2001)
	No change in CD11a, CD11b expression	Reduced phagocytosis	Fulop et al. (2004), Tseng et al. (2012)
		Impaired NET formation	Wenisch et al. (2000)
		Increased/decreased ROS formation	
		Impaired receptor recruitment into lipid rafts	

Source: Adapted from Hazeldine and Lord (2014).

Although the absolute and circulating numbers of neutrophils and monocytes/macrophages in the immune system are not typically affected by age, important changes including decrease phagocytosis, decreased chemotaxis, and decreased signaling molecule production are observed with age. In turn, these changes have the potential to negatively affect the host response to implanted biomaterials.

native stem cell populations (Sicari et al., 2014) for the organization of newly formed tissue will inevitably be affected by the aging process. Similar to changes associated with the innate immune system, aging does not appear to decrease the absolute number of stem cells, but instead, it impairs their capacity to produce and to differentiate into progenitor cells (Sharpless and DePinho, 2007). The effects of age on the host response to biomaterials is discussed more thoroughly in Chapter 11.

NUTRITIONAL STATUS

Malnutrition is a global problem with implications for the host–biomaterial interaction. Malnutrition can result in increased susceptibility to infections and comorbidities, impaired healing ability, altered metabolic state, and changes to the innate immune system that directly affect the interaction between the host and an implanted biomaterial (Table 1.3).

Table 1.3 Nutritional status-related changes to innate immune system
Effect of malnutrition in innate immunity

Parameter	References
Similar or elevated number of leukocytes	Hughes et al. (2009)
	Schopfer and Douglas (1976)
Elevated number of granulocytes	Najera et al. (2004)
	Schopfer and Douglas (1976)
Reduced granulocyte chemotaxis	Vasquez-Garibay et al. (2002)
	Vasquez-Garibay et al. (2004)
Reduced granulocyte adherence to foreign material	Goyal et al. (1981)
Reduced granulocyte microbicidal activity	Douglas and Schopfer (1974)
	Chhangani et al. (1985)
	Keusch et al. (1987)
Reduce leukocyte phagocytosis	Carvalho Neves Forte et al. (1984)
	Shousha and Kamel (1972)
	Schopfer and Douglas (1976)
Increased markers of apoptosis in leukocytes	Nassar et al. (2007)
Increased signs of DNA damage in leukocytes	Gonzalez et al. (2002)
Reduced levels or activity of complement system components	McFarlane (1971)
	Ozkan et al. (1993)
	Sakamoto et al. (1992)
	Kumar et al. (1984)
	Sirisinha et al. (1973)

Although malnutrition can increase the number of leukocytes and granulocytes, this phenomenon is attributed to an underlying chronic pro-inflammatory state due in part to increased susceptibility to infections. As with aging, malnutrition causes a decrease in functionality in the cells of the immune system. These changes affect the host–biomaterial interaction and include decreased chemotaxis, phagocytosis, and adherence among others.

ANATOMIC FACTORS

Biomaterials are used in virtually every anatomic location for a wide variety of clinical applications. Each anatomic site (e.g., vascular, musculotendinous, central nervous system, skin, GI tract, respiratory, pelvic floor reconstruction, bone and cartilage, and total joints) is associated with distinctive microenvironmental conditions such as an air interface, blood contact, and mechanical loading (Figure 1.2). In addition, tissue-specific physiologic requirements such as electrical conductivity, biosensing (e.g., glucose sensors, implantable cardioverter defibrillators), and load bearing will exist depending on the specific application. These environmental conditions affect the host response by providing stimuli (e.g., cyclic stretching, load bearing, laminar flow, presence of an interface, etc.) that directly affect cellular processes such as gene transcription, migration, and differentiation. These conditions necessarily dictate design parameters. For example, joint replacement implants must be strong enough to bear weight without breaking or deforming, vascular constructs should have luminal surfaces that prevent thrombus formation and improve blood flow, synthetic meshes used in hernia repair must possess

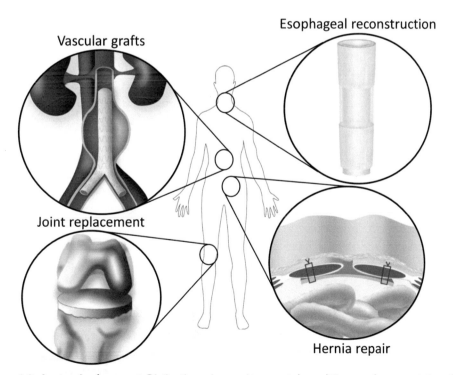

Figure 1.2 *Anatomic placement.* Distinctive microenvironmental conditions such as an air interface (esophagus), blood contact (vascular grafts), and mechanical loading (orthopedic and hernia repair applications) will dictate design parameters and play a role in the host response.

sufficient tensile strength to withstand the biomechanical forces exerted by and on the abdominal wall, and semipermeable membranes in dialysis and extra corporeal membrane oxygenation (ECMO) machines must selectively facilitate molecule traffic.

In addition to the different microenvironmental conditions, anatomic placement requirements include the state of the adjacent tissue (i.e., healthy and vascularized vs. contaminated and necrotic). Vascularized healthy tissue facilitates nutrient traffic and immune system access into the treatment site. Granulation tissue formation and angiogenesis are both important phases of the host response to biomaterials, and both processes depend on the state of the surrounding tissue and the microenvironment. Furthermore, contaminated biomaterials can often lead to a number of complications including abscess formation, sepsis, need for subsequent revisions, and ultimately failure of the application.

COMORBIDITIES

The host response is affected by a number of underlying pathologic conditions, particularly those which affect the immune system, wound healing ability, stem cell viability, and/or the state of the tissues adjacent to the treatment site.

Obesity

Data from the National Health and Nutrition Examination Survey, 2009–2010 (Flegal et al., 2012; Ogden et al., 2012) indicates that more than two in three adults are considered overweight or obese in the United States. Obesity is a risk factor for type 2 diabetes and cardiovascular disease, and both obesity and diabetes are now recognized as pro-inflammatory diseases (Osborn and Olefsky, 2012). Although the inflammatory state present in these conditions is distinct from that of acute inflammation (Kraakman et al., 2014), there are a number of implications for the field of biomaterial-mediated tissue repair that have been often ignored in preclinical and clinical studies.

Inflammation is a fundamental component of the host response to implanted biomaterials. The innate immune system modulates the wound healing response and is a key mediator and determinant of the clinical outcome of biomaterial implantation (Figure 1.1). Immune cells, particularly neutrophils and macrophages are the main effectors in most biomaterial applications. As first responders, neutrophils clear pathogens and establish chemical gradients that affect later stages of biomaterial–host interaction. Macrophages, on the other hand, display phenotypic heterogeneity and are responsible for both positive and negative events during biomaterial-mediated tissue repair. Macrophage phenotype has been shown to be predictive of clinical outcome in the context of biologically derived biomaterials. While the presence of M1 macrophages is associated with pro-inflammatory processes including foreign body reaction, cytotoxicity, and biomaterial encapsulation, M2 macrophages are associated with constructive tissue remodeling and site-appropriate tissue deposition. Obesity has been tightly associated with M1 macrophage accumulation within adipose tissue and other organs (Kraakman et al., 2014; Weisberg et al., 2003; Xu et al., 2003). In addition, obesity has also been shown to increase pro-inflammatory molecule production (Hotamisligil et al., 1993). Hence, obesity and other underlying conditions that may promote proinflammatory environments should be taken into account when considering biomaterials as possible treatment options. A thorough discussion of the role of inflammation in the host response can be found in Chapters 2, 3, 6, 7, and 8.

Diabetes

Diabetes mellitus, a condition that affects an estimated 29 million patients in the United States and an additional 86 million prediabetic patients (Centers for Disease Control and Prevention, 2014), is among the most overlooked factors that can affect the host–biomaterial interaction. Diabetes mellitus is considered a pro-inflammatory disease (Kraakman et al., 2014) that increases susceptibility to infections and bacteremia in the acute setting and can cause vascular deterioration and diabetic ulcers chronically.

Increased susceptibility to infections and bacteremia are risk factors for bacterial engraftment on artificial heart valves and in synthetic vascular grafts, and both conditions are independent risk factors for infective endocarditis (Chirouze et al., 2014; Klein and Wang, 2014). Once engrafted, bacteria can cause artificial heart valve dysfunction, abscess formation, and sepsis. In the case of degradable materials, bacterial contamination can affect degradation rates and compromise the biomechanical properties of the biomaterial. In fact, when the surgical field is contaminated, biomaterials derived from biologic sources are indicated for use over synthetic biomaterials due in part to their antimicrobial properties. If contamination persists, further interventions including revisions and abscess drainage are required. The clinical performance of biomaterials has consistently been suboptimal once these events have occurred.

CHEMOTHERAPY AND RADIATION THERAPY

Tissue defects resulting from neoplastic tissue resection are one of the indications for biomaterial use in tissue repair. A number of these applications rely on either endogenous or exogenous cell proliferation for the purposes of tissue repair and/or organ function restoration. However, due to the nature of neoplastic disease, both chemotherapy and radiation therapy target rapidly dividing cells populations at systemic and local levels, respectively. Thus, biomaterial-based therapies that rely on cell proliferation will inevitably be affected when used in conjunction with chemotherapy and/or radiation therapy. In addition to affecting rapidly dividing cell populations, there are a number of consequences that can result from these therapies that also affect the biomaterial–host interaction. While patients subjected to chemotherapy often present with anorexia and immune system dysfunction, localized radiation therapy affects the integrity of adjacent tissues and the microenvironment causing necrosis and scar tissue formation.

DESIGN CONSIDERATIONS

The distinctive microenvironmental conditions in the host and the clinical performance expectations of each application must be taken into consideration during biomaterial design. No biomaterial is biologically inert, and while it might be acceptable for constructs intended for temporary use to be merely biotolerable, biomaterials intended for use in more complex applications—including those requiring functional tissue/organ replacement and/or constructive tissue remodeling—will inevitably have to adhere to more stringent criteria.

The host response is the primary determinant of clinical success in all applications. Hence, the safety and efficacy of these technologies will be better served by placing emphasis upon understanding the host response and the dynamic interaction between biomaterial- and host-related factors that affect clinical outcomes.

REFERENCES

Anderson, J.M., Rodriguez, A., Chang, D.T., 2008. Foreign body reaction to biomaterials. Semin. Immunol. 20 (2), 86–100.

Badylak, S.F., 2014. Decellularized allogeneic and xenogeneic tissue as a bioscaffold for regenerative medicine: factors that influence the host response. Ann. Biomed. Eng. 42 (7), 1517–1527.

Badylak, S.F., Hoppo, T., Nieponice, A., Gilbert, T.W., Davison, J.M., Jobe, B.A., 2011. Esophageal preservation in five male patients after endoscopic inner-layer circumferential resection in the setting of superficial cancer: a regenerative medicine approach with a biologic scaffold. Tissue Eng. Part A 17 (11–12), 1643–1650.

Born, J., Uthgenannt, D., Dodt, C., Nunninghoff, D., Ringvolt, E., Wagner, T., et al., 1995. Cytokine production and lymphocyte subpopulations in aged humans. An assessment during nocturnal sleep. Mech. Ageing Dev. 84 (2), 113–126.

Butcher, S.K., Chahal, H., Nayak, L., Sinclair, A., Henriquez, N.V., Sapey, E., et al., 2001. Senescence in innate immune responses: reduced neutrophil phagocytic capacity and cd16 expression in elderly humans. J. Leukoc. Biol. 70 (6), 881–886.

Carey, L.E., Dearth, C.L., Johnson, S.A., Londono, R., Medberry, C.J., Daly, K.A., et al., 2014. In vivo degradation of 14c-labeled porcine dermis biologic scaffold. Biomaterials 35 (29), 8297–8304.

Centers for Disease Control and Prevention. 2014. National Diabetes Statistics Report: Estimates of Diabetes and Its Burden in the United States, 2014. Atlanta GA: U.S. Department of Health and Human Services; 2014.

Carvalho Neves Forte, W., Martins Campos, J.V., Carneiro Leao, R., 1984. Non specific immunological response in moderate malnutrition. Allergol. Immunopathol. (Madr) 12 (6), 489–496.

Chhangani, L., Sharma, M.L., Sharma, U.B., Joshi, N., 1985. In vitro study of phagocytic and bactericidal activity of neutrophils in cases of protein energy malnutrition. Indian J. Pathol. Microbiol. 28 (3), 199–203.

Chirouze, C., Hoen, B., Duval, X., 2014. Infective endocarditis epidemiology and consequences of prophylaxis guidelines modifications: the dialectical evolution. Curr. Infect. Dis. Rep. 16 (11), 440.

Douglas, S.D., Schopfer, K., 1974. Phagocyte function in protein-calorie malnutrition. Clin. Exp. Immunol. 17 (1), 121–128.

Flegal, K.M., Carroll, M.D., Kit, B.K., Ogden, C.L., 2012. Prevalence of obesity and trends in the distribution of body mass index among us adults, 1999–2010. JAMA 307 (5), 491–497.

Fulop, T., Larbi, A., Douziech, N., Fortin, C., Guerard, K.P., Lesur, O., et al., 2004. Signal transduction and functional changes in neutrophils with aging. Aging Cell 3 (4), 217–226.

Gonzalez, C., Najera, O., Cortes, E., Toledo, G., Lopez, L., Betancourt, M., et al., 2002. Hydrogen peroxide-induced DNA damage and DNA repair in lymphocytes from malnourished children. Environ. Mol. Mutagen. 39 (1), 33–42.

Goyal, H.K., Kaushik, S.K., Dhamieja, J.P., Suman, R.K., Kumar, K.K., 1981. A Study of granulocyte adherence in protein calorie malnutrition. Indian Pediatr. 18 (5), 287–292.

Hazeldine, J., Lord, J.M., 2014. Innate immunesenescence: underlying mechanisms and clinical relevance. Biogerontology.

Hearps, A.C., Martin, G.E., Angelovich, T.A., Cheng, W.J., Maisa, A., Landay, A.L., et al., 2012. Aging is associated with chronic innate immune activation and dysregulation of monocyte phenotype and function. Aging Cell 11 (5), 867–875.

Hotamisligil, G.S., Shargill, N.S., Spiegelman, B.M., 1993. Adipose expression of tumor necrosis factor-alpha: direct role in obesity-linked insulin resistance. Science 259 (5091), 87–91.

Hughes, S.M., Amadi, B., Mwiya, M., Nkamba, H., Tomkins, A., Goldblatt, D., 2009. Dendritic cell anergy results from endotoxemia in severe malnutrition. J. Immunol. 183 (4), 2818–2826.

Keusch, G.T., Cruz, J.R., Torun, B., Urrutia, J.J., Smith Jr., H., Goldstein, A.L., 1987. Immature circulating lymphocytes in severely malnourished guatemalan children. J. Pediatr. Gastroenterol. Nutr. 6 (2), 265–270.

Klein, M., Wang, A., 2014. Infective endocarditis. J. Intensive. Care Med.

Klinge, U., Klosterhalfen, B., Muller, M., Schumpelick, V., 1999. Foreign body reaction to meshes used for the repair of abdominal wall hernias. Eur. J. Surg. 165 (7), 665–673.

Kraakman, M.J., Murphy, A.J., Jandeleit-Dahm, K., Kammoun, H.L., 2014. Macrophage polarization in obesity and type 2 diabetes: weighing down our understanding of macrophage function? Front. Immunol. 5, 470.

Kumar, R., Kumar, A., Sethi, R.S., Gupta, R.K., Kaushik, A.K., Longia, S., 1984. A Study of complement activity in malnutrition. Indian Pediatr. 21 (7), 541–547.

Leber, G.E., Garb, J.L., Alexander, A.I., Reed, W.P., 1998. Long-term complications associated with prosthetic repair of incisional hernias. Arch. Surg. 133 (4), 378–382.

Londono, R., Badylak, S.F., 2014. Biologic scaffolds for regenerative medicine: mechanisms of in vivo remodeling. Ann. Biomed. Eng.

Ludke, A., Li, R.K., Weisel, R.D., 2014. The rejuvenation of aged stem cells for cardiac repair. Can. J. Cardiol.

McFarlane, H., 1971. Cell-mediated immunity in protein-calorie malnutrition. Lancet 2 (7734), 1146–1147.

McLachlan, J.A., Serkin, C.D., Morrey, K.M., Bakouche, O., 1995. Antitumoral properties of aged human monocytes. J. Immunol. 154 (2), 832–843.

Najera, O., Gonzalez, C., Toledo, G., Lopez, L., Ortiz, R., 2004. Flow cytometry study of lymphocyte subsets in malnourished and well-nourished children with bacterial infections. Clin. Diagn. Lab. Immunol. 11 (3), 577–580.

Nassar, M.F., Younis, N.T., Tohamy, A.G., Dalam, D.M., El Badawy, M.A., 2007. T-Lymphocyte subsets and thymic size in malnourished infants in egypt: a hospital-based study. East Mediterr. Health J. 13 (5), 1031–1042.

Nauseef, W.M., Borregaard, N., 2014. Neutrophils at work. Nat. Immunol. 15 (7), 602–611.

Nguyen, M., Pace, A.J., Koller, B.H., 2005. Age-induced reprogramming of mast cell degranulation. J. Immunol. 175 (9), 5701–5707.

Ogden, C.L., Carroll, M.D., Kit, B.K., Flegal, K.M., 2012. Prevalence of obesity and trends in body mass index among us children and adolescents, 1999–2010. JAMA 307 (5), 483–490.

Oh, J., Lee, Y.D., Wagers, A.J., 2014. Stem cell aging: mechanisms, regulators and therapeutic opportunities. Nat. Med. 20 (8), 870–880.

Osborn, O., Olefsky, J.M., 2012. The cellular and signaling networks linking the immune system and metabolism in disease. Nat. Med. 18 (3), 363–374.

Ozkan, H., Olgun, N., Sasmaz, E., Abacioglu, H., Okuyan, M., Cevik, N., 1993. Nutrition, immunity and infections: T lymphocyte subpopulations in protein--energy malnutrition. J. Trop. Pediatr. 39 (4), 257–260.

Qian, F., Wang, X., Zhang, L., Chen, S., Piecychna, M., Allore, H., et al., 2012. Age-associated elevation in Tlr5 leads to increased inflammatory responses in the elderly. Aging Cell 11 (1), 104–110.

Record, R.D., Hillegonds, D., Simmons, C., Tullius, R., Rickey, F.A., Elmore, D., et al., 2001. In Vivo degradation of 14c-labeled Small intestinal submucosa (Sis) when used for urinary bladder repair. Biomaterials 22 (19), 2653–2659.

Sakamoto, M., Nishioka, K., 1992. Complement system in nutritional deficiency. World Rev. Nutr. Diet. 67, 114–139.

Schopfer, K., Douglas, S.D., 1976. Neutrophil function in children with kwashiorkor. J. Lab. Clin. Med. 88 (3), 450–461.

Seidler, S., Zimmermann, H.W., Bartneck, M., Trautwein, C., Tacke, F., 2010. Age-dependent alterations of monocyte subsets and monocyte-related chemokine pathways in healthy adults. BMC Immunol. 11, 30.

Sharpless, N.E., DePinho, R.A., 2007. How stem cells age and why this makes us grow old. Nat. Rev. Mol. Cell Biol. 8 (9), 703–713.

Shousha, S., Kamel, K., 1972. Nitro blue tetrazolium test in children with kwashiorkor with a comment on the use of latex particles in the test. J. Clin. Pathol. 25 (6), 494–497.

Sicari, B.M., Rubin, J.P., Dearth, C.L., Wolf, M.T., Ambrosio, F., Boninger, M., et al., 2014. An acellular biologic scaffold promotes skeletal muscle formation in mice and humans with volumetric muscle loss. Sci. Transl. Med. 6 (234), 234ra58.

Sirisinha, S., Edelman, R., Suskind, R., Charupatana, C., Olson, R.E., 1973. Complement and C3-proactivator levels in children with protein-calorie malnutrition and effect of dietary treatment. Lancet 1 (7811), 1016–1020.

Slack, S.M., Bohnert, J.L., Horbett, T.A., 1987. The effects of surface chemistry and coagulation factors on fibrinogen adsorption from plasma. Ann. N.Y. Acad. Sci. 516, 223–243.

Tseng, C.W., Kyme, P.A., Arruda, A., Ramanujan, V.K., Tawackoli, W., Liu, G.Y., 2012. Innate Immune dysfunctions in aged mice facilitate the systemic dissemination of methicillin-resistant s. Aureus. PLoS One 7 (7), e41454.

van Duin, D., Mohanty, S., Thomas, V., Ginter, S., Montgomery, R.R., Fikrig, E., et al., 2007. Age-associated defect in human Tlr-1/2 function. J. Immunol. 178 (2), 970–975.

Vasquez-Garibay, E., Campollo-Rivas, O., Romero-Velarde, E., Mendez-Estrada, C., Garcia-Iglesias, T., Alvizo-Mora, J.G., et al., 2002. Effect of renutrition on natural and cell-mediated immune response in infants with severe malnutrition. J. Pediatr. Gastroenterol. Nutr. 34 (3), 296–301.

Vasquez-Garibay, E., Mendez-Estrada, C., Romero-Velarde, E., Garcia-Iglesias, M.T., Campollo-Rivas, O., 2004. Nutritional support with nucleotide addition favors immune response in severely malnourished infants. Arch. Med. Res. 35 (4), 284–288.

Wang, J., Arase, H., 2014. Regulation of immune responses by neutrophils. Ann. N.Y. Acad. Sci. 1319 (1), 66–81.

Weisberg, S.P., McCann, D., Desai, M., Rosenbaum, M., Leibel, R.L., Ferrante Jr., A.W., 2003. Obesity is associated with macrophage accumulation in adipose tissue. J. Clin. Invest. 112 (12), 1796–1808.

Wenisch, C., Patruta, S., Daxbock, F., Krause, R., Horl, W., 2000. Effect of age on human neutrophil function. J. Leukoc. Biol. 67 (1), 40–45.

Xu, H., Barnes, G.T., Yang, Q., Tan, G., Yang, D., Chou, C.J., et al., 2003. Chronic inflammation in fat plays a crucial role in the development of obesity-related insulin resistance. J. Clin. Invest. 112 (12), 1821–1830.

CHAPTER 2

Perspectives on the Inflammatory, Healing, and Foreign Body Responses to Biomaterials and Medical Devices

James Anderson[1] and Stephanie Cramer[2]
[1]Department of Pathology and Biomedical Engineering, Case Western Reserve University, Cleveland, OH, USA
[2]Department of Biomedical Engineering, Case Western Reserve University, Cleveland, OH, USA

Contents

INTRODUCTION

The host response to biomaterials, medical devices, and prostheses ultimately determines the success or failure and the downstream efficacy of the respective implant in the clinical setting. Table 2.1 provides a global perspective of *in vivo* complications of medical devices and provides both material-dependent and biologically dependent (i.e., host response-dependent) modes and mechanisms of failure, many of which are interactive and synergistic. Inflammation, healing, and foreign body reactions (FBRs) are the earliest host responses following implantation and provide the basis for determining host–device compatibility.

The most commonly used term to describe an appropriate host response to biomaterials in the form of a medical device is biocompatibility. A simplistic definition of biocompatibility is those materials which do not induce an adverse tissue reaction. A more helpful definition of biocompatibility is the ability of a material to perform with an appropriate host response in a specific application (Williams, 1987, 2008). This definition is helpful in that it links material properties or characteristics with performance

Host Response to Biomaterials.
DOI: http://dx.doi.org/10.1016/B978-0-12-800196-7.00002-5

Table 2.1 *In vivo* complications of medical devices

Heart valve prostheses	Vascular grafts/ stents	Cardiac assist/ replacement devices	Orthopedic devices	Dental implants
Thrombosis	Thrombosis	Thrombosis	Bone resorption	Adverse FBR
Embolism	Embolism	Embolism	Corrosion	Biocorrosion
Paravalvular leak	Infection	Endocarditis	Fatigue	Electrochemical galvanic coupling
Anticoagulation- related hemorrhage	Perigraft erosion	Extraluminal infection	Fixation failure	Fatigue
Infective endocarditis	Perigraft seroma	Component fracture	Fracture	Fixation failure
Extrinsic dysfunction	False aneurysm	Hemolysis	Incomplete osseous integration	Fracture
Incomplete valve closure	Anastomotic hyperplasia	Calcification	Infection	Infection
Cloth wear	Disintegration or degradation		Interface separation	Interface Separation
Hemolytic anemia	Proliferative restenosis		Loosening	Loss of mechanical force transfer
Component fracture	Strut-related inflammation		Mechanical mismatch	Loosening
Tissue valves	FBR		Motion and pain	FBR
Cusp tearing	Incomplete expansion		Particulate formation	Corrosion
Cusp calcification	Overexpansion		Surface wear	Particulate formation
	Malposition		Stress riser	Wear

(i.e., biological requirements, specific applications, specific medical device, or biomaterial used as a medical device). The "appropriate host response" implies identification and characterization of tissue reactions and responses that could prove harmful to the host and/or lead to ultimate failure of the biomaterial, medical device, or prosthesis through biological mechanisms. Viewed from the opposite perspective, the "appropriate host response" implies identification and characterization of the tissue reactions and responses critical for the successful use of the biomaterial or medical device. Biocompatibility assessment is considered to be a measure of the magnitude and duration of the adverse alterations in homeostatic mechanisms that determine the host response (Anderson, 2001). Safety assessment or biocompatibility assessment of a biomaterial or medical device is generally considered to be synonymous.

Table 2.2 Sequence/continuum of host reactions following implantation of medical devices

Injury
Blood–material interactions
Provisional matrix formation
Acute inflammation
Chronic inflammation
Granulation tissue
FBR
Fibrosis/fibrous capsule development

Inflammation, wound healing, and the FBR are generally considered part of the tissue or cellular host response to injury (Kumar et al., 2005). Table 2.2 lists the sequence/continuum of these events following injury. Overlap and simultaneous occurrence of these events should be considered (e.g., the FBR at the implant interface may be initiated with the onset of acute and chronic inflammation). From a biomaterials perspective, placing a biomaterial in an *in vivo* environment requires injection, insertion, or surgical implantation, all of which injure the tissue or organ involved.

The placement procedure initiates a response to injury by the tissue, organ, or body, and mechanisms are activated to maintain homeostasis. Obviously, the extent of injury varies with the implantation procedure. A more detailed description of the innate immune-response contribution to these initial events is provided in Chapters 6 and 7. The degrees to which the homeostatic mechanisms are perturbed, and the extent to which pathophysiologic conditions are created and undergo resolution, are a measure of the host response to the biomaterial and may ultimately determine its biocompatibility. Although it is conceptually convenient to separate homeostatic mechanisms into blood–material or tissue–material interactions, it must be remembered that the various components or mechanisms involved in homeostasis are present in both blood and tissue, are inextricably linked, and are a part of the physiologic continuum. Furthermore, it must be noted that the host response is tissue-dependent, organ-dependent, and species-dependent.

BLOOD–MATERIAL INTERACTIONS/PROVISIONAL MATRIX FORMATION

Immediately following injury, changes in vascular flow, caliber, and permeability occur. Fluid, proteins, and blood cells escape from the vascular system into the injured tissue in a process called exudation. The changes in the vascular system, which also include the hematologic alterations associated with acute inflammation, are followed by cellular events that characterize the inflammatory response. The chemical factors that mediate many of the vascular and cellular responses of inflammation and the initial host response are described in detail in numerous reviews and in Chapter 5.

Table 2.3 Cells and components of vascularized connective tissue

Intravascular (blood) cells	Connective tissue cells	ECM components
Neutrophils (PMNs)	Mast cells	Collagens
Monocytes	Fibroblasts	Elastin
Eosinophils	Macrophages	Proteoglycans
Lymphocytes	Lymphocytes	Fibronectin
		Laminin
Plasma cells		
Basophils		
Platelets		

Blood–material interactions and the inflammatory response are intimately linked; in fact, early responses to injury involve mainly blood and vasculature. Regardless of the implantation site, the initial inflammatory response is activated by injury to vascularized connective tissue (Table 2.3). Inflammation serves to contain, neutralize, dilute, or wall-off the injurious agent or process (Inflammation: Basic Principles and Clinical Correlates, 1999) In addition, the inflammatory response initiates a series of events that may heal and reconstitute the implant site through replacement of the injured tissue with native parenchymal cells, fibroblastic scar tissue, or a combination of the two. Since blood and its components are involved in the initial inflammatory response, blood clot formation and/or thrombosis also occur. Blood coagulation and thrombosis are generally considered humoral responses and are influenced by homeostatic mechanisms such as the extrinsic and intrinsic coagulation systems, the complement system, the fibrinolytic system, the kinin-generating system, and platelets. Thrombus or blood clot formation on the surface of a biomaterial is related to the well-known Vroman effect in which a hierarchical and dynamic series of collision, adsorption, and exchange processes, determined by protein mobility and concentration, regulate early time-dependent changes in blood protein adsorption. From a wound-healing perspective, blood protein deposition on a biomaterial surface is described as provisional matrix formation. Blood interactions with biomaterials are generally considered under the category of hematocompatibility. The complexity and interaction between blood/material interactions and tissue/material interactions are illustrated in Figure 2.1 which demonstrates the responses at the anastomosis of a vascular graft with an artery.

Injury to vascularized tissue during the implantation procedure leads to immediate development of the provisional matrix at the implant site. This provisional matrix consists of fibrin and inflammatory mediators produced by activation of the coagulation and thrombosis and complement systems, respectively, activated platelets, inflammatory cells, and endothelial cells. These events occur early, within minutes to hours following implantation of a medical device, and initiate the resolution, reorganization, and repair processes such as fibroblast recruitment. The provisional matrix provides both structural

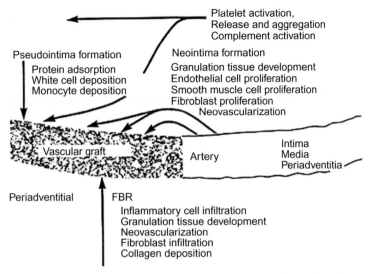

Figure 2.1 Blood and tissue interactions at the anastomosis of a vascular graft and artery. Provisional matrix forms at the periadventitial (tissue) interface and at the anastomosis (focal thrombosis) providing for inflammation and healing. Healing of the focal thrombus (organization) on the luminal side of the anastomosis is facilitated by both blood and artery components.

and biochemical components to the process of wound healing. The complex three-dimensional structure of the fibrin network with attached adhesive proteins provides a substrate for cell adhesion and migration. The presence of cytokines, chemokines, and growth factors within the provisional matrix provides a rich milieu of activating and inhibiting substances for cellular proliferative and synthetic processes, mitogenesis, and chemoattraction. The provisional matrix may be viewed as a naturally derived, biodegradable, sustained release system in which these various bioactive molecules are released to orchestrate subsequent wound-healing processes. Although our understanding of the provisional matrix and its capabilities has improved, our knowledge of the key molecular regulators of the formation of the provisional matrix and subsequent wound-healing events is poor. In part, this lack of knowledge is due to the fact that most studies have been conducted *in vitro*, and there is a paucity of *in vivo* studies that provide a more complex perspective. However, attractive hypotheses have been presented regarding the presumed ability of adsorbed materials to modulate cellular behavior.

The predominant cell type present in the inflammatory response varies with time as seen in Figure 2.2. In general, neutrophils predominate during the first several days following injury and exposure to a biomaterial and then are replaced by monocytes. Three factors account for this change in cell type: neutrophils are short-lived and disintegrate and disappear after 24–48 h, neutrophil emigration from the vasculature to the tissues is of short duration, and chemotactic factors for neutrophil migration are

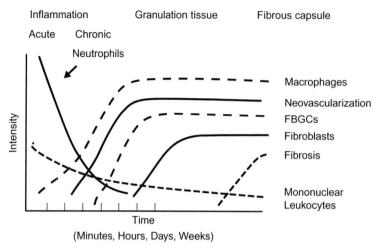

Figure 2.2 The temporal variation in the acute inflammatory response, chronic inflammatory response, granulation tissue development, and FBR to implanted biomaterials. The intensity and time variables are dependent upon the extent of injury created in the implantation and the size, shape, topography, and chemical and physical properties of the biomaterial.

activated early in the inflammatory response. Following emigration from the vasculature, monocytes differentiate into macrophages and these cells are very long-lived (up to months). Monocyte emigration may continue for days to weeks, depending on the extent of injury and type of implanted biomaterial. In addition, chemotactic factors for monocytes are produced over longer periods of time. In short-term (24h) implants in humans, administration of both H1 and H2 histamine receptor antagonists greatly reduced the recruitment of macrophages/monocytes and neutrophils on polyethylene terephthalate surfaces (Zdolsek et al., 2007). These studies also demonstrated that plasma–coated implants accumulated significantly more phagocytes than did serum-coated implants.

The temporal sequence of events following implantation of a biomaterial is illustrated in Figure 2.2. The size, shape, and chemical and physical properties of the biomaterial may be responsible for variations in the intensity and duration of the inflammatory or wound-healing process, and thus the host response to a biomaterial.

ACUTE INFLAMMATION

While injury initiates the inflammatory response, the chemicals released from plasma, cells, or injured tissues mediate the inflammatory response. Important chemical mediators of inflammation are presented in Table 2.4. Several points must be noted to understand the inflammatory response and its relationship to biomaterials. First, although chemical mediators are classified on a structural or functional basis, complex

Table 2.4 Important chemical mediators of inflammation derived from plasma, cells, or injured tissue

Mediators	Examples
Vasoactive agents	Histamines, serotonin, adenosine, endothelial-derived relaxing factor (EDRF), prostacyclin, endothelin, thromboxane α_2
Plasma proteases	
Kinin system	Bradykinin, kallikrein
Complement system	C3a, C5a, C3b, C5b–C9
Coagulation/fibrinolytic system	Fibrin degradation products, activated Hageman factor (FXIIA), tissue plasminogen activator (tPA)
Leukotrienes	Leukotriene B_4 (LTB_4), hydroxyeicosatetranoic acid (HETE)
Lysosomal proteases	Collagenase, elastase
Oxygen-derived free radicals	H_2O_2, superoxide anion
Platelet activating factors	Cell membrane lipids
Cytokines	IL-1, TNF
Growth factors	PDGF, fibroblast growth Factor (FGF), TGF-α or TGF-β, EGF

interactions provide a system of checks and balances regarding their respective activities and functions. Second, chemical mediators are quickly inactivated or destroyed, suggesting that their action is predominantly local (i.e., at the implant site). Third, generally the lysosomal proteases and the oxygen-derived free radicals produce the most significant damage or injury. These chemical mediators are also important in the degradation of certain biomaterials (Wiggins et al., 2001; Christenson et al., 2004a,b, 2007).

Acute inflammation is of relatively short duration, lasting for minutes to hours to days depending on the extent of injury and the type of implanted biomaterial. Its main characteristics are the exudation of fluid and plasma proteins (edema) and the emigration of leukocytes (predominantly neutrophils). Neutrophils (polymorphonuclear leukocytes, PMNs) and other motile white cells emigrate or move from the blood vessels into the perivascular tissues and the injury (implant) site. Leukocyte emigration is assisted by "adhesion molecules" present on leukocyte and endothelial surfaces. The surface expression of these adhesion molecules can be induced, enhanced, or altered by inflammatory agents and chemical mediators. White cell emigration is controlled, in part, by chemotaxis which is the unidirectional migration of cells along a chemical gradient. A wide variety of exogenous and endogenous substances have been identified as chemotactic stimuli. Specific receptors for chemotactic agents on the cell membranes of leukocytes are important in the emigration of leukocytes. These and other receptors also play a role in the transmigration of white cells across the endothelial lining of vessels and activation of leukocytes. Following localization of leukocytes at the injury (implant) site, phagocytosis and the release of proteolytic enzymes occur following activation of neutrophils and macrophages. The major role of the neutrophil in acute inflammation is to phagocytose microorganisms and foreign materials. Phagocytosis is seen as a three-step process in which the stimulus (e.g., damaged tissue, infectious agent, biomaterial) undergoes recognition and neutrophil attachment, engulfment, and killing or degradation. In regard to biomaterials, engulfment and degradation may or may not occur, depending on the properties of the biomaterial.

Although biomaterials are not generally phagocytosed by neutrophils or macrophages because of the disparity in size (i.e., the surface of the biomaterial is greater than the size of the cell), certain events in phagocytosis may occur. The process of recognition and attachment is expedited when the injurious agent is coated by naturally occurring serum factors called "opsonins." Two major opsonins are immunoglobulin G and the complement-activated fragment, C3b. Both of these plasma-derived proteins are known to adsorb to biomaterials, and neutrophils and macrophages have corresponding cell membrane receptors for these opsonins. These receptors may also play a role in the activation of the attached neutrophil or macrophage. Other blood proteins such as fibrinogen, fibronectin, and vitronectin may also facilitate cell adhesion to biomaterial surfaces. Owing to the disparity in size between the biomaterial surface and the attached cell, frustrated phagocytosis may occur—a process that does not involve engulfment of the biomaterial but does cause the extracellular release of leukocyte products in an attempt to degrade the biomaterial.

Henson has shown that neutrophils adherent to complement-coated and immunoglobulin-coated nonphagocytosable surfaces may release enzymes by direct extrusion or exocytosis from the cell (Henson, 1971). The amount of enzyme released during this process depends on the size of the polymer particle, with larger particles inducing greater amounts of enzyme release. This disparity suggests that the specific mode of cell activation depends, at least in part, upon the size of the implant and whether or not a material in a phagocytosable form. For example, a powder, particulate, or nanomaterial may provoke a different degree of inflammatory response than the same material in a nonphagocytosable form such as film. In general, materials greater than 5 μm are not phagocytosed, while materials less than 5 μm can be phagocytosed by inflammatory cells.

Acute inflammation normally resolves quickly, usually less than 1 week, depending on the extent of injury at the implant site. The presence of acute inflammation (i.e., PMNs) at the tissue/implant interface at time periods beyond 1 week (i.e., weeks, months, or years) suggests the presence of infection (Figure 2.3A).

CHRONIC INFLAMMATION

Chronic inflammation has a more heterogeneous histological appearance than acute inflammation. In general, chronic inflammation is characterized by the presence of macrophages, monocytes, and lymphocytes, with the proliferation of blood vessels and connective tissue. Many factors can modify the course and histologic appearance of chronic inflammation.

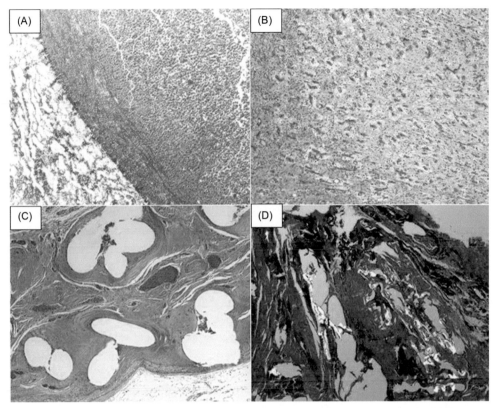

Figure 2.3 (A). Acute and chronic inflammation of an infected ePTFE vascular graft. Inflammatory cells are observed within the graft lumen, at the luminal graft surface, and infiltrating the porous graft interstices. H&E Stain, 16× original magnification. (B). Granulation tissue with extensive neo-vascularization in a healing, previously infected, total hip prosthesis. H&E Stain, 8.0× original magnification. (C). Fibrous FBR and fibrous encapsulation of polypropylene mesh fibers from a ventral hernia repair. H&E Stain, 8.0× original magnification. (D). Wear products from a total hip prosthesis. Polyethylene shards are seen as white materials with partial polarized light microscopy and metallosis (metal particles) are seen as black aggregates. An extensive FBR is also observed. H&E Stain, 8.0× original magnification.

Clinically, surgical pathologists commonly use the term chronic inflammation to describe the FBR. Caution is recommended in the use of this term as it demonstrates the breadth of histological findings that lead to the clinical diagnosis of chronic inflammation. Chronic inflammation predominantly composed of monocytes, macrophages, and lymphocytes is most commonly associated with toxicity or infection, whereas the FBR is most commonly composed of macrophages and foreign body giant cells (FBGCs).

Persistent inflammatory stimuli lead to chronic inflammation. While the chemical and physical properties of the biomaterial themselves may lead to chronic inflammation, *in situ* motion of the implant or infection may also produce chronic inflammation. The chronic inflammatory response to biomaterials is usually of short duration and is confined to the implant site. The presence of mononuclear cells, including FBR with the development of granulation tissue, is considered the normal wound-healing response to implanted biomaterials (i.e., the normal FBR). Chronic inflammation with the presence of collections of lymphocytes and monocytes at extended implant times (weeks, months, years) also may suggest the presence of a long-standing infection. The prolonged presence of acute and/or chronic inflammation also may be due to toxic leachables from a biomaterial (Marchant et al., 1986).

The following example illustrates this point. *In vivo* subcutaneous implantation studies were conducted in rats and rabbits with naltrexone sustained release preparations that included placebo (polymer-only) beads and naltrexone containing beads (Yamaguchi, 1992). Histopathological tissue reactions were determined at days 3, 7, 14, 21, and 28. The only significant histological finding in both rats and rabbits at any time period was the persistent chronic inflammation that occurred focally around the naltrexone containing beads. The focal inflammatory cell density in both rats and rabbits was higher for the naltrexone beads than for the placebo beads at days 14, 21, and 28, respectively. This difference in inflammatory response between naltrexone beads and placebo beads increased with increasing time of implantation. Considering the resolution of the inflammatory response for the placebo beads with implantation time in both rats and rabbits is the more severe inflammatory reaction suggested that the naltrexone drug itself was the causative agent of the focal chronic inflammation present surrounding the naltrexone beads in the implant sites.

This case study displays the importance of using an appropriate control material in experiments. If no negative control (i.e., placebo polymer-only material) had been used, the polymer in the naltrexone containing beads also would have been considered as a causative agent of the extended chronic inflammatory response. Similar chronic inflammatory responses have been identified with drugs, polymer plasticizers and other additives, fabrication and manufacturing aids, and sterilization residuals. Each case presents its own unique factors in a risk assessment process necessary for determining safety (biocompatibility) and benefit versus risk in clinical application.

Lymphocytes and plasma cells are involved principally in immune reactions and are key mediators of antibody production and delayed hypersensitivity responses. Although these cells may be present in nonimmunologic injuries and inflammation, their roles in such circumstances are largely unknown (Brodbeck et al., 2005; MacEwan et al., 2005). Little is known regarding humoral (or acquired) immune responses and cell-mediated immunity to synthetic biomaterials. The role of the acquired immune response to biomaterials is discussed in Chapter 8. The role of macrophages (cells of the innate

Table 2.5 Tissues and cells of MPS and RES

Tissues	Cells
Implant sites	Inflammatory macrophages
Liver	Kupffer cells
Lung	Alveolar macrophages
Connective tissue	Histiocytes
Bone marrow	Macrophages
Spleen and lymph nodes	Fixed and free macrophages
Serous cavities	Pleural and peritoneal macrophages
Nervous system	Microglial cells
Bone	Osteoclasts
Skin	Langerhans' cells
Lymphoid tissue	DCs

humoral response) must be considered in the possible development of acquired immune responses to synthetic biomaterials. Macrophages and dendritic cells (DCs) process and present the antigen to immunocompetent cells and thus are key mediators in the development of immune reactions. Chapters 6 and 7 discuss this topic at length.

Monocytes and macrophages belong to the mononuclear phagocytic system (MPS), also known as the reticuloendothelial system (RES). These systems consist of cells in the bone marrow, peripheral blood, and specialized tissues. Table 2.5 lists the tissues that contain cells belonging to the MPS or RES. The specialized cells in these tissues may be responsible for systemic effects in organs or tissues secondary to the release of components or products from implants through various tissue–material interactions (e.g., corrosion products, wear debris, degradation products) or the presence of implants (e.g., microcapsule or nanoparticle drug-delivery systems).

Over the past decade, increasing numbers of studies have identified significant differences in macrophage phenotypic expression. This difference in macrophage function or activation, dictated by different environmental cues, has been classified in various ways. Following on the T-cell literature, macrophages have been classified as M1 macrophages defined as classically activated or pro-inflammatory macrophages and M2 macrophages described as alternatively activated macrophages or anti-inflammatory/pro-wound-healing macrophages (Gordon, 2003; Gordon and Pluddemann, 2013; Mooney et al., 2010). Others have attempted to identify three different macrophage classifications: classically activated macrophages, wound-healing macrophages, and regulatory macrophages (Mosser and Edwards, 2008). In this classification, it is the regulatory macrophage that has anti-inflammatory activity whereas the wound-healing macrophage facilitates tissue repair. Attempts to classify macrophage activity are artificial and can be misleading given the wide variety of environmental cues that may activate macrophages and result in a wide variety of different forms of macrophage polarization (i.e., phenotypic expression). Mantovani best describes macrophage polarization, activity, or phenotypic expression as being a continuum ranging from M1 to M2 (Mantovani et al., 2002, 2004), and Chapter 6 describes the macrophage response to biomaterials in detail.

The macrophage is arguably the most important cell in chronic inflammation because of the great number of biologically active products it can produce. Important classes of products produced and secreted by macrophages include neutral proteases, chemotactic factors, arachidonic acid metabolites, reactive oxygen metabolites, complement components, coagulation factors, growth-promoting factors, cytokines, and acid. Phagolysosomes in macrophages can be very acidic with a pH as low as 4 and direct microelectrode studies of this acid environment have measured pH levels as low as 3.5. Moreover, only several hours are necessary to achieve these acidic levels following adhesion of macrophages (Haas, 2007; Jankowski et al., 2002; Klebanoff, 2005; Segal, 2005; Silver et al., 1988).

Growth factors such as platelet-derived growth factor (PDGF), fibroblast growth factor (FGF), transforming growth factor-β (TGF-β), TGF-α/epidermal growth factor (EGF), and interleukin-1 (IL-1) or tumor necrosis factor (TNF-α) are important to the growth of fibroblasts and blood vessels and the regeneration of epithelial cells. Effector molecules released by activated macrophages can initiate cell migration, differentiation, and tissue remodeling, and are involved in various stages of wound healing.

GRANULATION TISSUE

Within 1 day following implantation of a biomaterial (i.e., injury), the healing response is initiated by monocytes and macrophages. Fibroblasts and vascular endothelial cells in the implant site proliferate and begin to form granulation tissue, which is a specialized type of tissue that is the hallmark of healing inflammation. Granulation tissue derives its name from the pink, soft, granular appearance on the surface of healing wounds and its characteristic histological feature includes the proliferation of new small blood vessels and fibroblasts. Depending on the extent of injury, granulation tissue may be seen as early as 3–5 days following implantation of a biomaterial.

New small blood vessels are formed by the budding or sprouting of preexisting vessels in a process known as neovascularization or angiogenesis (Browder et al., 2000; Nguyen and D'Amore, 2001) (Figure 2.3B). This process involves proliferation, maturation, and organization of endothelial cells into capillary vessels. Fibroblasts also proliferate in developing granulation tissue and are active in synthesizing collagen and proteoglycans. In the early stages of granulation tissue development, proteoglycans predominate but later collagen, especially type III collagen, predominates and forms the fibrous capsule seen with most biomaterials. Some fibroblasts in developing granulation tissue may have the features of smooth muscle cells (e.g., actin microfilaments). These cells are called myofibroblasts and are considered to be responsible for the wound contraction seen during the development of granulation tissue. In addition to contraction, myofibroblasts can invade and repair injured tissues by secreting an organizing extracellular matrix (ECM) (Hinz et al., 2001). Recent studies indicate that myofibroblasts can originate from different precursor cells, the major contribution being from local recruitment of connective tissue fibroblasts; however, local mesenchymal stem cells, bone-marrow-derived mesenchymal stem cells (fibrocytes), and cells derived from the epithelial–mesenchymal transition process may be an alternative source of myofibroblasts (Micallef et al., 2012). Macrophages are almost always present in granulation tissue. Other cells may also be present if chemotactic stimuli are generated.

The wound-healing response is generally dependent on the extent or degree of injury or defect created by the implantation procedure (Broughton et al., 2006; Mustoe et al., 1987; Pierce, 2001; Clark, 1996; Hunt et al., 1984). Wound healing by primary union or first intention is the healing of clean, surgical incisions in which the wound edges have been approximated by surgical sutures. This term does not apply in the context of host response to biomaterials. Healing under these conditions occurs without significant bacterial contamination and with a minimal loss of tissue. Wound healing by secondary union or second intention occurs when there is a large tissue defect that must be filled or there is extensive loss of cells and tissue. In wound healing by secondary intention, regeneration of parenchymal cells cannot completely reconstitute the original architecture and much larger amounts of granulation tissue are formed that result in larger areas of fibrosis or scar formation. Under these conditions, different regions of tissue may show different stages of the wound-healing process simultaneously. Wound healing by second intention is commonly seen with biomaterials and is related to the extent of provisional matrix formed between the implant and tissue.

Granulation tissue is distinctly different from granulomas, which are small collections of modified macrophages called epithelioid cells. Langhans cells or FBGCs may surround nonphagocytosable particulate materials in granulomas. FBGCs are formed by the fusion of monocytes and macrophages in an attempt to phagocytose the material.

FOREIGN BODY REACTION

The FBR to biomaterials is composed of FBGCs and the components of granulation tissue (e.g., macrophages, fibroblasts, and capillaries, in varying amounts) depend upon the form and topography of the implanted material (Anderson, 2001; Anderson et al., 2008). Relatively flat and smooth surfaces such as that found on silicone breast prostheses have an FBR composed of a layer of macrophages and FBGCs one to two cells in thickness. Relatively rough surfaces such as those found on the outer surfaces of expanded polytetrafluoroethylene (ePTFE) or Dacron vascular prostheses have an FBR composed of macrophages and FBGCs at the surface. Fabric materials generally have a surface response composed of macrophages and FBGCs, with varying degrees of granulation tissue subjacent to the surface response (Figure 2.3C).

As previously discussed, the form and topography of the surface of the biomaterial determines the composition of the FBR (Bota et al., 2010). With biocompatible materials, the composition of the FBR in the implant site may be controlled by the surface properties of the biomaterial, the form of the implant, and the relationship between the surface area of the biomaterial and the volume of the implant. For example, high surface-to-volume implants such as fabrics, porous materials, particulate (Figure 2.3D), or microspheres will have higher ratios of macrophages and FBGCs in the implant site than smooth surface implants, which will have fibrosis as a significant component of the implant site (Charnley, 1970; Revell, 2008; Ney et al., 2006; Revell, 2008).

The FBR may persist at the tissue–implant interface for the lifetime of the implant (Figure 2.2). Generally, fibrosis (i.e., fibrous encapsulation) surrounds the biomaterial or implant with its interfacial FBR, isolating the implant and FBR from the local tissue environment. Early in the inflammatory and wound-healing response, macrophages are activated upon adherence to the material surface (Purdue, 2008).

Although it is generally felt that the chemical and physical properties of the biomaterial are responsible for macrophage activation, the subsequent events regarding the activity of macrophages at the surface are unclear. Tissue macrophages, derived from circulating blood monocytes, may coalesce to form multinucleated FBGC. It is not uncommon to see very large FBGC containing large numbers of nuclei on the surface of biomaterials. While these FBGC may persist for the lifetime of the implant, it is not known if they remain activated, releasing their lysosomal constituents, or become quiescent (Brodbeck and Anderson, 2009).

Figure 2.4 demonstrates the progression from circulating blood monocyte to tissue macrophage to FBGC development that is most commonly observed. Indicated in the figure are important biological responses that are considered to play an important role

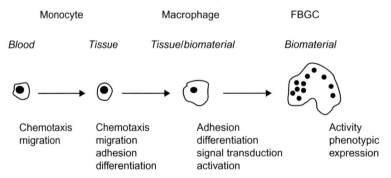

Figure 2.4 *In vivo* transition from blood-borne monocyte, to biomaterial adherent monocyte/macrophage, to FBGC at the tissue–biomaterial interface.

in FBGC development. Material surface chemistry may control adherent macrophage apoptosis (i.e., programmed cell death) which renders potentially harmful macrophages nonfunctional, while the surrounding environment of the implant remains unaffected. The level of adherent macrophage apoptosis appears to be inversely related to the ability of the surface to promote fusion of macrophages into FBGCs, suggesting a mechanism for macrophages to escape apoptosis.

Figure 2.5 demonstrates the sequence of events involved in inflammation and wound healing when medical devices (i.e., biomaterials) are implanted. In general, the PMN predominant acute inflammatory response and the lymphocyte/monocyte predominant chronic inflammatory response resolve quickly (i.e., within 2 weeks) depending on the type and location of the implant. Studies using IL-4 or IL-13, respectively, demonstrate the role for Th2 helper lymphocytes and/or mast cells in the development of the FBR at the tissue/material interface (McNally and Anderson, 1994; McNally et al., 1996). Integrin receptors of IL-4-induced FBGC are characterized by the early constitutive expression of $\alpha V\beta1$ and the later induced expression of $\alpha5\beta1$ and $\alpha X\beta2$, which indicate potential interactions with adsorbed complement C3, fibrin(ogen), fibronectin, Factor X, and vitronectin (McNally and Anderson, 1994, 2002; McNally et al., 1996, 2007, 2008; Hynes and Zhao, 2000; Nilsson et al., 2007; Jenney and Anderson, 2000). Interactions through indirect (paracrine) cytokine

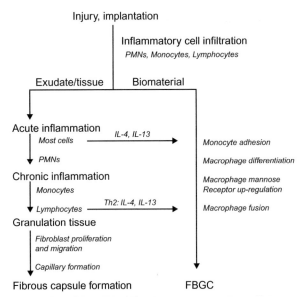

Figure 2.5 Sequence of events involved in inflammatory and wound-healing responses leading to FBGC formation. This shows the potential importance of mast cells in the acute inflammatory phase and Th2 lymphocytes in the transient chronic inflammatory phase with the production of IL-4 and IL-13, which can induce monocytes/macrophage fusion to form GBGCs.

and chemokine signaling have shown a significant effect in enhancing adherent mac-rophage/FBGC activation at early times, whereas interactions via direct (juxtacrine) cell-to-cell mechanisms dominate at later times (Chang et al., 2009; Jones et al., 2004, 2007; Anderson and Jones, 2007). Th2 helper lymphocytes have been described as "anti-inflammatory" based on their cytokine profile, of which IL-4 is a significant component.

FIBROSIS/FIBROUS ENCAPSULATION

Generally, the end-stage healing response to biomaterials is fibrosis or fibrous encapsu-lation; however, there may be exceptions to this general statement (e.g., porous mate-rials inoculated with parenchymal cells or porous materials implanted into tissue or bone). As previously stated, the tissue response to biomaterials is in part dependent upon the extent of injury or defect created in the implantation procedure and the amount of provisional matrix.

The ultimate goal of tissue engineering and regenerative medicine is the replace-ment of injured tissue by cells that reconstitute normal tissue and organ structures. Numerous approaches, including stem cells, scaffolds, and growth factors, are currently being investigated. The relatively rapid responses of inflammation, wound healing, and the FBR, as well as other significant factors in tissue regeneration, present major chal-lenges to the successful achievement of this goal. This is especially significant with the use of scaffold materials where migration and integration of the scaffold porosity is necessary in tissue engineering approaches.

Repair of biomaterial implant sites can involve two distinct processes: construc-tive remodeling, which is the replacement of injured tissue by parenchymal cells of the same type, and replacement by connective tissue that constitutes the fibrous cap-sule. These processes are generally controlled by either (Williams, 1987) the prolifera-tive capacity of the cells in the tissue or organ receiving the implant and the extent of injury as it relates to the destruction, or (Williams, 2008) persistence of the tissue framework (i.e., ECM) of the implant site.

The regenerative capacity of cells allows them to be classified into three groups: labile, stable (or expanding), and permanent (or static) cells. Labile cells continue to pro-liferate throughout life, stable cells retain this capacity but do not continuously repli-cate, and permanent cells cannot reproduce after birth. Perfect repair with restitution of normal structure can theoretically occur only in tissues consisting of stable and labile cells, whereas all injuries to tissues composed of permanent cells may give rise to fibrosis and fibrous capsule formation with very little restitution of the normal tissue or organ structure. Tissues composed of permanent cells (e.g., nerve cells and cardiac muscle cells) most commonly undergo an organization of the inflammatory exudate, leading to fibrosis. Tissues of stable cells (e.g., parenchymal cells of the liver, kidney, and pancreas), mesenchymal cells (e.g., fibroblasts, smooth muscle cells, osteoblasts, and chondroblasts), and vascular endothelial and labile cells (e.g., epithelial cells and lymphoid and hematopoietic cells) may also follow this pathway to fibrosis or may undergo resolution of the inflammatory exudate, leading to restitution of the normal tissue structure.

The condition of the underlying framework or supporting ECM of the parenchymal cells following an injury plays an important role in the restoration of normal tissue structure. Retention of the framework ECM with injury may lead to restitution of the normal tissue structure, whereas destruction of the framework most commonly leads to fibrosis. It is important to consider the species-dependent nature of the regenerative capacity of cells. For example, cells from the same organ or tissue but from different species may exhibit different regenerative capacities and/or connective tissue repair, as with endothelialization with vascular grafts and stents.

Local and systemic factors play a role in the wound-healing response to biomaterials or implants. Local factors include the anatomic site (tissue or organ) of implantation, the adequacy of blood supply, and the potential for infection. Systemic factors include nutrition, hematologic derangements, glucocorticoid administration, and pre-existing diseases such as atherosclerosis, diabetes, and infection.

The end stage of wound-healing/tissue repair with implanted medical devices is the fibrous capsule. Initially believed to be produced by infiltrating fibroblasts, it is now known that myofibroblasts and fibrocytes (resident and circulating mesenchymal progenitor cells) play a significant role in producing collagenous fibrosis, the main constituent of the fibrous capsule (Hinz et al., 2001; Bucala, 2012; Wynn, 2008; Wynn and Ramalingam, 2012; Hinz, 2007).

The implantation of biomaterials or medical devices may be best viewed from the perspective that the implant provides an impediment or hindrance to appropriate (normal) tissue or organ regeneration and healing. The fibrous capsule surrounding drug-delivery devices has also been suggested to be a barrier to drug diffusion and inhibition of the function of drug-delivery systems and biosensors (e.g., glucose sensors). That view may be short-sighted, however, as recent studies with a wireless controlled drug-delivery microchip for the delivery of an osteoporosis inhibitor of approximately 4000 molecular weight has been shown to produce clinically relevant blood levels for inhibition of osteoporosis (Farra et al., 2012). Given the limited ability to control the sequence of events following injury in the implantation procedure, restitution of normal tissue structures with function is rare. Current studies directed toward developing a better understanding of the modification of the inflammatory response, stimuli providing for appropriate proliferation of permanent and stable cells, and the appropriate application of growth factors may provide keys to the control of inflammation, wound healing, and fibrous encapsulation of biomaterials.

Table 2.6 Common components in the inflammatory (innate) and adaptive immune responses

Components	Cellular components
Complement cascade components Immunoglobulins	Macrophages NK (natural killer) cells DCs Cells with dual phagocytic and antigen-presenting capabilities

INNATE AND ADAPTIVE IMMUNE RESPONSES

With the advent of tissue engineering, the importance of immune response and immunotoxicity evaluation has increased significantly (Jones et al., 2008; Sefton et al., 2008). Evaluation of the immune response is especially challenging given the unique nature of the respective medical devices and the delayed presentation of a response. Differences in animal versus human immune responses provide additional complexity to this issue. The following presents an overview and guidance to immune-response evaluation.

The inflammatory (innate) and immune (adaptive) responses have common components. It is possible to have inflammatory responses only with no adaptive immune response. In this situation, both humoral and cellular components that are shared by both types of responses may only participate in the inflammatory response. Table 2.6 indicates the common components to the inflammatory and immune responses. Macrophages and DCs are known as professional antigen–presenting cells responsible for the initiation of the adaptive immune response.

DISCUSSION AND PERSPECTIVES

In spite of the significant advances that have been made in mechanistic understanding of the inflammatory, healing, and FBRs to biomaterials and medical devices over the past two decades, numerous challenges which limit projection to clinical application still exist. The purpose of this section is to identify several of these problems that offer challenges/opportunities for the future.

Differences in the responses to the implantation of a biomaterial or medical device still exist between species. This is a significant concern given that animal studies are a required precursor to clinical application. Current thought regarding the source of macrophages and their fused entity (i.e., FBGCs) suggest that differentiated macrophages may be present due to self-renewal (Sieweke and Allen, 2013). That is, resident macrophages are capable of proliferation. Studies that support this hypothesis have been conducted in nonhuman mammals and many major macrophage populations have been found to be derived from embryonic progenitors and are capable of renewal independent of hematopoietic stem cells. From a clinical applications perspective, this is a significant question as implant retrieval studies have identified macrophages and

FBGCs in the FBR to biomaterials and medical devices to be present at the tissue/ material interface for approximately 30 years. As there is no compelling evidence that the macrophages in the FBR to implanted biomaterials and medical devices are capable of self-renewal (i.e., proliferation), the turnover rate of these cells at the interface and the precursor cells that continue to populate the surface of the biomaterial or medical device (Sieweke and Allen, 2013; Jenkins et al., 2011; Hashimoto et al., 2013) remain unanswered questions. An example of significant interspecies differences is the fact that human vascular grafts do not endothelialize their luminal surface whereas higher vertebrates, including chimpanzees and baboons, do provide an endothelial lining in the healing response of vascular grafts. While putative evidence focuses on circulating stem cells in the blood to provide an endothelial lining, no evidence exists today to support this hypothesis.

The lack of a host response to an implanted biomaterial may be desirable in some applications; however, the holy grail of a biomaterial surface that does not allow adherence of proteins or cells remains elusive. As noted earlier, almost immediately upon implantation, the humoral and cellular components of blood come in contact with implanted biomaterials or medical devices resulting in a provisional matrix. Recent studies have focused on inhibition of biomaterial-induced complement activation to reduce the protein adhesion phenomenon on the surface (Kourtzelis et al., 2013; Ekdahl et al., 2011; Morais et al., 2010). Inhibition of biomaterial-induced complement activation would be expected to lead to a reduction in monocyte/macrophage adhesion to the biomaterial (McNally and Anderson, 1994, 2002). However, the adhesion of monocytes/macrophages to biomaterial surfaces is far more complex as monocytes/macrophages express protein adhesion receptors (integrins) with at least three different types of beta chains ($\beta1$, $\beta2$, $\beta3$) that in turn can bind to a wide variety of proteins present in the provisional matrix. These blood-derived proteins include complement C3b fragments, fibrin, fibrinogen, fibronectin, factor X, and vitronectin. Moreover, integrin expression by monocytes/macrophages is time-dependent and $\beta1$ integrins are not initially detected on adherent monocytes but begin to appear during macrophage development and are strongly expressed on fusing macrophages that form FBGCs (McNally and Anderson, 2002). Thus, monocyte/macrophage adhesion with subsequent macrophage fusion to form FBGCs at the interface is far more complex given the relatively large number of adhesion proteins, their respective monocyte/macrophage receptors, and the time-dependent nature of receptor up-regulation on adherent macrophages and FBGCs. Other mechanisms such as apoptosis or anoikis of adherent cells may be considered to reduce the adherent monocyte/macrophage/ FBGC adhesion to biomaterial surfaces. Apoptosis is a programmed cell death while anoikis is a term for apoptosis induced by cell detachment from its supportive matrix. Various biomaterial surface chemistries have identified apoptosis of adherent macrophages both *in vitro* and *in vivo* (Jones et al., 2004; Brodbeck et al., 2001, 2003; Shive et al., 2002). These potential mechanisms for reducing cellular adhesion have been poorly studied and offer an opportunity for controlled and down-regulation of monocyte/macrophage/FBGCs adhesion to biomaterial surfaces.

Regarding development of the fibrous capsule surrounding implants, fibrocytes, a subpopulation of circulating mesenchymal progenitor cells, have been identified as augmenting wound repair as well as producing different fibrosing disorders in humans (Bucala, 2012). Blood circulating fibrocytes can be recruited to sites of tissue or implant injury and differentiate into fibroblasts and myofibroblasts. Myofibroblasts are now considered to be a major contributor to fibrosis and may be responsible for the remodeling of granulation tissue collagen to fibrosis-dependent collagen (i.e., collagen type I). Recent studies have suggested that the mechanical properties of the biomaterial substrate can influence the contractile nature of myofibroblasts (Hinz, 2007; Hinz et al., 2012; Hinz and Gabbiani, 2010; Klingberg et al., 2013).

A successful approach to the inhibition of inflammatory adhesion and activation has been the modification of biomaterial surfaces with CD47, a transmembrane molecular marker of "self." As inflammatory cells do not recognize these surfaces as being foreign, inflammatory cell adhesion is reduced with a down-regulation of expressed cytokines, an up-regulation of matrix metalloproteinases, and involvement of JAK/STAT signaling mechanisms (Stachelek et al., 2011; Finley et al., 2013). These findings suggest that both biomaterial degradation and fibrous capsule formation can be reduced with CD47 modification of biomaterial surfaces. Strict control of biomedical polymer morphology and porosity has also provided a means to down-regulate FBGC and fibrous capsule formation (Bota et al., 2010; Madden et al., 2010; Fukano et al., 2010). These approaches can be expected to be useful in the development of scaffolds for clinical use.

Ultimately, the success or failure of a medical device and implant is modulated by the interaction between the characteristics of the biomaterial or medical device, patient conditions or factors, and surgical technique. Table 2.7 identifies patient

Table 2.7 Patient conditions and other factors influencing implant failure

Orthopedic	Cardiovascular
Polyarthritis syndromes	Atherosclerosis
Connective tissue disorders	Diabetes
Osteoarthritis	Infection
Trauma	Ventricular hypertrophy
Infection	Hypertension
Metabolic disease	Arrhythmias
Endocrine disease	Coagulation abnormalities
Tumor	Cardiac function
Primary joint disease	Recipient activity level
Osteonecrosis	
Recipient activity level	

conditions that can influence the success or failure of orthopedic and cardiovascular devices. These conditions may modulate the inflammatory, healing, and FBRs resulting in the eventual failure of the biomaterials or medical device. Infection remains a significant factor leading to implant failure. Recent studies suggest that individual patient genomic factors may predispose the patient to implant failure. Other chapters in this text discuss the role of age (Chapter 11) and body system location (Chapters 12 and 13) upon the host response to implanted materials.

REFERENCES

Anderson, J.M., 2001. Biological responses to materials. Ann. Rev. Mater. Res. 31, 81–110.

Anderson, J.M., Jones, J.A., 2007. Phenotypic dichotomies in the foreign body reaction. Biomaterials 28 (34), 5114–5120.

Anderson, J.M., Rodriguez, A., Chang, D.T., 2008. Foreign body reaction to biomaterials. Semin. Immunol. 20 (2), 86–100.

Bota, P.C., Collie, A.M., Puolakkainen, P., Vernon, R.B., Sage, E.H., Ratner, B.D., et al., 2010. Biomaterial topography alters healing *in vivo* and monocyte/macrophage activation *in vitro*. J. Biomed. Mater. Res. A. 95 (2), 649–657.

Brodbeck, W.G., Anderson, J.M., 2009. Giant cell formation and function. Curr. Opin. Hematol. 16 (1), 53–57.

Brodbeck, W.G., Shive, M.S., Colton, E., Nakayama, Y., Matsuda, T., Anderson, J.M., 2001. Influence of biomaterial surface chemistry on the apoptosis of adherent cells. J. Biomed. Mater. Res. 55 (4), 661–668.

Brodbeck, W.G., Colton, E., Anderson, J.M., 2003. Effects of adsorbed heat labile serum proteins and fibrinogen on adhesion and apoptosis of monocytes/macrophages on biomaterials. J. Mater. Sci. Mater. Med. 14 (8), 671–675.

Brodbeck, W.G., Macewan, M., Colton, E., Meyerson, H., Anderson, J.M., 2005. Lymphocytes and the foreign body response: lymphocyte enhancement of macrophage adhesion and fusion. J. Biomed. Mater. Res. A. 74 (2), 222–229.

Broughton II, G., Janis, J.E., Attinger, C.E., 2006. The basic science of wound healing. Plast. Reconstr. Surg. 117 (7 Suppl.), 12S–34S.

Browder, T., Folkman, J., Pirie-Shepherd, S., 2000. The hemostatic system as a regulator of angiogenesis. J. Biol. Chem. 275 (3), 1521–1524.

Bucala, R., 2012. Review series—inflammation & fibrosis. Fibrocytes and fibrosis. QJM 105 (6), 505–508.

Chang, D.T., Colton, E., Anderson, J.M., 2009. Paracrine and juxtacrine lymphocyte enhancement of adherent macrophage and foreign body giant cell activation. J. Biomed. Mater. Res. A. 89 (2), 490–498.

Charnley, J., 1970. The reaction of bone to self-curing acrylic cement. A long-term histological study in man. J. Bone Joint Surg. Br. 52 (2), 340–353.

Christenson, E.M., Anderson, J.M., Hiltner, A., 2004a. Oxidative mechanisms of poly(carbonate urethane) and poly(ether urethane) biodegradation: *in vivo* and *in vitro* correlations. J. Biomed. Mater. Res. A. 70A (2), 245–255.

Christenson, E.M., Dadsetan, M., Wiggins, M., Anderson, J.M., Hiltner, A., 2004b. Poly(carbonate urethane) and poly(ether urethane) biodegradation: *in vivo* studies. J. Biomed. Mater. Res. A. 69 (3), 407–416.

Christenson, E., Anderson, J.M., Hiltner, A., 2007. Biodegradation mechanisms of polyurethan elastomers. Corrosion Eng., Sci. Technol. 69 (3), 312–323.

Clark, R.A.F. (Ed.), 1996. The molecular and cellular biology of wound repair, 2nd ed. Plenum Press, New York.

Ekdahl, K.N., Lambris, J.D., Elwing, H., Ricklin, D., Nilsson, P.H., Teramura, Y., et al., 2011. Innate immunity activation on biomaterial surfaces: a mechanistic model and coping strategies. Adv. Drug Deliv. Rev. 63 (12), 1042–1050.

Farra, R., Sheppard Jr., N.F., McCabe, L., Neer, R.M., Anderson, J.M., Santini Jr., J.T., et al., 2012. First-in-human testing of a wirelessly controlled drug delivery microchip. Sci. Transl. Med. 4 (122), 122ra21.

Finley, M.J., Clark, K.A., Alferiev, I.S., Levy, R.J., Stachelek, S.J., 2013. Intracellular signaling mechanisms associated with CD47 modified surfaces. Biomaterials 34 (34), 8640–8649.

Fukano, Y., Usui, M.L., Underwood, R.A., Isenhath, S., Marshall, A.J., Hauch, K.D., et al., 2010. Epidermal and dermal integration into sphere-templated porous poly(2-hydroxyethyl methacrylate) implants in mice. J. Biomed. Mater. Res. A. 94 (4), 1172–1186.

Gordon, S., 2003. Alternative activation of macrophages. Nat. Rev. Immunol. 3 (1), 23–35.

Gordon, S., Pluddemann, A., 2013. Tissue macrophage heterogeneity: issues and prospects. Semin. Immunopathol. 35 (5), 533–540.

Haas, A., 2007. The phagosome: compartment with a license to kill. Traffic 8 (4), 311–330.

Hashimoto, D., Chow, A., Noizat, C., Teo, P., Beasley, M.B., Leboeuf, M., et al., 2013. Tissue-resident macrophages self-maintain locally throughout adult life with minimal contribution from circulating monocytes. Immunity 38 (4), 792–804.

Henson, P.M., 1971. The immunologic release of constituents from neutrophil leukocytes. II. Mechanisms of release during phagocytosis, and adherence to nonphagocytosable surfaces. J. Immunol. 107 (6), 1547–1557.

Hinz, B., 2007. Formation and function of the myofibroblast during tissue repair. J. Invest. Dermatol. 127 (3), 526–537.

Hinz, B., Gabbiani, G., 2010. Fibrosis: recent advances in myofibroblast biology and new therapeutic perspectives. F1000 Biol. Rep. 2, 78.

Hinz, B., Mastrangelo, D., Iselin, C.E., Chaponnier, C., Gabbiani, G., 2001. Mechanical tension controls granulation tissue contractile activity and myofibroblast differentiation. Am. J. Pathol. 159 (3), 1009–1020.

Hinz, B., Phan, S.H., Thannickal, V.J., Prunotto, M., Desmouliere, A., Varga, J., et al., 2012. Recent developments in myofibroblast biology: paradigms for connective tissue remodeling. Am. J. Pathol. 180 (4), 1340–1355.

Hunt, T.K., Heppenstall, R.B., Pines, E., Rovee, D. (Eds.), 1984. Soft and hard tissue repair. Praeger Scientific, New York.

Hynes, R.O., Zhao, Q., 2000. The evolution of cell adhesion. J. Cell Biol. 150 (2), F89–F96.

Inflammation: Basic Principles and Clinical Correlates. third ed. Elsevier, New York, NY. 1999.

Jankowski, A., Scott, C.C., Grinstein, S., 2002. Determinants of the phagosomal pH in neutrophils. J. Biol. Chem. 277 (8), 6059–6066.

Jenkins, S.J., Ruckerl, D., Cook, P.C., Jones, L.H., Finkelman, F.D., van Rooijen, N., et al., 2011. Local macrophage proliferation, rather than recruitment from the blood, is a signature of TH2 inflammation. Science 332 (6035), 1284–1288.

Jenney, C.R., Anderson, J.M., 2000. Adsorbed serum proteins responsible for surface dependent human macrophage behavior. J. Biomed. Mater. Res. 49 (4), 435–447.

Jones, J.A., Dadsetan, M., Collier, T.O., Ebert, M., Stokes, K.S., Ward, R.S., et al., 2004. Macrophage behavior on surface-modified polyurethanes. J. Biomater. Sci. Polym. Ed. 15 (5), 567–584.

Jones, J.A., Chang, D.T., Meyerson, H., Colton, E., Kwon, I.K., Matsuda, T., et al., 2007. Proteomic analysis and quantification of cytokines and chemokines from biomaterial surface-adherent macrophages and foreign body giant cells. J. Biomed. Mater. Res. A. 83 (3), 585–596.

Jones, J.A., McNally, A.K., Chang, D.T., Qin, L.A., Meyerson, H., Colton, E., et al., 2008. Matrix metalloproteinases and their inhibitors in the foreign body reaction on biomaterials. J. Biomed. Mater. Res. A. 84 (1), 158–166.

Klebanoff, S.J., 2005. Myeloperoxidase: friend and foe. J. Leukoc. Biol. 77 (5), 598–625.

Klingberg, F., Hinz, B., White, E.S., 2013. The myofibroblast matrix: implications for tissue repair and fibrosis. J. Pathol. 229 (2), 298–309.

Kourtzelis, I., Rafail, S., DeAngelis, R.A., Foukas, P.G., Ricklin, D., Lambris, J.D., 2013. Inhibition of biomaterial-induced complement activation attenuates the inflammatory host response to implantation. FASEB J. 27 (7), 2768–2776.

Kumar, V., Abbas, A.K., Fausto, N., Robbins, S.L., Cotran, R.S., 2005. Robbins and Cotran pathologic basis of disease, seventh ed. Elsevier Saunders, Philadelphia, PA.

MacEwan, M.R., Brodbeck, W.G., Matsuda, T., Anderson, J.M., 2005. Student Research Award in the Undergraduate Degree Candidate Category, 30th Annual Meeting of the Society for Biomaterials, Memphis, TN, April 27–30, 2005. Monocyte/lymphocyte interactions and the foreign body response: *in vitro* effects of biomaterial surface chemistry. J. Biomed. Mater. Res. A. 74 (3), 285–293.

Madden, L.R., Mortisen, D.J., Sussman, E.M., Dupras, S.K., Fugate, J.A., Cuy, J.L., et al., 2010. Proangiogenic scaffolds as functional templates for cardiac tissue engineering. Proc. Natl. Acad. Sci. U.S.A. 107 (34), 15211–15216.

Mantovani, A., Sozzani, S., Locati, M., Allavena, P., Sica, A., 2002. Macrophage polarization: tumor-associated macrophages as a paradigm for polarized M2 mononuclear phagocytes. Trends. Immunol. 23 (11), 549–555.

Mantovani, A., Sica, A., Sozzani, S., Allavena, P., Vecchi, A., Locati, M., 2004. The chemokine system in diverse forms of macrophage activation and polarization. Trends. Immunol. 25 (12), 677–686.

Marchant, R.E., Anderson, J.M., Dillingham, E.O., 1986. *In vivo* biocompatibility studies. VII. Inflammatory response to polyethylene and to a cytotoxic polyvinylchloride. J. Biomed. Mater. Res. 20 (1), 37–50.

McNally, A.K., Anderson, J.M., 1994. Complement C3 participation in monocyte adhesion to different surfaces. Proc. Natl. Acad. Sci. U.S.A. 91 (21), 10119–10123.

McNally, A.K., Anderson, J.M., 2002. Beta1 and beta2 integrins mediate adhesion during macrophage fusion and multinucleated foreign body giant cell formation. Am. J. Pathol. 160 (2), 621–630.

McNally, A.K., DeFife, K.M., Anderson, J.M., 1996. Interleukin-4-induced macrophage fusion is prevented by inhibitors of mannose receptor activity. Am. J. Pathol. 149 (3), 975–985.

McNally, A.K., Macewan, S.R., Anderson, J.M., 2007. Alpha subunit partners to beta1 and beta2 integrins during IL-4-induced foreign body giant cell formation. J. Biomed. Mater. Res. A. 82 (3), 568–574.

McNally, A.K., Jones, J.A., Macewan, S.R., Colton, E., Anderson, J.M., 2008. Vitronectin is a critical protein adhesion substrate for IL-4-induced foreign body giant cell formation. J. Biomed. Mater. Res. A. 86 (2), 535–543.

Micallef, L., Vedrenne, N., Billet, F., Coulomb, B., Darby, I.A., Desmouliere, A., 2012. The myofibroblast, multiple origins for major roles in normal and pathological tissue repair. Fibrogenesis Tissue Repair 5, S5. (Suppl. 1), In: Petrides, P.E., Brenner, D. (Eds.), Proceedings of the Fibroproliferative Disorders: From Biochemical Analysis to Targeted Therapies).

Mooney, J.E., Rolfe, B.E., Osborne, G.W., Sester, D.P., van Rooijen, N., Campbell, G.R., et al., 2010. Cellular plasticity of inflammatory myeloid cells in the peritoneal foreign body response. Am. J. Pathol. 176 (1), 369–380.

Morais, J.M., Papadimitrakopoulos, F., Burgess, D.J., 2010. Biomaterials/tissue interactions: possible solutions to overcome foreign body response. AAPS J. 12 (2), 188–196.

Mosser, D.M., Edwards, J.P., 2008. Exploring the full spectrum of macrophage activation. Nat. Rev. Immunol. 8 (12), 958–969.

Mustoe, T.A., Pierce, G.F., Thomason, A., Gramates, P., Sporn, M.B., Deuel, T.F., 1987. Accelerated healing of incisional wounds in rats induced by transforming growth factor-beta. Science 237 (4820), 1333–1336.

Ney, A., Xia, T., Madler, L., Li, N., 2006. Toxic potential of materials at the nano level. Science 311 (5761), 622–627.

Nguyen, L.L., D'Amore, P.A., 2001. Cellular interactions in vascular growth and differentiation. Int. Rev. Cytol. 204, 1–48.

Nilsson, B., Ekdahl, K.N., Mollnes, T.E., Lambris, J.D., 2007. The role of complement in biomaterial-induced inflammation. Mol. Immunol. 44 (1-3), 82–94.

Pierce, G.F., 2001. Inflammation in nonhealing diabetic wounds: the space–time continuum does matter. Am. J. Pathol. 159 (2), 399–403.

Purdue, P.E., 2008. Alternative macrophage activation in periprosthetic osteolysis. Autoimmunity 41 (3), 212–217.

Revell, P.A., 2008. Biological causes of prosthetic joint failure. In: Revell, P.A. (Ed.), Join Replacement technology Woodhead Publishing, Cambridge, UK.

Revell, P.A., 2008. The combined role of wear particles, macrophages and lymphocytes in the loosening of total joint prostheses. J. R. Soc. Interface. 5 (28), 1263–1278.

Sefton, M., Babensee, J.E., Woodhouse, K.A. (Eds.) 2008. Special issue on innate and adhesion dynamics. Seminars in Immunology 20, 83–156.

Segal, A.W., 2005. How neutrophils kill microbes. Annu. Rev. Immunol. 23, 197–223.

Shive, M.S., Brodbeck, W.G., Anderson, J.M., 2002. Activation of caspase 3 during shear stress-induced neutrophil apoptosis on biomaterials. J. Biomed. Mater. Res. 62 (2), 163–168.

Sieweke, M.H., Allen, J.E., 2013. Beyond stem cells: self-renewal of differentiated macrophages. Science 342 (6161), 1242974.

Silver, I.A., Murrills, R.J., Etherington, D.J., 1988. Microelectrode studies on the acid microenvironment beneath adherent macrophages and osteoclasts. Exp. Cell. Res. 175 (2), 266–276.

Stachelek, S.J., Finley, M.J., Alferiev, I.S., Wang, F., Tsai, R.K., Eckells, E.C., et al., 2011. The effect of CD47 modified polymer surfaces on inflammatory cell attachment and activation. Biomaterials 32 (19), 4317–4326.

Wiggins, M.J., Wilkoff, B., Anderson, J.M., Hiltner, A., 2001. Biodegradation of polyether polyurethane inner insulation in bipolar pacemaker leads. J. Biomed. Mater. Res. 58 (3), 302–307.

Williams, D.F., 1987. European Society for Biomaterials, Definitions in Biomaterial. Elsevier, Amsterdam/ New York.

Williams, D.F., 2008. On the mechanisms of biocompatibility. Biomaterials 29 (20), 2941–2953.

Wynn, T.A., 2008. Cellular and molecular mechanisms of fibrosis. J. Pathol. 214 (2), 199–210.

Wynn, T.A., Ramalingam, T.R., 2012. Mechanisms of fibrosis: therapeutic translation for fibrotic disease. Nat. Med. 18 (7), 1028–1040.

Yamaguchi, KaAJ, 1992. Biocompatibility studies of naltrexone sustained release formulations. J. Control. Release 19, 299–314.

Zdolsek, J., Eaton, J.W., Tang, L., 2007. Histamine release and fibrinogen adsorption mediate acute inflammatory responses to biomaterial implants in humans. J. Transl. Med. 5, 31.

CHAPTER 3

The Biocompatibility of Implant Materials

Buddy D. Ratner
Department of Bioengineering, University of Washington, Seattle, WA, USA

Contents

Introduction	37
The Meaning of Biocompatibility	38
Biocompatibility: Historical Thinking	38
Biocompatibility Today	39
Toxicology	41
Organisms colonizing biomaterials and their impact on bioreaction	42
Mechanical effects	42
Cell–biomaterials interactions	43
Changing the Paradigm of Biocompatibility	45
Relevance to Biocompatibility	47
Conclusions	48
References	49

INTRODUCTION

The term "biocompatibility" is used so widely and so casually in so many fields that the meaning and significance of the word have been obscured and diluted. But, there is no question that biocompatibility is central to all medical implants, synthetic or natural. Evolving concepts in biology are shifting the thinking related to biocompatibility, and this chapter will consider biocompatible biomaterials in this new light.

The focus here will be on implanted materials for medical applications. The chapter will provide an overview of "biocompatibility" (i.e., what does biocompatibility mean?), a historical perspective on biocompatibility, and the central role of biocompatibility in the clinical outcome of implantable materials. The chapter will address how the body responds to various classes of biomaterials including synthetic, naturally occurring and biodegradable, and the significance of structural (morphological) and compositional aspects of a biomaterial in the host response.

Host Response to Biomaterials.
DOI: http://dx.doi.org/10.1016/B978-0-12-800196-7.00003-7
© 2015 Elsevier Inc.
All rights reserved.

THE MEANING OF BIOCOMPATIBILITY

When we say a biomaterial is biocompatible, several questions come to mind:

- Is biocompatibility "yes" or "no," or is there a continuum of biocompatibilities ranging from "good" to "bad?"
- How can we measure biocompatibility? Can we quantify biocompatibility?
- Are toxicology and biocompatibility the same thing?
- How can we improve or enhance the biocompatibility of a biomaterial?

To address these questions, a historical perspective will be presented. Then, biocompatibility today, i.e., biocompatibility as viewed by regulatory agencies and researchers, will be introduced. Finally, new concepts that will change our thinking on biocompatibility and our definition of the word will be presented and discussed.

BIOCOMPATIBILITY: HISTORICAL THINKING

Some examples of "biocompatibility" have been observed through much of history. Although early examples were not scientifically based, empirical observation and functional performance suggest that materials whose *in vivo* performance would today qualify as biocompatible have been seen and used since the earliest days of human civilization.

In the state of Washington (United States), near the town of Kennewick, the remains of a male human dated to over 8000 years ago were found. Embedded within the pelvis was a spear point, apparently well healed into the bone. One speculation was that he went through a good portion of his life with that spear point in his body. It is likely that the spear point was healed in a collagenous capsule (the foreign body reaction, FBR) and thus isolated from the individual's body in a manner similar to the way a contemporary medical implant might heal.

Two examples from the first 600 years of the modern era of humanity also illustrate early "successes" with biocompatibility. In 1931, during an archeological excavation in Honduras, the skull of a Mayan woman dated to about AD 600 was found with three seashell dental implants (Vukovic et al., 2009). Later radiological examination revealed that these implants were bonded to the bone of the jaw (osseointegrated). Around 1998, a wrought iron dental implant of an upper premolar was found in a skull in a Gallo–Roman necropolis at Chantambre, France, dated in the period AD 100–200 (Crubezy et al., 1998). Radiological evidence also demonstrated that osseointegration is consistent with modern criteria for a well-placed dental implant. Both examples demonstrate evidence of ancient attempts to replace anatomical structures with prosthetic substitutes and suggest there was some level of success, even without a scientific basis for the materials or an understanding of biocompatibility.

As early as 1891, German surgeon Themistocles Glück fashioned a hip prosthesis from ivory and nickel-plated hardware. Also around this time, Czech surgeon Vitezlav

Chlumsky experimented with hip joint interpositional materials including celluloid, silver, rubber, magnesium, zinc, glass, and celluloid. Many other material experiments from this era can be cited, particularly in the areas of orthopedics, cardiovascular medicine, and ophthalmology. The probability is low that these early material implantation experiments could have succeeded as there was no understanding of toxicology or biocompatibility.

An important observation was made during World War II by British ophthalmologic surgeon, Harold Ridley. Dr. Ridley examined aviators who, due to machine gunfire shattering the aircraft windshield, had unintentional implantations of shards of windshield in their eyes (Apple and Sims, 1996). The windshield was made of poly(methyl methacrylate) (PMMA) and Dr. Ridley noted that the shards resided in the globe of eye for years with little reaction. Although Ridley never used the term "biocompatibility," his observation of inertness and lack of reaction were consistent with modern ideas of biocompatibility. Thus, he decided to make the first human intraocular lens (IOL) out of PMMA. The first implantation was in 1949 and today about 10,000,000 IOLs are implanted each year although PMMA has, since the 1990s, been supplanted by softer acrylic polymers.

The term "biocompatibility" evolved around 1970, possibly in a seminal paper by C.A. Homsy. Therein, the concepts of toxicology and its relationship to biocompatibility were clarified (Homsy, 1970). Homsy demonstrated that organic leachables, as measured by infrared spectroscopy, could be correlated with the impact of these leachables on cells in culture. In a paper published in 1971, Homsy's ideas were integrated into a series of tests to assess the suitability of materials for a National Institutes of Health (NIH)-sponsored artificial heart program (Homsy et al., 1971). Since these early explorations around the ideas of biocompatibility, thousands of papers have been published using the term "biocompatibility." In fact, GOOGLE Scholar lists more than 17,000 papers using this term in 2014 alone. There is much variability in how the term is used and what it means. The next section of this chapter will bring biocompatibility ideas to a modern context.

BIOCOMPATIBILITY TODAY

In an effort to harmonize the terminology that was evolving in the nascent biomaterials/medical device field, a consensus conference was held in Chester, UK, in 1985. In 1987, a book was published offering a definition of biocompatibility that was arrived at by consensus of the participants, including many leading figures in the field at that time:

"the ability of a material to perform with an appropriate host response in a specific application (Williams, 1987)"

This definition, though accurate and historically important in the design, development, and application of biomaterials in medicine, nevertheless offers no insights into the mechanisms of biocompatibility, how to test the biocompatibility of a material, or how to optimize or enhance the biocompatibility of a material. Nor does it attempt to integrate new discoveries in cell and molecular biology that impact the biological reaction to implanted materials. The following text will expand the definition and explore the philosophical and scientific ideas surrounding biocompatibility.

There are many biological, medical, and engineering background concepts that impact biocompatibility. It would be impossible to review all this material in detail in this chapter. A reference volume that provides extensive background reading on this subject is the textbook, *Biomaterials Science: An introduction to Materials in Medicine*, 3rd edition (Ratner et al., 2013). Particular subjects found in this textbook and important to understanding modern ideas about biocompatibility include inflammation, wound healing, the foreign body response, *in vitro* assessment of tissue compatibility, *in vivo* assessment of tissue compatibility, regulatory issues associated with medical device development, and standards organizations and their thinking on this subject. Some of these subjects will be briefly reviewed here in overviewing biocompatibility and additional discussion of biocompatibility can be found in Chapters 2 and 14.

Biocompatibility can be assessed using *in vitro* and *in vivo* assays. First, *in vitro* assays will be discussed and further elaborated upon in the toxicology section of this chapter. Although a variety of direct chemical and physical interactions may also be important in *in vitro* assessment, e.g., mechanical "interrogation" of a surface by cells (Mammoto et al., 2013) or bioreceptor "lock-and-key" interactions driving specific biological processes (Lutolf and Hubbell, 2005), measurement of the consequences of leachable or secreted substances from biomaterials to cells in culture is a key starting point in *in vitro* biocompatibility assays. For example, inhibition of cell proliferation or cell death induced by substances leaching from a solid biomaterial are negative outcomes in such assays and would be characteristic of materials that are not biocompatible. No material can be "biocompatible" if it leaches cytotoxic substances (except perhaps a drug delivery system intended to deliver cytotoxic substances specifically to cancerous cells).

The *in vivo* (implantation) response to synthetic biomaterials that have no toxic leachables measured *in vitro* and are virtually free of endotoxin is generally described as a mild inflammatory reaction. After approximately 2–3 weeks, this reaction resolves into a thin fibrous capsule surrounding the implant with macrophages and giant cells present at the implant surface that persist for the life of the implant (Figure 3.1). Overall, however, after about 3 weeks, the reaction site is relatively quiescent and there is otherwise no indication of an active or progressive adverse local or systemic response. The composite reaction is termed the FBR. An uncomplicated FBR with a thin, nonadherent capsule surrounding the implant is considered today to be the hallmark of a "biocompatible" biomaterial. Many details of the biology associated with the FBR are described in review papers (Anderson et al., 2008; Luttikhuizen et al., 2006) and in Chapters 2, 5, and 9.

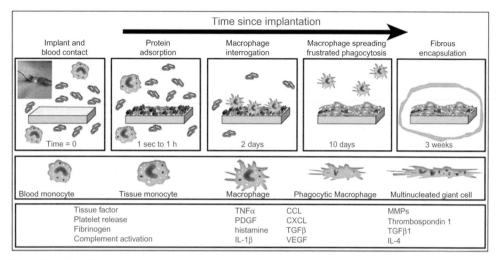

Figure 3.1 The FBR: time course, monocyte/macrophage phenotypes, and some of the key proteins involved at each stage.

The primary reaction observed with most implanted synthetic materials is the FBR. Materials and implants that show behavior upon implantation different from the FBR will be discussed toward the end of this chapter. Five factors that impact the FBR are:

1. Toxicology (the measurement and study of the effects of material leaching from biomaterials).
2. Reactions related to products from extrinsic microbiologic organisms colonizing the biomaterial (e.g., endotoxin contamination).
3. Mechanical effects such as rubbing, irritation, compression, and modulus mismatch.
4. Size of the implant impacts the FBR including its size comparable to the organism receiving the implant and relative to the size of macrophages.
5. A broad range of biospecific interactions with surrounding proteins and cells that might direct long-term *in vivo* bioreaction.

Points 1–4 above are well understood and often applied in the design of biocompatible biomaterials—we understand the principles and have the ability to measure their impact. Importantly, we can design devices using clearly defined principles to achieve appropriate outcomes. Point 5 is less well developed and considerations are discussed below.

Toxicology

Polymeric materials often contain extractable (leachable) components such as unreacted monomer, oligomers, initiator fragments, stabilizers, and other processing additives. Metals, glasses, and ceramics can release ions and other processing components. If these substances negatively impact cells (*in vitro*), adjacent tissues (*in vivo*), or affect an organism systemically, these are toxicology considerations. Biomaterials researchers, standards organizations, and government regulatory agencies have developed reliable methods to measure and identify leachates. There are sensitive and standardized methods to characterize the reaction of tissues and cells to these leached substances. The ISO (International Organization for Standardization) 10993 standards provide many specific, defined tests for toxicity associated with leachables.

Organisms colonizing biomaterials and their impact on bioreaction

Bacteria and their cell wall components are intense inflammatory activators. Fungi such as *Candida* are also inflammatory activators (Kojic and Darouiche, 2004). In the case of implants contaminated with fungi, bacteria, or bacterial cell wall endotoxin (lipopolysaccharide), an intense and usually long-term biological reaction is seen, characterized by large numbers of leukocytes (mostly neutrophils and macrophages, collectively called "pus") in the vicinity of the implant. Pain, redness and heat are associated with this response and can often lead to an exceptionally thick foreign body capsules. High concentrations of extravascular white blood cells and thick, dense foreign body capsules are characteristics of poor biocompatibility. Surface endotoxin can convert a "biocompatible" biomaterial to one that is not biocompatible. Extreme reactions to devices with contaminating organisms have been documented with breast implants (Pajkos et al., 2003) and with other implant devices. This response is distinct from *infection* with live microbiologic organisms, such as bacteria or fungi, in which the organisms may proliferate and cause ongoing local tissue destruction and potentially systemic effects. Though infection with live organisms shares some observed characteristics with "poor biocompatibility" and can occasionally look like "poor biocompatibility," we generally refer to this not as a biocompatibility issue, but rather a sterilization issue. Endotoxin, on the other hand, can lead to "poor biocompatibility." Endotoxin can be measured on biomaterials using a limulus amoebocyte lysate (LAL) assay (Young et al., 1972; Gorbet and Sefton, 2005). Although there may be a low level of endotoxin on most all biomaterials, if levels are sufficiently low, the endotoxin may not impact the reaction to implanted biomaterials (Gorbet and Sefton, 2005). Water supplies can contaminate biomaterials with endotoxin and water, even from a high-quality water purification system and should be routinely assayed for endotoxin.

Mechanical effects

If an implant is rubbing, abrading or moving in contact with tissue, or has sharp edges, undesirable reactions that may appear as "nonbiocompatible" will be observed. Mechanical mismatch between a hard biomaterial and a soft tissue can lead to damage or irritation to the soft tissue. Cell responses to mechanical forces are well known and usually quite significant (Stamenović and Ingber, 2009). An excellent example of the mechanical effect on *in vivo* bioreaction was seen in 1976 when scientists implanted in rat muscle medical grade "biocompatible" materials having circular, triangular, and pentagonal shapes (Matlaga et al., 1976). The degree of reaction increased in the order: circle (lowest reaction), pentagon, and triangle. The effect was attributed to micromotion associated with the acute angle of the triangle leading to the greatest tissue irritation. Mechanical effects on implants and the biological reaction to implants have been reviewed (Helton et al., 2011a,b). Interestingly, when implant dimensions are less than a few microns, the FBR may disappear (Sanders et al., 2000). In general, it is the role of the implant designer to ensure that the device does not excessively rub or irritate tissue (rounded edges are better than sharp edges, for example). It is the role of the surgeon to appropriately place and anchor the device in the implant site to minimize such rubbing and irritation.

Cell–biomaterials interactions

Hundreds of articles are published each year on cell–biomaterial interactions, a theme prominent in biomaterials scientific literature. For 100 years or more, it has been clear that living cells interact with and attach to different materials in different ways. The nature of that interaction profoundly influences cell attachment, spreading, proliferation, differentiation, activation, secretion, detachment, and apoptosis. It is also well established that the protein adsorption event preceding cell interaction with surfaces directs and modulates the cellular response. Since inflammatory cells such as neutrophils and macrophages "interrogate" implanted materials shortly after implantation, and since different surfaces interact in different ways with proteins, we would expect the nature (i.e., surface chemistry) of the biomaterial immersed in proteinaceous medium (e.g., serum, plasma) to impact the cell-driven *in vivo* reaction. However, let us examine this expectation. *In vitro*, profound differences are seen in cell interactions between different materials. For example, a poly(2-hydroxyethyl methacrylate) (polyHEMA) hydrogel will not permit macrophages to adhere in cell culture, while a tissue culture polystyrene (TCPS) surface readily adheres those same cells. Yet, if the polyHEMA and the TCPS are implanted *in vivo*, both will heal similarly with an avascular, collagenous foreign body capsule. In fact, all "biocompatible" materials, whether hydrophilic, hydrophobic, metallic, polymeric, or ceramic, will heal similarly with a classic (and largely quiescent) FBR if there are (1) no leachables, (2) no contaminating products from extrinsic organisms, and (3) minimal mechanical irritation. Biodegradable polymers such as poly(lactic acid) (PLA) can produce an FBR, but when they degrade to small, metabolizable molecules, the foreign body capsule may eventually be remodeled (resorbed) by the body. This striking difference between *in vitro* response and *in vivo* response has yet to be explained, but it does highlight the multifactorial complexity of the *in vivo* environment in comparison to the relatively simple *in vitro* environment where just one cell type at a time is studied.

The phenomena of "frustrated phagocytosis" and cytokine release are important. Macrophages have evolved to be efficient at engulfing and digesting foreign, aberrant and nonliving material. Examples include bacteria, dead cells, fragments of dead tissue, and synthetic particles with dimensions in the nano and macro ranges. Phagocytosis occurs when the foreign body has surface molecules that trigger receptors on the surface of the macrophage. Such trigger molecules include mannose sugar moieties, complement molecules, the Fc portion of antibodies, and denatured proteins (Hespanhol and Mantovani, 2002). The macrophage then engulfs the foreign body. Once inside this phagocyte, the foreign particle is trapped in a lipid–membrane compartment called a lysosome in which a battery of chemicals attempts to degrade the foreign material.

"Frustrated phagocytosis" occurs when the macrophage is incapable of engulfing and consuming some mass of material considerably larger than its size (certainly true for a macroscopic medical device implant). The macrophage is spread thin on the surface of the implant as it tries to engulf it and, in the process, the macrophage may release the contents of lysosomes or other vacuoles into the adjacent tissues. The diffusible components released may cause local tissue damage and inflammation. In trying to spread over this large surface (i.e., the implant), a macrophage might fuse with other adjacent macrophages and form multinucleated foreign body giant cells (FBGCs), often considered a marker of the FBR. Such FBGC can be a millimeter in size or larger. Macrophages also release cytokines (diffusible signaling proteins) in response to biomaterials (Bonfield et al., 1992). Cytokines can be considered as pro-inflammatory (e.g., IL-1, tissue necrosis factor alpha (TNF-α)) or anti-inflammatory (e.g., IL-4, IL-10). Measurements of the enzymatic release and cytokine shower from an implanted biomaterial may offer insights to biocompatibility (Marchant et al., 1983; Rodriguez et al., 2009).

A summary of some key ideas about biocompatibility from the preceding discussion is provided below:

1. Leachable chemical substances, products of extrinsic organism surface contamination (particularly endotoxin), and/or micromotion can lead to undesirable outcomes upon implantation (i.e., the implant does not appear to be biocompatible).
2. If leachables, extrinsic organism surface contamination, and micromotion are not impacting the reaction, most all materials will exhibit a similar bioreaction *in vivo*. This bioreaction is referred to as the FBR and is composed of a thin fibrous capsule with mild but persistent inflammation.
3. When the foreign body capsule is thin and the reaction site, after approximately 1 month, is relatively quiescent, this is an acceptable FBR and the implant can be considered "biocompatible."

4. The commonly observed interface between a long-term implanted medical device and the surrounding tissues is a thin, dense, collagenous capsule that isolates the implant from the body. Regulatory agencies consider this capsule, and a relatively quiescent reaction around the implant, as an acceptable reaction to an implant.

CHANGING THE PARADIGM OF BIOCOMPATIBILITY

Millions of devices made of biocompatible biomaterials are implanted in humans every year, largely with success. However, there are concerns with the way implants heal (the FBR). A new generation of biomaterials is needed to achieve integrated, vascularized, nonfibrotic healing. Such implant healing would reduce complications and make possible new applications for long-term implants.

For example, a dense fibrous capsule can inhibit diffusion of analytes to implanted sensors, interfere with release of drugs from implanted controlled drug release devices, and raise the resistance of an electrical interface with the body, thereby inhibiting communication with tissues for implanted electrodes. Capsular contraction is a problem for some devices such as breast implants, where the scar contraction distorts the mitigate implant. Moreover, the lack of vascularity near the implant–tissue interface can slow the body's response to bacterial invasion and related biofilm formation. Also, the capsule associated with the FBR can create surgical problems for device removal and revision. In many cases, a vascularized, integrated tissue reconstruction (more resembling normal tissue reconstruction) would be preferable to the avascular, dense capsule.

The potential for vascularized, nonfibrotic healing is now being realized. Such reconstructive healing can be achieved with extracellular matrix (ECM) components, with inert biomaterials that have engineered porosity, with materials that are exceptionally nonfouling and materials decorated with biomimetic receptors that "fool" the body into thinking the implant is "self."

ECMs derived from a number of tissues (e.g., small intestinal submucosa (SIS) and urinary bladder matrix (UBM)), have been found to remodel within the body with little or no fibrosis, appropriate vascularity, and general tissue reconstruction (Badylak, 2007). SIS and other ECMs have been used in millions of human surgeries largely with good results. Many review articles elaborate on these decellularized tissues as biomaterials (Badylak et al., 2011; Hoshiba et al., 2010; Arenas-Herrera et al., 2013; Andrée et al., 2013; Teodori et al., 2014). If the decellularized tissue is chemically cross-linked, it will heal in a more pro-inflammatory manner with a foreign body capsule and a classical FBR (Badylak et al., 2008; Brown et al., 2009). The excellent healing of these decellularized matrices is attributed to the ability of macrophages to degrade the ECM to bioactive peptides that actively promote healing (Vorotnikova et al., 2010). Chemical cross-linking slows degradation and inhibits this small molecule release.

Importantly, the ECM structure is heavily infused with macrophages in the early stage of healing and those macrophages have been shown to express a phenotype (frequently referred to as a polarization) conducive to healing (M2), in contrast to the pro-inflammatory, pro-fibrotic M1 phenotype (Mantovani, 2006; Badylak et al., 2008) (see Chapters 4 and 6). Note that these decellularized tissues (i.e., ECM scaffolds), often in sheet form, induce or guide a pro-reconstructive healing and then degrade. There are also suggestions that soluble ECMs derived from neonatal cell culture might be used as coating for implants to aid in healing and integration (Naughton and Kellar, 2008).

The second example presented here of materials that generate an implant reaction that is different from the classic FBR involves porous polymers. Certain porous synthetic biomaterials will also heal in a minimally fibrotic, angiogenic fashion. Observations on the special characteristics of the healing of porous structures in body were first noted in the 1970s (Karp et al., 1973; Klawitter et al., 1976). Many studies observed this porosity effect, and an article published in 1995 focused on the importance of pore size to healing (Brauker et al., 1995). The concern with all these studies was that the implant materials used had a broad distribution of pore sizes making it difficult to ascertain the effect of a specific pore size on healing. A method was developed to make materials with a single, consistent pore size based on using solvent-soluble microspheres as templates to create uniform, interconnected pores (Figure 3.2). When such materials were implanted subcutaneously, it was noted that when pores were in the size range 30–40 μm, vascularized healing and reconstruction with little fibrosis was observed (Marshall et al., 2004; Madden et al., 2010). These materials were heavily infused with macrophages during healing and more of the macrophages were in the M2 phenotype (Madden et al., 2010; Sussman et al., 2014). These same materials with 30–40 μm pores healed well in skin percutaneous sites (with dermal and epidermal reconstruction) (Fukano et al., 2010), heart muscle (Madden et al., 2010), and other tissues.

Another example of a new class of materials that heal in a manner differently from the classic FBR considers nonfouling materials (i.e., materials that resist protein adsorption and cellular interaction) (Ratner and Hoffman, 2013; Blaszykowski et al., 2012). Though many protein-resistant (nonfouling) surfaces have been developed, largely hydrogels and hydrophilic coatings, upon implantation, these materials usually show the classic FBR. In fact, it has been demonstrated that upon exposure to high protein concentrations (as are found in body fluids), surfaces that showed resistance to protein adsorption with low protein solution concentrations became adsorptive to proteins (Zhang et al., 2008). If adsorbed proteins are the first step in triggering the FBR (as is suggested in Figure 3.1), then perhaps by completely eliminating the adsorbed proteins a material that is not recognized by the body can be made? This hypothesis was tested with implants of an exceptionally protein-resistant hydrogel biomaterial, poly(carboxybetaine methacrylate) (Zhang et al., 2013). After 3 months of subcutaneous implantation, no measurable FBR was noted. In this study, M2 macrophages were again seen to be present at the implant site.

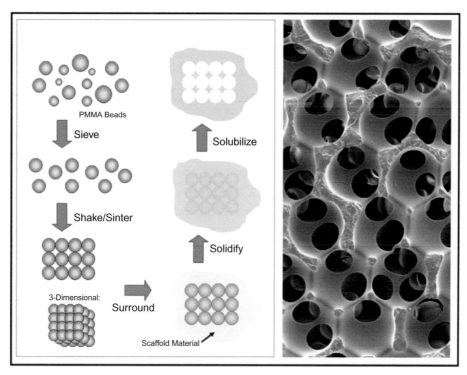

Figure 3.2 A schematic illustration of the sphere-templating process for preparing porous biomaterials with uniform-sized pores. The scanning electron microscopic image shows the uniformity of the material and the interconnect "throats" between pores.

A fourth strategy to inhibit the FBR involves immobilizing to biomaterial surfaces the cell surface receptors found on many body cells that indicate "self" and prevent the body from attacking the cells. The extracellular domain of a recombinant form of receptor protein CD47 (found on red blood cells) was immobilized to polyurethane and poly(vinyl chloride) (Stachelek et al., 2011). Upon implantation, reduced inflammatory cell interaction with the surfaces was noted.

RELEVANCE TO BIOCOMPATIBILITY

With relevance to biocompatibility, consider this example. A synthetic hydrogel is fabricated as a solid slab, or as a porous structure with 30–40 μm interconnected pores. The chemical compositions of both are identical. Also, they have similar mechanical properties, no leachables, and no endotoxin or bacteria. Yet one heals in a capsule with the classic FBR while the other heals in a vascularized, reconstructed manner with little fibrosis. It seems challenging to use the word "biocompatible" for both given the sharp differences in *in vivo* biological reaction despite identical chemistries. This dichotomy has led the author of this chapter to propose two new definitions relating to biocompatibility.

For the biocompatibility observed in the four examples presented here where we observe an integrated, vascularized reconstructive outcome, this definition is proposed:

> **BIOCOMPATIBILITY: the ability of materials to locally trigger and guide normal wound healing, reconstruction and tissue integration.**

For the "biocompatibility" associated with today's commercialized implants that are approved by regulatory agencies and work satisfactorily in many applications in medicine, the term "biocompatibility" is replaced by "biotolerability."

> **BIOTOLERABILITY: the ability of materials to reside in the body for long periods of time with only low degrees of inflammatory reaction.**

CONCLUSIONS

Biomaterials as we know them today were first introduced to medical practice in the late 1940s and early 1950s. Since then there has been an evolution in sophistication and functionality of biomaterials (Williams, 2008). First generation biomaterials were considered to be "inert" (e.g., silicones, titanium, Teflon, polyethylene) although the tissue response to the same biomaterials today is considered anything but inert. Second generation biomaterials (1970s, 1980s) interacted with and changed, in a controlled manner, the biological environment. For example, the biodegradability of PLA, the bone integration, and bone formation as seen with bioactive glasses, the induction of a controlled thrombotic deposit, such as occurs with a textured polymer on the internal surface of a left ventricular assist device. Third generation biomaterials (1990+) biospecifically orchestrate biological processes and can direct regeneration and restore functionality, and/or respond to the environment in a proactive manner to favorably influence a tissue reaction. Examples include engineered ECMs (Lutolf and Hubbell, 2005), sphere templated biomaterials (Madden et al., 2010), decellularized ECMs (Badylak, 2007), and "smart" biomaterials (Reyes et al., 2007). Also, consider the published debate on the effectiveness of biomaterials guided by specific peptide signals (Williams, 2011). As biomaterials evolve, so, too must the definition of biocompatibility. This chapter traced biocompatibility ideas from early history, discussed the roots of today's accepted biocompatibility ideas, and illustrated how new developments have made the existing definition of biocompatibility unwieldy and inaccurate.

The way we define biocompatibility will evolve over the next few years. Examples that challenge the present paradigm of biocompatibility are published and materials that show unique healing are being applied in clinical medicine (Pourjavan et al., 2014; Badylak et al., 2011). Recent discoveries on the diversity of macrophage phenotypes and understanding of resident tissue stem cell pools in the body may permit engineered "biocompatibility" with control of the extent and rate of biointegration. These new developments strengthen the science of biocompatibility and bring biomaterials and tissue engineering closer together. Precision control of biocompatibility can lead to new biomaterials-based therapies with profound advantages for the patient.

To answer the questions posed at the beginning of this chapter:

- Is biocompatibility "yes" or "no," or is there a continuum of biocompatibilities ranging from "good" to "bad?"
  Answer: The extremes, good biocompatibility and bad biocompatibility, can be easily defined by histological appearance of the implant site. Intermediate levels of biocompatibility may be defined in the future by a ratio of M1/M2 macrophages, by cytokine profiles or by quantification of vascularity and angiogenesis.
- How can we measure biocompatibility? Can we quantify biocompatibility?
  Answer: At the present time, we can quantify toxicology by measuring leachables. In the future we may quantify M1/M2 ratio, vascularity, cytokines, and other factors to arrive at a quantitative assessment, perhaps to be called "the biocompatibility parameter."
- Are toxicology and biocompatibility the same thing?
  Answer: Toxicology is routine and accurately defined. Biocompatibility, by the new definition presented here, is distinct from toxicology and certainly more complex to qualitatively and quantitatively express.
- How can we improve or enhance the biocompatibility of a biomaterial?
  Answer: Four examples have been presented here for improving biocompatibility (based on the new definition). Other paths to improved biocompatibility will, no doubt, be described in the future.

For now, the medical device regulatory agencies subscribe almost exclusively to definition of biocompatibility that we have been using, a definition that traces its roots to the first functionally successful implants in the 1950s. In reality, it is important to appreciate the accepted standards for biomaterials (ISO 10993). These standards are used by the $300B+ worldwide medical device industry and these standards impact millions of patients. Still, there is a shift in thinking about this subject in the biomaterials and tissue engineering research communities. Driven by discoveries in basic cell and molecular biology and embraced by biomaterials and tissue engineering researchers, newer ideas are being generated and these ideas shift the way we think about the word "biocompatibility."

REFERENCES

Anderson, J.M., Rodriguez, A., Chang, D.T., 2008. Foreign body reaction to biomaterials. Semin. Immunol. 20, 86–100.

Andrée, B., Bär, A., Haverich, A., Hilfiker, A., 2013. Small intestinal submucosa segments as matrix for tissue engineering: review. Tissue Eng. Part B: Rev. 19 (4), 279–291.

Apple, D.J., Sims, J., 1996. Harold Ridley and the invention of the intraocular lens. Surv. Ophthalmol. 40 (4), 279–292.

Arenas-Herrera, J.E., Ko, I.K., Atala, A., Yoo, J.J., 2013. Decellularization for whole organ bioengineering. Biomed. Mater. 8 (1), 014106.

Badylak, S., Valentin, J., Ravindra, A., Mccabe, G., Stewart-Akers, A., 2008. Macrophage phenotype as a determinant of biologic scaffold remodeling. Tissue. Eng. Part. A. 14 (11), 1835–1842.

Badylak, S.F., 2007. The extracellular matrix as a biologic scaffold material. Biomaterials 28 (25), 3587–3593.

Badylak, S.F., Hoppo, T., Nieponice, A., Gilbert, T.W., Davison, J.M., Jobe, B.A., 2011. Esophageal preservation in five male patients after endoscopic inner-layer circumferential resection in the setting of superficial cancer: a regenerative medicine approach with a biologic scaffold. Tissue Eng.: Part A 17 (11–12), 1643–1650.

Badylak, S.F., Taylor, D., Uygun, K., 2011. Whole-organ tissue engineering: decellularization and recellularization of three-dimensional matrix scaffolds. Annu. Rev. Biomed. Eng. 13 (1), 27–53.

Blaszykowski, C., Sheikh, S., Thompson, M., 2012. Surface chemistry to minimize fouling from blood-based fluids. Chem. Soc. Rev. 41 (17), 5599–5612.

Bonfield, T.L., Colton, E., Marchant, R.E., Anderson, J.M., 1992. Cytokine and growth factor production by monocyte/macrophages on protein preadsorbed polymers. J. Biomed. Mater. Res. 26, 837–850.

Brauker, J.H., Carr-Brendel, V.E., Martinson, L.A., Crudele, J., Johnston, W.D., Johnson, R.C., 1995. Neovascularization of synthetic membranes directed by membrane microarchitecture. J. Biomed. Mater. Res. 29, 1517–1524.

Brown, B., Valentin, J., Stewartakers, A., Mccabe, G., Badylak, S., 2009. Macrophage phenotype and remodeling outcomes in response to biologic scaffolds with and without a cellular component. Biomaterials 30 (8), 1482–1491.

Crubezy, E., Murail, P., Girard, L., Bernadou, J.-P., 1998. False teeth of the roman world. Nature 391, 29.

Fukano, Y., Usui, M.L., Underwood, R.A., Isenhath, S., Marshall, A.J., Hauch, K.D., et al., 2010. Epidermal and dermal integration into sphere-templated porous poly(2-hydroxyethyl methacrylate) implants in mice. J. Biomed. Mater. Res. A. 94 (4), 1172–1186.

Gorbet, M.B., Sefton, M.V., 2005. Endotoxin: the uninvited guest. Biomaterials 26 (34), 6811–6817.

Helton, K.L., Ratner, B.D., Wisniewski, N.A., 2011a. Biomechanics of the sensor–tissue interface—effects of motion, pressure, and design on sensor performance and foreign body response—Part II: Examples and application. J. Diabetes Sci. Technol. 5 (3), 647–656.

Helton, K.L., Ratner, B.D., Wisniewski, N.A., 2011b. Biomechanics of the sensor–tissue interface—effects of motion, pressure, and design on sensor performance and the foreign body response—Part I: Theoretical framework. J. Diabetes Sci. Technol. 5 (3), 632–646.

Hespanhol, M.R., Mantovani, B., 2002. Phagocytosis by macrophages mediated by receptors for denatured proteins—dependence on tyrosine protein kinases. Braz. J. Med. Biol. Res. 35 (3), 383–389.

Homsy, C.A., 1970. Bio-compatibility in selection of materials for implantation. J. Biomed. Mater. Res. 4, 341–356.

Homsy, C.A., Ansevin, K.D., O'Bannon, W., Thompson, S.A., Hodge, R., Estrella, M.A., 1971. Rapid in vitro screening of polymers for biocompatibility. In: Rembaum, A., Shen, M. (Eds.), Biomedical Polymers Marcel Dekker, New York, NY, pp. 121–140.

Hoshiba, T., Lu, H., Kawazoe, N., Chen, G., 2010. Decellularized matrices for tissue engineering. Expert. Opin. Biol. Ther. 10 (12), 1717–1728.

Karp, R.D., Johnson, K.H., Buoen, L.C., Ghobrial, H.K.G., Brand, I., Brand, K.G., 1973. Tumorigenesis by millipore filters in mice: histology and ultrastructure of tissue reactions as related to pore size. J. Nat. Cancer Inst. 51 (4), 1275–1279.

Klawitter, J.J., Bagwell, J.G., Weinstein, A.M., Sauer, B.W., Pruitt, J.R., 1976. An evaluation of bone growth into porous high density polyethylene. J. Biomed. Mater. Res. 10 (2), 311–323.

Kojic, E.M., Darouiche, R.O., 2004. Candida infections of medical devices. Clin. Microbiol. Rev. 17 (2), 255–267.

Lutolf, M.P., Hubbell, J.A., 2005. Synthetic biomaterials as instructive extracellular microenvironments for morphogenesis in tissue engineering. Nat. Biotechnol. 23 (1), 47–55.

Luttikhuizen, D.T., Harmsen, M.C., Van Luyn, M.J.A., 2006. Cellular and molecular dynamics in the foreign body reaction. Tiss. Eng. 12 (7), 1955–1970.

Madden, L.R., Mortisen, D.J., Sussman, E.M., Dupras, S.K., Fugate, J.A., Cuy, J.L., et al., 2010. Proangiogenic scaffolds as functional templates for cardiac tissue engineering. Proc. Natl. Acad. Sci. U.S.A. 107 (34), 15211–15216.

Mammoto, T., Mammoto, A., Ingber, D.E., 2013. Mechanobiology and developmental control. Annu. Rev. Cell. Dev. Biol. 29, 27–61.

Mantovani, A., 2006. Macrophage diversity and polarization: *in vivo* veritas. Blood 108 (2), 408–409.

Marchant, R., Hiltner, A., Hamlin, C., Rabinovitch, A., Slobodkin, R., Anderson, J.M., 1983. *In vivo* bio-compatibility studies. I. The cage implant system and a biodegradable hydrogel. J. Biomed. Mater. Res. 17, 301–325.

Marshall, A.J., Irvin, C.A., Barker, T., Sage, E.H., Hauch, K.D., Ratner, B.D., 2004. Biomaterials with tightly controlled pore size that promote vascular in-growth. ACS Polym. Preprints 45 (2), 100–101.

Matlaga, B.F., Yasenchak, L.P., Salthouse, T.N., 1976. Tissue response to implanted polymers: the significance of sample shape. J. Biomed. Mater. Res. 10 (3), 391–397.

Naughton, G., Kellar, R., 2008. Human ECM for devices and therapeutics. MD & DI (May), 102–109.

Pajkos, A., Deva, A.K., Vickery, K., Cope, C., Chang, L., Cossart, Y.E., 2003. Detection of subclinical infection in significant breast implant capsules. Plast. Reconstr. Surg. 111 (5), 1605–1611.

Pourjavan, S., Collignon, N.J.M., De Groot, V., Eiferman, R.A., Marshall, A.J., Roy, C.J., 2014. STARflo™: a suprachoroidal drainage implant made from STAR biomaterial. In: Samples, J.R., Ahmed, I.I.K. (Eds.), Surgical Innovations in Glaucoma Springer Publishers, New York, NY, pp. 235–251.

Ratner, B.D., Hoffman, A.S., 2013. Non-fouling surfaces. In: Ratner, B.D., Hoffman, A.S., Schoen, F., Lemons, J. (Eds.), Biomaterials Science: An Introduction to Materials in Medicine, third ed Elsevier, Inc., Amsterdam, pp. 241–247.

Ratner, B.D., Hoffman, A.S., Schoen, F., Lemons, J. (Eds.), 2013. Biomaterials Science: An Introduction to Materials in Medicine, third ed. Elsevier, Inc., Amsterdam.

Reyes, C.D., Petrie, T.A., Burns, K.L., Schwartz, Z., García, A.J., 2007. Biomolecular surface coating to enhance orthopaedic tissue healing and integration. Biomaterials 28 (21), 3228–3235.

Rodriguez, A., Meyerson, H., Anderson, J.M., 2009. Quantitative *in vivo* cytokine analysis at synthetic biomaterial implant sites. J. Biomed. Mater. Res. A 89A, 152–159.

Sanders, J.E., Stiles, C.E., Hayes, C.L., 2000. Tissue response to single polymer fibers of varying diameters: evaluation of fibrous encapsulation and macrophage density. J. Biomed. Mater. Res. 52, 231–237.

Stachelek, S.J., Finley, M.J., Alferiev, I.S., Wang, F., Tsai, R.K., Eckells, E.C., et al., 2011. The effect of CD47 modified polymer surfaces on inflammatory cell attachment and activation. Biomaterials 32 (19), 4317–4326.

Stamenović, D., Ingber, D.E., 2009. Tensegrity-guided self assembly: from molecules to living cells. Soft. Matter. 5 (6), 1137–1145.

Sussman, E.M., Halpin, M.C., Muster, J., Moon, R.T., Ratner, B.D., 2014. Porous implants modulate healing and induce shifts in local macrophage polarization in the foreign body reaction. Ann. Biomed. Eng. 42 (7), 1508–1516.

Teodori, L., Costa, A., Marzio, R., Perniconi, B., Coletti, D., Adamo, S., et al., 2014. Native extracellular matrix: a new scaffolding platform for repair of damaged muscle. Front. Physiol. 5, 218.

Vorotnikova, E., McIntosh, D., Dewilde, A., Zhang, J., Reing, J.E., Zhang, L., et al., 2010. Extracellular matrix-derived products modulate endothelial and progenitor cell migration and proliferation *in vitro* and stimulate regenerative healing *in vivo*. Matrix. Biol. 29 (8), 690–700.

Vukovic, A., Bajsman, A., Zukic, S., Secic, S., 2009. Cosmetic dentistry in ancient time—short review. Bull. Int. Assoc. Paleodontol. 3 (2), 9–13.

Williams, D.F., 1987. Definitions in Biomaterials. Progress in Biomedical Engineering, 4. Elsevier, Amsterdam.

Williams, D.F., 2008. On the mechanisms of biocompatibility. Biomaterials 29 (20), 2941–2953.

Williams, D.F., 2011. The role of short synthetic adhesion peptides in regenerative medicine; The debate. Biomaterials 32 (18), 4195–4197.

Young, N.S., Levin, J., Prendergast, R.A., 1972. An invertebrate coagulation system activated by endotoxin: evidence for enzymatic mediation. J. Clin. Invest. 51 (7), 1790–1797.

Zhang, L., Cao, Z., Bai, T., Carr, L., Ella-Menye, J.-R., Irvin, C., et al., 2013. Zwitterionic hydrogels implanted in mice resist the foreign-body reaction. Nat. Biotechnol. 31 (6), 553–556.

Zhang, Z., Zhang, M., Chen, S., Horbett, T., Ratner, B., Jiang, S., 2008. Blood compatibility of surfaces with superlow protein adsorption. Biomaterials 29 (32), 4285–4291.

CHAPTER 4

Host Response to Naturally Derived Biomaterials

Samuel T. Lopresti and Bryan N. Brown
Department of Bioengineering, McGowan Institute for Regenerative Medicine, University of Pittsburgh, Pittsburgh, PA, USA

Contents

INTRODUCTION

The use of naturally derived materials in clinical and preclinical settings offers a number of advantages over the use of synthetic materials. First and foremost is the native ligand landscape and inherent bioactivity present within naturally derived materials. These ligands are often highly conserved when naturally derived materials are sourced from mammalian tissues; however, it should be noted that certain other natural materials derived from plant, insect, or crustacean sources have chemical compositions which are similar to mammalian proteins and are reported to offer similar advantages. Second

Host Response to Biomaterials.
DOI: http://dx.doi.org/10.1016/B978-0-12-800196-7.00004-9

is the ability of the host to degrade and process the material efficiently, avoiding aspects of the foreign body response observed with many synthetic polymers. However, a number of disadvantages are also associated with the use of naturally derived materials. These disadvantages include potential immunogenicity, biologic variability among source tissues, and significant complexity with respect to the mechanisms associated with either success or failure of the material in medical applications.

The history of the use of naturally derived biomaterials in medical applications is long. The use of xenogeneic skin grafts was mentioned in the Papyrus of Ebers from the fifteenth century BC. Later, Egyptians reported using animal sinew as suture material. While these materials were acceptable more than two millennia ago, the success of xenogeneic and allogeneic tissue-derived materials was limited due to the immune response following implantation (Watson and Dark, 2012). Poor outcomes, and other practical considerations, provided the impetus for further development and refinement of biomaterials, both synthetic and natural in origin, for use in surgical reconstructive applications as well as in engineered tissues and organs intended to replace transplants with laboratory grown tissues.

Commonly, the naturally derived materials used in current medical applications are derived from the extracellular matrix (ECM) of mammalian tissue. However, others are sourced from the exoskeletons of crustaceans or from bacterial sources. Table 4.1 lists a variety of naturally derived materials which are currently in clinical use, though many of the materials listed are intended for temporary or topical use as opposed to implantation.

The present chapter focuses upon the host response to naturally derived materials, both in common clinical applications and in more recent and novel tissue engineering and regenerative medicine applications. It is now increasingly clear that, regardless of the application in which naturally derived biomaterials are used, the host response elicited following implantation is an integral part of the remodeling process and a critical determinant of success. Though beyond the scope of this chapter to provide a full discussion of the differences between the host response to multiple classes of metallic, polymeric, and naturally derived materials and the implications of such responses for clinical outcomes, this chapter will outline the distinct aspects of the host response which are associated with the success of naturally derived materials. It is important to note that the host response to each naturally derived material is unique and based upon the composition, ligand landscape, and processing methods inherent to the source material used for production. Thus, though biomaterials have been derived from multiple natural sources including mammalian tissues as well as insect, crustacean, and plant sources we focus upon one class of natural biomaterial—those derived through the decellularization of mammalian tissues and organs. These materials have now been used in millions of human patients to date, with both positive and poor outcomes having been reported. Therefore, tissue-derived materials represent an effective case study.

Table 4.1 Examples of medical products composed of naturally derived materials

Material	Source	Properties	Use/example
Alginate	Algae (Kelp)	Anionic polysaccharide, limited degradation unless modified, forms hydrogels	Wound dressing (Phytacare®)
Chitosan	Crustacean exoskeletons	Positively charged, enzymatic degradation, can form hydrogels	Hemostat/ wound dressing (HemCon®)
Silk	Synthesized by spider or silk worms	Physiologic function is as a protective cocoon, strong and can be woven, slow, or minimal degradation	Suture (Perma-Hand®)
Collagen	Animal tissues/cell culture/bacterial fermentation	Abundant ECM protein, triple helix structure, provide cell attachment sites	Injectable dermal filler (CosmoDerm®)
Gelatin	Denatured collagen	Inexpensive, used for cell attachment in cell culture	Sterile absorbable sponge (Gelfoam®)
Fibrin/ fibrinogen	Animal tissues or plasma	Fibrin results from polymerization of fibrinogen with thrombin, crucial for clot formation	Fibrin sealant (Evicel®)
Hyaluronic acid	Animal tissues/ bacterial fermentation	Lubricating polymer, only nonsulfated GAG, negatively charged, can form hydrogels	Dermal filler (Restylane®)
Heparin	Animal tissues/ plasma	Strongly negatively charged GAG, binds to numerous growth factors, anticoagulant activity, used to coat stents	Stent and catheter coating (TyCo®)
Decellularized tissue	Animal tissues	Complex mixture of proteins and GAGs in tissue-specific composition and architecture	Surgical mesh (see Table 4.2 for multiple examples)

Source: Distinctive properties and an example of a currently available, FDA-approved product are listed. Adapted from Ratner (2013).

The focus upon decellularized tissue-derived biomaterials presented in this chapter is not intended to imply that other sources are inferior or less successful, but rather to provide a focused discussion of the many factors which affect the host response to a single class of naturally derived material as well as provide a contrast to other chapters describing the host response to multiple types of synthetic material. Many of the concepts which are described herein are easily applied to other natural biomaterial sources.

THE USE OF DECELLULARIZED TISSUE AS A BIOMATERIAL FOR SURGICAL RECONSTRUCTION AND CONSTRUCTIVE REMODELING

Mesh materials derived through the decellularization of human or animal tissue sources are commonly used in surgical repair and reconstruction. There are more than 30 commercially available, FDA-approved products with indications commonly including wound care, soft tissue reconstruction, and orthopedic applications, among others. These materials vary in their source tissue, methods of processing, and methods of sterilization (Badylak, 2004; Brown and Badylak, 2014). Table 4.2 provides examples of currently available decellularized scaffold materials available for clinical use, their tissue source, and clinical indications.

These materials have been used for more than a decade and in millions of human patients to date. Their success in promoting positive remodeling outcomes following placement, however, has been reported to be variable depending upon the source of the material, methods of preparation, and application. As an example, a rodent abdominal defect model was used to evaluate the host remodeling response following the implantation of five commonly used materials for orthopedic applications. The results demonstrated that those materials which were effectively decellularized and exhibited more rapid degradation were associated with increased cellular infiltration at early time points and improved histologic appearance downstream (Valentin et al., 2006). These reports appear to be consistent with those observed in multiple human clinical applications.

Positive outcomes with tissue-derived biomaterials can be described as a process of "constructive" or "inductive" remodeling, particularly when applied to tissue engineering and regenerative medicine applications wherein desired outcomes include the formation of new, site-appropriate, functional host tissue in addition to surgical repair (Badylak et al., 2011a). These constructive and inductive outcomes are in contrast to surgical "repair" in that they result in new, functional tissue formation. For example, multiple recent animal and human clinical studies have demonstrated that placement of an acellular tissue-derived scaffold can result in the formation of functional skeletal muscle (Daly et al., 2011; Valentin et al., 2010; Sicari et al., 2012a, 2014a; Turner and Badylak, 2012; Mase et al., 2010). Briefly, though the full set of mechanisms which lead to this type of constructive remodeling are not known, the early response to scaffold placement includes a robust infiltration by immune cells followed by material degradation, recruitment of local and circulating progenitor cells, and eventual formation of new tissue (Badylak et al., 2011a; Badylak, 2014). Constructive remodeling has now been observed following the placement of acellular tissue-derived biomaterials in musculoskeletal tissue, esophagus, cartilage, and cardiovascular applications among numerous others (Sicari et al., 2014a; Badylak et al., 2011b; Brown et al., 2011b, 2012a; Wainwright et al., 2012; Remlinger et al., 2010). Whether used

Table 4.2 Examples of currently available decellularized tissue-based products

Product	Company	Material	Cross-linking	Form	Use
AlloDerm®	LifeCell	Human skin	Natural	Dry sheet	Abdominal wall, breast, ENT/head and neck reconstruction, grafting
AlloPatch HD®	Musculoskeletal Transplant Foundation	Human dermis	Cross-linked	Dry sheet	Orthopedic applications
Axis™	Coloplast	Human dermis	Natural	Dry sheet	Pelvic organ prolapse
Biodesign®	Cook Biotech	Porcine SIS	Natural	Dry sheet	Repair of cranial or spinal dura
CollaMend™ FM	CR Bard	Porcine dermis	Cross-linked	Dry sheet	Soft tissue repair
Durepair®	Medtronic	Fetal bovine skin	Natural	Dry sheet	Repair of cranial or spinal dura
Graft Jacket®	Wright Medical Tech	Human skin	Cross-linked	Dry sheet	Foot ulcers
MatriStem®	ACell	Porcine urinary bladder	Natural	Dry sheet	Soft tissue repair and reinforcement, burns, gynecologic
Oasis®	Healthpoint Biotherapeutics	Porcine SIS	Natural	Dry sheet	Partial and full thickness wounds; superficial and second-degree burns
Peri-Guard®	Baxter	Bovine pericardium	Cross-linked	Hydrated sheet	Pericardial and soft tissue repair
Permacol™	Covidien	Porcine skin	Cross-linked	Hydrated sheet	Soft connective tissue repair
Restore®	DePuy	Porcine SIS	Natural	Sheet	Reinforcement of soft tissues
SurgiMend®	TEI Biosciences	Fetal bovine skin	Natural	Dry sheet	Surgical repair of damaged or ruptured soft tissue membranes
Suspen®	Coloplast	Human fascia lata	Natural	Dry sheet	Urethral sling
TissueMend®	Stryker	Fetal bovine skin	Natural	Dry sheet	Surgical repair and reinforcement of soft tissue in rotator cuff
Vascu-Guard®	Baxter	Bovine pericardium	Cross-linked	Hydrated sheet	Reconstruction of blood vessels in neck, legs, and arms

Source: Adapted from Ratner (2013).

in surgical reconstruction or as an inductive template for constructive remodeling, the host response to such materials is now known to be a clear determinant of successful outcomes (Brown and Badylak, 2013, 2014; Badylak et al., 2008, 2011a; Brown et al., 2012b; Badylak and Gilbert, 2008). The factors which affect the host response and subsequent ability to promote constructive remodeling following the placement of tissue-derived materials are discussed in more detail below.

IMMUNE REJECTION

Discussion of the host immune response to tissue-derived biomaterials would be incomplete without first discussing briefly the mechanisms of immune rejection to viable tissues and organs. Using xenogeneic or allogeneic tissues as materials for tissue repair or transplantation without any processing of the material or immunosuppression of the patient will uniformly lead to immune rejection by the adaptive immune response. T- and B-lymphocytes will be activated in response to non-self-antigenic epitopes on cells in these tissues with a subsequent activation of an antibody-mediated response resulting in rejection (Vadori and Cozzi, 2014; Fox et al., 2001). Early attempts to solve this problem revolved around immunosuppressive therapies and were partially successful (Sachs et al., 2001). Improvements in the number and combination of immunosuppressive therapies and human leukocyte antigen (HLA) matching have helped to inhibit rejection (Susal and Opelz, 2013; Opelz et al., 1999). Xenogeneic tissue and organ transplants are currently unavailable due to ineffective immunosuppressive therapy (Scalea et al., 2012). However, there are efforts utilizing both pharmacological and genetic approaches to create xenogeneic organs suitable for human transplantation.

While immunosuppressive drugs can inhibit the immune rejection of xenogeneic and allogeneic tissues, this therapeutic approach leaves the patient susceptible to infection and other diseases. An effective approach to the use of xenogeneic and allogeneic tissues is decellularization. Such an approach removes the cellular content from these tissues and, thereby, many of the epitopes recognized by the host as foreign. Decellularization leaves behind the ECM of these tissues, many components of which are highly conserved across mammalian species (van der Rest and Garrone, 1991). Due to this genetic preservation, xenogeneic and allogeneic materials can be safely implanted into patients without an adverse adaptive immune reaction if properly decellularized (Gilbert et al., 2006).

DECELLULARIZATION PROCESSES

As stated above, decellularization is necessary to remove the cellular components of tissues that elicit an adverse host response. Decellularization is the process of using various methods, physical, enzymatic, or chemical, to lyse cells and remove the intra-cellular components from a tissue while preserving the native extracellular components (Freytes et al., 2004; Lin et al., 2004; Dahl et al., 2003; Vyavahare et al., 1997; De Filippo et al., 2002; Falke et al., 2003). In theory, the goal of an effective decellularization process is to remove the cellular epitopes and antigens that elicit potentially destructive immune responses resulting in implant failure while preserving the composition and configuration of ECM macromolecules. As discussed in the following sections, preservation of the native microenvironment by maintaining the integrity of ECM proteins and related molecules is important in triggering a beneficial host response resulting in constructive remodeling.

Each tissue has a unique composition and organization of cells and ECM. As a result, the decellularization protocol must be optimized for each tissue to maximize cellular content removal while preserving the beneficial ECM proteins, glycosaminoglycans, and growth factors in their native state. Table 4.3 details briefly different methods of decellularization and their mechanism for removal of specific tissue constituents.

While optimized decellularization strategies remove most of the molecules that elicit an adaptive immune response to xenogeneic or allogeneic materials, it is logical that some cell-derived components will remain due to the decellularization processes which generally promote lysis and uncontrolled release of cellular components. There have been few studies which determine the consequences of these remnant molecules upon the host response and tissue remodeling process; however, paradoxically, those studies which have investigated their presence have clearly demonstrated the potential for both positive and negative effects of cellular remnants. In the following section, three cellular constituents known to affect the host response and subsequent remodeling of tissue-derived biomaterials are described.

α-GAL EPITOPE

A major consideration of deriving biomaterials from xenogeneic sources is the α-Gal epitope. As described in detail in Chapter 10, this carbohydrate moiety consisting of Galα1-3Galβ1-4GlcNAc-R or Galα1-3Galβ1-3GlcNAc-R is found in nonprimate mammals, as well as New World monkeys, and is produced by the glycosylation enzyme α1,3galactosyltransferase. This enzyme is absent in humans; therefore, the sugar moiety is also absent in human tissues. Instead, humans produce large amounts of antibodies to the α-Gal epitope following exposure which is common shortly after birth as part of the normal gut flora (Galili, 2005). A full review of the α-Gal epitope and its effects upon the host response and tissue remodeling can be found in Chapter 10 and is therefore only mentioned briefly here in the context of tissue-derived biomaterials. Analysis of decellularized porcine tissues including heart valve, anterior cruciate ligament, and small intestinal submucosa has shown the α-Gal epitope to be present

Table 4.3 Overview of strategies used in tissue decellularization

Method	Mode of action	Effects on ECM	References
Physical			
Snap freezing	Intracellular ice crystals disrupt cell membrane	ECM can be disrupted or fractured during rapid freezing	Jackson et al. (1987a,b, 1988, 1991, 1990), Roberts et al. (1991), Gulati (1988)
Mechanical force	Pressure can burst cells and tissue removal eliminates cells	Mechanical force can cause damage to ECM	Freytes et al. (2004), Lin et al. (2004)
Mechanical agitation	Can cause cell lysis, but more commonly used to facilitate chemical exposure and cellular material removal	Aggressive agitation or sonication can disrupt ECM as the cellular material is removed	Freytes et al. (2004), Lin et al. (2004), Dahl et al. (2003), Schenke–Layland et al. (2003)
Chemical			
Alkaline; acid	Solubilizes cytoplasmic components of cells; disrupts nucleic acids	Removes GAGs	Freytes et al. (2004), De Filippo et al. (2002), Falke et al. (2003), Probst et al. (1997), Yoo et al. (1998)
Nonionic detergents			
Triton X-100	Disrupts lipid–lipid and lipid–protein interactions, while leaving protein–protein interactions intact	Mixed results; efficiency dependent on tissue, removes GAGs	Lin et al. (2004), Dahl et al. (2003), De Filippo et al. (2002), Chen et al. (2000), Cartmell and Dunn (2000), Woods and Gratzer (2005), Grauss et al. (2003)
Ionic detergents			
Sodium dodecyl sulfate (SDS)	Solubilize cytoplasmic and nuclear cellular membranes; tend to denature proteins	Removes nuclear remnants and cytoplasmic proteins; tends to disrupt native tissue structure, remove GAGs and damage collagen	Lin et al. (2004), Woods and Gratzer (2005), Rieder et al. (2004), Chen et al. (2004), Hudson et al. (2004a,b)
Sodium deoxycholate		More disruptive to tissue structure than SDS	Lin et al. (2004), Woods and Gratzer (2005), Rieder et al. (2004), Chen et al. (2004), Hudson et al. (2004a,b)

Agent	Mechanism	Effect	References
Triton X-200		Yielded efficient cell removal when used with zwitterionic detergents	Lin et al. (2004), Woods and Gratzer (2005), Rieder et al. (2004), Chen et al. (2004) Hudson et al. (2004a,b)
Zwitterionic detergents			
CHAPS	Exhibit properties of nonionic and ionic detergents	Efficient cell removal with ECM disruption similar to that of Triton X-100	Dahl et al. (2003)
Sulfobetaine-10 and −16 (SB-10, SB-16)		Yielded cell removal and mild ECM disruption with Triton X-200	Lin et al. (2004), Woods and Gratzer (2005), Rieder et al. (2004), Chen et al. (2004), Hudson et al. (2004a,b)
Tri(*n*-butyl) phosphate	Organic solvent that disrupts protein–protein interactions	Variable cell removal; loss of collagen content, although effect on mechanical properties was minimal	Dahl et al. (2003), Woods and Gratzer (2005)
Hypotonic and hypertonic solutions	Cell lysis by osmotic shock	Efficient for cell lysis, but does not effectively remove the cellular remnants	Dahl et al. (2003) Vyavahare et al. (1997), Woods and Gratzer (2005) Goissis et al. (2000)
EDTA, EGTA	Chelating agents that bind divalent metallic ions, thereby disrupting cell adhesion to ECM	No isolated exposure, typically used with enzymatic methods (e.g., trypsin)	Bader et al. (1998) Gamba et al. (2002), McFetridge et al. (2004), Teebken et al. (2000)
Enzymatic			
Trypsin	Cleaves peptide bonds on the C-side of Arg and Lys	Prolonged exposure can disrupt ECM structure, removes laminin, fibronectin, elastin, and GAGs	Bader et al. (1998), Gamba et al. (2002), McFetridge et al. (2004), Teebken et al. (2000)
Endonucleases	Catalyze the hydrolysis of the interior bonds of ribonucleotide and deoxyribonucleotide chains	Difficult to remove from the tissue and could invoke an immune response	Dahl et al. (2003), Woods and Gratzer (2005), Rieder et al. (2004), Courtman et al. (1994)
Exonucleases	Catalyze the hydrolysis of the terminal bonds of ribonucleotide and deoxyribonucleotide chains		

Source: Adapted from Gilbert et al. (2006).

following decellularization processes and recognized by the recipient (McPherson et al., 2000; Konakci et al., 2005; Yoshida et al., 2012). This recognition, along with the presence of source tissue-derived DNA within biologic scaffold materials, has led to suggestions for immune-mediated causes of poor outcomes. However, more than 15 years of clinical experience in several million recipients have resulted in no documented cases of rejection or sensitization in patients, even those receiving multiple implants. α-Gal knockout tissue sources do exist, and ECM scaffold materials have been derived from these animals. However, derivation of ECM from α-Gal knockout sources appears to have no impact upon the downstream remodeling outcomes (Daly et al., 2009). Additional processing steps using recombinant α-Gal are possible and have been shown to reduce the T-lymphocyte reaction to implanted porcine tissues (Xu et al., 2009). However, the use of α-Gal in ECM-based materials is not commonly employed due to cost and previous studies demonstrating that small quantities of the α-Gal epitope do not affect remodeling outcomes.

DNA CONTENT AND DEGREE OF DECELLULARIZATION

While the exact mechanisms by which nucleic acids may affect the host response to biologic scaffold materials are unknown, it is logical that the presence of nucleic acids due to lysis of xenogeneic and allogeneic cells is inevitable. Intact nuclei and DNA remnants have been shown to be present in commercially available products (Gilbert et al., 2009). If ECM composition is to be maintained, that it is likely impossible to fully remove all DNA, or any other cellular component, from a source tissue, even with thorough decellularization methods. Alternatively, the use of harsh decellularization processes can limit the ability to promote constructive remodeling of the scaffold material. Despite the presence of DNA within ECM-based materials, few adverse clinical effects directly attributed to its presence have been observed (Gilbert et al., 2006; Crapo et al., 2011).

The reduction of both the quantity and size of remnant DNA has been shown to be beneficial to the host response which occurs following implantation in preclinical studies (Keane et al., 2012; Brown et al., 2009). Analysis of tissue-derived biomaterials has shown a correlation between DNA content and fragment size and the host response. Ineffectively decellularized scaffolds trigger a prolonged inflammatory response following implantation. Keane et al. (2012) analyzed the *in vivo* host response to ECM materials of varying degrees of decellularization of small intestinal submucosa using peracetic acid (PAA). ECM scaffolds decellularized using phosphate-buffered saline (PBS), 1 h 0.1% PAA or 2 h 0.1% PAA were implanted into a rat abdominal wall reconstruction model. Scaffolds treated with PBS or 1 h PAA were ineffectively cleared of DNA while the 2 h PAA treatment fragmented and removed DNA to a greater degree. The macrophage response to ineffectively decellularized scaffolds was predominately pro-inflammatory while the response to adequately decellularized scaffolds predominantly anti-inflammatory (Keane et al., 2012). This study suggests that there may be a threshold amount of these components required to elicit adverse effects, and further investigation is warranted. At present, a standard for DNA content less than 50 ng/mg dry weight of ECM and less than 200 base pairs in length has been suggested to prevent an adverse inflammatory reaction and to prevent disease transmission.

DAMAGE-ASSOCIATED MOLECULAR PATTERN MOLECULES

Damage-associated molecular pattern molecules (DAMPs) are multifunctional modulators of the immune system (Kang et al., 2014; Tang et al., 2012). These molecules consist of multiple heat shock proteins, S100 molecules, and HMGB1, among others, which have functional roles in the intracellular environment. DAMPs are also commonly released into the extracellular microenvironment following cellular damage, including necrotic or programmed cell death. Within the extracellular space, they are recognized through similar pathways to pathogen-associated molecular pattern molecules (PAMPs). That is, DAMPs are predominantly recognized through the Toll-like receptor (TLR) system (Piccinini and Midwood, 2010; Tian et al., 2007). Of note, DAMPs can have both pro- and anti-inflammatory effects as well as chemotactic, mitogenic, and tissue remodeling effects depending upon the context in which they are recognized by the host (Lolmede et al., 2009; Ranzato et al., 2009; Limana et al., 2005; De Mori et al., 2007). DAMPs are increasingly studied for their roles in multiple disease processes as well as in tissue remodeling outcomes following injury.

It is logical to assume that ECM scaffold materials contain DAMPs as they are derived through the lysis of the cells which reside within each tissue and organ and that these molecules may have important implications for the host response to tissue-derived scaffolds. Further, as DNA and RNA (which are also considered DAMPs by some) are present in cells and tissues, these molecules and other DAMPs are naturally retained within ECM scaffold materials to varying degrees. Little work has been done to identify the effect of DAMPs present within ECM scaffold materials upon the host response. However, based upon reports in the literature, even small amounts of these molecules could have a potent effect.

High mobility group box 1, an intracellular DNA binding protein, is among the best recognized and most studied DAMPs (Kang et al., 2014). A recent study demonstrated that HMGB1 was present within ECM-based scaffold materials following decellularization of multiple tissues (Daly et al., 2012a). When macrophages were seeded onto ECM scaffolds which were chemically cross-linked, preventing recognition of HMGB1, or when an inhibitor of HMGB1 recognition was supplied in the macrophage culture media, an increase in pro-inflammatory gene expression as well as increased cell death were observed. These findings suggest that the presence of HMGB1 within biologic scaffolds is potentially important to modulation of the host response and improve tissue remodeling outcomes. This outcome is in contrast to the presence of DNA and the α-Gal epitope, both of which are associated with detrimental downstream effects when present in significant quantities. A better understanding of the role of individual cellular components in determining the overall host response to ECM materials is clearly needed.

CHEMICAL CROSS-LINKING OF ECM SCAFFOLDS

The use of chemicals to cross-link tissue-derived biomaterials is a commonly employed strategy for the prevention of degradation and/or masking of cellular epitope remaining within the decellularized material (Badylak, 2004; Jarman-Smith et al., 2004; Liang et al., 2004). Cross-linking reagents include glutaraldehyde, carbodiimide, and hexamethylene diisocyanate, among others (Vasudev et al., 2000). Due to the rapid degradation which has been observed following *in vivo* placement of many ECM-derived materials and subsequent loss of mechanical integrity, chemical cross-linking has been used to prevent or retard degradation and thereby the loss of mechanical integrity. The lack of degradation, while often purported to be an advantage in certain applications, is now recognized to prevent the process of constructive remodeling (Valentin et al., 2006, 2009, 2010; Brown et al., 2012b). Chemical cross-linking has also been employed to mask potentially immunogenic elements within nondecellularized and decellularized tissue-based grafts, and is commonly employed in the manufacture of porcine heart valves for human applications (Huelsmann et al., 2012). However, and as described above, not all cellular components within an ECM scaffold material have been associated with poor outcomes, particularly if present only in small amounts. The chemical changes to biological ligands caused by cross-linking can remove much of the beneficial bioactivity which is a major advantage of these biomaterials (Brown et al., 2010). Further, and as discussed in the following section, chemical cross-linking prevents the release of growth factors and bioactive peptides generated by parent molecule degradation.

RESPONSE TO INDIVIDUAL ECM COMPONENTS AND DEGRADATION PRODUCTS

ECM-derived materials are composed of a heterogeneous network of different ECM proteins, glycosaminoglycans, and growth factors. Individual ECM components possess unique bioactivity through ligands which are recognized by different receptors. This receptor recognition of ECM components leads to specific signaling pathways that affect the cellular response to a material following implantation (Yeh et al.,

2011; Rao et al., 2000; Boilard et al., 2010; Cheresh et al., 1989; Suehiro et al., 1997; Belkin et al., 2005; Turley et al., 2002; Hall et al., 1994; Jiang et al., 2005). The contributions of a heterogeneous mixture of ECM ligands to multiple receptors are complex and confounding to interpretation and are beyond the scope of the present chapter. However, the response to individually isolated ECM components has been studied extensively. Among the main constituents of most tissue-derived biomaterials are collagen, fibrin, laminin, and glycosaminoglycans. Additionally, bioactive growth factors contained within source tissues are commonly detectable in decellularized materials as well (Brown et al., 2011a; Crapo et al., 2012; Wolf et al., 2012; Reing et al., 2010; Keane et al., 2013). While the presence and configuration of these components within the initial material will dictate the initial host response, ECM scaffolds are known to degrade rapidly upon implantation. Several studies have shown that peptides produced from the degradation of these materials have inherent bioactivity, suggesting that degradation products influence the host response.

DEGRADATION OF NATURALLY DERIVED BIOMATERIALS

Individual ECM components affect the host response following implantation not only through ligands on their initial form but also through the small peptides and polysaccharides resulting from their degradation. As stated above, degradation is a key characteristic for the success of ECM-derived materials.

Protease-mediated degradation

Matrix degradation is an integral part of the remodeling process associated with the response to injury and to implanted materials. Circulatory immune cells rely upon matrix degradation for extravasation into tissues to propagate the inflammatory response to materials. Such cells release enzymes such as matrix metalloproteases (MMPs) into inflammatory zones to prepare tissues for macrophage and T-cell binding, to release membrane and ECM-bound cytokines, and to increase access to extravascular tissues. Neutrophils secrete MMP-8 and -9 while macrophages secrete MMP-1, -2, -3, -7, -9, and -12 (Weiss, 1989; Sorsa et al., 1994; Shapiro et al., 1993; Shapiro, 1994; Horton et al., 1999; Campbell et al., 1991; Schwartz et al., 1998). T-cells mainly secrete the gelatinases MMP-2 and -9 following stimulation by β1-integrin or vascular cell adhesion molecule-mediated binding (Leppert et al., 1995; Zhou et al., 1993; Montgomery et al., 1993). Inflammatory mediators such as TNF-α/β and interleukin-1 (IL-1) α/β also stimulate expression of MMPs in macrophages (Unemori et al., 1991; Hanemaaijer et al., 1997; Johnatty et al., 1997; Leber and Balkwill, 1998; Vaday et al., 2000, 2001). Many of the cytokines that impact MMP expression are associated with the ECM and are released upon ECM molecule degradation or conformation change. In turn, these cytokines are subject to further activation or degradation by MMPs (Nelson et al., 2000).

These MMPs are present throughout the normal wound healing process following injury. They are upregulated during the inflammatory phase of tissue remodeling. Transforming growth factor-β (TGF-β) in turn inhibits MMPs in the resolution phase to assist with new matrix stabilization (Kerr et al., 1988; Overall et al., 1991). Macrophages secrete tissue inhibitors of metalloproteases (TIMPs) to control MMP activity and prevent destructive tissue degradation (Hernandez-Barrantes et al., 2002).

It is logical that natural biomaterials, such as those composed of ECM, are recognized by the same MMPs involved in matrix degradation during wound healing. Degradation of these materials via MMP-mediated inflammatory responses leads to the natural resolution of the inflammatory response. When these materials cannot degrade, e.g., due to processing with cross-linking agents, the materials are subject to a chronic inflammatory response and subsequent scar tissue or encapsulation outcomes in place of constructive remodeling (Brown et al., 2012b).

ECM fragments

It is presumed that, at least in part, the mechanisms by which ECM scaffold materials modulate the host response resulting in constructive remodeling include the release of cryptic peptides derived from degradation of the intact parent ECM molecules. There are now a number of known "matricryptins" or "matrikines" within native ECM (Davis, 2010; Davis et al., 2000; Maquart et al., 2005). These matricryptins are exposed either through conformational changes of the intact ECM proteins or through degradation resulting in new recognition sites with potent bioactivity. Interactions of cells with these matrix fragments have been shown to influence cell behavior through a number of mechanisms including integrin, TLR, and scavenger receptor signaling. The result is diverse bioactivity including angiogenesis, anti-angiogenesis, chemotaxis, adhesion, and antimicrobial effects among others (McFetridge et al., 2004; Davis, 2010; Davis et al., 2000; Maquart et al., 2005; Brennan et al., 2006, 2008; Haviv et al., 2005; Ramchandran et al., 1999; Vlodavsky et al., 2002).

In vitro models of ECM scaffold degradation have identified a few of these matricryptic peptides. Reing et al. digested urinary bladder matrix (UBM) with pepsin or papain and exposed them to both multipotent progenitor cells and endothelial cells to the resultants solubilized matrix. The UBM degradation products possessed both chemotactic and mitogenic properties for multipotent progenitor cells but inhibited chemotaxis and proliferation of differentiated endothelial cells (Reing et al., 2009). Agrawal et al. (2011b) identified a matricryptic peptide derived from the α subunit of collagen type III present within a tissue-derived biologic scaffold that is chemotactic for perivascular stem cells, human cortical neural stem cells, rat adipocyte stem cells, C2C12 myoblast cells, and rat Schwann cells. This same peptide was shown to promote osteogenesis and bone formation as measured by calcium deposition, alkaline phosphatase activity, and osteogenic gene expression induced in perivascular stem cells (Agrawal et al., 2011a).

Brennan et al. investigated the impact of age and species on the chemoattractant properties of skin ECM degradation products on keratinocyte progenitor cells. Enzymatically prepared digestion products from human fetal skin, human adult skin, and porcine adult skin were assayed for chemotactic responses by keratinocyte progenitor and stem cells harvested from adult humans. The porcine adult ECM showed greater chemotaxis of the keratinocyte progenitors than human adult ECM, while the human fetal ECM showed the greatest chemotactic response. These data suggest that both the age and species of the ECM source animal can affect the host response (Brennan et al., 2008). The topic of age-related effects upon the host response to ECM-based scaffold materials is described in the next section.

A recent study by Sicari et al. investigated the effects of degradation products derived from porcine small intestinal submucosa upon macrophage phenotype. Briefly, macrophages treated with ECM degradation products were found to promote an M2 anti-inflammatory phenotype which was similar to that induced by IL-4. Additional work demonstrated that the macrophages treated with ECM degradation products produced factors which were chemotactic for both myoblasts and perivascular progenitor cell populations. The secreted products of ECM degradation product-treated macrophages were also shown to promote myogenesis of skeletal muscle progenitor cells (Sicari et al., 2014b). The results of this study and those described above demonstrate the potential effects of ECM degradation upon the host response, with important implications for recruitment of progenitor cells to sites of tissue remodeling and downstream remodeling outcomes. The link between the unique profile of the host response to ECM scaffold materials and tissue remodeling outcomes is discussed in more depth in the following sections.

EFFECT OF SOURCE ANIMAL AGE ON NATURAL BIOMATERIAL HOST RESPONSE

ECM materials are dependent upon the characteristics of the animal and organ from which they are derived. The age of source animals used for the production of ECM-derived biomaterials has proven to affect the host response to these scaffolds. It has been shown that the ECM changes in composition, cytoarchitecture, and ability to support stem cells as the organism ages or undergoes stress (Kurtz and Oh, 2012). In addition to changes in ECM composition, increased modification of ECM proteins has been identified with increased age. Specifically, the accumulation of advanced glycation end products (AGEs) on ECM molecules is implicated in age-related changes in physiology and host response (Brownlee, 1995; Dyer et al., 1991; Ulrich and Cerami, 2001). These AGEs form molecular cross-links which can alter the degradation, mechanics, and signaling of the ECM, which can change the cellular phenotypes in an organism. It is logical, therefore, that scaffolds derived from aged tissue sources will elicit different host responses compared to those derived from younger source tissues.

Brennan et al. described that fetal human skin ECM degradation products possessed greater chemotactic properties for human keratinocyte progenitor cells than those derived from adult human skin. Tottey et al. investigated characteristics of porcine small intestine submucosa (SIS) derived from different source animal age, and showed that older SIS had higher tensile strength, elastic moduli, and thickness. Older SIS also degraded slower when exposed to collagenase. Decreasing amounts of basic fibroblast growth factor (bFGF), vascular endothelial growth factor (VEGF), and sulfated glycosamingoglycans (sGAG) were present with increasing source animal age ECM. Older ECM caused increased proliferation and metabolism of perivascular stem cells, while decreasing the migration of these cells in comparison to younger source animal age ECM (Tottey et al., 2011). All of these changes in the characteristics of ECM-derived biomaterials appear to have an impact upon the host response upon implantation.

Sicari et al. investigated the *in vivo* remodeling characteristics of SIS derived from different age source animal pigs (3, 12, 26, and 52 weeks old) using a rat abdominal wall reconstruction model. Explanted tissue showed that all of the implanted ECM test articles elicited a strong infiltration by mononuclear cells, were degraded completely, and induced angiogenesis by 2 weeks of implantation. SIS scaffolds derived from young pigs, however, showed an increased anti-inflammatory, pro-healing response; an effect which decreased with increasing source animal age. The young-derived implants elicited formation of functional muscle fibers and nerves, which was not seen in the old age source animal ECM, and scaffolds harvested from young animals also showed reduced cellularity at 28 and 120 days, indicating a resolution of the inflammatory response. Explants from animals treated with young source animal age SIS had the highest uniaxial tensile strength, indicating improved functional tissue formation (Sicari et al., 2012b). The accumulated changes to ECM as an organism ages can critically affect the host response to ECM-derived scaffolds and the potential to promote constructive remodeling.

THE HOST RESPONSE TO ECM BIOMATERIALS

The preceding sections discuss multiple aspects of the sourcing and production of decellularized tissue-derived biomaterials which have an impact upon the overall host response and the tissue remodeling outcomes associated with their use. In the following section, the specific cellular constituents of the host response and their phenotype following placement are discussed. As has been described, placement of biologic scaffolds can result in either constructive remodeling and encapsulation or scar tissue formation. Those scaffold materials which promote constructive remodeling have been consistently associated with a distinct host response including specific T-cell and macrophage populations.

In general, the host response to decellularized tissues includes early infiltration of a neutrophil population (24–48 h) followed by an intense accumulation of mononuclear cells by 72 h postimplantation. These cells include a significant population of macrophages, but also T-cells, B-cells, eosinophils, and mast cells (Brown et al., 2009; Allman et al., 2001). In the absence of large amounts of cellular material remaining within the scaffold material following decellularization, chemical cross-linking, or contaminants such as endotoxin, this response will diminish over time, leading to constructive remodeling outcomes (Valentin et al., 2006, 2010; Brown et al., 2009, 2012b; Keane et al., 2012; Daly et al., 2012b). Of note, however, the early host response to chemically cross-linked materials has a similar characteristic appearance in the first 14–28 days postimplantation, with little to no evidence of a constructive remodeling outcome thereafter. This population of cells is histologically indistinguishable between materials which either do or do not promote constructive remodeling. Further, such a response when observed in the context of most naturally and synthetically derived materials has conventionally been interpreted as either acute or chronic inflammation associated with negative implications including downstream encapsulation and fibrosis (Anderson, 1988). This has provided the impetus for further investigation of cellular phenotypes within the sites of tissue remodeling. In particular, distinct T-cell and macrophage subsets have been shown to be elicited by those materials which promote constructive remodeling outcomes.

Th1- AND Th2-LYMPHOCYTE RESPONSE

Thymocytes (T-cells) of the adaptive immune system play a critical role in the inflammatory response present in the days to weeks following biomaterial implantation. A specific subset of T-cells which are CD4 positive, termed T-helper cells, are crucial in this response. They are known to exist along a spectrum between T-helper 1 (Th1) and T-helper 2 (Th2) cells, which release pro-inflammatory and anti-inflammatory cytokines, respectively. The theory suggested that T-helper cells polarized into distinct phenotypes resulting in a select cytokine expression pattern. Originally this was described as the balance between Th1 and Th2 subsets. The T-helper cell subset is responsible for amplifying the immune response and directing cell responses to better fight off specific types of infection or foreign bodies. Th1-cells mediate cellular immunity to incite cytotoxicity of virally infected cells and cancer cells. Th2-cells mediate humoral immunity, leading to the production of antibodies to fight extracellular pathogens. Th1-cells primarily secrete interferon-γ (IFN-γ) and to a lesser extent IL-2 and -12. Th2-cells secrete IL-4 as well as IL-5 (Bluestone et al., 2009). These cytokines influence the response of other immune and host cells. Th2 responses are associated with xenogeneic graft tolerance while Th1 responses are responsible for graft rejection (Badylak and Gilbert, 2008). While a full description of the role of T-cell subtypes in the host response to implantable materials is beyond the scope of the present chapter, it can clearly be understood that, given their xenogeneic or allogeneic origin, T-cells may play an important role in the response to ECM scaffold materials. Readers are referred to Chapter 8 for a full review of the role of T-cells in the host response in general.

T-helper cells are present in the inflammatory response to ECM scaffold materials (Allman et al., 2001, 2002). In one study, a mouse model was used to examine the T-cell response to subcutaneously implanted xenogeneic muscle, syngeneic muscle, or decellularized small intestinal submucosa. All implants elicited a response which was histologically similar. However, the results demonstrated that the xenogeneic tissue implant elicited a response which was consistent with rejection. In comparison, both the syngeneic tissue and the SIS implants elicited an early inflammatory response which resolved and led to organized, site-appropriate, tissue remodeling at the site of implantation. Analysis of the cytokine profile within the remodeling site revealed that the ECM group was associated with the expression of IL-4 and suppression of IFN-γ as compared to the xenogeneic tissue implant group. In the same study, it was demonstrated that the animals produced an ECM-specific antibody response due to a degree of nonhomologous protein sequences between species. However, it was demonstrated that this response was restricted to the IgG1 isotype with no adverse outcome. Reimplantation of the same mice with a second ECM scaffold led to an enhanced anti-ECM antibody response, also restricted to the IgG1 isotype, but no formation of a Th1-type response. Further investigations determined that the observed responses in this study were T-cell dependent. However, it was also shown that while both T- and B-cells participate in the response to implanted ECM materials, they are not required for constructive tissue remodeling, suggesting a more important role for other cell types.

MACROPHAGE POLARIZATION

Macrophages are considered among the most important cells within the host response to biomaterials as they are the predominant immune cell present from a few days to several weeks or years postimplantation depending on the nature of the material implanted. As is described in Chapter 6, a spectrum of macrophage phenotypes has been described. Definition of these phenotypes utilizes the T-helper polarization scheme, with pro-inflammatory macrophages being described as M1 and anti-inflammatory macrophages as M2. M1 macrophages are defined as being activated by cytokines such as IFN-γ and bacterial components such as lipopolysaccharide (LPS). M1 macrophages are associated with pathogen clearance and classical inflammatory responses, as well as secretion of inflammatory mediators such as IL-12 and TNF-α (MacMicking et al., 1997). M2 macrophages are defined as being activated by anti-inflammatory cytokines such as IL-4, -10, and -13 (Mantovani et al., 2004). M2 macrophages are associated with immunoregulation and constructive tissue remodeling (Brown and Badylak, 2013). These are simplified, theoretical definitions of macrophage polarization with the reality that macrophages can be activated by many factors and will have unique phenotypes along this spectrum based upon the stimuli they encounter. Macrophage polarization has now been associated with functional tissue formation outcomes downstream of biomaterial implantation in multiple settings (Mantovani et al., 2013).

Macrophages, unlike T- and B-cells, have been demonstrated to be an essential determinant of constructive remodeling following implantation of ECM-based materials (Valentin et al., 2009). A recent study depleted the circulating mononuclear phagocyte population in a rat model by utilizing injection of clodronate containing liposomes (Valentin et al., 2009). The results of this study demonstrated that the ECM scaffold material was not degraded or remodeled in the absence of a circulating monocyte population suggesting that, unlike T- and B-cells, macrophages are required for ECM scaffold remodeling. Subsequent investigations have focused upon the phenotype of the macrophages responding to ECM implants and their role in constructive remodeling downstream (Brown et al., 2009, 2012b; Badylak et al., 2008; Sicari et al., 2014b; Wolf et al., 2014). A recent study investigated the macrophage response to 15 commercially available ECM-based surgical mesh materials when placed into a partial thickness defect of the rat abdominal wall (Brown et al., 2012b). The results of the study showed that, despite a similarity in the early histologic response, each of the materials was associated with a distinct outcome downstream. When a validated histologic scoring system and immunofluorescent labeling of macrophage phenotype was employed, it was determined that the number of M2 macrophages and the ratio of M2:M1 cells within the site of remodeling at 14 days was predictive of downstream histologic outcomes, with the early host response accounting for more than 65% of the variation in downstream outcomes.

Further studies have demonstrated individual factors which influence the polarization profile of the macrophages responding to implantation of ECM scaffolds. Brown et al. analyzed the differences in the host response to cellular and acellular ECM scaffolds prepared from xenogeneic and allogeneic sources (Brown et al., 2009). The test articles evaluated in this study included a cellular muscle autograft, decellularized allogeneic abdominal wall tissue, cellular xenogenic UBM, and decellularized UBM. Both cellular autografts and xenografts elicited a macrophage polarization profile skewed toward a pro-inflammatory, M1-type response as assessed by immunohistochemistry and gene expression analysis and were associated with disorganized tissue deposition and scarring. Acellular grafts were shown to be associated with an increase in the anti-inflammatory profile as assessed by the same measures as well as improved remodeling outcomes.

Other studies have demonstrated the effects of chemical cross-linking upon the host response to ECM scaffolds. Valentin et al examined the host response to materials derived from small intestinal scaffold that either were or were not cross-linked (Valentin et al., 2010). The results of this study demonstrated that those materials which were chemically cross-linked elicited a predominantly M1-type macrophage response and were associated with remodeling outcomes consistent with a foreign body reaction. Non-cross-linked materials were associated with a shift to the M2 phenotype and constructive tissue remodeling. While the exact mechanisms by which ECM scaffolds modulate the host response are not yet known, these results coupled with those described above demonstrating that ECM degradation products promote an M2 phenotype and strongly suggest that ECM scaffold degradation is a necessary event.

Further evidence for the role of ECM degradation products in modulating the host response is provided by studies which have utilized ECM degradation products as coatings for materials which are known to induce a strong M1 response and downstream foreign body reaction (Wolf et al., 2014; Faulk et al., 2014). Wolf et al. (2014) analyzed the macrophage polarization response to ECM-coated and -uncoated polypropylene surgical mesh. Using immunofluorescent staining for M1 and M2 macrophages, the study analyzed the macrophage polarization profile of mesh explants from a rat abdominal wall defect repair model at 3, 7, 14, and 35 days. A robust macrophage presence was observed as early as 7 days and lasted until 35 days postimplantation in all cases. Uncoated polypropylene meshes were associated with an M1, pro-inflammatory environment surrounding the implant site. ECM coating was shown to reduce the M1 pro-inflammatory response. This change in the M2:M1 ratio was associated with reduced foreign body reaction and fibrotic tissue formation surrounding the mesh material both in short- and long-term studies (Wolf et al., 2014; Faulk et al., 2014).

CONCLUSION

Naturally derived biomaterials differ from their synthetic counterparts due in part to an inherent biologically active ligand landscape which elicits a unique host response depending upon the nature and preparation of the material. It is now well accepted that the host response and the involved immune cells play a determinant role in tissue remodeling outcomes following their placement. ECM scaffolds are naturally derived materials obtained through the decellularization of mammalian tissues and organs. These scaffold materials, when appropriately decellularized and prepared, can promote a process of constructive remodeling, leading to formation of new, site-appropriate, functional host tissues. The preparation and degradation of the material implicate the host response, and if tuned appropriately, the material can promote a beneficial, anti-inflammatory, pro-remodeling response.

While ECM-based materials represent only one example of naturally derived material, the phenomena described herein are easily applied to other naturally derived materials. That is, naturally derived materials must be prepared carefully in order to reduce any potentially immunogenic content related to their source, the natural bioactivity must be preserved throughout processing, and the material must be allowed to degrade. Those materials which are prepared in this manner, and which are able to shift the host response toward a more M2 macrophage phenotype, will meet with improved success in both preclinical and clinical applications.

REFERENCES

Agrawal, V., Kelly, J., Tottey, S., Daly, K.A., Johnson, S.A., Siu, B.F., et al., 2011. An isolated cryptic peptide influences osteogenesis and bone remodeling in an adult mammalian model of digit amputation. Tissue Eng. Part A 17 (23-24), 3033–3044.

Agrawal, V., Tottey, S., Johnson, S.A., Freund, J.M., Siu, B.F., Badylak, S.F., 2011. Recruitment of progenitor cells by an extracellular matrix cryptic peptide in a mouse model of digit amputation. Tissue Eng. Part A 17 (19-20), 2435–2443.

Allman, A.J., McPherson, T.B., Badylak, S.F., Merrill, L.C., Kallakury, B., Sheehan, C., et al., 2001. Xenogeneic extracellular matrix grafts elicit a TH2-restricted immune response. Transplantation 71 (11), 1631–1640.

Allman, A.J., McPherson, T.B., Merrill, L.C., Badylak, S.F., Metzger, D.W., 2002. The Th2-restricted immune response to xenogeneic small intestinal submucosa does not influence systemic protective immunity to viral and bacterial pathogens. Tissue Eng. 8 (1), 53–62.

Anderson, J.M., 1988. Inflammatory response to implants. ASAIO Trans. 34 (2), 101–107.

Bader, A., Schilling, T., Teebken, O.E., Brandes, G., Herden, T., Steinhoff, G., et al., 1998. Tissue engineering of heart valves--human endothelial cell seeding of detergent acellularized porcine valves. Eur. J. Cardiothorac. Surg. 14 (3), 279–284.

Badylak, S.F., 2004a. Xenogeneic extracellular matrix as a scaffold for tissue reconstruction. Transpl. Immunol. 12 (3-4), 367–377.

Badylak, S.F., 2014b. Decellularized allogeneic and xenogeneic tissue as a bioscaffold for regenerative medicine: factors that influence the host response. Ann. Biomed. Eng. 42 (7), 1517–1527.

Badylak, S.F., Gilbert, T.W., 2008. Immune response to biologic scaffold materials. Semin. Immunol. 20 (2), 109–116.

Badylak, S.F., Valentin, J.E., Ravindra, A.K., McCabe, G.P., Stewart-Akers, A.M., 2008. Macrophage phenotype as a determinant of biologic scaffold remodeling. Tissue Eng. Part A 14 (11), 1835–1842.

Badylak, S.F., Hoppo, T., Nieponice, A., Gilbert, T.W., Davison, J.M., Jobe, B.A., 2011a. Esophageal preservation in five male patients after endoscopic inner-layer circumferential resection in the setting of superficial cancer: a regenerative medicine approach with a biologic scaffold. Tissue Eng. Part A 17 (11-12), 1643–1650.

Badylak, S.F., Brown, B.N., Gilbert, T.W., Daly, K.A., Huber, A., Turner, N.J., 2011b. Biologic scaffolds for constructive tissue remodeling. Biomaterials 32 (1), 316–319.

Belkin, A.M., Tsurupa, G., Zemskov, E., Veklich, Y., Weisel, J.W., Medved, L., 2005. Transglutaminase-mediated oligomerization of the fibrin(ogen) alphaC domains promotes integrin-dependent cell adhesion and signaling. Blood 105 (9), 3561–3568.

Bluestone, J.A., Mackay, C.R., O'Shea, J.J., Stockinger, B., 2009. The functional plasticity of T cell subsets. Nat. Rev. Immunol. 9 (11), 811–816.

Boilard, E., Nigrovic, P.A., Larabee, K., Watts, G.F., Coblyn, J.S., Weinblatt, M.E., et al., 2010. Platelets amplify inflammation in arthritis via collagen-dependent microparticle production. Science 327 (5965), 580–583.

Brennan, E.P., Reing, J., Chew, D., Myers-Irvin, J.M., Young, E.J., Badylak, S.F., 2006. Antibacterial activity within degradation products of biological scaffolds composed of extracellular matrix. Tissue Eng. 12 (10), 2949–2955.

Brennan, E.P., Tang, X.H., Stewart-Akers, A.M., Gudas, L.J., Badylak, S.F., 2008. Chemoattractant activity of degradation products of fetal and adult skin extracellular matrix for keratinocyte progenitor cells. J. Tissue Eng. Regen. Med. 2 (8), 491–498.

Brown, B.N., Badylak, S.F., 2013. Expanded applications, shifting paradigms and an improved understanding of host-biomaterial interactions. Acta Biomater 9 (2), 4948–4955.

Brown, B.N., Badylak, S.F., 2014. Extracellular matrix as an inductive scaffold for functional tissue reconstruction. Transl. Res. 163 (4), 268–285.

Brown, B.N., Valentin, J.E., Stewart-Akers, A.M., McCabe, G.P., Badylak, S.F., 2009. Macrophage phenotype and remodeling outcomes in response to biologic scaffolds with and without a cellular component. Biomaterials 30 (8), 1482–1491.

Brown, B.N., Barnes, C.A., Kasick, R.T., Michel, R., Gilbert, T.W., Beer-Stolz, D., et al., 2010. Surface characterization of extracellular matrix scaffolds. Biomaterials 31 (3), 428–437.

Brown, B.N., Freund, J.M., Han, L., Rubin, J.P., Reing, J.E., Jeffries, E.M., et al., 2011a. Comparison of three methods for the derivation of a biologic scaffold composed of adipose tissue extracellular matrix. Tissue Eng. Part C Methods 17 (4), 411–421.

Brown, B.N., Chung, W.L., Pavlick, M., Reppas, S., Ochs, M.W., Russell, A.J., et al., 2011b. Extracellular matrix as an inductive template for temporomandibular joint meniscus reconstruction: a pilot study. J. Oral Maxillofac. Surg. 69 (12), e488–e505.

Brown, B.N., Londono, R., Tottey, S., Zhang, L., Kukla, K.A., Wolf, M.T., et al., 2012a. Macrophage phenotype as a predictor of constructive remodeling following the implantation of biologically derived surgical mesh materials. Acta Biomater. 8 (3), 978–987.

Brown, B.N., Chung, W.L., Almarza, A.J., Pavlick, M.D., Reppas, S.N., Ochs, M.W., et al., 2012b. Inductive, scaffold-based, regenerative medicine approach to reconstruction of the temporomandibular joint disk. J. Oral Maxillofac. Surg. 70 (11), 2656–2668.

Brownlee, M., 1995. Advanced protein glycosylation in diabetes and aging. Annu. Rev. Med. 46, 223–234.

Campbell, E.J., Cury, J.D., Shapiro, S.D., Goldberg, G.I., Welgus, H.G., 1991. Neutral proteinases of human mononuclear phagocytes. Cellular differentiation markedly alters cell phenotype for serine proteinases, metalloproteinases, and tissue inhibitor of metalloproteinases. J. Immunol. 146 (4), 1286–1293.

Cartmell, J.S., Dunn, M.G., 2000. Effect of chemical treatments on tendon cellularity and mechanical properties. J. Biomed. Mater. Res. 49 (1), 134–140.

Chen, F., Yoo, J.J., Atala, A., 2000. Experimental and clinical experience using tissue regeneration for urethral reconstruction. World J. Urol. 18 (1), 67–70.

Chen, R.N., Ho, H.O., Tsai, Y.T., Sheu, M.T., 2004. Process development of an acellular dermal matrix (ADM) for biomedical applications. Biomaterials 25 (13), 2679–2686.

Cheresh, D.A., Berliner, S.A., Vicente, V., Ruggeri, Z.M., 1989. Recognition of distinct adhesive sites on fibrinogen by related integrins on platelets and endothelial cells. Cell 58 (5), 945–953.

Courtman, D.W., Pereira, C.A., Kashef, V., McComb, D., Lee, J.M., Wilson, G.J., 1994. Development of a pericardial acellular matrix biomaterial: biochemical and mechanical effects of cell extraction. J. Biomed. Mater. Res. 28 (6), 655–666.

Crapo, P.M., Gilbert, T.W., Badylak, S.F., 2011. An overview of tissue and whole organ decellularization processes. Biomaterials 32 (12), 3233–3243.

Crapo, P.M., Medberry, C.J., Reing, J.E., Tottey, S., van der Merwe, Y., Jones, K.E., et al., 2012. Biologic scaffolds composed of central nervous system extracellular matrix. Biomaterials 33 (13), 3539–3547.

Dahl, S.L., Koh, J., Prabhakar, V., Niklason, L.E., 2003. Decellularized native and engineered arterial scaffolds for transplantation. Cell Transplant. 12 (6), 659–666.

Daly, K.A., Stewart-Akers, A.M., Hara, H., Ezzelarab, M., Long, C., Cordero, K., et al., 2009. Effect of the alphaGal epitope on the response to small intestinal submucosa extracellular matrix in a nonhuman primate model. Tissue Eng. Part A 15 (12), 3877–3888.

Daly, K.A., Wolf, M., Johnson, S.A., Badylak, S.F., 2011. A rabbit model of peripheral compartment syndrome with associated rhabdomyolysis and a regenerative medicine approach for treatment. Tissue Eng. Part C Methods 17 (6), 631–640.

Daly, K.A., Liu, S., Agrawal, V., Brown, B.N., Huber, A., Johnson, S.A., et al., 2012a. The host response to endotoxin-contaminated dermal matrix. Tissue Eng. Part A 18 (11-12), 1293–1303.

Daly, K.A., Liu, S., Agrawal, V., Brown, B.N., Johnson, S.A., Medberry, C.J., et al., 2012b. Damage associated molecular patterns within xenogeneic biologic scaffolds and their effects on host remodeling. Biomaterials 33 (1), 91–101.

Davis, G.E., 2010. Matricryptic sites control tissue injury responses in the cardiovascular system: relationships to pattern recognition receptor regulated events. J. Mol. Cell. Cardiol. 48 (3), 454–460.

Davis, G.E., Bayless, K.J., Davis, M.J., Meininger, G.A., 2000. Regulation of tissue injury responses by the exposure of matricryptic sites within extracellular matrix molecules. Am. J. Pathol. 156 (5), 1489–1498.

De Filippo, R.E., Yoo, J.J., Atala, A., 2002. Urethral replacement using cell seeded tubularized collagen matrices. J. Urol. 168 (4 Pt 2), 1789–1792. discussion 1792-1783.

De Mori, R., Straino, S., Di Carlo, A., Mangoni, A., Pompilio, G., Palumbo, R., et al., 2007. Multiple effects of high mobility group box protein 1 in skeletal muscle regeneration. Arterioscler. Thromb. Vasc. Biol. 27 (11), 2377–2383.

Dyer, D.G., Blackledge, J.A., Katz, B.M., Hull, C.J., Adkisson, H.D., Thorpe, S.R., et al., 1991. The Maillard reaction in vivo. Z. Ernahrungswiss. 30 (1), 29–45.

Falke, G., Yoo, J.J., Kwon, T.G., Moreland, R., Atala, A., 2003. Formation of corporal tissue architecture in vivo using human cavernosal muscle and endothelial cells seeded on collagen matrices. Tissue Eng. 9 (5), 871–879.

Faulk, D.M., Londono, R., Wolf, M.T., Ranallo, C.A., Carruthers, C.A., Wildemann, J.D., et al., 2014. ECM hydrogel coating mitigates the chronic inflammatory response to polypropylene mesh. Biomaterials 35 (30), 8585–8595.

Fox, A., Mountford, J., Braakhuis, A., Harrison, L.C., 2001. Innate and adaptive immune responses to non-vascular xenografts: evidence that macrophages are direct effectors of xenograft rejection. J. Immunol. 166 (3), 2133–2140.

Freytes, D.O., Badylak, S.F., Webster, T.J., Geddes, L.A., Rundell, A.E., 2004. Biaxial strength of multilaminated extracellular matrix scaffolds. Biomaterials 25 (12), 2353–2361.

Galili, U., 2005. The alpha-gal epitope and the anti-Gal antibody in xenotransplantation and in cancer immunotherapy. Immunol. Cell Biol. 83 (6), 674–686.

Gamba, P.G., Conconi, M.T., Lo Piccolo, R., Zara, G., Spinazzi, R., Parnigotto, P.P., 2002. Experimental abdominal wall defect repaired with acellular matrix. Pediatr. Surg. Int. 18 (5-6), 327–331.

Gilbert, T.W., Sellaro, T.L., Badylak, S.F., 2006. Decellularization of tissues and organs. Biomaterials 27 (19), 3675–3683.

Gilbert, T.W., Freund, J.M., Badylak, S.F., 2009. Quantification of DNA in biologic scaffold materials. J. Surg. Res. 152 (1), 135–139.

Goissis, G., Suzigan, S., Parreira, D.R., Maniglia, J.V., Braile, D.M., Raymundo, S., 2000. Preparation and characterization of collagen-elastin matrices from blood vessels intended as small diameter vascular grafts. Artif. Organs 24 (3), 217–223.

Grauss, R.W., Hazekamp, M.G., van Vliet, S., Gittenberger-de Groot, A.C., DeRuiter, M.C., 2003. Decellularization of rat aortic valve allografts reduces leaflet destruction and extracellular matrix remodeling. J. Thorac. Cardiovasc. Surg. 126 (6), 2003–2010.

Gulati, A.K., 1988. Evaluation of acellular and cellular nerve grafts in repair of rat peripheral nerve. J. Neurosurg. 68 (1), 117–123.

Hall, C.L., Wang, C., Lange, L.A., Turley, E.A., 1994. Hyaluronan and the hyaluronan receptor RHAMM promote focal adhesion turnover and transient tyrosine kinase activity. J. Cell Biol. 126 (2), 575–588.

Hanemaaijer, R., Sorsa, T., Konttinen, Y.T., Ding, Y., Sutinen, M., Visser, H., et al., 1997. Matrix metalloproteinase-8 is expressed in rheumatoid synovial fibroblasts and endothelial cells. Regulation by tumor necrosis factor-alpha and doxycycline. J. Biol. Chem. 272 (50), 31504–31509.

Haviv, F., Bradley, M.F., Kalvin, D.M., Schneider, A.J., Davidson, D.J., Majest, S.M., et al., 2005. Thrombospondin-1 mimetic peptide inhibitors of angiogenesis and tumor growth: design, synthesis, and optimization of pharmacokinetics and biological activities. J. Med. Chem. 48 (8), 2838–2846.

Hernandez-Barrantes, S., Bernardo, M., Toth, M., Fridman, R., 2002. Regulation of membrane type-matrix metalloproteinases. Semin. Cancer Biol. 12 (2), 131–138.

Horton, M.R., Shapiro, S., Bao, C., Lowenstein, C.J., Noble, P.W., 1999. Induction and regulation of macrophage metalloelastase by hyaluronan fragments in mouse macrophages. J. Immunol. 162 (7), 4171–4176.

Hudson, T.W., Liu, S.Y., Schmidt, C.E., 2004a. Engineering an improved acellular nerve graft via optimized chemical processing. Tissue Eng. 10 (9-10), 1346–1358.

Hudson, T.W., Zawko, S., Deister, C., Lundy, S., Hu, C.Y., Lee, K., et al., 2004b. Optimized acellular nerve graft is immunologically tolerated and supports regeneration. Tissue Eng. 10 (11-12), 1641–1651.

Huelsmann, J., Gruen, K., El Amouri, S., Hornung, K., Holzfuß, C., Lichtenberg, A., et al., 2012. Residual alpha-gal epitope content and elasticity of crosslinked vs. decellularized bovine pericardium. Thorac. cardiovasc. Surg. 60 (01), P70.

Jackson, D.W., Grood, E.S., Arnoczky, S.P., Butler, D.L., Simon, T.M., 1987a. Cruciate reconstruction using freeze dried anterior cruciate ligament allograft and a ligament augmentation device (LAD). An experimental study in a goat model. Am. J. Sports Med. 15 (6), 528–538.

Jackson, D.W., Grood, E.S., Arnoczky, S.P., Butler, D.L., Simon, T.M., 1987b. Freeze dried anterior cruciate ligament allografts. Preliminary studies in a goat model. Am. J. Sports Med. 15 (4), 295–303.

Jackson, D.W., Grood, E.S., Wilcox, P., Butler, D.L., Simon, T.M., Holden, J.P., 1988. The effects of processing techniques on the mechanical properties of bone-anterior cruciate ligament-bone allografts. An experimental study in goats. Am. J. Sports Med. 16 (2), 101–105.

Jackson, D.W., Windler, G.E., Simon, T.M., 1990. Intraarticular reaction associated with the use of freeze-dried, ethylene oxide-sterilized bone-patella tendon-bone allografts in the reconstruction of the anterior cruciate ligament. Am. J. Sports Med. 18 (1), 1–10. discussion 10-11.

Jackson, D.W., Grood, E.S., Cohn, B.T., Arnoczky, S.P., Simon, T.M., Cummings, J.F., 1991. The effects of in situ freezing on the anterior cruciate ligament. An experimental study in goats. J. Bone Joint Surg. Am. 73 (2), 201–213.

Jarman-Smith, M.L., Bodamyali, T., Stevens, C., Howell, J.A., Horrocks, M., Chaudhuri, J.B., 2004. Porcine collagen crosslinking, degradation and its capability for fibroblast adhesion and proliferation. J. Mater. Sci. Mater. Med. 15 (8), 925–932.

Jiang, D., Liang, J., Fan, J., Yu, S., Chen, S., Luo, Y., et al., 2005. Regulation of lung injury and repair by Toll-like receptors and hyaluronan. Nat. Med. 11 (11), 1173–1179.

Johnatty, R.N., Taub, D.D., Reeder, S.P., Turcovski-Corrales, S.M., Cottam, D.W., Stephenson, T.J., et al., 1997. Cytokine and chemokine regulation of proMMP-9 and TIMP-1 production by human peripheral blood lymphocytes. J. Immunol. 158 (5), 2327–2333.

Kang, R., Chen, R., Zhang, Q., Hou, W., Wu, S., Cao IIIrd, L., et al., 2014. HMGB1 in health and disease. Mol. Aspects Med.

Keane, T.J., Londono, R., Turner, N.J., Badylak, S.F., 2012. Consequences of ineffective decellularization of biologic scaffolds on the host response. Biomaterials 33 (6), 1771–1781.

Keane, T.J., Londono, R., Carey, R.M., Carruthers, C.A., Reing, J.E., Dearth, C.L., et al., 2013. Preparation and characterization of a biologic scaffold from esophageal mucosa. Biomaterials 34 (28), 6729–6737.

Kerr, L.D., Olashaw, N.E., Matrisian, L.M., 1988. Transforming growth factor beta 1 and cAMP inhibit transcription of epidermal growth factor- and oncogene-induced transin RNA. J. Biol. Chem. 263 (32), 16999–17005.

Konakci, K.Z., Bohle, B., Blumer, R., Hoetzenecker, W., Roth, G., Moser, B., et al., 2005. Alpha-Gal on bioprostheses: xenograft immune response in cardiac surgery. Eur. J. Clin. Invest. 35 (1), 17–23.

Kurtz, A., Oh, S.J., 2012. Age related changes of the extracellular matrix and stem cell maintenance. Prev. Med. 54, S50–S56.

Leber, T.M., Balkwill, F.R., 1998. Regulation of monocyte MMP-9 production by TNF-alpha and a tumour-derived soluble factor (MMPSF). Br. J. Cancer 78 (6), 724–732.

Leppert, D., Waubant, E., Galardy, R., Bunnett, N.W., Hauser, S.L., 1995. T cell gelatinases mediate basement membrane transmigration in vitro. J. Immunol. 154 (9), 4379–4389.

Liang, H.C., Chang, Y., Hsu, C.K., Lee, M.H., Sung, H.W., 2004. Effects of crosslinking degree of an acellular biological tissue on its tissue regeneration pattern. Biomaterials 25 (17), 3541–3552.

Limana, F., Germani, A., Zacheo, A., Kajstura, J., Di Carlo, A., Borsellino, G., et al., 2005. Exogenous high-mobility group box 1 protein induces myocardial regeneration after infarction via enhanced cardiac C-kit+ cell proliferation and differentiation. Circ. Res. 97 (8), e73–e83.

Lin, P., Chan, W.C., Badylak, S.F., Bhatia, S.N., 2004. Assessing porcine liver-derived biomatrix for hepatic tissue engineering. Tissue Eng. 10 (7-8), 1046–1053.

Lolmede, K., Campana, L., Vezzoli, M., Bosurgi, L., Tonlorenzi, R., Clementi, E., et al., 2009. Inflammatory and alternatively activated human macrophages attract vessel-associated stem cells, relying on separate HMGB1- and MMP-9-dependent pathways. J. Leukoc. Biol. 85 (5), 779–787.

MacMicking, J., Xie, Q.W., Nathan, C., 1997. Nitric oxide and macrophage function. Annu. Rev. Immunol. 15, 323–350.

Mantovani, A., Sica, A., Sozzani, S., Allavena, P., Vecchi, A., Locati, M., 2004. The chemokine system in diverse forms of macrophage activation and polarization. Trends Immunol. 25 (12), 677–686.

Mantovani, A., Biswas, S.K., Galdiero, M.R., Sica, A., Locati, M., 2013. Macrophage plasticity and polarization in tissue repair and remodelling. J. Pathol. 229 (2), 176–185.

Maquart, F.X., Bellon, G., Pasco, S., Monboisse, J.C., 2005. Matrikines in the regulation of extracellular matrix degradation. Biochimie 87 (3-4), 353–360.

Mase Jr., V.J., Hsu, J.R., Wolf, S.E., Wenke, J.C., Baer, D.G., Owens, J., et al., 2010. Clinical application of an acellular biologic scaffold for surgical repair of a large, traumatic quadriceps femoris muscle defect. Orthopedics 33 (7), 511.

McFetridge, P.S., Daniel, J.W., Bodamyali, T., Horrocks, M., Chaudhuri, J.B., 2004. Preparation of porcine carotid arteries for vascular tissue engineering applications. J. Biomed. Mater. Res. A 70 (2), 224–234.

McPherson, T.B., Liang, H., Record, R.D., Badylak, S.F., 2000. Galalpha(1,3)Gal epitope in porcine small intestinal submucosa. Tissue Eng. 6 (3), 233–239.

Montgomery, A.M., Sabzevari, H., Reisfeld, R.A., 1993. Production and regulation of gelatinase B by human T-cells. Biochim. Biophys. Acta 1176 (3), 265–268.

Nelson, A.R., Fingleton, B., Rothenberg, M.L., Matrisian, L.M., 2000. Matrix metalloproteinases: biologic activity and clinical implications. J. Clin. Oncol. 18 (5), 1135–1149.

Opelz, G., Wujciak, T., Dohler, B., Scherer, S., Mytilineos, J., 1999. HLA compatibility and organ transplant survival. Collaborative Transplant Study. Rev. Immunogenet. 1 (3), 334–342.

Overall, C.M., Wrana, J.L., Sodek, J., 1991. Transcriptional and post-transcriptional regulation of 72-kDa gelatinase/type IV collagenase by transforming growth factor-beta 1 in human fibroblasts. Comparisons with collagenase and tissue inhibitor of matrix metalloproteinase gene expression. J. Biol. Chem. 266 (21), 14064–14071.

Piccinini, A.M., Midwood, K.S., 2010. DAMPening inflammation by modulating TLR signalling. Mediators Inflamm., 2010.

Probst, M., Dahiya, R., Carrier, S., Tanagho, E.A., 1997. Reproduction of functional smooth muscle tissue and partial bladder replacement. Br. J. Urol. 79 (4), 505–515.

Ramchandran, R., Dhanabal, M., Volk, R., Waterman, M.J., Segal, M., Lu, H., et al., 1999. Antiangiogenic activity of restin, NC10 domain of human collagen XV: comparison to endostatin. Biochem. Biophys. Res. Commun. 255 (3), 735–739.

Ranzato, E., Patrone, M., Pedrazzi, M., Burlando, B., 2009. HMGb1 promotes scratch wound closure of HaCaT keratinocytes via ERK1/2 activation. Mol. Cell. Biochem. 332 (1-2), 199–205.

Rao, W.H., Hales, J.M., Camp, R.D., 2000. Potent costimulation of effector T lymphocytes by human collagen type I. J. Immunol. 165 (9), 4935–4940.

Ratner, B.D., 2013. Biomaterials science : an introduction to materials in medicine. Elsevier/Academic Press, Amsterdam ; Boston.

Reing, J.E., Zhang, L., Myers-Irvin, J., Cordero, K.E., Freytes, D.O., Heber-Katz, E., et al., 2009. Degradation products of extracellular matrix affect cell migration and proliferation. Tissue Eng. Part A 15 (3), 605–614.

Reing, J.E., Brown, B.N., Daly, K.A., Freund, J.M., Gilbert, T.W., Hsiong, S.X., et al., 2010. The effects of processing methods upon mechanical and biologic properties of porcine dermal extracellular matrix scaffolds. Biomaterials 31 (33), 8626–8633.

Remlinger, N.T., Czajka, C.A., Juhas, M.E., Vorp, D.A., Stolz, D.B., Badylak, S.F., et al., 2010. Hydrated xenogeneic decellularized tracheal matrix as a scaffold for tracheal reconstruction. Biomaterials 31 (13), 3520–3526.

Rieder, E., Kasimir, M.T., Silberhumer, G., Seebacher, G., Wolner, E., Simon, P., et al., 2004. Decellularization protocols of porcine heart valves differ importantly in efficiency of cell removal and susceptibility of the matrix to recellularization with human vascular cells. J. Thorac. Cardiovasc. Surg. 127 (2), 399–405.

Roberts, T.S., Drez Jr., D., McCarthy, W., Paine, R., 1991. Anterior cruciate ligament reconstruction using freeze-dried, ethylene oxide-sterilized, bone-patellar tendon-bone allografts. Two year results in thirty-six patients. Am. J. Sports Med. 19 (1), 35–41.

Sachs, D.H., Sykes, M., Robson, S.C., Cooper, D.K., 2001. Xenotransplantation. Adv. Immunol. 79, 129–223.

Scalea, J., Hanecamp, I., Robson, S.C., Yamada, K., 2012. T-cell-mediated immunological barriers to xeno-transplantation. Xenotransplantation 19 (1), 23–30.

Schenke-Layland, K., Vasilevski, O., Opitz, F., Konig, K., Riemann, I., Halbhuber, K.J., et al., 2003. Impact of decellularization of xenogeneic tissue on extracellular matrix integrity for tissue engineering of heart valves. J. Struct. Biol. 143 (3), 201–208.

Schwartz, J.D., Monea, S., Marcus, S.G., Patel, S., Eng, K., Galloway, A.C., et al., 1998. Soluble factor(s) released from neutrophils activates endothelial cell matrix metalloproteinase-2. J. Surg. Res. 76 (1), 79–85.

Shapiro, S.D., 1994. Elastolytic metalloproteinases produced by human mononuclear phagocytes. Potential roles in destructive lung disease. Am. J. Respir. Crit. Care Med. 150 (6 Pt 2), S160–S164.

Shapiro, S.D., Kobayashi, D.K., Ley, T.J., 1993. Cloning and characterization of a unique elastolytic metalloproteinase produced by human alveolar macrophages. J. Biol. Chem. 268 (32), 23824–23829.

Sicari, B.M., Agrawal, V., Siu, B.F., Medberry, C.J., Dearth, C.L., Turner, N.J., et al., 2012a. A murine model of volumetric muscle loss and a regenerative medicine approach for tissue replacement. Tissue Eng. Part A 18 (19-20), 1941–1948.

Sicari, B.M., Johnson, S.A., Siu, B.F., Crapo, P.M., Daly, K.A., Jiang, H., et al., 2012b. The effect of source animal age upon the in vivo remodeling characteristics of an extracellular matrix scaffold. Biomaterials 33 (22), 5524–5533.

Sicari, B.M., Dziki, J.L., Siu, B.F., Medberry, C.J., Dearth, C.L., Badylak, S.F., 2014a. The promotion of a constructive macrophage phenotype by solubilized extracellular matrix. Biomaterials 35 (30), 8605–8612.

Sicari, B.M., Rubin, J.P., Dearth, C.L., Wolf, M.T., Ambrosio, F., Boninger, M., et al., 2014b. An acellular biologic scaffold promotes skeletal muscle formation in mice and humans with volumetric muscle loss. Sci. Transl. Med. 6 (234), 234ra258.

Sorsa, T., Ding, Y., Salo, T., Lauhio, A., Teronen, O., Ingman, T., et al., 1994. Effects of tetracyclines on neutrophil, gingival, and salivary collagenases. A functional and western-blot assessment with special reference to their cellular sources in periodontal diseases. Ann. N.Y. Acad. Sci. 732, 112–131.

Suehiro, K., Gailit, J., Plow, E.F., 1997. Fibrinogen is a ligand for integrin alpha5beta1 on endothelial cells. J. Biol. Chem. 272 (8), 5360–5366.

Susal, C., Opelz, G., 2013. Current role of human leukocyte antigen matching in kidney transplantation. Curr. Opin. Organ Transplant. 18 (4), 438–444.

Tang, D., Kang, R., Coyne, C.B., Zeh, H.J., Lotze, M.T., 2012. PAMPs and DAMPs: signal 0s that spur autophagy and immunity. Immunol. Rev. 249 (1), 158–175.

Teebken, O.E., Bader, A., Steinhoff, G., Haverich, A., 2000. Tissue engineering of vascular grafts: human cell seeding of decellularised porcine matrix. Eur. J. Vasc. Endovasc. Surg. 19 (4), 381–386.

Tian, J., Avalos, A.M., Mao, S.Y., Chen, B., Senthil, K., Wu, H., et al., 2007. Toll-like receptor 9-dependent activation by DNA-containing immune complexes is mediated by HMGB1 and RAGE. Nat. Immunol. 8 (5), 487–496.

Tottey, S., Johnson, S.A., Crapo, P.M., Reing, J.E., Zhang, L., Jiang, H., et al., 2011. The effect of source animal age upon extracellular matrix scaffold properties. Biomaterials 32 (1), 128–136.

Turley, E.A., Noble, P.W., Bourguignon, L.Y., 2002. Signaling properties of hyaluronan receptors. J. Biol. Chem. 277 (7), 4589–4592.

Turner, N.J., Badylak, S.F., 2012. Regeneration of skeletal muscle. Cell Tissue Res. 347 (3), 759–774.

Ulrich, P., Cerami, A., 2001. Protein glycation, diabetes, and aging. Recent Prog. Horm. Res. 56, 1–21.

Unemori, E.N., Hibbs, M.S., Amento, E.P., 1991. Constitutive expression of a 92-kD gelatinase (type V collagenase) by rheumatoid synovial fibroblasts and its induction in normal human fibroblasts by inflammatory cytokines. J. Clin. Invest. 88 (5), 1656–1662.

Vaday, G.G., Hershkoviz, R., Rahat, M.A., Lahat, N., Cahalon, L., Lider, O., 2000. Fibronectin-bound TNF-alpha stimulates monocyte matrix metalloproteinase-9 expression and regulates chemotaxis. J. Leukoc. Biol. 68 (5), 737–747.

Vaday, G.G., Schor, H., Rahat, M.A., Lahat, N., Lider, O., 2001. Transforming growth factor-beta suppresses tumor necrosis factor alpha-induced matrix metalloproteinase-9 expression in monocytes. J. Leukoc. Biol. 69 (4), 613–621.

Vadori, M., Cozzi, E., 2014. Immunological challenges and therapies in xenotransplantation. Cold Spring Harb. Perspect. Med. 4 (4), a015578.

Valentin, J.E., Badylak, J.S., McCabe, G.P., Badylak, S.F., 2006. Extracellular matrix bioscaffolds for orthopaedic applications. A comparative histologic study. J. Bone Joint Surg. Am. 88 (12), 2673–2686.

Valentin, J.E., Stewart-Akers, A.M., Gilbert, T.W., Badylak, S.F., 2009. Macrophage participation in the degradation and remodeling of extracellular matrix scaffolds. Tissue Eng. Part A 15 (7), 1687–1694.

Valentin, J.E., Turner, N.J., Gilbert, T.W., Badylak, S.F., 2010. Functional skeletal muscle formation with a biologic scaffold. Biomaterials 31 (29), 7475–7484.

van der Rest, M., Garrone, R., 1991. Collagen family of proteins. Faseb. J. 5 (13), 2814–2823.

Vasudev, S.C., Chandy, T., Sharma, C.P., Mohanty, M., Umasankar, P.R., 2000. Effects of double cross-linking technique on the enzymatic degradation and calcification of bovine pericardia. J. Biomater. Appl. 14 (3), 273–295.

Vlodavsky, I., Goldshmidt, O., Zcharia, E., Atzmon, R., Rangini-Guatta, Z., Elkin, M., et al., 2002. Mammalian heparanase: involvement in cancer metastasis, angiogenesis and normal development. Semin. Cancer Biol. 12 (2), 121–129.

Vyavahare, N., Hirsch, D., Lerner, E., Baskin, J.Z., Schoen, F.J., Bianco, R., et al., 1997. Prevention of bioprosthetic heart valve calcification by ethanol preincubation. Efficacy and mechanisms. Circulation 95 (2), 479–488.

Wainwright, J.M., Hashizume, R., Fujimoto, K.L., Remlinger, N.T., Pesyna, C., Wagner, W.R., et al., 2012. Right ventricular outflow tract repair with a cardiac biologic scaffold. Cells Tissues Organs 195 (1-2), 159–170.

Watson, C.J., Dark, J.H., 2012. Organ transplantation: historical perspective and current practice. Br. J. Anaesth. 108 (1), i29–i42.

Weiss, S.J., 1989. Tissue destruction by neutrophils. N. Engl. J. Med. 320 (6), 365–376.

Wolf, M.T., Daly, K.A., Reing, J.E., Badylak, S.F., 2012. Biologic scaffold composed of skeletal muscle extracellular matrix. Biomaterials 33 (10), 2916–2925.

Wolf, M.T., Dearth, C.L., Ranallo, C.A., LoPresti, S.T., Carey, L.E., Daly, K.A., et al., 2014. Macrophage polarization in response to ECM coated polypropylene mesh. Biomaterials 35 (25), 6838–6849.

Woods, T., Gratzer, P.F., 2005. Effectiveness of three extraction techniques in the development of a decellularized bone-anterior cruciate ligament-bone graft. Biomaterials 26 (35), 7339–7349.

Xu, H., Wan, H., Zuo, W., Sun, W., Owens, R.T., Harper, J.R., et al., 2009. A porcine-derived acellular dermal scaffold that supports soft tissue regeneration: removal of terminal galactose-alpha-(1,3)-galactose and retention of matrix structure. Tissue Eng. Part A 15 (7), 1807–1819.

Yeh, Y.C., Wu, C.C., Wang, Y.K., Tang, M.J., 2011. DDR1 triggers epithelial cell differentiation by promoting cell adhesion through stabilization of E-cadherin. Mol. Biol. Cell 22 (7), 940–953.

Yoo, J.J., Meng, J., Oberpenning, F., Atala, A., 1998. Bladder augmentation using allogenic bladder submucosa seeded with cells. Urology 51 (2), 221–225.

Yoshida, R., Vavken, P., Murray, M.M., 2012. Decellularization of bovine anterior cruciate ligament tissues minimizes immunogenic reactions to alpha-gal epitopes by human peripheral blood mononuclear cells. Knee 19 (5), 672–675.

Zhou, H., Bernhard, E.J., Fox, F.E., Billings, P.C., 1993. Induction of metalloproteinase activity in human T-lymphocytes. Biochim. Biophys. Acta 1177 (2), 174–178.

CHAPTER 5

Molecular Events at Tissue–Biomaterial Interface

Themis R. Kyriakides

Department of Biomedical Engineering, Yale University, New Haven, CT, USA

Contents

Host Response to Biomaterials.
DOI: http://dx.doi.org/10.1016/B978-0-12-800196-7.00005-0

GENERAL PRINCIPLES GUIDING PROTEIN INTERACTIONS AT THE BIOMATERIAL INTERFACE

Introduction

Biomaterial implantation induces focal hemorrhage and edema formation that lead to enrichment of interstitial fluid with plasma proteins. Within seconds of implantation, proteins interact with the biomaterial surface and over time create a proteinaceous coating (Horbett, 2012). The interactions of proteins with surfaces are complex and are governed by numerous parameters including protein composition, protein properties, and the chemistry, geometry, and topography of the biomaterial (Wilson et al., 2005). It is appreciated that specific protein properties such as size, diffusion coefficient, and affinity for the surface are critical in determining the final composition of the protein coating. Similarly, biomaterial surface properties including wettability, charge, topographical features, among others, also influence the final composition. Finally, the outcome is also tissue-specific based on the nature of the interstitial fluid and the presence of specialized inflammatory cells in different regions of the body. And while different tissues somewhat predictably elicit different responses to the presence of foreign implants, overarching principles exist and are discussed herein.

Protein adsorption at the biomaterial interface

Native proteins coat biomaterials in a process that is both rapid and competitive. When plasma-based protein adsorption occurs on an implanted material, a large number of proteins compete for surface-binding sites based upon their respective concentration gradients and surface affinities (Wilson et al., 2005; Horbett, 2012; Fabrizius–Homan and Cooper, 1991). Adsorption is driven primarily by the accumulation of numerous noncovalent bonds at the surface–protein interface, the redistribution of charged groups at the interface, and conformational changes to protein structure. From a protein perspective, size, charge, structure, stability, and unfolding rate all contribute to surface interactions. From a biomaterial perspective, topography, composition, hydrophobicity, and charge are key determinants of protein adsorption.

Hydrophobic interactions

Protein adsorption thermodynamics have been extensively studied and have been shown to involve the energetic interactions between proteins and various material surfaces (Wilson et al., 2005). On hydrophobic surfaces, heavily polar water molecules near the surface display increased association with neighboring water molecules. This leads to energetically unfavorable losses in entropy. To compensate, dehydration of protein structure causes hydrophobic moieties within the protein structure to form weak hydrophobic interactions with the surface at the exclusion of water molecules. This, in turn, leads to a favorable increase in the entropy of water in solution while driving the adsorption of proteins to the biomaterial surface. While individual hydrophobic interactions, or van der Waal forces, are relatively weak, collectively they contribute a huge driving force for overall adsorption of proteins to hydrophobic and weakly hydrophilic surfaces, particularly when one considers that 40–50% of the surface of most small proteins is nonpolar.

Protein adsorption on hydrophilic surfaces also occurs, with some studies somewhat surprisingly reporting similar amounts of adsorption regardless of whether a surface is hydrophobic or hydrophilic (Wilson et al., 2005). Despite the fact that the displacement of water from the surface of a hydrophilic material represents a large energy barrier to adsorption by proteins, the processes of charge interactions and changes in protein conformation provide adequate favorable energetic changes to drive adsorption.

Charge–charge interactions

Global charges on proteins and surfaces play a pivotal role in eletrostatically driven adsorption. Specifically, opposite charges attract and therefore are expected to influence charge–charge interactions between surface atoms and protein structures. However, it is important to appreciate the complexity of such interactions in aqueous solutions where charges on both surface and protein moieties are altered by pH, small ion interactions, and strong hydration bonds formed by water molecules. Even when adsorption would appear to be unfavorable, as is the case with like charges at a given pH, the presence of these other factors can provide adequate favorable energy change to push adsorption, particularly when the isoelectric point of a protein is achieved within the system.

Protein conformation changes

Adsorption can be rendered energetically favorable when upon contact; structural changes within the protein increase the overall entropy of the system. For instance,

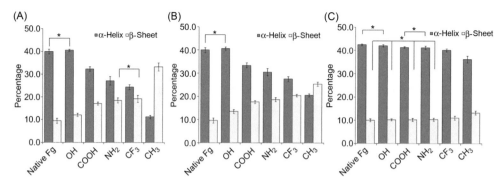

Figure 5.1 Changes in secondary structure of adsorbed human fibrinogen (Fg) adsorbed at (A) 0.1, (B) 1.0, and (C) 10.0 mg/mL on SAM surfaces determined by CD compared to its native conformation. ($n = 6$, mean $\pm$ 95% CI). * denotes not significant, all other values are significantly different from one another; $P < 0.05$. *Reprinted with permission from Sivaraman and Latour (2010).*

it has been demonstrated that at low concentrations, fibrinogen preferentially loses α-helix secondary structures and adopts an unfolded β-sheet conformation when adsorbing to more hydrophobic surfaces as shown in Figure 5.1 (Sivaraman and Latour, 2010).

More importantly, the ability of unfolded, flexible molecules to form noncovalent bonds with a surface in a rapid manner results in enhanced adsorption kinetics. Due to changes in protein conformation, many surfaces that would normally not favor proteins adsorption acquire a protein layer. Thus, conformational changes in proteins can overcome unfavorable global charges or hydrophobicity. However, this process does not necessarily result in fully denatured or unfolded proteins. Other factors, including the number and strength of a protein's internal structures as well as surface hydrophobicity, dictate the extent of conformational change upon adsorption and the ability of a protein to regain native structure and function upon desorption from a surface. For example, structurally stable, yet flexible proteins such as bovine serum albumin are able to assume a different conformation upon adsorption to hydrophilic surfaces such as silica but readily regain native structure and function when they desorb back into solution (Norde and Giacomelli, 2000).

Rearrangements of protein structure during adsorption proceed in a stepwise manner with varying kinetics. This means that at any given time, there is a heterogeneous distribution of varying structural conformations among adsorbed proteins on a surface. These different structural "populations" covering the biomaterial surface landscape vary in their rate of desorption and exchange with similar molecules in solution. More importantly, they differ in their respective binding site availability for cell adhesion and activation. For example, fibrinogen molecules are known to adsorb at different rates while forming a spectrum of conformations depending on concentration and surface chemistry (Keselowsky et al., 2003; Sivaraman and Latour, 2010). At low fibrinogen concentrations, more hydrophobic surfaces mediate larger percentages of conformational unraveling of α-helices within its native structure. In turn, higher amounts of platelet adhesion to surfaces is seen under these conditions, likely because these conformation changes within fibrinogen result in the exposure of integral platelet-binding motifs that are otherwise not available to platelet receptors when this protein is in its native state. Thus, by undergoing conformational changes, adsorbed proteins enhance cell adhesion and activity, which contribute to protein-mediated modulation of cellular activity.

Protein characteristics at the biomaterial surface

As discussed in the previous section, thermodynamic favorability drives structural changes within proteins to facilitate protein to surface adsorption. Whether or not these structural changes also result in increased cell adhesion and activation is largely protein-specific. Protein-mediated cellular responses are largely dependent on two conditions. First, on the overall adsorption profile on an implanted surface, which is defined by which proteins are adsorbed and in what quantity. Second, on the protein monolayer's bioactivity, which is the ability of adsorbed proteins to induce specific cellular responses (Horbett, 2012). The following discussion will focus on the effects that different surface characteristics have on the adsorption profile and bioactivity of the protein monolayer at the tissue–biomaterial interface.

Hydrophilic versus hydrophobic surfaces

Hydrophilic surface modifications of biomaterials are widely considered to enhance cell adhesion and activity when compared with more hydrophobic counterparts. This is likely due to an array of protein conformations that reside on surfaces of varying hydrophilicity. As mentioned above, the loss of compact secondary structure and exposure of normally sequestered moieties can enhance cellular binding to certain proteins, as in the case of plasma fibrinogen, for which binding of platelets from solution is enhanced with loss of secondary structure. However, the opposite may actually be true for other proteins. Cases in which protein adsorption occurs while restricting surface-induced conformational changes has been shown to more effectively preserve native biological activity for specific plasma proteins such as fibronectin (Keselowsky et al., 2003, 2005; Lan et al., 2005). Thus, conformational changes appear to variably impact the binding potential of different proteins and such considerations must be taken into account when delving deeper into the complex mechanisms through which protein adsorption is modulated on implanted surfaces.

Furthermore, the ability of surface characteristics to dictate the reversibility of adsorption also plays a role in subsequent cell–surface interactions. For many cell types, proliferation and activity are highly dependent on the extracellular matrix (ECM), which in the case of implanted materials is represented by the adsorbed protein mono-layer. On heavily hydrophobic surfaces in which the protein monolayer is tightly fixed to the surface, cell proliferation is often impaired. Specifically, the role of surface-adsorbed fibronectin on surface-mediated cell proliferation has been demonstrated. It has been shown that with increasing hydrophobicity of implanted surfaces, an upper limit of fibronectin adsorption strength exists beyond which cells are unable to effectively reorganize this surface-bound matrix and are compromised in their ability to proliferate and function normally (Keselowsky et al., 2005). Therefore, the reversibility of protein adsorption, or more simply, the tightness to which proteins adhere to a given surface, impacts not only the ability of cells to bind but also their ability to function properly once in contact with a foreign surface.

Surface charge effects

While many studies have demonstrated that the dominant variable in protein adsorption is material hydrophobicity, alterations to protein–protein interactions on implanted surfaces are also impacted by surface charge effects and become an important consideration given that nearly all interfaces are charged in aqueous solution (Grinnell and Feld, 1982). Ultimately, the impact of surface polarity on protein adsorption, much like hydrophobicity effects, has a downstream effect on the biological response to implanted biomaterials. This is due to a direct impact on protein pattern-ing and composition within the protein monolayer that occurs with altered protein–surface interactions in the presence of charged ion functional groups on the surface landscape.

Protein composition of the adsorbed monolayer can be altered with varying surface charges. For example, differing ratios of fibronectin to vitronectin were observed with increasing positively charged surfaces (Altankov and Groth, 1994). In addition, prefer-ential adsorption of vitronectin on charged, rather than nonpolar regions of patterned surfaces has been demonstrated (Shelton et al., 1988). Taken together, these observa-tions suggest that the charged environment intimately influences protein monolayer formation and impacts cellular responses. Furthermore, ionic content within the sys-tem also affects protein composition in the adsorbed layer; the presence of counterions within solution can serve as stabilizers of protein structure thereby altering adsorption dynamics at the interface (Wilson et al., 2005).

The role of surface topography

Surface topography has been shown to influence cell–biomaterial interactions and there is significant interest in how these interactions are modulated by adsorbed pro-teins. However, the lack of standards for characterizing different surface morpholo-gies complicates the interpretation of numerous studies. For example, surface area changes that accompany surface topography changes are often not corrected for and the unintended creation of confined spaces during surface fabrication could result in regions that behave different structurally from the rest of the material. In addition, various methods used to fabricate different surface textures also alter the surface chemistry properties, thereby making it difficult to ascertain cause and effect. Nevertheless, there is evidence that differences in surface roughness can cause differential protein adsorption. Specifically, studies examining grooved silicone have shown that different surface textures altered serum fibronectin and vitronectin deposition (den Braber et al., 1998). In addition, studies looking at protein adsorption from single-protein buffers onto surfaces of increasing roughness showed an increased fibronectin deposition, though correction for surface area increases was shown to potentially reverse this trend (François et al., 1997). While the effects are difficult to measure, there is evidence for modulation of protein adsorption through alteration of surface topography, making this yet another consideration when designing biomaterial surfaces. Depending on the ultimate goal of an implant, whether it be increased cellular adhesion and proliferation as in the case of many tissue engineering applications or the prevention of foreign body response (FBR) for biological implants, the cellular response could potentially be modified depending upon the topographical characteristics of the surface.

Summary

While the FBR to implanted biomaterials is ultimately mediated by cell activity at the tissue–material interface, it is important to appreciate that these processes would not be possible without an initial, rapid protein-mediated response. This response results in an adsorbed protein layer whose composition and bioactivity directly translates a foreign surface into a biologically understandable language to which cells are able to respond. Therefore, the distribution and availability of adhesion proteins along with the surface characteristics that modulate their adsorption become major considerations for any biomaterial application.

Though the role of surface characteristics on protein adsorption is complex, several trends seem to hold true. Moderately hydrophilic surfaces tend to enhance protein adsorption in a manner that more faithfully preserves native structure and thus bioactivity. Moreover, charged surface groups can provide a driving force for protein adsorption and influence the selectivity for different proteins within the protein layer. However, despite the presence of evidence suggesting a role for surface topography in modulating protein adsorption, it is likely to be minor when compared with surface chemistry characteristics such as hydrophilicity and surface charge. Regardless of the application, it is important to recognize that formation and composition of an initial protein-mediated response provides the essential link through which a biological system responds to the presence of a biomaterial. Therefore, the key to tailoring the FBR may ultimately reside in the modulation of this protein-mediated response.

CELL–PROTEIN INTERACTIONS AT THE INTERFACE

Introduction

As discussed in the previous section, understanding cell–protein interactions at the tissue–biomaterial interface must first be grounded in the understanding that cells generally do not make direct contact with the biomaterial itself. Instead, because the adsorption of proteins on the biomaterial surface is much more rapid than cell migration to the surface, cells at the interface depend more on the adsorbed native proteins rather than on the material itself to dictate their response. Protein adsorption converts biomaterial surfaces into a biologically recognizable entity that is capable of interacting with cells' native receptors. Thus, while properties of the biomaterial such as surface chemistry and topography all affect cellular response, this response is translated into biological signals via the adsorbed proteins. Here we will focus primarily on key cell–protein interactions that guide the local response to biomaterials. Additionally, we will discuss how cell–protein interactions at the tissue–biomaterial interface affect more systemic responses.

Understanding of cell–protein interactions is essential as the phenomenon can be harnessed to artificially manipulate cellular response to a biomaterial. Just as the native adsorbed proteins affect cell behavior, so can proteins introduced via the biomaterial itself. As researchers have sought to understand how specific adhesion proteins on biomaterials affect particular cellular responses, they have also attempted to alter cellular responses by introducing biomaterials coated with particular proteins. While this field is still relatively young, progress that has been made demonstrates the potential clinical applications and improvements on current standards of care that may be achieved by gaining an even deeper understanding of cell–protein interactions.

From the simplest perspective, there are three basic phases to cellular interaction at the tissue–biomaterial interface: (i) cellular adhesion, (ii) changes in cell morphology and motility, and (iii) modulation of cellular functions. While it is convenient to separate the interaction into these three phases, it is important to understand that cellular adhesion is really the governing process that goes on to affect the next two phases, as well as to ultimately elicit systemic cellular responses to biomaterials. In this chapter, we will focus on the basic principles governing cell–protein interaction and how this initial interaction leads to a more persistent effect known as the FBR. In addition, we will look at multicomponent signaling complexes called inflammasomes, which assemble in response to cellular stress and activate inflammatory cascades and how recent studies show that inflammasomes have the potential to influence the nature of both the acute and chronic inflammatory phases of tissue–biomaterial interactions.

Cellular adhesion principles

For most cell types, adhesion to some type of ECM is essential to their survival. Without attachment, cells will eventually undergo apoptosis (Frisch et al., 1996). Not only are these interactions with the ECM necessary, but they are also functional as cellular behavior can be regulated by the nature of its adhesive interactions (Frisch et al., 1996). There are two basic approaches to studying cell–protein interactions at the tissue–biomaterial interface. The more intuitive approach would involve implanting a biomaterial *in situ*, and after a period of time, removing the biomaterial and analyzing its surface. While this is the most translatable form of experiment since it actually studies what happens *in situ*, this type of analysis would be extremely complex and difficult to break down into single component studies. Thus, most researchers begin their investigations by studying biomaterials in a more controlled, *in vitro* setting. The most commonly used *in vitro* setup for studying cell–protein adhesion interactions is in a culture dish containing a serum-supplemented medium. As serum proteins are the abundant sources of adhesion proteins involved in cellular interaction *in vivo*, supplementing culture medium with serum proteins is a simple way of recreating these interactions *in vitro*.

Integrins

It has been shown that the primary interaction between cells and adhesion proteins occurs via heterodimeric receptors in the cell membranes called integrins (Winograd-Katz et al., 2014). Integrins bind to specific short peptide sequences presented by the adsorbed proteins. A decrease in cell attachment can be observed when antibodies that target integrin ligands are introduced into the medium. Similarly, changes in integrin expression affect change in the degree of cellular attachment. Integrins are made up of an α and β subunit, and over 18α and 8β subunits have been identified and can pair to produce numerous different receptor types. Specific peptide sequences facilitate their interactions with ECM proteins and this phenomenon has been exploited in many biomaterial and tissue engineering applications. For example, the peptide sequence RGD, which is present in fibronectin, laminin, vitronectin, and collagen, has been used to facilitate cell adhesion via multiple integrins (Carson and Barker, 2009; Shekaran and Garcia, 2011). Cells cultured *in vitro* adhere to culture dish, which is most commonly made from tissue culture polystyrene (TCP) and are dependent on fibronectin and vitronectin for attachment. Thus, a large number of studies have focused on these two integrin ligands. It should be noted that integrin activity is not limited to cellular attachment, but it has also been shown to be involved in a wide range of intracellular signaling and thus affect a variety of cellular functions such as cytoskeletal organization, cell proliferation, differentiation, apoptosis, and migration.

Cell adhesive proteins

Numerous serum proteins including fibronectin, vitronectin, fibrinogen, and components of complement like complement protein 3 (C3) have been shown to enhance cell adhesion to surfaces in numerous *in vitro* studies. Thus, investigators have focused on determining their adsorption to surfaces and contribution to cell adhesion and have made some novel discoveries. For example, C3 has been shown to enhance the adhesion of macrophages to polyurethane (PU) (Kao et al., 1996). Depletion of C3 from serum completely abolishes cell adhesion to PU, whereas depletion of fibronectin has no effect. Despite the demonstrated role of C3 in cell adhesion to PU, subsequent studies showed that it did not form covalent bonds with the surface (Wettero et al., 2002). In fact, it was shown that albumin and immunoglobulin (Ig) G but not fibrinogen allowed C3 binding and activation (Andersson et al., 2005). Therefore, other adsorbed proteins are critical in generating bioactive C3 on the surface. Interestingly, even though albumin does not support cell adhesion, it has been shown to modulate fibronectin-mediated cell adhesion (Lewandowska et al., 1992). Specifically, it was shown that fibronectin does not support extensive cell adhesion on polystyrene or self-assembled monolayers (SAMs) unless albumin is present.

Fibrinogen is another serum protein that has been implicated in mediating cell–biomaterial interactions *in vitro* and *in vivo*. Extensive work has demonstrated that this is mediated by a conformational change that occurs when fibrinogen interacts with surfaces, which allows the exposure of cryptic epitopes that serve as integrin-binding sites (Hu et al., 2001). Use of specific peptides and monoclonal antibodies allowed the characterization of these sites and confirmed the significance of fibrinogen unfolding in cell adhesion. Unfolding and exposure of these epitopes was greater on polyethylene terephthalate (PET), polyethylene (PE), and poly(vinyl chloride) (PVC), which support greater adhesion of monocytes and neutrophils. In contrast, these observations were dampened on polyether urethane (PEU) and polydimethylsiloxane (PDMS) because of reduced exposure of the cryptic epitopes.

Analysis of platelet interactions with modified SAMs has shed more light on this phenomenon. In trying to address the impact of conformational changes in fibrinogen versus overall levels, investigators discovered that platelet adhesion was enhanced only on surfaces that induced conformational changes and was independent of overall fibrinogen levels (Sivaraman and Latour, 2010). Specifically, alkanethiol SAMs were modified to contain one of the following terminal functional groups: CH3, OCH2CF3, NH2, COOH, or OH, which resulted in variable hydrophobicity. Changes in fibrinogen conformation, measured as the overall ratio of α-helix to β-sheet, was greatest on CH3- and lowest on OH-modified SAMs. Similarly, platelet adhesion was highest and lowest on the CH3- and OH-modified SAMs, respectively. As mentioned above, platelet adhesion was not dependent on the overall amount of adsorbed fibrinogen. This somewhat paradoxical observation could be explained by the possible inhibition of unfolding on high fibrinogen concentrations where tight packing of adsorbed molecules could prevent unfolding. Consistent with this suggestion, a similar study showed that, in comparison to OH-SAM, a far greater amount of fibronectin was required to support cell adhesion on CH3-SAM (Keselowsky et al., 2003). In this case, changes in the conformation of fibronectin would result in loss of adhesive function. This phenomenon might also explain the ability of albumin to enhance the cell adhesive properties of fibronectin on certain surfaces; by occupying sites on the surface, albumin could prevent fibronectin unfolding.

The advent of high throughput techniques has allowed the more systematic evaluation of adhesive protein adsorption and the identification of novel and more complex cell–biomaterial interactions. For example, proteomic analysis of serum proteins adsorbed to polypropylene (PP), PET, and PDMS revealed high levels of serum amyloid P, which as a single coating was shown to enhance the adhesion of granulocytes and monocytes on these biomaterials (Kim et al., 2005). Figure 5.2 shows two-dimensional (2D) gel electrophoresis analysis of adsorbed proteins. Other proteins identified by this method included fibrinogen, Ig light chain κ, α_2 macroglobulin, complement C4, and α_1 antitrypsin.

Using a similar proteomic approach, investigators analyzed the adsorption of proteins onto bare titanium, nickel titanium, and chitosan film, and identified the serum proteins adiponectin, thrombospondin (TSP) 1, fibronectin, and coagulation factor 2 as being critical for endothelial cell adhesion and spreading in a highly orchestrated temporal fashion (Yang et al., 2013).

These studies represent a small sample that highlights the complexity of findings involving multiple biomaterials and cell types. It is therefore difficult to reach overarching conclusions regarding the importance of specific protein–cell interactions in the FBR. Nevertheless, some principles have been defined in the case of blood platelets and they could apply to other cell types (Horbett, 2012). These include the observation that biomaterials acquire bioactivity due to adsorbed proteins, which depends on the intrinsic surface activity and bulk phase concentration of proteins. In addition, specific patterns of adsorption concentrate and immobilize adhesive proteins and thus enhance interactions with cells.

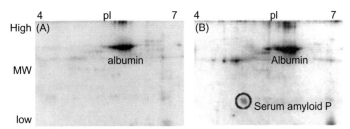

Figure 5.2 PP tubes were incubated with 1% bovine serum albumin in PBS for 1 h, followed by incubation with 5% human serum for (A) 4 h or (B) 24 h. The substrates were washed three times with 10 mL of PBS and adsorbed proteins were removed from the surface with elution buffer. The proteins were analyzed by 2D electrophoresis. After 4 h, albumin was the most prominent band on the 2D gel. After 24 h, more proteins were found on the surface, including serum amyloid P, which was identified by ion trap mass spectrometry. *Reprinted with permission from Kim et al. (2005).*

Dynamic environment

While we have emphasized thus far the need for adhesion proteins on the surface of the biomaterial before cells can adhere, it is important to keep in mind that this is a dynamic system. Cells are capable of secreting adhesion proteins such as fibronectin thus altering the properties of their attachment. Additionally, cells are capable of adapting to their environment, even once initial adhesion has occurred. Researchers have shown that cells can manipulate the population of integrin receptors based on the surface ligands on the biomaterial available for cellular binding. In addition, as discussed above, cells undergo cytoskeletal remodeling and activation due to activation of multiple signaling pathways. In the case of endothelial cells, this involves activation of the transforming growth factor (TGF)-β pathway following binding to TSP1.

Cell types involved in adhesion

While there are numerous types of cells that are affected by a total systemic tissue–biomaterial response, this section will focus only on the cells directly involved in cell–protein interactions or immediately located at the tissue–biomaterial interface. These cell types include platelets, macrophages (which form foreign body giant cells (FBGCs)), and fibroblasts. While the participation of other cells types such as neutrophils and endothelial cells should not be discounted, this triad of cells makes up the bulk of the FBR, which results in a collagenous capsule isolating the biomaterial from the surrounding tissue. Functionally, this capsule is often responsible for the failure of implanted biomaterials, thus it is important to keep in mind that minimizing this response is often the goal of optimizing biomaterials for efficacious use. It should be noted that even though this category only consists of a few distinct cell types, these cells and their interactions with adsorbed proteins on the biomaterial surface are responsible for the wide diversity of downstream effects that can be caused by biomaterial implantation. The extent of the response at each of these steps can be affected by the properties of the implanted biomaterial and the implantation site.

Platelets

Platelets are one of the first cells involved in the FBR to a biomaterial. Once a biomaterial is exposed to blood, it is coated with serum proteins, and platelets begin to aggregate around the surface and release chemoattractants (such as TGF-β, platelet-derived growth factor (PDGF), chemokine (C-X-C motif) ligand 4 (CXCL4), leukotriene B(4) (LTB4), and interleukin (IL)-4), which recruit macrophages to the site of implantation. In addition, platelets can release proteins such as fibrinogen that could serve as provisional matrix for recruited cells.

Macrophages and FBGCs

Once macrophages are recruited to the surface, they begin to assemble, which leads to further release of chemoattractive signals by the macrophages themselves (such as tumor necrosis factor (TNF)-α, IL-1β, IL-6, and monocyte chemotactic protein (MCP)-1/CCL2) and thus propagate macrophage assembly at the interface. Once macrophages are bound via their integrin receptors, downstream signal transduction can affect cytoskeletal rearrangement and formation of more adhesion structures allowing macrophages to undergo cytoskeletal remodeling that results in "spreading" over the biomaterial surface. This spreading is partially facilitated by "podosomes," which are specialized macrophage adhesion structures consisting of a central core of actin surrounded by a ring of proteins that regulate actin polymerization. These podosomes are associated with both initial macrophage adhesion and subsequent cytoskeleton remodeling that allow macrophage fusion to form FBGCs. *In vitro* studies have shown that the latter involves extensive lamellipodia formation that promotes contact between adjacent cells.

Fibroblasts and fibrotic encapsulation

While fibroblasts do not necessarily adhere directly to the adsorbed proteins on the surface, they are extremely important in the surrounding tissue's interaction with an implanted biomaterial. The long-term outcome of the FBR is the fibrotic encapsulation of the implanted biomaterial. This fibrotic encapsulation is mediated by two main mechanisms. First, the activated macrophages have been shown to overexpress ECM proteins such as fibronectin, which is deposited during the healing portion of the FBR and is critical for the assembly of collagen fibrils. Second, activated macrophages stimulate fibrogenesis by fibroblasts. It is important to note that this function is in direct opposition to classically activated macrophages, which actually inhibit fibrogenesis. Fibroblasts are recruited to the site of the implanted biomaterial and deposit ECM components around the biomaterial, which contribute to the formation of the fibrous capsule.

Lymphocytes in the FBR

While not covered in our brief overview of the FBR above, it is important to touch on the presence of lymphocytes at the tissue–biomaterial interface. It has long been noted that lymphocytes appear to adhere to biomaterial surface *in vitro*. It has also been observed that lymphocytes associate with both macrophages and FBGCs in cell culture. This association has been demonstrated to be a mutually beneficial interaction in which lymphocytes enhance macrophage adhesion and fusion, and the presence of macrophages stimulates lymphocytic proliferation. However, like fibroblasts, lymphocytes do not adhere to the biomaterial surface itself, but rather associate with the macrophages or FBGCs.

Summary

We began this section by discussing how an understanding of cell–protein interactions at the tissue–biomaterial interface is key in understanding what interactions could be targeted in order to minimize harmful cellular responses to biomaterials. We discussed the basic principles of cellular adhesion to biomaterials via the integrin receptors and the involvement of specific proteins. Despite the plethora of *in vitro* studies demonstrating the importance of specific proteins in mediating cell–surface interactions, approaches that target single proteins have not been successful *in vivo*. This highlights both the ability of multiple proteins to support cell adhesion and the need to create surfaces that resist the adsorption of multiple proteins. Or, as we discuss in the next section, it might be more efficacious to target cellular processes that occur post adhesion.

MOLECULAR PATHWAYS IN THE REGULATION OF CELL ACTIVATION AND CELL–CELL INTERACTIONS

Introduction

Numerous cell types including inflammatory cells, fibroblasts, endothelial cells, smooth muscle cells, osteoblasts, and various stem cells have been the focus of detailed analysis in the context of biomaterial interactions. However, it is appreciated that in *in vivo* settings, especially in soft tissues, the key cell type that dictates the progression of the FBR is the macrophage. Whether recruited as monocytes or present as resident macrophages, these cells dominate the interface in both the short- and long-term and display novel activation and remarkable plasticity. For example, macrophages undergo homotypic fusion to form multinucleate FBGCs and differentiation to form fibrogenic cells (McNally and Anderson, 2011; Helming and Gordon, 2009; Mooney et al., 2014). By adopting specific phenotypes, macrophages orchestrate the ensuing fibrogenic response leading to encapsulation.

Biomaterials and inflammasome activation

Due to tissue damage associated with implantation, recruited monocytes encounter chemoattractant signals and cytokines that induce their differentiation to macrophages and subsequent activation. Conceivably, resident macrophages encounter the same signals and undergo similar activation. Numerous *in vitro* and *in vivo* studies have shown that exposure of macrophages to biomaterials induces the secretion of the potent proinflammatory cytokine IL-1β. Synthesis of IL-1β is induced by multiple signals that activate the Toll-like receptor (TLR)-4 and cause the upregulation of the IL-1β gene and the production of inactive pro-IL-1β. Conversion of pro-IL-1β to the active form depends on cleavage by caspase-1, which depends on the formation of the inflammasome as shown in Figure 5.3 (Strowig et al., 2012; Latz et al., 2013; Bryant and Fitzgerald, 2009). The inflammasome is a high molecular weight protein complex that consists of a nucleotide-binding domain and leucine-rich repeat-containing type (NLRP), apoptosis-associated speck-like protein-containing CARD (ASC), and caspase-1.

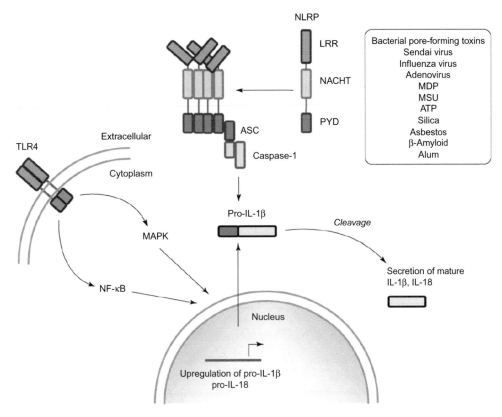

Figure 5.3 Mechanisms regulating IL-1β production. Generation of IL-1β requires a priming signal, often from pathogen recognition receptors (PRRs) such as TLRs that activate NF-κB and NF-κB-dependent transcription of pro-IL-1β. The pro-IL-1β is then cleaved into the active, mature 17 kDa cytokine by caspase-1. NLR-containing inflammasomes activate caspase-1. NLRs such as NLRP3 oligomerize upon activation (by danger signals such as those shown in the box) and recruit the adapter molecule ASC that subsequently recruits and activates caspase-1. *Reprinted with permission from Bryant and Fitzgerald. (2009).*

As stated above, formation of the complex leads to activation of caspase-1, a phenomenon that can be induced by various stimuli including disruption of cellular integrity, ATP, silica, or uric acid (Henao-Mejia et al., 2012; Bryant and Fitzgerald, 2009). More recently, investigators showed that the inflammasome is activated in the context of cell–biomaterial interactions (Malik et al., 2011). Specifically, poly-methyl methacrylate (PMMA) microspheres (150 μm in diameter, which exceeds the upper limit of macrophage phagocytosis) induced inflammasome activation and IL-1β secretion *in vitro* and *in vivo* in a mouse intraperitoneal model. Moreover, short-term studies in mice deficient for caspase-1, NLRP3, or ASC demonstrated that IL-1β production in response to PMMA was dependent on the inflammasome. Of note, investigators have made the observation that large PMMA microspheres can induce inflammasome activation in the absence of serum. Therefore, it is possible to consider that direct contact between PMMA and macrophages can initiate inflammation as shown in Figure 5.4.

An explanation for this observation was provided by experiments where depletion of cholesterol or inhibition of spleen tyrosine kinase (Syk) signaling diminished IL-1β production. These results suggested that the physical contact between microspheres and the plasma membrane induces inflammasome activation. However, due to the large number of proteins, it is unclear if such interactions occur *in vivo*.

In a subcutaneous PDMS implantation model in genetically modified mice, caspase-1 and ASC were found to be required for the full progression of the FBR and formation of collagenous capsules (Malik et al., 2011). Specifically, capsule thickness was reduced in the FBR of caspase-1KO and ASC KO mice despite normal levels of FBGC formation. Interestingly, NLRP3 KO mice displayed normal formation of collagenous capsule suggesting that other NLRPs are involved in the progression of the FBR. These recent findings have the potential to be very powerful, as they offer some insight into the vaguely understood mechanism of cell–biomaterial interactions and subsequent formation of FBGC and development of the FBR.

Macrophage priming and adhesion in the FBR

Other chemokines and cytokines, like MCP-1and IL-4, are induced in the FBR and influence macrophage adhesion, activation, and function. As mentioned above, macrophages encounter protein-coated surfaces in a "primed" state. It is critical to appreciate that in the context of the FBR, both proteins and cells are altered. First, multiple proteins are at different stages of denaturation. Second, cells are "primed" due to exposure to multiple exogenous and endogenous signals. Therefore, the ensuing macrophage adhesion represents a unique scenario that is not reproduced in other pathologies. Moreover, macrophages proceed to undergo homotypic fusion and form FBGC, a hallmark of the FBR. *In vitro* studies have implicated the partial contribution of multiple integrins including αMβ2, αXβ2, α5β1, αVβ1, α3βb1, and α2β1 to macrophage adhesion (McNally and Anderson, 2011). Consistent with integrin engagement, proline-rich tyrosine kinase-2 (PYK2) and focal adhesion kinase (FAK) have been shown to be induced and activated in IL-4-treated fusing macrophages (McNally and Anderson, 2011). These specific integrins can interact with serum proteins such as C3, fibrinogen, and plasma fibronectin, and ECM proteins including fibronectin, vitronectin, collagen, and laminin, all of which are present in the FBR. However, it should be noted that only vitronectin could support the formation of FBGC as an *in vitro* substrate on TCP. Thus, macrophages display remarkable specificity in their interactions with biomaterials and this fact may explain why they do not form FBGC in wound environments despite the presence of multiple integrin ligands. The importance and specificity of these interactions has also been demonstrated in *in vitro* studies where

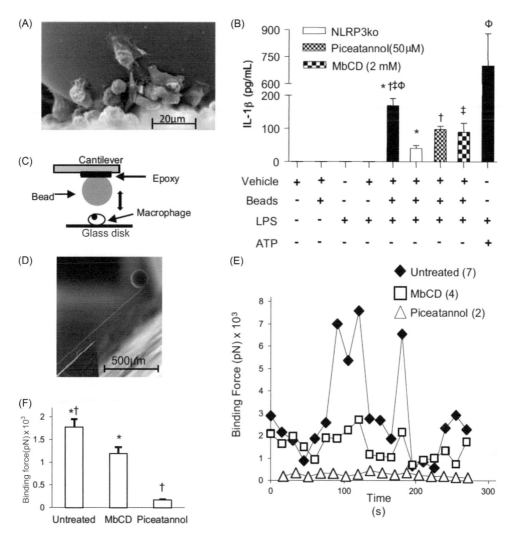

Figure 5.4 PMMA microspheres induce IL-1β production from peritoneal macrophages in a membrane lipid- and Syk-dependent manner. (A) Single microsphere, which is much larger than attached macrophages and cannot be phagocytosed. (B) Microspheres induce IL-1β, which is significantly less in the absence of Nlrp3 and can be reduced in wild-type macrophages by the cholesterol inhibitor MbCD (50 μm), and the Syk inhibitor piceatannol (2 mM). (C) Experimental design for measuring the binding force between a single microsphere and a single macrophage using an AFM. (D) Single microsphere on the cantilever of the AFM. (E) Binding force between a single microsphere and cell over a period in the presence and absence of MbCD or piceatannol. (F) Readings of binding affinity in all experiments depicted in (E) are averaged. *†‡ϕ$P \leq 0.05$. *Reprinted with permission from Malik et al. (2011).*

surfaces that do not support monocyte adhesion and macrophage development were shown to be nonpermissive for FBGC formation (McNally and Anderson, 2011).

Molecular regulators of macrophage activation and fusion

Macrophage activation on the surface of biomaterials is a complex process that does not fit into the archetypical categories of classical (M1), alternative (M2), and their subsets. Despite the dominant role of IL-4 in FBGC formation, which is a prototypical M2 cytokine, macrophages in the FBR do not assume an exclusive M2 phenotype (Mooney et al., 2014). It is also worth considering that the initial signals that activate monocytes, such as MCP-1 and IL-1β, are primarily M1-associated. Therefore, macrophages are able to integrate multiple activation cues and undergo unique activation characterized by features of both M1 and M2. Consistent with this suggestion, several molecules have been implicated in the formation of FBGC including cell receptors (IL-4R, cluster of differentiation (CD) 36, triggering receptor expressed on myeloid cells (TREM)-2, signal regulatory protein (SIRP)-1α, CD47, P2X purinoceptor (P2X)-7, CD9/CD81), membrane-associated proteins (DNAX activating protein 12 (DAP12), dendritic cell-specific transmembrane protein (DC-STAMP), E-cadherin), cytoskeleton-associated molecules (Rac1, DOCK180), and secreted molecules (MCP-1, TNF-α, matrix metalloproteinase (MMP)-9) (Helming and Gordon, 2009).

JAK/STAT pathway and macrophage activation/fusion

Based on studies in MCP-1 KO mice, which display diminished FBGC formation, the existence of at least two distinct pathways have been shown to be required for FBGC formation. The first pathway involves the IL-4-mediated induction of the Janus kinase (JAK)/signal transducer and activator of transcription (STAT)-6 pathway leading to translocation of STAT6 to the nucleus and transcription of E-cadherin, β-catenin. The cellular source of IL-4 in the biomaterial milieu is not clear but could be mast cells, eosinophils, basophils, and/or natural killer cells. Nevertheless, E-cadherin and β-catenin are expressed at the cell membrane prior to fusion and appear to facilitate cell–cell interactions. Upon fusion, both proteins are lost from the membrane and appear in the cytoplasm. The importance of E-cadherin in FBGC formation has been demonstrated in *in vitro* experiments where anti-E-cadherin antibodies inhibited fusion (Moreno et al., 2007). Despite its demonstrated importance for fusion, this pathway is intact in MCP-1-null macrophages that fail to fuse. Therefore, the existence of a second pathway downstream of MCP-1 has been suggested. Specifically, macrophages lacking MCP-1 are deficient in Rac1-dependent cytoskeletal remodeling, lamellipodia formation, do not induce TNF-α, and do not secrete MMP-9 (Skokos et al., 2011). These events occur in IL-4-treated wild-type macrophages and are all required in the formation of FBGC. Details of these pathways are summarized in Figure 5.5.

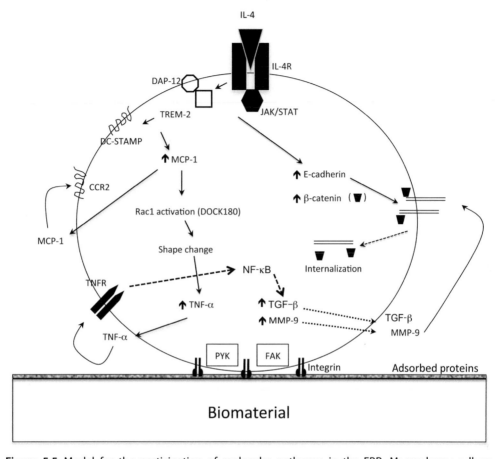

Figure 5.5 Model for the participation of molecular pathways in the FBR. Macrophages adhere to adsorbed proteins via integrins that activate PYK and FAK. In parallel, IL-4 induces activation of at least two pathways including the JAK/STAT pathway, leading to the induction of E-cadherin, β-catenin, and an unknown pathway that induces MCP-1 and TNF-α. TNF-α interacts with its receptors and induces the canonical activation of the NF-κB pathway leading to induction of MMP-9 and TGF-β. Studies in DAP12-null macrophages suggest that DAP12 signaling is essential for programming macrophages into a fusion-competent state. MCP-1-null macrophages are deficient in cytoskeletal remodeling and have low levels of TNF-α and MMP-9 but induce E-cadherin and β-catenin normally. This implies that part of the JAK/STAT pathway is intact in MCP-1-null cells and that at least two divergent pathways are involved in fusion. Addition of TNF-α to MCP-1-null macrophages in a fusion experiment induces MMP-9 expression and restores the fusion defect, conceivably by cleaving E-cadherin at the surface. It is suggested that a link between the two pathways exists based on the effects of MCP-1 and MMP-9 deficiency on the subcellular localization of E-cadherin and β-catenin. *Reprinted with permission from Skokos et al. (2011).*

Even though the exact signaling pathway that links MCP-1 binding to TNF-α induction and MMP-9 secretion has not been established, it is assumed that this is mediated by activation of either p38 mitogen-activated protein kinase (MAPK) or extracellular signal-regulated protein kinases 1 and 2 (ERK1/2). Previous studies have shown that MCP-1 induces chemotaxis via the activation of p38MAPK and modulates adhesion via an ERK1/2-dependent mechanism (Ashida et al., 2001; Arefieva et al., 2005).

NF-κB pathway and macrophage activation/fusion

Despite the fact that IL-4 is known to induce alternative (M2) polarization of macrophages, a number of classical (M1) molecules are induced in the FBR including MCP-1 and TNF-α. The induction of the latter is intriguing because it is a key cytokine in many inflammatory responses. Following activation of the TNF receptor, a series of complex interactions leads to the activation of the nuclear factor-κB (NF-κB) signaling pathway. The pathway involves NF-κB/Rel proteins including p52/p100, p50/p105, c-Rel, RelA/p65, and RelB (Hayden and Ghosh, 2008). Two types of activation have been described, the canonical (p50/RelA) and noncanonical (p52/RelB). In the cytoplasm, these proteins are bound and inhibited by inhibitor of κB (IκB) proteins, which are ubiquinated and targeted for degradation in inflammatory settings. When that occurs, NF-κB/Rel complexes are freed, become activated by phosphorylation, and translocate to the nucleus where they drive transcription of target genes. Recently, it was demonstrated that the canonical NF-κB pathway is engaged in macrophage fusion *in vitro* and *in vivo*. Specifically, *in vitro* studies showed that p50 and RelA were induced and translocated to the nucleus in response to IL-4. Temporally, this event was prominent on day 3, which is consistent with the pattern of TNF-α induction. More importantly, pharmacological inhibition of the pathway resulted in the formation of smaller FBGC with fewer nuclei indicating that p50/RelA are not critical for the initiation of fusion but play a critical role in its progression. Consistent with this suggestion, *in vivo* experiments showed the nuclear translocation of p50 and RelA in implant-associated macrophages 4 days after implantation. Moreover, this was not observed in fusion-deficient MCP-1 KO macrophages. As mentioned above, these cells are capable of activating JAK/STAT6 and inducing and localizing E-cadherin at the surface. Therefore, it is concluded that the NF-κB and JAK/STAT6 pathways are activated independently.

Additional pathways in FBGC formation

Integration of additional activation pathways is also suggested by studies in mice lacking DAP12 (Helming et al., 2008). When this transmembrane protein is activated, it undergoes phosphorylation and recruits kinases such as SYK, which has been implicated in macrophage fusion. The primary role of DAP12 is thought to be regulation of transcription of fusion mediators such as DC-STAMP, MMP-9, and E-cadherin. Moreover, DAP12 interacts with the receptor TREM-2 and this interaction, similar to the activation of transcription, is thought to be important for macrophage programming. Finally, loss of DAP12 is associated with a reduction in the expression of DC-STAMP, a receptor-associated signaling protein that has been shown to be critical for macrophage fusion. Other significant molecular events in fusion include interaction of the scavenger receptor CD36 with exposed phosphatidylserine (Helming et al., 2009; Helming and Gordon, 2009). Recent evidence suggests that this lipid, which is normally confined to the inner leaflet, is exposed on the surface of fusing macrophages. The mechanism for changes in lipid distribution during fusion is not clear but studies have implicated the ATP-gated receptor P2X7 (Lemaire et al., 2012). Specifically, activation of this receptor leads to the formation of large pores on the plasma membrane and phosphatidylserine exposure on the cell surface where it can interact with CD36.

As mentioned above, a complex set of exogenous and endogenous signals regulate the progression of the FBR. These include adsorbed proteins on the surface, signals generated as part of the inflammatory response, and signals induced by these entities in cells in the vicinity of implants. However, the relative contribution of these signals has been difficult to determine. For example, the importance of IL-4 in the activation and fusion of macrophages has been shown in numerous *in vitro* and *in vivo* studies. Specifically, it was shown that monocytes isolated from mice lacking the IL-4 receptor (IL-4Rα) were unable to fuse (Helming and Gordon, 2007). Moreover, neutralizing anti-IL-4 antibodies were able to inhibit macrophage fusion on poly(etherurethane urea) (PEUU) in a cage implant model (Kao et al., 1995). However, FBGC formation progressed normally in IL-4Rα-deficient mice, suggesting that additional macrophage fusion-inducing cytokines can mediate FBGC formation (Yang et al., 2014). These findings highlight the difficulty in developing strategies to limit FBGC formation.

Summary

The existence of multiple pathways highlights the complexity of the macrophage activation and fusion process and is consistent with the unique polarization phenotype exhibited by these cells when in contact with biomaterials. Conceivably, these molecular pathways contribute to macrophage activation and fusion leading to the normal progression of the FBR. One possible molecular mechanism that could signify convergence between at least two of these pathways involves the putative cleavage of E-cadherin by MMP-9 at the cell surface. Upon cleavage, macrophages that are in close contact could initiate fusion. It should be noted that cleavage of E-cadherin by MMP-9 has been shown in tumor cells (Symowicz et al., 2007). Regardless of the mechanism involved, the formation of FBGC can be detrimental for biomaterials because these cells can damage surfaces (McNally and Anderson, 2011). In addition, because they are a hallmark of the FBR, FBGCs were thought to contribute to its progression and be responsible for encapsulation. While they are capable of generating pro-fibrotic signals, many studies have shown that a reduction in FBGC formation is not associated with a reduction in capsule thickness. Therefore, it is now appreciated that macrophage-derived signals are critical for driving the full progression of the FBR.

MOLECULAR PATHWAYS MEDIATING TISSUE REMODELING AT THE INTERFACE

Introduction

Progression of the FBR involves the deposition of ECM leading to the eventual encapsulation of implants. As mentioned earlier in this chapter, the FBR involves aspects of wound healing due to the injury to tissues during implantation. It is helpful then to consider similarities and differences between these two processes. Similar to wound healing, the FBR generally initiates as an inflammatory response and progresses to matrix deposition and remodeling. However, the FBR is distinguished by a striking paucity of blood vessels in the largely avascular collagenous capsules. Moreover, matrix deposition displays highly ordered alignment of collagen fibers within which reside elongated thin fibroblasts. In fact, the tight packing of collagen fibers and fibroblasts in the FBR is often similar to that of tendons and ligaments. Thus, the eventual outcome of the FBR does not resemble the loosely organized and vascularized ECM of wounds. Based on the assumption that macrophages are key determinants of the FBR, it is possible that a uniquely activated macrophage population provides the signals for ordered matrix deposition and inhibition of blood vessel formation.

Extracellular matrix

ECM is the noncellular component of tissues and organs that functions, in part, as structural support for tissues and scaffold for cells. The ECM also provides critical biochemical and biomechanical cues that play important roles in tissue morphogenesis, differentiation, and homeostasis (Ozbek et al., 2010). Although the basic structure and function of all ECMs are the same, the physical and biochemical properties can vary depending on the tissue (Frantz et al., 2010). Tissue specificity is critical for defining the mechanical properties of different tissues and organs, including tensile strength, compressive strength, and elasticity (Faulk et al., 2014). Even though the ECM is not composed of cells, it interacts with cells to regulate important functions. Cells can adhere to the ECM via integrin proteins and these interactions influence cell attachment, shape, and motility (Walters and Gentleman, 2015). Growth factors and other molecular mediators are also able to bind the ECM, which helps to bring them into contact with adjacent cells and initiate downstream signal transduction.

ECM is composed of three primary components: proteoglycans, adhesive glycoproteins, and fibrous proteins, which provide an environment that regulates cell proliferation, differentiation, and function (Halper and Kjaer, 2014). Proteoglycans are heavily glycosylated proteins consisting of a core protein and one or more covalently attached glycosaminoglycan chains. Because of their unique buffering, hydration, and binding properties, proteoglycans interact with other ECM components and form hydrated gels that resist compressive forces. Fibrous proteins in the ECM include collagen and elastin that are responsible for tensile strength and elasticity. Collagen fibrils form an organized structure of aligned fibers that make up the primary structural component of the ECM. In addition to determining mechanical properties of the ECM, collagens regulate cell adhesion, support chemotaxis and migration, and direct tissue development. Elastin fibers are much more elastic than collagen fibers and allow the ECM and surrounding tissues to stretch and recoil. Adhesive glycoproteins, such as fibronectin and laminin, support cell attachment to the ECM and mediate cell function. Fibroblasts secrete and organize two types of collagens (type I and type III collagens), elastin, and fibronectin. These proteins are critical for maintaining the structural integrity of the ECM. In addition to these major components, the ECM contains matricellular proteins that are important for tissue remodeling at the tissue–biomaterial interface. Matricellular proteins are ECM proteins that act primarily as mediators of cell–matrix interactions rather than as structural components (Murphy-Ullrich and Helene Sage, 2014). A number of proteins belong to this group including TSP1, TSP2, secreted *protein* acidic and rich in cysteine (SPARC), tenascin-C, and osteopontin, all of which have been implicated in the FBR (Morris and Kyriakides, 2014).

Biomaterials and fibrogenic responses

Matrix deposition and remodeling in response to biomaterials occurs in the form of fibrosis, which is characterized by proliferation of ECM-producing fibroblasts and excessive deposition of collagen-rich ECM. The process whereby the fibrous tissues develop is called fibrogenesis, and it is common to both wound healing and the FBR; however, the exact mechanisms and final outcomes are different. As mentioned previously, one of the initial events in the FBR is the infiltration of macrophages to the site of the biomaterial–tissue interaction. Once macrophages are activated, they are able to produce pro-fibrogenic growth factors, including TGF-β. It is assumed that fibroblasts respond to this and other growth factors and initiate fibrogenesis. Researchers have studied this phenomenon using macrophages cultured *in vitro*: after macrophages are exposed to biomedical polymers, they become activated and stimulate fibroblast activity (Holt et al., 2010; Pan et al., 2011; Zeng and Chen, 2010). Both macrophages and fibroblasts play key roles in tissue remodeling during the FBR. After the initial phase of inflammation, fibrotic tissue begins to form around the biomaterial and this process involves the increased proliferation and activation of fibroblasts that upregulate collagen production. Hyperactivity of fibroblasts creates a dense, highly ordered collagenous tissue with low cellular content that lacks both vascularization and permeability. Dependence of the FBR on increased collagen production was shown in studies where inhibition of collagen synthesis resulted in reduced capsule thickness (Rujitanaroj et al., 2013). As stated above, it is important to consider why the formation of dense highly ordered collagenous matrix is not observed in wound healing. This could be due to the continuous presence of the biomaterial that could chronically disrupt the homeostatic environment and generate sustained cellular responses. Conceivably, synthesis and release of pro-inflammatory and pro-fibrotic molecules could persist and contribute to the unique phenotype of the FBR. In parallel, the process could be sustained by the lack of anti-inflammatory and anti-fibrotic signals that are observed in the latter phases of wound healing. Despite the significance of encapsulation, little is known about this process at the molecular level.

Additional cell types have been implicated in the encapsulation process including mast cells. Specifically, it was shown that collagen levels in the FBR were reduced in mast cell-deficient mice (WBB6F1/J-Kit(W)/Kit(W-v)) due to reduced responses in fibrocytes and myofibroblasts (Thevenot et al., 2011). This observation suggested that mast cell degranulation, in addition to stimulating inflammation, contributes to fibrosis. Interestingly, PEU and PET implantation studies in these mice showed normal FBGC formation (Yang et al., 2014). From these studies, and studies in MCP-1-null mice, it can be concluded that FBGC formation can be uncoupled from implant encapsulation.

Molecular determinants of biomaterial-induced fibrogenic responses

Several experimental studies have demonstrated the significance of specific proteins in biomaterial encapsulation. For example, mice that lack the matricellular protein TSP2 display loose organization of collagen fibers but no change in capsule thickness (Kyriakides et al., 1999, 2001b). At the molecular level, this is due, in part, to the ability of TSP2 to bind matrix-degrading enzymes such as MMP-2 and MMP-9 and facilitate their uptake and degradation. Therefore, TSP2-null mice have excess MMPs that could act on the collagenous matrix and alter its deposition pattern. Interestingly, MMP-9-null mice display reduced collagen and fibronectin deposition in the FBR suggesting a critical role for this enzyme in ECM production (MacLauchlan et al., 2009b). Other studies have shown that mice that lack another matricellular protein, SPARC, form thinner foreign body capsules (Puolakkainen et al., 2003). This observation is consistent with a role for SPARC in collagen fibrillogenesis. Little is known about the participation of proteoglycans in the FBR except that they can be detected in collagenous capsules. For example, the expression of the proteoglycan decorin, which participates in collagen fibrillogenesis, and other proteoglycans such as perlecan, were detected in the FBR (Ward et al., 2008; Farrugia et al., 2014). Perhaps more suggestive of a role for this class of molecules was the finding that modification of cross-linked collagen matrices via attachment of glycosaminoglycans resulted in reduced FBR (Pieper et al., 2000).

Inflammation and fibrogenesis

As mentioned above, the concept that biomaterial-induced inflammation is a critical determinant of the FBR is well established. Therefore, several anti-inflammatory strategies have been successful in reducing capsule thickness including the treatment of experimental animals with anti-inflammatory drugs (i.e., prednisolone, dexamethasone), administration of pulsed acoustic cellular expression (PACE), and other methods (Bridges and Garcia, 2008; Reichenberger et al., 2014; Vacanti et al., 2012; Morais et al., 2010). Moreover, targeted deletion of plasma fibronectin in mice was associated with increased capsule thickness (Keselowsky et al., 2007). From a biomaterial perspective, several studies have shown that with increasing size (implant thickness or fiber diameter), inflammation and encapsulation are enhanced (Sanders and Rochefort, 2003; Ward et al., 2002). These studies highlight the significance of the inflammatory response in the development of fibrosis.

Macrophage activation and implant fibrosis

Our current understanding of the inflammatory response has expanded to include specific types of macrophage activation. Therefore, it is now appreciated that the presence of alternatively activated (M2) macrophages is often associated with less fibrogenic responses (Brown et al., 2012; Wolf et al., 2015). In fact, as shown in Figure 5.6, a mouse implantation study with low protein adsorbing zwitterion-based hydrogels showed loss of capsule formation associated with an M2 macrophage phenotype (Zhang et al., 2013).

In addition, other studies of macrophage phenotype have suggested that a higher percentage of M2 macrophages is inversely proportional to scar tissue formation and implant encapsulation (Brown et al., 2012). Finally, M2 macrophages were observed in the FBR to porous materials that elicit tissue integration and increased neovascularization (Sussman et al., 2014).

While it is attractive to associate M2 macrophages with better FBR outcomes, this is not always the case. As discussed in the section "Cell–Protein Interactions at the Interface," macrophage activation is complex and is perhaps better described as a continuum instead of distinct phases (Mosser and Edwards, 2008; Mantovani et al., 2013) (see Chapter 6). In addition, tissue-specific factors could also dictate the macrophage response and overall FBR. For example, studies in mice lacking MCP-1 showed normal and almost complete attenuation of encapsulation in subcutaneous and intraperitoneal implant models, respectively (Kyriakides et al., 2004; Skokos et al., 2011). Therefore, even in the same experimental model, the FBR outcomes differed depending on the site of implantation. The almost complete loss of encapsulation of

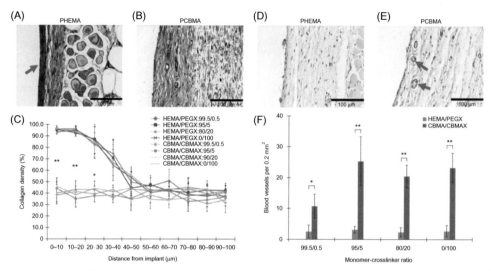

Figure 5.6 (A, B) Three months after subcutaneous implantation of hydrogels, tissues were stained with Masson's trichome. Blue staining indicates collagen capsule surrounding pHEMA hydrogel with 5% cross-linking density (A) and PCBMA hydrogel with 5% cross-linking density (B). Hydrogels are located on the left side of the images. The collagen capsule is indicated by the red arrow. Scale bars, 100 μm. (C) Collagen density. Data were collected in the tissue within 100 μm from the interface (at 10 μm increments). (D, E) Three months after subcutaneous implantation of hydrogels, tissues were stained with MECA-32 antibody, which binds to blood vessel endothelial cells (red arrows). Brown staining indicates blood vessel endothelial cells near pHEMA hydrogel with 5% cross-linking density (D) and PCBMA hydrogel with 5% cross-linking density (E). Scale bars, 100 μm. (F) Blood vessel density in the tissue surrounding hydrogels made with indicated monomer/cross-linker ratios. Two sections at different positions of each hydrogel disk were used and at least five different fields were randomly examined in each section. All data are presented as mean of biological replicates (six mice per type of hydrogel) from individual experiments ± s.d. *P < 0.05; **P < 0.01. *Reprinted with permission from Zhang et al. (2013).*

intraperitoneal implants in MCP-1-null mice prompted detailed analysis of macrophage activation. In comparison to wild-type mice, these mice failed to induce TNF-α. Surprisingly, all other aspects of macrophage activation appeared to be similar to control and included both features of M1 and M2. Moreover, *in vivo* studies showed that lack of induction of TNF-α was associated with reduced NF-κB signaling and reduced levels of TGF-β. Despite the fact that these observations are limited to the intraperitoneal model, they provide insight into the molecular pathways that link macrophage recruitment/activation and production of pro-fibrogenic signals.

Distinct outcomes based on the site of implantation have also been reported in the case of cross-linked bovine type I collagen disks (Luttikhuizen et al., 2006; van Amerongen et al., 2006). Specifically, these disks undergo extensive degradation when implanted on the epicardium but not in the subcutaneous space. It was also shown that implant degradation correlated with a higher and lower gene expression of pro- (IL-1, IL-6) inflammatory (IL-10) cytokines, respectively (Luttikhuizen et al., 2006). In addition, the expression and activity of MMP-8, MMP-13, and MMP-9 were higher in the epicardium implant model. Moreover, epicardial implants using the same disks showed deposition of vascularized ECM in the epicardium (van Amerongen et al., 2006). Therefore, differences in the microenvironment can dictate the fate of some implants and the outcome of the FBR.

Angiogenic responses

New blood vessels typically arise via the process of angiogenesis, in which new microvessels sprout from preexisting vessels (Potente et al., 2011). In addition, blood vessels can be formed *de novo* via vasculogenesis. In their normal, quiescent state, endothelial cells have a very slow turnover rate. However, when activated in wound healing and the FBR, endothelial cells change their phenotype to initiate angiogenesis. The angiogenic process can be divided into several phases: (i) Preexisting vessels are activated and an endothelia cell (tip cell) leads sprout formation. (ii) Stalk cells, which are endothelia cells neighboring the tip cells, undergo proliferation, change shape, and begin to form lumens. (iii) Mural cells such as pericytes or smooth muscle cells are recruited from the surrounding stroma and interact with the newly formed vessels in order to stabilize them. (iv) Successful maturation of the new formed vessels involves fusion with existing vessels and perfusion of blood (Eilken and Adams, 2010). At the molecular level, vascular endothelial growth factors (VEGFs) and Notch signaling regulate the early sprouting process and neovessel formation (Jakobsson et al., 2009). Subsequent recruitment of pericytes is stimulated by PDGF produced by endothelia cells. However, the process is much more complex and is coordinated by the expression of several other molecular mediators that regulate the development of functional vasculature. For example, angiogenesis is tightly regulated *in vivo* via the interplay between pro-angiogenic (VEGF, angiopoietins, PDGF) and anti-angiogenic (angiostatin, endostatin, anti-thrombin III, TSP1 and TSP2) stimuli that can suppress endothelial cell proliferation and migration or lumen formation.

Biomaterials and angiogenesis

In the context of the angiogenesis and biomaterials, a distinction is made between angiogenesis, which is used to describe the development of vessels in the peri-implant tissue, and neovascularization referring to the new, functional vascular networks that develop within an implant as a result of the migration of endothelia cells. In the context of the FBR, unique circumstances may limit both processes, resulting in lack of functional vessels. First, the encapsulation of solid implants is associated with a striking paucity of vessels and this is detrimental to many biomaterials and devices. Second, in the case of porous implants and hydrogels, the vascular networks that form are often leaky and lack functionality due to insufficient maturation. As mentioned above, these processes are regulated by the coordinated expression of both pro- and anti-angiogenic factors. In the case of peri-implant tissue, the lack of vessels could be attributed to an imbalance between these factors. Formation of functional vascular networks within constructs and hydrogels is more complicated (Park and Gerecht, 2014). These entities appear to induce angiogenesis and perhaps vasculogenesis, but the newly formed vessels fail to anastomose with the existing vasculature and remain immature and leaky. Conceivably, this is due to the lack of signals, such as PDGF, that promote interaction of supporting mural cells with endothelial cells.

Inflammation and mediators of angiogenic responses

During wound healing, multiple factors contribute to the stimulation of angiogenesis, including an increase in the permeability of existing vessels to allow for extravasation proteins that give rise to a provisional matrix, and the secretion of numerous angiogenic factors by the inflammatory cells at the site of injury (Tonnesen et al., 2000). Activated monocytes and macrophages move into the wound during the first 24–48 h and secrete factors such as basic fibroblast growth factor (bFGF), VEGF, PDGF, and MCP-1, all of which have been shown to stimulate cells involved in angiogenesis. Macrophages also secrete proteases capable of degrading the ECM, altering its structure and composition, and release growth factors that induce angiogenic processes in endothelial cells. However, macrophages subsequently undergo a switch from this pro-angiogenic state to an angio-inhibitory phenotype to mediate regression of capillaries that is typical in the later stages of wound healing (Novak and Koh, 2013). It is unclear if vessel formation is regulated in a similar manner in the FBR, but it is clear that following resolution the number of vessels in foreign body capsules is much lower than that in wounds. In addition, the large influx of capillaries observed in wound granulation tissue is not observed in the FBR. Although the specific mechanisms driving neovascularization in the FBR have not been fully elucidated, it is accepted that neovascularization relies on sprouting angiogenesis at the site of implantation and possibly the recruitment of bone-marrow-derived endothelial progenitor cells that incorporate into vessels and differentiate into endothelial cells. These cells encounter limited pro-angiogenic signals and perhaps an excess of anti-angiogenic signals and thus are unable to mount significant responses. Consistent with this suggestion, immunohistochemical analysis of capsules revealed high levels of TSP2 (Kyriakides et al., 1999). More importantly, capsules and porous implants were excessively vascularized in mice that lack TSP2, suggesting that this protein plays a critical role in limiting angiogenesis in the FBR (Kyriakides et al., 1999; 2001b). As mentioned above, TSP2 could influence the levels of MMPs and alter collagen remodeling. In addition, loss of TSP2 has been associated with increased levels of soluble VEGF in a wound model (Maclauchlan et al., 2009a). Finally, TSP2 can directly bind endothelial cells via multiple receptors including CD36 and CD47 and interfere with pro-angiogenic signaling (Calabro et al., 2014). Therefore, its absence could lead to enhanced angiogenesis via multiple pathways.

Biomaterial properties and angiogenesis

Lack of vascularization in the context of the FBR results in limited or inadequate transport of molecules, which in turn limits the utility of implanted sensors, drug-delivery systems, immunoisolation devices, and tissue engineered constructs. Therefore, it is essential to understand the mechanisms controlling angiogenesis in the context of the FBR and develop strategies for facilitating transport to implants (Park and Gerecht, 2014). Studies have shown that the geometry and topography of implanted biomaterials (including pore size and related parameters such as fibril length and intermodal distance) affect the FBR and can facilitate the formation of microvasculature when optimized. For example, membranes with pore sizes of 5–15 μm consistently resulted in vascularized capsules containing blood vessels in direct contact with the membrane surface, regardless of chemical composition (Brauker et al., 1995). Furthermore, the number of vessels was relatively stable for almost a year following subcutaneous implantation in rats. Subsequent studies based on sphere-templated poly(2-hydroxy-ethyl methacrylate) (pHEMA) scaffolds showed that 34 μm pore size was associated with reduced fibrosis and increased angiogenesis (Sussman et al., 2014). Interestingly, in the same study, investigators observed distinct macrophage polarization patterns. Specifically, within and on the surface of implants, macrophages displayed predominantly M1 phenotype whereas within the capsule they were M2. In addition, and consistent with other studies, the investigators reported significant overlap between M1 and M2 markers. It should be noted that other physiochemical properties of biomaterials, such as composition and surface chemistry, also play important roles in either stimulating or inhibiting an angiogenic response.

Biomaterial-based strategies and angiogenic responses

Biomaterials can be modified via surface coatings with biologically active compounds such as growth factors or ECM proteins that encourage endothelial cell adhesion and the formation of vascular structures. Potential growth factors for use in this capacity include those that have been implicated in vascular development and angiogenesis such as bFGF, VEGFs, PDGF, and TGF-β. There are numerous studies describing their controlled release from a variety of biomaterial-based systems. Mimicking the ECM has also been an attractive strategy for enhancing angiogenesis. Endothelial cells in vessels are supported by a basement membrane composed primarily of fibronectin, laminin, collagen, and hyaluronic acid. Therefore, several studies have attempted to include one or more of these proteins in biomaterials. In addition, coating of porous PE scaffolds with collagen resulted in increases in the expression of pro-inflammatory

(IL-1α, IL-1β) and pro-angiogenic genes (VEGF, MMP-9) based on microarray analysis (Ehashi et al., 2014).

An alternative approach to the presentation of pro-angiogenic signals includes the targeting of angiostatic factors with the aim of shifting the angiogenic balance as was described above in the case of TSP2. Other approaches include vascular cell transplantation, where endothelial cells alone or in combination with supporting cells such as pericytes were delivered with implanted scaffolds (Chang et al., 2013). Molecular cross-talk between these two cell types resulted in increased pericyte investment of neovessels and improved vessel function. In addition, gene delivery approaches, achieved via the overexpression of angiogenic factors by cells transfected *in situ*, have shown enhanced angiogenesis. However, a common issue with both growth factor and cell transplantation approaches is the lack of immediate anastomoses to the host vasculature, which limits perfusion of the constructs.

Bio-functionalized materials, often modified with ECM-derived peptides to guide angiogenesis, can also be used to mobilize and capture endogenous endothelial cells within the biomaterial and stimulate neovascularization. Moreover, some biomaterials have the capacity to induce angiogenesis by themselves in the absence of added cells, growth factors, or ECM cues. Mimicking biological patterning may be especially useful to control neovascularization, given that unguided or uncontrolled growth can lead to pathological or deformed vessels.

Molecular strategies to enhance angiogenic responses

Specific applications, such as glucose sensors and tissue engineered constructs, have increased dependence on angiogenesis. Interestingly, prolonged inflammation is often associated with persistent angiogenic responses but this is not the case with implanted biomaterials. Conceivably, this relative decrease in angiogenesis is due to loss of production of pro-angiogenic factors by late stage macrophages or sequestration of these factors outside of the avascular fibrous capsule, where an increased angiogenic response is often seen. Alternatively, excessive deposition of angiogenesis inhibitors during matrix production could also negatively influence angiogenesis. Regardless of the mechanism, the result is inefficient transport of molecules from microcirculation to the implant. Several groups have attempted to increase the number and stability of vessels in the FBR. Such strategies include delivery of pro-angiogenic factors such as VEGF, PDGF, and MCP-1, which constitute the majority of neovascularization approaches (Jay et al., 2010; Richardson et al., 2001; Brudno et al., 2013; Klueh et al., 2005). Furthermore, the secretion and sequestration of angiogenic factors by the ECM can be replicated closely by modulating their release. This controlled release could be accomplished by engineering chemical or enzymatic susceptibilities that allow for spatial and temporal control of release. In addition, engineered enzyme (MMP)-sensitive hydrogel systems were shown to stimulate vascular formation (Seliktar et al., 2004;

Kraehenbuehl et al., 2008). Alternatively, targeting the expression of anti-angiogenic factors, such as TSP2 or prolyl hydroxylase domain protein 2 (PHD2), was shown to enhance vessel density in the FBR (Kyriakides et al., 2001a; Nelson et al., 2014). Specifically, it was shown that gene-activated matrix delivery of an antisense TSP2 cDNA enhanced blood vessel formation and altered collagen fibrillogenesis in mouse subcutaneous implant models. Similarly, Figure 5.7 shows delivery of PHD2-specific siRNA from a porous polyester urethane (PEUR) scaffold that resulted in sustained increased blood vessel formation associated with increased VEGF and bFGF.

Summary

Morphological assessment of the FBR indicates novel processes including FBGC formation, deposition of dense and highly oriented collagenous matrix, and paucity of blood vessels. Recent evidence has implicated the unique activation of macrophages in the development of these processes in the context of biomaterials. Molecular signals derived from macrophages, including TGF-β, induce fibrogenesis. Moreover, the sustained presence of the biomaterial is considered a persistent stimulus for macrophages that either continue to secrete pro-fibrogenic or failed to produce anti-fibrogenic

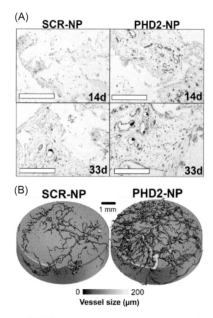

Figure 5.7 Sustained silencing of PHD2 increases angiogenesis within PEUR tissue scaffolds. CD31 staining was significantly increased within PHD2 scaffolds at day 14 and day 33 (scale = 200 μm, vessels appear red, nuclei are counterstained purple with hematoxylin, and the white space represents residual PEUR scaffold). (F) Micro-CT images visually demonstrate the increased vasculature within the PHD2-NP scaffolds. *Reprinted with permission from Nelson et al. (2014).*

factors. Numerous studies have attributed these phenomena to specific macrophage polarization phenotypes, but recent analyses suggest that macrophages in the FBR have distinct activation states with features of both M1 and M2. It is also worth considering that implantation injures the surrounding ECM and most likely produces additional stimulatory signals for macrophages and fibroblasts. Despite intense research, difficulties in reducing fibrosis and increasing blood vessel density in the FBR remain. While delivery of pro-angiogenic factors such as VEGF can stimulate angiogenesis, the stability and viability of the resulting vessels is not optimal. Strategies to deliver more than one factor, such as VEGF and PDGF, have shown improvement in stability but are more difficult to control. Similarly, inhibition of negative regulators of angiogenesis, such as TSP2, is a promising approach. However, current inhibition strategies are cumbersome and not suitable for many biomaterial applications. Therefore, more research is needed to develop specific and efficient strategies to reduce fibrosis and enhance angiogenesis. Moreover, certain biomaterials show promise in modulating macrophage activation and subsequent aspects of the FBR. Even though the molecular basis for these findings is not understood, such materials hold promise in elucidating the key mechanisms that drive the FBR.

ACKNOWLEDGMENTS

I would like to thank Aaron Morris, Nina Kristofik, Jittisa Ketkaew, Shihan Khan, Ramak Khosravi, Amanda Pellowe, and all the graduate students in my biomaterial–tissue interactions course for helpful discussions and assistance.

REFERENCES

Altankov, G., Groth, T., 1994. Reorganization of substratum-bound fibronectin on hydrophilic and hydrophobic materials is related to biocompatibility. J. Mater. Sci. Mater. Med. 5, 732–737.

Andersson, J., Ekdahl, K.N., Lambris, J.D., Nilsson, B., 2005. Binding of C3 fragments on top of adsorbed plasma proteins during complement activation on a model biomaterial surface. Biomaterials 26, 1477–1485.

Arefieva, T.I., Kukhtina, N.B., Antonova, O.A., Krasnikova, T.L., 2005. MCP-1-stimulated chemotaxis of monocytic and endothelial cells is dependent on activation of different signaling cascades. Cytokine 31, 439–446.

Ashida, N., Arai, H., Yamasaki, M., Kita, T., 2001. Distinct signaling pathways for MCP-1-dependent integrin activation and chemotaxis. J. Biol. Chem. 276, 16555–16560.

Brauker, J.H., Carr-Brendel, V.E., Martinson, L.A., Crudele, J., Johnston, W.D., Johnson, R.C., 1995. Neovascularization of synthetic membranes directed by membrane microarchitecture. J. Biomed. Mater. Res. 29, 1517–1524.

Bridges, A.W., Garcia, A.J., 2008. Anti-inflammatory polymeric coatings for implantable biomaterials and devices. J. Diabetes. Sci. Technol. 2, 984–994.

Brown, B.N., Ratner, B.D., Goodman, S.B., Amar, S., Badylak, S.F., 2012. Macrophage polarization: an opportunity for improved outcomes in biomaterials and regenerative medicine. Biomaterials 33, 3792–3802.

Brudno, Y., Ennett-Shepard, A.B., Chen, R.R., Aizenberg, M., Mooney, D.J., 2013. Enhancing microvascular formation and vessel maturation through temporal control over multiple pro-angiogenic and pro-maturation factors. Biomaterials 34, 9201–9209.

Bryant, C., Fitzgerald, K.A., 2009. Molecular mechanisms involved in inflammasome activation. Trends. Cell Biol. 19, 455–464.

Calabro, N.E., Kristofik, N.J., Kyriakides, T.R., 2014. Thrombospondin-2 and extracellular matrix assembly. Biochim. Biophys. Acta. 1840, 2396–2402.

Carson, A.E., Barker, T.H., 2009. Emerging concepts in engineering extracellular matrix variants for directing cell phenotype. Regen. Med. 4, 593–600.

Chang, W.G., Andrejecsk, J.W., Kluger, M.S., Saltzman, W.M., Pober, J.S., 2013. Pericytes modulate endothelial sprouting. Cardiovasc. Res. 100, 492–500.

Den Braber, E.T., De Ruijter, J.E., Ginsel, L.A., Von Recum, A.F., Jansen, J.A., 1998. Orientation of ECM protein deposition, fibroblast cytoskeleton, and attachment complex components on silicone microgrooved surfaces. J. Biomed. Mater. Res. 40, 291–300.

Ehashi, T., Takemura, T., Hanagata, N., Minowa, T., Kobayashi, H., Ishihara, K., et al., 2014. Comprehensive genetic analysis of early host body reactions to the bioactive and bio-inert porous scaffolds. PLoS ONE 9, e85132.

Eilken, H.M., Adams, R.H., 2010. Dynamics of endothelial cell behavior in sprouting angiogenesis. Curr. Opin. Cell Biol. 22, 617–625.

Fabrizius-Homan, D.J., Cooper, S.L., 1991. Competitive adsorption of vitronectin with albumin, fibrinogen, and fibronectin on polymeric biomaterials. J. Biomed. Mater. Res. 25, 953–971.

Farrugia, B.L., Whitelock, J.M., Jung, M., Mcgrath, B., O'grady, R.L., Mccarthy, S.J., et al., 2014. The localisation of inflammatory cells and expression of associated proteoglycans in response to implanted chitosan. Biomaterials 35, 1462–1477.

Faulk, D.M., Johnson, S.A., Zhang, L., Badylak, S.F., 2014. Role of the extracellular matrix in whole organ engineering. J. Cell. Physiol. 229, 984–989.

François, P., Vaudaux, P., Taborelli, M., Tonetti, M., Lew, D.P., Descouts, P., 1997. Influence of surface treatments developed for oral implants on the physical and biological properties of titanium. (II) Adsorption isotherms and biological activity of immobilized fibronectin. Clin. Oral. Implants. Res. 8, 217–225.

Frantz, C., Stewart, K.M., Weaver, V.M., 2010. The extracellular matrix at a glance. J. Cell. Sci. 123, 4195–4200.

Frisch, S.M., Vuori, K., Ruoslahti, E., Chan-Hui, P.Y., 1996. Control of adhesion-dependent cell survival by focal adhesion kinase. J. Cell. Biol. 134, 793–799.

Grinnell, F., Feld, M.K., 1982. Fibronectin adsorption on hydrophilic and hydrophobic surfaces detected by antibody-binding and analyzed during cell-adhesion in serum-containing medium. J. Biol. Chem. 257, 4888–4893.

Halper, J., Kjaer, M., 2014. Basic components of connective tissues and extracellular matrix: elastin, fibrillin, fibulins, fibrinogen, fibronectin, laminin, tenascins and thrombospondins. Adv. Exp. Med. Biol. 802, 31–47.

Hayden, M.S., Ghosh, S., 2008. Shared principles in NF-kappaB signaling. Cell 132, 344–362.

Helming, L., Gordon, S., 2007. Macrophage fusion induced by IL-4 alternative activation is a multistage process involving multiple target molecules. Eur. J. Immunol. 37, 33–42.

Helming, L., Gordon, S., 2009. Molecular mediators of macrophage fusion. Trends. Cell. Biol. 19, 514–522.

Helming, L., Tomasello, E., Kyriakides, T.R., Martinez, F.O., Takai, T., Gordon, S., et al., 2008. Essential role of DAP12 signaling in macrophage programming into a fusion-competent state. Sci. Signal. 1, ra11.

Helming, L., Winter, J., Gordon, S., 2009. The scavenger receptor CD36 plays a role in cytokine-induced macrophage fusion. J. Cell. Sci. 122, 453–459.

Henao-Mejia, J., Elinav, E., Strowig, T., Flavell, R.A., 2012. Inflammasomes: far beyond inflammation. Nat. Immunol. 13, 321–324.

Holt, D.J., Chamberlain, L.M., Grainger, D.W., 2010. Cell–cell signaling in co-cultures of macrophages and fibroblasts. Biomaterials 31, 9382–9394.

Horbett, T.A., 2012. Adsorbed proteins on biomaterials. In: Ratner, B.D. (Ed.), Biomaterials Science: An Introduction to Materials in Medicine, third ed. Academic Press.

Hu, W.J., Eaton, J.W., Ugarova, T.P., Tang, L., 2001. Molecular basis of biomaterial-mediated foreign body reactions. Blood 98, 1231–1238.

Jakobsson, L., Bentley, K., Gerhardt, H., 2009. VEGFRs and Notch: a dynamic collaboration in vascular patterning. Biochem. Soc. Trans. 37, 1233–1236.

Jay, S.M., Shepherd, B.R., Andrejecsk, J.W., Kyriakides, T.R., Pober, J.S., Saltzman, W.M., 2010. Dual delivery of VEGF and MCP-1 to support endothelial cell transplantation for therapeutic vascularization. Biomaterials 31, 3054–3062.

Kao, W.J., Mcnally, A.K., Hiltner, A., Anderson, J.M., 1995. Role for interleukin-4 in foreign-body giant cell formation on a poly(etherurethane urea) in vivo. J. Biomed. Mater. Res. 29, 1267–1275.

Kao, W.J., Sapatnekar, S., Hiltner, A., Anderson, J.M., 1996. Complement-mediated leukocyte adhesion on poly(etherurethane ureas) under shear stress in vitro. J. Biomed. Mater. Res. 32, 99–109.

Keselowsky, B.G., Bridges, A.W., Burns, K.L., Tate, C.C., Babensee, J.E., Laplaca, M.C., et al., 2007. Role of plasma fibronectin in the foreign body response to biomaterials. Biomaterials 28, 3626–3631.

Keselowsky, B.G., Collard, D.M., Garcia, A.J., 2003. Surface chemistry modulates fibronectin conformation and directs integrin binding and specificity to control cell adhesion. J. Biomed. Mater. Res. A. 66, 247–259.

Keselowsky, B.G., Collard, D.M., Garcia, A.J., 2005. Integrin binding specificity regulates biomaterial surface chemistry effects on cell differentiation. Proc. Natl. Acad. Sci. USA. 102, 5953–5957.

Kim, J.K., Scott, E.A., Elbert, D.L., 2005. Proteomic analysis of protein adsorption: serum amyloid P adsorbs to materials and promotes leukocyte adhesion. J. Biomed. Mater. Res. A. 75, 199–209.

Klueh, U., Dorsky, D.I., Kreutzer, D.L., 2005. Enhancement of implantable glucose sensor function in vivo using gene transfer-induced neovascularization. Biomaterials 26, 1155–1163.

Kraehenbuehl, T.P., Zammaretti, P., Van Der Vlies, A.J., Schoenmakers, R.G., Lutolf, M.P., Jaconi, M.E., et al., 2008. Three-dimensional extracellular matrix-directed cardioprogenitor differentiation: systematic modulation of a synthetic cell-responsive PEG-hydrogel. Biomaterials 29, 2757–2766.

Kyriakides, T.R., Foster, M.J., Keeney, G.E., Tsai, A., Giachelli, C.M., Clark-Lewis, I., et al., 2004. The CC chemokine ligand, CCL2/MCP1, participates in macrophage fusion and foreign body giant cell formation. Am. J. Pathol. 165, 2157–2166.

Kyriakides, T.R., Hartzel, T., Huynh, G., Bornstein, P., 2001a. Regulation of angiogenesis and matrix remodeling by localized, matrix-mediated antisense gene delivery. Mol. Ther. 3, 842–849.

Kyriakides, T.R., Leach, K.J., Hoffman, A.S., Ratner, B.D., Bornstein, P., 1999. Mice that lack the angiogenesis inhibitor, thrombospondin 2, mount an altered foreign body reaction characterized by increased vascularity. Proc. Natl. Acad. Sci. USA. 96, 4449–4454.

Kyriakides, T.R., Zhu, Y.H., Yang, Z., Huynh, G., Bornstein, P., 2001b. Altered extracellular matrix remodeling and angiogenesis in sponge granulomas of thrombospondin 2-null mice. Am. J. Pathol. 159, 1255–1262.

Lan, M.A., Gersbach, C.A., Michael, K.E., Keselowsky, B.G., Garcia, A.J., 2005. Myoblast proliferation and differentiation on fibronectin-coated self assembled monolayers presenting different surface chemistries. Biomaterials 26, 4523–4531.

Latz, E., Xiao, T.S., Stutz, A., 2013. Activation and regulation of the inflammasomes. Nat. Rev. Immunol. 13, 397–411.

Lemaire, I., Falzoni, S., Adinolfi, E., 2012. Purinergic signaling in giant cell formation. Front. Biosci. (Elite Ed) 4, 41–55.

Lewandowska, K., Pergament, E., Sukenik, C.N., Culp, L.A., 1992. Cell-type-specific adhesion mechanisms mediated by fibronectin adsorbed to chemically derivatized substrata. J. Biomed. Mater. Res. 26, 1343–1363.

Luttikhuizen, D.T., Van Amerongen, M.J., De Feijter, P.C., Petersen, A.H., Harmsen, M.C., Van Luyn, M.J., 2006. The correlation between difference in foreign body reaction between implant locations and cytokine and MMP expression. Biomaterials 27, 5763–5770.

Maclauchlan, S., Skokos, E.A., Agah, A., Zeng, J., Tian, W., Davidson, J.M., et al., 2009a. Enhanced angiogenesis and reduced contraction in thrombospondin-2-null wounds is associated with increased levels of matrix metalloproteinases-2 and -9, and soluble VEGF. J. Histochem. Cytochem. 57, 301–313.

Maclauchlan, S., Skokos, E.A., Meznarich, N., Zhu, D.H., Raoof, S., Shipley, J.M., et al., 2009b. Macrophage fusion, giant cell formation, and the foreign body response require matrix metalloproteinase 9. J. Leukoc. Biol. 85, 617–626.

Malik, A.F., Hoque, R., Ouyang, X., Ghani, A., Hong, E., Khan, K., et al., 2011. Inflammasome components Asc and caspase-1 mediate biomaterial-induced inflammation and foreign body response. Proc. Natl. Acad. Sci. USA. 108, 20095–20100.

Mantovani, A., Biswas, S.K., Galdiero, M.R., Sica, A., Locati, M., 2013. Macrophage plasticity and polarization in tissue repair and remodelling. J. Pathol. 229, 176–185.

Mcnally, A.K., Anderson, J.M., 2011. Macrophage fusion and multinucleated giant cells of inflammation. Adv. Exp. Med. Biol. 713, 97–111.

Mooney, J.E., Summers, K.M., Gongora, M., Grimmond, S.M., Campbell, J.H., Hume, D.A., et al., 2014. Transcriptional switching in macrophages associated with the peritoneal foreign body response. Immunol. Cell. Biol. 92, 518–526.

Morais, J.M., Papadimitrakopoulos, F., Burgess, D.J., 2010. Biomaterials/tissue interactions: possible solutions to overcome foreign body response. AAPS J. 12, 188–196.

Moreno, J.L., Mikhailenko, I., Tondravi, M.M., Keegan, A.D., 2007. IL-4 promotes the formation of multinucleated giant cells from macrophage precursors by a STAT6-dependent, homotypic mechanism: contribution of E-cadherin. J. Leukoc. Biol. 82, 1542–1553.

Morris, A.H., Kyriakides, T.R., 2014. Matricellular proteins and biomaterials. Matrix. Biol.

Mosser, D.M., Edwards, J.P., 2008. Exploring the full spectrum of macrophage activation. Nat. Rev. Immunol. 8, 958–969.

Murphy-Ullrich, J.E., Helene Sage, E., 2014. Revisiting the matricellular concept. Matrix. Biol.

Nelson, C.E., Kim, A.J., Adolph, E.J., Gupta, M.K., Yu, F., Hocking, K.M., et al., 2014. Tunable delivery of siRNA from a biodegradable scaffold to promote angiogenesis *in vivo*. Adv. Mater. 26, 607–614. 506.

Norde, W., Giacomelli, C.E., 2000. BSA structural changes during homomolecular exchange between the adsorbed and the dissolved states. J. Biotechnol. 79, 259–268.

Novak, M.L., Koh, T.J., 2013. Phenotypic transitions of macrophages orchestrate tissue repair. Am. J. Pathol. 183, 1352–1363.

Ozbek, S., Balasubramanian, P.G., Chiquet-Ehrismann, R., Tucker, R.P., Adams, J.C., 2010. The evolution of extracellular matrix. Mol. Biol. Cell. 21, 4300–4305.

Pan, H., Jiang, H., Kantharia, S., Chen, W., 2011. A fibroblast/macrophage co-culture model to evaluate the biocompatibility of an electrospun Dextran/PLGA scaffold and its potential to induce inflammatory responses. Biomed. Mater. 6, 065002.

Park, K.M., Gerecht, S., 2014. Harnessing developmental processes for vascular engineering and regeneration. Development 141, 2760–2769.

Pieper, J.S., Van Wachem, P.B., Van Luyn, M.J.A., Brouwer, L.A., Hafmans, T., Veerkamp, J.H., et al., 2000. Attachment of glycosaminoglycans to collagenous matrices modulates the tissue response in rats. Biomaterials 21, 1689–1699.

Potente, M., Gerhardt, H., Carmeliet, P., 2011. Basic and therapeutic aspects of angiogenesis. Cell 146, 873–887.

Puolakkainen, P., Bradshaw, A.D., Kyriakides, T.R., Reed, M., Brekken, R., Wight, T., et al., 2003. Compromised production of extracellular matrix in mice lacking secreted protein, acidic and rich in cysteine (SPARC) leads to a reduced foreign body reaction to implanted biomaterials. Am. J. Pathol. 162, 627–635.

Reichenberger, M.A., Heimer, S., Lass, U., Germann, G., Kollensperger, E., Mueller, W., et al., 2014. Pulsed acoustic cellular expression (PACE) reduces capsule formation around silicone implants. Aesthetic. Plast. Surg. 38, 244–251.

Richardson, T.P., Peters, M.C., Ennett, A.B., Mooney, D.J., 2001. Polymeric system for dual growth factor delivery. Nat. Biotechnol. 19, 1029–1034.

Rujitanaroj, P.O., Jao, B., Yang, J., Wang, F., Anderson, J.M., Wang, J., et al., 2013. Controlling fibrous capsule formation through long-term down-regulation of collagen type I (COL1A1) expression by nanofiber-mediated siRNA gene silencing. Acta. Biomater. 9, 4513–4524.

Sanders, J.E., Rochefort, J.R., 2003. Fibrous encapsulation of single polymer microfibers depends on their vertical dimension in subcutaneous tissue. J. Biomed. Mater. Res. A. 67, 1181–1187.

Seliktar, D., Zisch, A.H., Lutolf, M.P., Wrana, J.L., Hubbell, J.A., 2004. MMP-2 sensitive, VEGF-bearing bioactive hydrogels for promotion of vascular healing. J. Biomed. Mater. Res. A. 68, 704–716.

Shekaran, A., Garcia, A.J., 2011. Extracellular matrix—mimetic adhesive biomaterials for bone repair. J. Biomed. Mater. Res. A. 96, 261–272.

Shelton, R.M., Rasmussen, A.C., Davies, J.E., 1988. Protein adsorption at the interface between charged polymer substrata and migrating osteoblasts. Biomaterials 9, 24–29.

Sivaraman, B., Latour, R.A., 2010. The relationship between platelet adhesion on surfaces and the structure versus the amount of adsorbed fibrinogen. Biomaterials 31, 832–839.

Skokos, E.A., Charokopos, A., Khan, K., Wanjala, J., Kyriakides, T.R., 2011. Lack of TNF-alpha-induced MMP-9 production and abnormal E-cadherin redistribution associated with compromised fusion in MCP-1-null macrophages. Am. J. Pathol. 178, 2311–2321.

Strowig, T., Henao-Mejia, J., Elinav, E., Flavell, R., 2012. Inflammasomes in health and disease. Nature 481, 278–286.

Sussman, E.M., Halpin, M.C., Muster, J., Moon, R.T., Ratner, B.D., 2014. Porous implants modulate healing and induce shifts in local macrophage polarization in the foreign body reaction. Ann. Biomed. Eng. 42, 1508–1516.

Symowicz, J., Adley, B.P., Gleason, K.J., Johnson, J.J., Ghosh, S., Fishman, D.A., et al., 2007. Engagement of collagen-binding integrins promotes matrix metalloproteinase-9-dependent E-cadherin ectodomain shedding in ovarian carcinoma cells. Cancer. Res. 67, 2030–2039.

Thevenot, P.T., Baker, D.W., Weng, H., Sun, M.W., Tang, L., 2011. The pivotal role of fibrocytes and mast cells in mediating fibrotic reactions to biomaterials. Biomaterials 32, 8394–8403.

Tonnesen, M.G., Feng, X., Clark, R.A., 2000. Angiogenesis in wound healing. J. Investig. Dermatol. Symp. Proc. 5, 40–46.

Vacanti, N.M., Cheng, H., Hill, P.S., Guerreiro, J.D., Dang, T.T., Ma, M., et al., 2012. Localized delivery of dexamethasone from electrospun fibers reduces the foreign body response. Biomacromolecules 13, 3031–3038.

Van Amerongen, M.J., Harmsen, M.C., Petersen, A.H., Kors, G., Van Luyn, M.J., 2006. The enzymatic degradation of scaffolds and their replacement by vascularized extracellular matrix in the murine myocardium. Biomaterials 27, 2247–2257.

Walters, N.J., Gentleman, E., 2015. Evolving insights in cell–matrix interactions: elucidating how nonsoluble properties of the extracellular niche direct stem cell fate. Acta. Biomater. 11, 3–16.

Ward, W.K., Li, A.G., Siddiqui, Y., Federiuk, I.F., Wang, X.J., 2008. Increased expression of interleukin-13 and connective tissue growth factor, and their potential roles during foreign body encapsulation of subcutaneous implants. J. Biomater. Sci. Polym. Ed. 19, 1065–1072.

Ward, W.K., Slobodzian, E.P., Tiekotter, K.L., Wood, M.D., 2002. The effect of microgeometry, implant thickness and polyurethane chemistry on the foreign body response to subcutaneous implants. Biomaterials 23, 4185–4192.

Wettero, J., Askendal, A., Bengtsson, T., Tengvall, P., 2002. On the binding of complement to solid artificial surfaces in vitro. Biomaterials 23, 981–991.

Wilson, C.J., Clegg, R.E., Leavesley, D.I., Pearcy, M.J., 2005. Mediation of biomaterial–cell interactions by adsorbed proteins: a review. Tissue Eng. 11, 1–18.

Winograd-Katz, S.E., Fassler, R., Geiger, B., Legate, K.R., 2014. The integrin adhesome: from genes and proteins to human disease. Nat. Rev. Mol. Cell. Biol. 15, 273–288.

Wolf, M.T., Vodovotz, Y., Tottey, S., Brown, B., Badylak, S.F., 2015. Predicting in vivo responses to biomaterials via combined in vitro and in silico analysis. Tissue Eng. Part C Methods. 21, 148–159.

Yang, D., Lu, X., Hong, Y., Xi, T., Zhang, D., 2013. The molecular mechanism of mediation of adsorbed serum proteins to endothelial cells adhesion and growth on biomaterials. Biomaterials 34, 5747–5758.

Yang, J., Jao, B., Mcnally, A.K., Anderson, J.M., 2014. In vivo quantitative and qualitative assessment of foreign body giant cell formation on biomaterials in mice deficient in natural killer lymphocyte subsets, mast cells, or the interleukin-4 receptoralpha and in severe combined immunodeficient mice. J. Biomed. Mater. Res. A. 102, 2017–2023.

Zeng, Q., Chen, W., 2010. The functional behavior of a macrophage/fibroblast co-culture model derived from normal and diabetic mice with a marine gelatin-oxidized alginate hydrogel. Biomaterials 31, 5772–5781.

Zhang, L., Cao, Z., Bai, T., Carr, L., Ella-Menye, J.R., Irvin, C., et al., 2013. Zwitterionic hydrogels implanted in mice resist the foreign-body reaction. Nat. Biotechnol. 31, 553–556.

CHAPTER 6

Macrophage Plasticity and Polarization: Relevance to Biomaterials

Maria Rosaria Galdiero[1,2] and Alberto Mantovani[1,3]
[1]Humanitas Clinical and Research Hospital, Rozzano, Milan, Italy
[2]Division of Clinical Immunology and Allergy, University of Naples Federico II, Naples, Italy
[3]Humanitas University, Rozzano, Milan, Italy

Contents

MACROPHAGE DIVERSITY AND PLASTICITY

Macrophages are an essential component of innate immunity and play a central role in host defense and inflammation (Gordon and Martinez, 2010). Beyond defense, these cells display homeostatic functions in orchestration of metabolic functions and tissue remodeling (Gordon and Martinez, 2010; Sica and Mantovani, 2012).

From the classical point of view, macrophages develop from a common myeloid progenitor stem cell in the bone marrow (Gordon and Taylor, 2005). Cytokines and growth factors induce differentiation of the common myeloid progenitor to monocytes, which leave the bone marrow and enter the bloodstream where they may reside before entering tissues to become macrophages. Once within the tissue, macrophages may undergo differentiation into a number of distinct phenotypes depending on the tissue type, microenvironmental conditions, and the immunologic milieu (Gordon and Taylor, 2005).

Diversity and plasticity are distinctive hallmarks of cells of the monocyte–macrophage lineage. Already at the short-lived stage of circulating precursor monocytes, distinct subsets have been characterized for instance in man based on differential expression of the CD16 (FcγRIII receptor) and chemokine receptors (CCR2, CX3CR1, and CCR8) and by different properties (Geissmann et al., 2010).

Host Response to Biomaterials.
DOI: http://dx.doi.org/10.1016/B978-0-12-800196-7.00006-2
117

Moreover, the classical point of view of the origin of macrophages from hematopoietic stem cells has been put into question by recent evidence. Indeed, in mice resident macrophages (e.g., microglia) have been found to originate from the yolk sac in a colony-stimulating factor-1 receptor (CSF/1R)-dependent and Myb-independent way (Schulz et al., 2012) and recent evidence suggests that macrophage accumulation can be sustained by local proliferation in particular during type II inflammation (Jenkins et al., 2011; Liddiard et al., 2011), even though the existence and relevance of distinct origins and proliferative capacity in the human setting need to be further investigated.

Macrophage plasticity is demonstrated by the capability of mononuclear phagocytes to respond to various environmental signals (microbial products, damaged cells, activated lymphocytes) with the acquisition of distinct functional phenotypes in tissues. Following the TH1–TH2 paradigm, it is now widely accepted that macrophages go through M1 (classical) or M2 (alternative) activation, in response to Toll-like receptor (TLR) ligands and interferon-gamma (IFNγ) or interleukin-4 (IL-4)/IL-13, respectively (Biswas and Mantovani, 2010).

However, it has been shown that unlike lymphocytes, where cellular phenotype is relatively fixed upon differentiation, macrophages have dynamic and plastic phenotypes that change with time, concentration, and duration of the polarizing signals (Stout et al., 2009; Porcheray et al., 2005).

The concept of macrophage polarization has been extensively studied in the fields of the host response against pathogens and cancer. However, in this chapter, we focus on a novel application of the M1/M2 paradigm in translational medicine. We will describe the characteristics and functions of macrophage polarization and plasticity in tissue repair and biomaterials implantation and their roles in regenerative medicine.

MACROPHAGE POLARIZATION: M1 AND M2 AS EXTREMES OF A CONTINUUM. LIMITATIONS OF THE PARADIGM

As aforementioned, signals derived from the microenvironment, such as microbes, damaged tissues, or activated lymphocytes, activate functional reprogramming of macrophages that give rise to a spectrum of distinct functional phenotypes (Biswas and Mantovani, 2010; Sica and Mantovani, 2012).

Specifically, IFNγ alone, or together with microbial stimuli (e.g., lipopolysaccharides (LPS)) or cytokines (e.g., tumor necrosis factors (TNF) and granulocyte macrophage colony-stimulating factor (GM-CSF)), induces classically activated proinflammatory M1 macrophages. In contrast, this classical activation is inhibited by IL-4 and IL-13, that in turn induce the alternative M2 form of macrophage activation (Gordon and Taylor, 2005) (Figure 6.1). Moreover, IL-33 and IL-21 are associated with Th2 and M2 polarization (Pesce et al., 2006; Kurowska-Stolarska et al., 2009).

The M1 phenotype is characterized by the expression of high levels of pro-inflammatory cytokines and high production of reactive nitrogen and oxygen intermediates. M1 macrophages show a pro-inflammatory profile, characterized by the production of high levels of IL-12 and IL-23, and inflammatory cytokines such as IL-1β, TNF, IL-6, and low production of immunosuppressive cytokines such as IL-10. M1 macrophages are classically involved in polarized Th1 responses and show strong microbicidal and tumoricidal activity, thus acting as effectors of host resistance against tumors and intracellular parasites (Sica and Mantovani, 2012; Tseng et al., 2013). According to their Th1-promoting roles, M1 macrophages release chemokines such as CXCL9 and CXCL10 which attract Th1 lymphocytes and efficiently produce effector molecules (e.g., reactive oxygen and nitrogen intermediates) (Sica and Mantovani, 2012) (Figure 6.1).

In contrast, M2 macrophages generally express low levels of the pro-inflammatory cytokines IL-12 and IL-23, while expressing high levels of IL-10, and show a variable

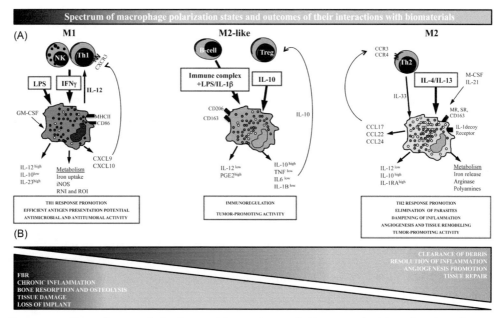

Figure 6.1 *Macrophage polarization and interaction with biomaterials.* (A) Under the influence of various stimuli, macrophages may acquire distinct phenotypes, with M1 and M2 at the extreme and many variations on the theme between the two extremes, known as M2-like phenotypes. For each polarization state, the main cytokine and chemokine profile, membrane receptors, metabolic aspects, and functional properties are described. (B) Following the interaction with biomaterials, FBR, chronic inflammation, bone resorption, osteolysis, and loss of function of the implants are described in a predominant M1 response. Resolution of inflammation, angiogenesis, tissue repair, and a good functional outcome of the implant have been described when a timely shift toward the M2 phenotype occurs.

ability to release inflammatory cytokines. M2 macrophages are characterized by high expression of scavenging, mannose, and galactose receptors, production of ornithine and polyamines through the arginase pathway (Gordon and Martinez, 2010; Biswas and Mantovani, 2010). In contrast to pro-inflammatory M1 macrophages, M2 cells retain a poor antigen presenting potential and have immunoregulatory functions such as the suppression of Th1 adaptive immunity, actively scavenging debris, contributing to the dampening of inflammation, promotion of wound healing, angiogenesis, tissue remodeling, and tumor progression (Biswas and Mantovani, 2010) (Figure 6.1). M2 macrophages participate in the Th2 response and thus in the elimination of parasites (Noel et al., 2004). Compared to M1 cells, M2 cells express and produce lower amounts of IL-1β, and higher amounts of IL-1ra and decoy type II receptor (Garlanda et al., 2013; Dinarello, 2005). According to their Th2-promoting phenotype, M2 macrophages release chemokines such as CCL17, CCL22, and CCL24, and are involved in regulatory T cell (Treg), Th2, eosinophil, and basophil recruitment (Mantovani et al., 2008; Martinez et al., 2006) (Mantovani et al., 2002; Martinez et al., 2006; Romagnani et al., 1999). Interestingly, M1- and M2-polarized macrophages have distinct features in terms of the metabolism of iron, folate, and glucose (Puig-Kroger et al., 2009; Recalcati et al., 2010).

The M1/M2 paradigm is actually an oversimplified representation with M1 and M2 macrophages, representing only the extremes of a continuum in a universe of activation states. In fact, beyond classical M1/M2 inducers, many other stimuli, such as antibody immune complexes together with LPS or IL-1, glucocorticoids, apoptotic cells, transforming growth factor-beta (TGF-β), and IL-10, also polarize macrophages toward a phenotype sharing some similarities with IL-4-activated macrophages and displaying immunoregulatory and protumoral functions, then defined as "M2-like" phenotypes (Biswas and Mantovani, 2010). To this regard, placenta and embryo, helminth or Listeria infection, obesity, and cancer represent *in vivo* examples of variations on the theme of M2 polarization (Rae et al., 2007).

The most relevant feature of macrophage plasticity consists in their potential to be reprogrammed by some stimuli, such as IFNγ or IFNα, and revert from immunosuppressive M2 macrophages into immunostimulatory M1 cells (De Palma et al., 2008; Duluc et al., 2009).

MACROPHAGES IN THE ORCHESTRATION OF TISSUE REPAIR

Resolution of inflammation has emerged as an active process in which macrophages are an essential component. As mentioned before, M2 or M2-like cells exert important roles in tissue repair and remodeling through the production of anti-inflammatory cytokines (e.g., IL-10, IL-1ra, and the IL-1 type II decoy receptor) (Biswas and Mantovani, 2012).

Lipid mediators also play a key role in the orchestration of resolution of inflammation (Serhan et al., 2008; Lawrence et al., 2002). Mononuclear phagocytes are an important source of lipid mediators (Titos et al., 2011; Uderhardt et al., 2012). Resolution (of inflammation) is now considered to be a distinct process separate from anti-inflammatory processes. Resolution of inflammation is characterized by an active switch in the mediators that predominate at the inflammatory sites. Initially, the arachidonic acid pathway gives rise to mediators such as prostaglandins and leukotrienes which activate and amplify many aspects of the inflammatory cascade. Next, prostaglandin E2 and prostaglandin D2 gradually give way to mediators exerting both anti-inflammatory and pro-resolution activities such as the lipoxins, resolvins, and protectins. These families of endogenous pro-resolution molecules are not immunosuppressive, but instead function in resolution by activating specific mechanisms to promote homeostasis. For example, specific lipoxins and members of the resolvin and protectin families are potent stimuli that actively and selectively stop neutrophil infiltration, stimulate nonphlogistic recruitment of monocytes, activate macrophage phagocytosis of microorganisms and apoptotic cells, increase lymphatic removal of phagocytes, and stimulate expression of antimicrobial defense mechanisms (Bystrom et al., 2008; Serhan et al., 2008). Although the role of macrophages in the pro-inflammatory response to implanted biomaterials has been extensively documented, their role in resolution of the host response (homeostasis) and as an anti-inflammatory influence has not been described.

M1 and M2 macrophages present a differential gene regulation of arachidonate metabolism-related enzymes (Martinez et al., 2006). M1 macrophages show a marked up-regulation of cyclooxygenase-2 (COX2), and down-regulation of COX1, and arachidonate 5-lipoxygenase (ALOX5). Conversely, M2 macrophages show up-regulation of ALOX15 and COX1. LPS and other inflammatory M1 signals induce the microsomal isoform of PGE synthase (mPGES), the terminal enzyme in the pathway for PGE2 production, and are functionally associated to COX2 expression. In contrast, mPGES is down-regulated by M2 stimuli such as IL-4 and IL-13 (Mosca et al., 2007).

In inflamed adipose tissue from high-fat-diet-induced obese mice, resolvin D1 markedly attenuated IFNγ/LPS-induced Th1 cytokines and up-regulated arginase-1 expression in macrophages. Moreover, it stimulated nonphlogistic phagocytosis and reduced the reactive oxygen species production in adipose macrophages, thus suggesting the elicitation of an M2-like activation state (Titos et al., 2011). Thus, under conditions of polarized inflammation, macrophages modulate the expression and activation of various enzymes involved in lipid metabolism, thus finely tuning their lipid mediators profile and essentially actively contributing to the fine modulation of the diverse phases of resolution of inflammation.

In a mouse model of peritonitis, a new hybrid macrophage population was found in the resolving phase of acute inflammation, aptly termed resolution-phase macrophages (rM).

These cells expressed an alternatively activated phenotype with weaker bactericidal properties but, similarly with classically activated pro-inflammatory M1 cells, expressed elevated markers of M1 cells including inducible COX2 and nitric oxide synthase (iNOS). This phenotype was controlled by cyclic adenosine monophosphate (cAMP), which, when inhibited, transformed rM to M1 cells. Thus, resolution-phase macrophages are neither classically nor alternatively activated, but instead are a hybrid of both, with a role in mediating restoration of tissue homeostasis (Bystrom et al., 2008).

Similarly, during the resolution of murine peritonitis, the emergence of pro-resolving CD11b$^{(low)}$ macrophages was observed. These macrophages were distinct from the majority of peritoneal macrophages in terms of their protein expression profile and pro-resolving properties, such as apoptotic leukocyte engulfment, indifference to TLR ligands, and emigration to lymphoid organs. Interaction with apoptotic cells *ex vivo* was also found to convert macrophages from the CD11b$^{(high)}$ to the CD11b$^{(low)}$ phenotype, thus suggesting that efferocytosis may give rise to CD11b$^{(low)}$ macrophages which are essential for complete nonphlogistic containment of inflammatory agents and the termination of acute inflammation (Schif-Zuck et al., 2011).

Macrophages exert distinct functions during the diverse phases of skin repair (Gordon and Martinez, 2010; Biswas and Mantovani, 2010). In a mouse model of conditional depletion of macrophages during the sequential stages of the repair response, it was found that in the early stage of the repair response (inflammatory phase), depletion of macrophages significantly reduced the formation of granulation tissue, impaired epithelialization, and resulted in minimized scar formation. The consecutive phase of tissue formation depletion of macrophages resulted in severe hemorrhage in the wound tissue, and the transition into the last phase of tissue maturation and wound closure was significantly impaired. Macrophage depletion in the late phase of tissue maturation did not significantly impact the outcome of the repair response. Overall it was discovered that macrophages undergo dynamic changes during different phases of wound healing and sequentially regulate and orchestrate the diverse phases of tissue repair events (Lucas et al., 2010). It is therefore logical to expect that variations in macrophage phenotype would be found over time following the implantation of biomaterials, but that the spatial and temporal patterns of these variations would depend upon the type of biomaterial, its degradability, and the anatomic site of placement.

In humans, chronic venous ulcers (CVUs) represent a failure to resolve a chronic inflammatory condition. In human and mouse models of CVUs, it was found that iron overloading induced a macrophage population with a pro-inflammatory M1 activation state, unable to switch in an M2 phenotype, perpetuating inflammation through enhanced TNFα and hydroxyl radical release, leading to impaired wound healing (Sindrilaru et al., 2011).

In ischemic heart disease and kidney pathology, monocytes recruited to the injured tissue undergo dynamic changes from a primarily M1 to a predominantly M2 phenotype (Swaminathan and Griffin, 2008; Lambert et al., 2008; Troidl et al., 2009). In models of acute ischemic heart pathology, the macrophage was identified as a primary responder cell type involved in the regulation of post-myocardial infarction wound healing. At the injury site, macrophages remove necrotic cardiac myocytes and apoptotic neutrophils, secrete soluble mediators, and regulate the angiogenic response (Lambert et al., 2008). Modulations in the phenotype of recruited mononuclear phagocytes have been observed in ischemic heart and kidney disease, thus suggesting a primary role for macrophage polarization in the natural history of tissue repair. It should be recognized that the implantation of any biomaterial is associated with tissue injury. Therefore, the host must respond not only to the biomaterial, but also to the initial tissue insult (See Chapters 2 and 3).

Fibrosis is a common feature of lung, liver, and other parenchymal organ diseases. Activated macrophages may exert a dual function in the orchestration of matrix deposition and remodeling. On the one hand, the classical M2-polarizing stimuli IL-4 and IL-13 exert pro-fibrotic activity by inducing alternative M2 activation. In particular, IL-13 directly stimulates collagen synthesis (Chiaramonte et al., 1999; Oriente et al., 2000) and induces the production of TGFβ as well as its activation via matrix metallopeptidase-9 (MMP9) (Lee et al., 2001), making macrophages a prime source of this pro-fibrotic cytokine (Karlmark et al., 2009). In the liver, activated resident and recruited macrophages also produce growth factors such as insulin-like growth factor 1 (IGF1) and platelet-derived growth factors, cytokines, and chemokines (e.g., CCL2), which recruit circulating monocytes and affect the function of fibroblasts (Sica et al., 2014). In general, polarized myeloid cells play a major role in orchestrating liver fibrosis in response to parasites (Beschin et al., 2013). In lung fibrosis, M2 macrophages also play a critical role taking part into TGFβ-dependent fibrotic pathways (Murray et al., 2011). In mouse models of Duchenne muscular dystrophy (DMD), it was found that fibrinogen-Mac-1 receptor binding induces IL-1β and drives the synthesis of TGFβ by macrophages, which in turn induces collagen production in fibroblasts and amplifies the pro-fibrotic network through the activation of M2 macrophages (Vidal et al., 2008).

On the other hand, macrophages can also exert anti-fibrotic activity and promote resolution of fibrosis. Macrophages are in fact an important source of collagenases (e.g., MMP13) which degrade fibrous tissue (Hironaka et al., 2000). Serum amyloid P component (SAP), an acute-phase protein present in circulation and extracellular matrix (ECM), has been shown to inhibit fibrosis in different models by regulating macrophage function (Murray et al., 2010; Castano et al., 2009; Murray et al., 2011). Thus, positive and negative regulators may modulate the pro- versus anti-fibrotic functions of macrophages accounting for their potential dual role in tissue fibrosis (Sica et al., 2014). A comprehensive discussion of fibrosis in response to biomaterials can be found in Chapters 5 and 9.

MACROPHAGE POLARIZATION IN THE RESPONSE TO BIOMATERIALS

As previously discussed in this chapter, there is strong evidence for a critical role of macrophages in the tissue repair and healing process, and a strong association exists between immune responses, inflammation, and macrophage activation. The host response to biomaterial implants is closely related to the host response to injury. Indeed, because of the *in vivo* implantation of biomaterials in to viable tissue, to some extent, an inevitable amount of tissue injury will occur. Therefore, the host response to injury is an important part of the host response to biomaterials and is a component of both the classical and emerging perspective (Brown and Badylak, 2013).

From the point of view accepted in the late 1980s, the host response to biomaterials included a number of stages such as injury, acute and chronic inflammation, foreign body reaction (FBR), granulation tissue formation, and encapsulation. From the early 1960s to the 1990s, the most desirable implantable biomaterial had, firstly, to be inert. It should be recognized that no biomaterial is inert. All biomaterials elicit a host response, much of which is mediated by macrophages. Intense scientific efforts over the last 30 years have led to a series of new concepts in the field of biomaterials and regenerative medicine, shifting paradigms from permanent "inert" biomaterials to short-term degradable materials serving as a scaffold for cell and tissue repair. Thus, biocompatibility has been newly defined as "the ability of biomaterials to perform a desired specific function with respect to medical therapy, without eliciting any undesirable local or systemic effects in the recipient, but generating the most appropriate beneficial cellular or tissue response in that specific situation" (Williams, 2008). Biocompatibility was distinguished from biotolerability. Biocompatibility refers to the ability of a material to specifically induce a local host response aimed at functional tissue reconstruction and repair while biotolerability refers to the ability of a material to rest in the host without inducing a harmful host response (Ratner, 2011) (See Chapter 3).

This dramatic change in the paradigms of biomaterials and regenerative medicine has led to a renewed interest in considering the role of immune cells in the host response to biomaterials. In the classical point of view, the interaction of immune cells with biomaterial inevitably led to ECM deposition, angiogenesis, and granulation tissue formation, with negative implications for implantation outcome. In the context of the Hippocratic "*primum non nocere*" point of view, this concept has led to a number of strategies aimed at avoiding the activation of the host immune response.

Recent advances on the characteristics of immune cells and their role in tissue repair has shed new light on the interaction between biomaterials and the host, and new strategies are currently in development to modulate and encourage the host immune response, rather than avoid it. Macrophages play a central role in this new paradigm.

In particular, it has been shown that the host macrophage response is not only fully acceptable but in fact it has been reevaluated as an essential component of a reconstructive tissue remodeling process following the implantation of certain biologically derived scaffold materials (Badylak et al., 2008; Brown et al., 2009, 2012a). The amount of new knowledge in macrophage plasticity and polarizing properties has led to a "revisited" role for macrophages in the host interaction with biomaterials.

When a material is implanted in soft tissue, skeletal tissue, or whole organs, it induces a host response and the M1/M2 paradigm plays an important role in orientating the outcome of implantation. The appropriate macrophage polarization and the capacity to switch and resolve polarized responses are critical in determining the outcome (Brown et al., 2012b). An initial M1 response is required in the first phases of implantation to eliminate potential pathogens and to remove dead cells and tissue debris from the wound site. Tissue remodeling requires a transition to a M2 phenotype which results in scar tissue or constructive remodeling depending on the timing of the macrophage phenotype switch. In fact, the lack of polarization, or an excessive and uncontrolled M2 polarization, may be responsible for excessive scarring or a delay in wound healing, respectively (Brown and Badylak, 2013). To this regard, a distinction between nondegradable biomaterials and degradable biomaterials is helpful.

Materials intended for long-term implantation, including metallic and polymeric materials designed to replace an organ or tissue, must be mechanically robust and functional without inducing deleterious responses from the host. Biological processes at the host–tissue interface for such materials typically result in an FBR. A common example of a nondegradable biomaterial device is the total joint replacement (TJR). TJR is a widely practiced and successful intervention for patients suffering from arthritis and degenerative articular diseases. Daily activities subject the implants to continuous wear and may give rise to the release of biologically active products which consist of metallic ions, polymeric particulates, and similar molecules that can activate monocyte/macrophages. Activated macrophages produce pro-inflammatory factors and cytokines that induce an inflammatory reaction that may result in chronic synovitis, osteoclasts activation, and resorption of periprosthetic bone, which may seriously compromise the functionality of the implant. Macrophages play a key role in determining the functional outcome of the inflammatory reaction that arises from the interaction between the biomaterial and the host periprosthetic microenvironment. Rao et al. retrieved periprosthetic tissues from patients with radiographic evidence of osteolysis and found a higher M1 macrophage infiltration in synovial tissues when compared to nonimplanted synovial tissues. The nonimplanted synovial tissues displayed a higher M2 phenotype, suggesting an important role for macrophage polarization in determining the functional outcome of TJR (Rao et al., 2012). Moreover, these data suggest that the modulation of macrophage phenotypes could be a potential therapeutic tool for reducing the possible inflammation-derived damages and optimizing the patient outcome following TJR (Rao et al., 2012). Further discussion of the host response to biomaterials used for orthopedic applications can be found in Chapter 12.

In contrast to nondegradable materials, degradable biomaterials are generally designed to function as "temporary scaffolds" for the host cells and tissues to promote the recovery of normal and functional structure of the tissue or organ of interest. These devices are usually manufactured from either synthetic or natural materials and combined with bioactive molecules or living cells. For these reasons, even though an initial inflammatory reaction occurs, the final host response to these degradable materials is completely different from the host response to permanent implants (Brown et al., 2012b).

The implantation of nondegradable synthetic biomaterials gives rise to an inflammatory response and activation of macrophages. Cells may undergo "frustrated phagocytosis" and fuse to one another becoming giant multinucleated cells which, together with the activation of resident fibroblasts, result in fibrous connective tissue deposition and encapsulation similar to the FBR (Anderson et al., 2008). Some studies have been aimed at investigating whether manipulation of synthetic biomaterials would be useful to modify the host response. Convincing evidence showed that the morphology and topography of the biomaterial is a crucial point in orientating the patient immune response through redirecting macrophage phenotypes (Saino et al., 2011; Bota et al., 2010). Madden et al. investigated an interesting cardiac tissue engineering strategy by using synthetic biomaterials in *in vitro* and *in vivo* models of reconstitution of cardiac tissue. In this system, the authors demonstrated that cardiac implantation of acellular scaffolds with pore diameters of 30–40 µm showed enhanced angiogenesis and reduced fibrotic response. Moreover, the majority of the activated macrophages in the reconstituted tissue expressed iNOS, indicating the activation of pro-inflammatory pathways. Macrophage mannose receptor (MMR) expression increased significantly at porous implants, and this increase was associated with improved neovascularization for implants with pores greater than 20 µm, thus supporting the hypothesis that M2-polarized macrophages (which express high levels of MMR) supported the enhanced neovascularization (Madden et al., 2010). Thus, topography and morphology of synthetic biomaterials may account for the success of the implantation through macrophage recruitment and phenotype modulation. This topic is further discussed in Chapters 3 and 5.

Naturally derived biomaterials are manufactured from mammalian tissues and display a wide range of biological molecules that potentially interact with ligands in the recipient thus eliciting a unique inflammatory response. Scaffold materials composed of ECM have been shown to promote a switch from M1 to M2 cell population following implantation (Badylak et al., 2008; Brown et al., 2009, 2012a).

In an *in vivo* model of ECM biomaterial implantation in rodents, a strong correlation was found between the early macrophage response to implanted materials and the outcome of tissue remodeling. Increased M2 macrophage infiltration with a higher M2:M1 ratio at the site of remodeling at 14 days postimplantation was associated with more positive downstream remodeling outcomes. This result suggests that the constructive remodeling success may be due to the recruitment and survival of different cell populations associated with materials that elicit an M1 or M2 response (Brown et al., 2012a).

Badylak et al. used an *in vivo* rodent model to investigate the impact of macrophage phenotype upon the remodeling outcome following the implantation of a wide variety of ECM-based devices. It was found that although macrophage infiltration occurred early in all grafts, the macrophage phenotype predicted the success of implantation. An M2 profile displayed constructive remodeling and the prevalence of the M1 phenotype was characterized by chronic inflammation (Badylak et al., 2008). The materials characterized by chronic inflammation and higher M1 infiltration had often been chemically treated to induce protein cross-links suggesting that chemical manipulation of naturally occurring biomaterials can notably modulate macrophage phenotype and influence the success or failure of the biomaterial. A more in-depth understanding of these mechanisms affecting the macrophage response to biomaterials will allow the design of next generation biomaterials and the development of regenerative medicine strategies aimed at ensuring functional host tissues.

CONCLUDING REMARKS

Plasticity is a well-known feature of the mononuclear phagocytes. Within the tissue microenvironment, the complex integration of tissue-derived signals, soluble mediators, and microbial factors regulate genetic reprogramming and result in differential activation and phenotypic changes of these cells.

Beyond the well-known properties of macrophage phenotypes and plasticity in the host's defense against pathogens and in cancer development, growing evidence suggests an emerging role in the host response to biomaterials. In particular, the time-dependent modulation from M1 to M2 phenotype seems to play a central role in the tissue remodeling process. Indeed, inappropriate polarization toward either an M1 or M2 extreme may result in pathologic consequences.

It is also suggested that macrophage phenotype may be directly modulated by biomaterials resulting in various functional outcomes of the implants. Accordingly, biomaterial design is now aimed at enhancing controlled macrophage recruitment and phenotype modulation, rather than preventing macrophage infiltration or focusing on their elimination (Mokarram and Bellamkonda, 2014). A better understanding of the biological mechanisms which underlie the macrophage polarization switching in response to biomaterials is essential for the development of macrophage-targeted strategies aimed at promoting functional tissue restoration rather than harmful, uncontrolled inflammation.

ACKNOWLEDGMENTS

Alberto Mantovani is supported by the Italian Ministry of Health and by ERC. Maria Rosaria Galdiero is supported by a fellowship from P.O.R. Campania FSE 2007-2013, Project CREMe.

REFERENCES

Anderson, J.M., Rodriguez, A., Chang, D.T., 2008. Foreign body reaction to biomaterials. Semin. Immunol. 20 (2), 86–100.

Badylak, S.F., Valentin, J.E., Ravindra, A.K., McCabe, G.P., Stewart-Akers, A.M., 2008. Macrophage phenotype as a determinant of biologic scaffold remodeling. Tissue Eng. Part A 14 (11), 1835–1842.

Beschin, A., De Baetselier, P., Van Ginderachter, J.A., 2013. Contribution of myeloid cell subsets to liver fibrosis in parasite infection. J. Pathol. 229 (2), 186–197.

Biswas, S.K., Mantovani, A., 2010. Macrophage plasticity and interaction with lymphocyte subsets: cancer as a paradigm. Nat. Immunol. 11 (10), 889–896.

Biswas, S.K., Mantovani, A., 2012. Orchestration of metabolism by macrophages. Cell. Metab. 15 (4), 432–437.

Bota, P.C., Collie, A.M., Puolakkainen, P., Vernon, R.B., Sage, E.H., Ratner, B.D., et al., 2010. Biomaterial topography alters healing *in vivo* and monocyte/macrophage activation *in vitro*. J. Biomed. Mater. Res. A. 95 (2), 649–657.

Brown, B.N., Badylak, S.F., 2013. Expanded applications, shifting paradigms and an improved understanding of host–biomaterial interactions. Acta. Biomater. 9 (2), 4948–4955.

Brown, B.N., Valentin, J.E., Stewart-Akers, A.M., McCabe, G.P., Badylak, S.F., 2009. Macrophage phenotype and remodeling outcomes in response to biologic scaffolds with and without a cellular component. Biomaterials 30 (8), 1482–1491.

Brown, B.N., Londono, R., Tottey, S., Zhang, L., Kukla, K.A., Wolf, M.T., et al., 2012a. Macrophage phenotype as a predictor of constructive remodeling following the implantation of biologically derived surgical mesh materials. Acta. Biomater. 8 (3), 978–987.

Brown, B.N., Ratner, B.D., Goodman, S.B., Amar, S., Badylak, S.F., 2012b. Macrophage polarization: an opportunity for improved outcomes in biomaterials and regenerative medicine. Biomaterials 33 (15), 3792–3802.

Bystrom, J., Evans, I., Newson, J., Stables, M., Toor, I., van Rooijen, N., et al., 2008. Resolution-phase macrophages possess a unique inflammatory phenotype that is controlled by cAMP. Blood 112 (10), 4117–4127.

Castano, A.P., Lin, S.L., Surowy, T., Nowlin, B.T., Turlapati, S.A., Patel, T., et al., 2009. Serum amyloid P inhibits fibrosis through Fc gamma R-dependent monocyte–macrophage regulation *in vivo*. Sci. Transl. Med. 1 (5), 5ra13.

Chiaramonte, M.G., Donaldson, D.D., Cheever, A.W., Wynn, T.A., 1999. An IL-13 inhibitor blocks the development of hepatic fibrosis during a T-helper type 2-dominated inflammatory response. J. Clin. Invest. 104 (6), 777–785.

De Palma, M., Mazzieri, R., Politi, L.S., Pucci, F., Zonari, E., Sitia, G., et al., 2008. Tumor-targeted interferon-alpha delivery by Tie2-expressing monocytes inhibits tumor growth and metastasis. Cancer Cell. 14 (4), 299–311.

Dinarello, C.A., 2005. Blocking IL-1 in systemic inflammation. J. Exp. Med. 201 (9), 1355–1359.

Duluc, D., Corvaisier, M., Blanchard, S., Catala, L., Descamps, P., Gamelin, E., et al., 2009. Interferon-gamma reverses the immunosuppressive and protumoral properties and prevents the generation of human tumor-associated macrophages. Int. J. Cancer 125 (2), 367–373.

Garlanda, C., Dinarello, C.A., Mantovani, A., 2013. The interleukin-1 family: back to the future. Immunity 39 (6), 1003–1018.

Geissmann, F., Manz, M.G., Jung, S., Sieweke, M.H., Merad, M., Ley, K., 2010. Development of monocytes, macrophages, and dendritic cells. Science 327 (5966), 656–661.

Gordon, S., Martinez, F.O., 2010. Alternative activation of macrophages: mechanism and functions. Immunity 32 (5), 593–604.

Gordon, S., Taylor, P.R., 2005. Monocyte and macrophage heterogeneity. Nat. Rev. Immunol. 5 (12), 953–964.

Hironaka, K., Sakaida, I., Matsumura, Y., Kaino, S., Miyamoto, K., Okita, K., 2000. Enhanced interstitial collagenase (matrix metalloproteinase-13) production of Kupffer cell by gadolinium chloride prevents pig serum-induced rat liver fibrosis. Biochem. Biophys. Res. Commun. 267 (1), 290–295.

Jenkins, S.J., Ruckerl, D., Cook, P.C., Jones, L.H., Finkelman, F.D., van Rooijen, N., et al., 2011. Local macrophage proliferation, rather than recruitment from the blood, is a signature of TH2 inflammation. Science 332 (6035), 1284–1288.

Karlmark, K.R., Weiskirchen, R., Zimmermann, H.W., Gassler, N., Ginhoux, F., Weber, C., et al., 2009. Hepatic recruitment of the inflammatory Gr1+ monocyte subset upon liver injury promotes hepatic fibrosis. Hepatology 50 (1), 261–274.

Kurowska-Stolarska, M., Stolarski, B., Kewin, P., Murphy, G., Corrigan, C.J., Ying, S., et al., 2009. IL-33 amplifies the polarization of alternatively activated macrophages that contribute to airway inflammation. J. Immunol. 183 (10), 6469–6477.

Lambert, J.M., Lopez, E.F., Lindsey, M.L., 2008. Macrophage roles following myocardial infarction. Int. J. Cardiol. 130 (2), 147–158.

Lawrence, T., Willoughby, D.A., Gilroy, D.W., 2002. Anti-inflammatory lipid mediators and insights into the resolution of inflammation. Nat. Rev. Immunol. 2 (10), 787–795.

Lee, C.G., Homer, R.J., Zhu, Z., Lanone, S., Wang, X., Koteliansky, V., et al., 2001. Interleukin-13 induces tissue fibrosis by selectively stimulating and activating transforming growth factor beta(1). J. Exp. Med. 194 (6), 809–821.

Liddiard, K., Rosas, M., Davies, L.C., Jones, S.A., Taylor, P.R., 2011. Macrophage heterogeneity and acute inflammation. Eur. J. Immunol. 41 (9), 2503–2508.

Lucas, T., Waisman, A., Ranjan, R., Roes, J., Krieg, T., Muller, W., et al., 2010. Differential roles of macrophages in diverse phases of skin repair. J. Immunol. 184 (7), 3964–3977.

Madden, L.R., Mortisen, D.J., Sussman, E.M., Dupras, S.K., Fugate, J.A., Cuy, J.L., et al., 2010. Proangiogenic scaffolds as functional templates for cardiac tissue engineering. Proc. Natl. Acad. Sci. U.S.A. 107 (34), 15211–15216.

Mantovani, A., Sozzani, S., Locati, M., Allavena, P., Sica, A., 2002. Macrophage polarization: tumor-associated macrophages as a paradigm for polarized M2 mononuclear phagocytes. Trends. Immunol. 23 (11), 549–555.

Mantovani, A., Allavena, P., Sica, A., Balkwill, F., 2008. Cancer-related inflammation. Nature 454 (7203), 436–444.

Martinez, F.O., Gordon, S., Locati, M., Mantovani, A., 2006. Transcriptional profiling of the human monocyte-to-macrophage differentiation and polarization: new molecules and patterns of gene expression. J. Immunol. 177 (10), 7303–7311.

Mokarram, N., Bellamkonda, R.V., 2014. A perspective on immunomodulation and tissue repair. Ann. Biomed. Eng. 42 (2), 338–351.

Mosca, M., Polentarutti, N., Mangano, G., Apicella, C., Doni, A., Mancini, F., et al., 2007. Regulation of the microsomal prostaglandin E synthase-1 in polarized mononuclear phagocytes and its constitutive expression in neutrophils. J. Leukoc. Biol. 82 (2), 320–326.

Murray, L.A., Rosada, R., Moreira, A.P., Joshi, A., Kramer, M.S., Hesson, D.P., et al., 2010. Serum amyloid P therapeutically attenuates murine bleomycin-induced pulmonary fibrosis via its effects on macrophages. PLoS. One. 5 (3), e9683.

Murray, L.A., Chen, Q., Kramer, M.S., Hesson, D.P., Argentieri, R.L., Peng, X., et al., 2011. TGF-beta driven lung fibrosis is macrophage dependent and blocked by serum amyloid P. Int. J. Biochem. Cell. Biol. 43 (1), 154–162.

Noel, W., Raes, G., Hassanzadeh Ghassabeh, G., De Baetselier, P., Beschin, A., 2004. Alternatively activated macrophages during parasite infections. Trends. Parasitol. 20 (3), 126–133.

Oriente, A., Fedarko, N.S., Pacocha, S.E., Huang, S.K., Lichtenstein, L.M., Essayan, D.M., 2000. Interleukin-13 modulates collagen homeostasis in human skin and keloid fibroblasts. J. Pharmacol. Exp. Ther. 292 (3), 988–994.

Pesce, J., Kaviratne, M., Ramalingam, T.R., Thompson, R.W., Urban Jr., J.F., Cheever, A.W., et al., 2006. The IL-21 receptor augments Th2 effector function and alternative macrophage activation. J Clin. Invest. 116 (7), 2044–2055.

Porcheray, F., Viaud, S., Rimaniol, A.C., Leone, C., Samah, B., Dereuddre-Bosquet, N., et al., 2005. Macrophage activation switching: an asset for the resolution of inflammation. Clin. Exp. Immunol. 142 (3), 481–489.

Puig-Kroger, A., Sierra-Filardi, E., Dominguez-Soto, A., Samaniego, R., Corcuera, M.T., Gomez-Aguado, F., et al., 2009. Folate receptor beta is expressed by tumor-associated macrophages and constitutes a marker for M2 anti-inflammatory/regulatory macrophages. Cancer. Res. 69 (24), 9395–9403.

Rae, F., Woods, K., Sasmono, T., Campanale, N., Taylor, D., Ovchinnikov, D.A., et al., 2007. Characterisation and trophic functions of murine embryonic macrophages based upon the use of a Csf1r-EGFP transgene reporter. Dev. Biol. 308 (1), 232–246.

Rao, A.J., Gibon, E., Ma, T., Yao, Z., Smith, R.L., Goodman, S.B., 2012. Revision joint replacement, wear particles, and macrophage polarization. Acta. Biomater. 8 (7), 2815–2823.

Ratner, B.D., 2011. The biocompatibility manifesto: biocompatibility for the twenty-first century. J Cardiovasc. Transl. Res. 4 (5), 523–527.

Recalcati, S., Locati, M., Marini, A., Santambrogio, P., Zaninotto, F., De Pizzol, M., et al., 2010. Differential regulation of iron homeostasis during human macrophage polarized activation. Eur. J. Immunol. 40 (3), 824–835.

Romagnani, P., De Paulis, A., Beltrame, C., Annunziato, F., Dente, V., Maggi, E., et al., 1999. Tryptase–chymase double-positive human mast cells express the eotaxin receptor CCR3 and are attracted by CCR3-binding chemokines. Am. J. Pathol 155 (4), 1195–1204.

Saino, E., Focarete, M.L., Gualandi, C., Emanuele, E., Cornaglia, A.I., Imbriani, M., et al., 2011. Effect of electrospun fiber diameter and alignment on macrophage activation and secretion of proinflammatory cytokines and chemokines. Biomacromolecules 12 (5), 1900–1911.

Schif-Zuck, S., Gross, N., Assi, S., Rostoker, R., Serhan, C.N., Ariel, A., 2011. Saturated-efferocytosis generates pro-resolving CD11b low macrophages: modulation by resolvins and glucocorticoids. Eur. J. Immunol. 41 (2), 366–379.

Schulz, C., Gomez Perdiguero, E., Chorro, L., Szabo-Rogers, H., Cagnard, N., Kierdorf, K., et al., 2012. A lineage of myeloid cells independent of Myb and hematopoietic stem cells. Science 336 (6077), 86–90.

Serhan, C.N., Chiang, N., Van Dyke, T.E., 2008. Resolving inflammation: dual anti-inflammatory and pro-resolution lipid mediators. Nat. Rev. Immunol. 8 (5), 349–361.

Sica, A., Mantovani, A., 2012. Macrophage plasticity and polarization: in vivo veritas. J. Clin. Invest. 122 (3), 787–795.

Sica, A., Invernizzi, P., Mantovani, A., 2014. Macrophage plasticity and polarization in liver homeostasis and pathology. Hepatology 59 (5), 2034–2042.

Sindrilaru, A., Peters, T., Wieschalka, S., Baican, C., Baican, A., Peter, H., et al., 2011. An unrestrained proinflammatory M1 macrophage population induced by iron impairs wound healing in humans and mice. J. Clin. Invest. 121 (3), 985–997.

Stout, R.D., Watkins, S.K., Suttles, J., 2009. Functional plasticity of macrophages: in situ reprogramming of tumor-associated macrophages. J. Leukoc. Biol. 86 (5), 1105–1109.

Swaminathan, S., Griffin, M.D., 2008. First responders: understanding monocyte-lineage traffic in the acutely injured kidney. Kidney. Int. 74 (12), 1509–1511.

Titos, E., Rius, B., Gonzalez-Periz, A., Lopez-Vicario, C., Moran-Salvador, E., Martinez-Clemente, M., et al., 2011. Resolvin D1 and its precursor docosahexaenoic acid promote resolution of adipose tissue inflammation by eliciting macrophage polarization toward an M2-like phenotype. J. Immunol. 187 (10), 5408–5418.

Troidl, C., Mollmann, H., Nef, H., Masseli, F., Voss, S., Szardien, S., et al., 2009. Classically and alternatively activated macrophages contribute to tissue remodelling after myocardial infarction. J. Cell. Mol. Med. 13 (9B), 3485–3496.

Tseng, D., Volkmer, J.P., Willingham, S.B., Contreras-Trujillo, H., Fathman, J.W., Fernhoff, N.B., et al., 2013. Anti-CD47 antibody-mediated phagocytosis of cancer by macrophages primes an effective antitumor T-cell response. Proc. Natl. Acad. Sci. USA. 110 (27), 11103–11108.

Uderhardt, S., Herrmann, M., Oskolkova, O.V., Aschermann, S., Bicker, W., Ipseiz, N., et al., 2012. 12/15-lipoxygenase orchestrates the clearance of apoptotic cells and maintains immunologic tolerance. Immunity 36 (5), 834–846.

Vidal, B., Serrano, A.L., Tjwa, M., Suelves, M., Ardite, E., De Mori, R., et al., 2008. Fibrinogen drives dystrophic muscle fibrosis via a TGFbeta/alternative macrophage activation pathway. Genes Dev. 22 (13), 1747–1752.

Williams, D.F., 2008. On the mechanisms of biocompatibility. Biomaterials 29 (20), 2941–2953.

CHAPTER 7

Role of Dendritic Cells in Response to Biomaterials

Jamal S. Lewis and Benjamin G. Keselowsky

J. Crayton Pruitt Family Department of Biomedical Engineering, University of Florida, Gainesville, FL, USA

Contents

INTRODUCTION

Classically, biomaterials have been defined as "*substance other than foods or drugs contained in therapeutic or diagnostic systems that are in contact with tissue or biological fluids*" (Langer and Tirrell, 2004) and indeed, throughout history biomaterials have been critical for the successful treatment of disease. From the earliest (circa AD 1) biomaterials, such as wooden teeth and glass eyes, to more contemporary examples such as nitinol stents and Dacron blood vessels, the influence of biomaterials on medicine has been revolutionary (Langer and Tirrell, 2004). This impact is, perhaps, even more evident in biomaterials-based tissue engineering.

Tissue engineering is an interdisciplinary field aimed at restoring physiologic function(s) by regenerating or replacing lost/damaged cells, tissues, and organs

Host Response to Biomaterials.
DOI: http://dx.doi.org/10.1016/B978-0-12-800196-7.00007-4

(Langer and Vacanti, 1993). A prominent strategy used in the field is to combine cells of interest with a biocompatible support material and ultimately implant these combinations to ameliorate tissue and organ loss or dysfunction. This support material or tissue scaffold is hypothesized to facilitate cells of interest toward the formation and integration of functional target tissue. More recently, these materials have been adapted, with the inclusion of tissue inductive factors (Sakiyama-Elbert and Hubbell, 2000; Schense and Hubbell, 2000), proteins (Lu et al., 2007; Yoneno et al., 2005; Mauney et al., 2007), and cells (Quint et al., 2012; Pei et al., 2009; Arinzeh et al., 2003), to make the biomaterial scaffold more bioactive and drive microenvironments beneficial to the development of functional tissues/organs. During the last two decades, advances in biomaterials-based tissue engineering have generated clinical alternatives to organ transplantation and reconstructive surgery. For instance, tissue-engineered skin substitutes are commercially available for wound healing applications (Capo et al., 2014; Han et al., 2014). Further, clinical trials are ongoing on tissue-engineered substitutes for cornea (www.clinicaltrials.gov and NCT01765244, 2014), cartilage (www.clinicaltrials.gov and NCT01242618, 2014), and bone (www.clinicaltrials.gov and NCT01958502, 2014).

Even with these successes in clinical translation, modern biomaterial combination products still face a number of challenges following implantation which limit their functionality and durability, and ultimately may lead to their failure. The greatest of these challenges, perhaps, is the interaction with the host immune system.

It has long been recognized that implantation of bulk biomaterials often triggers a profound reaction of host immune responses, collectively referred to as the foreign body reaction (Anderson et al., 2008; Anderson, 2001). The physical injury due to implantation of biomaterials in itself elicits an inflammatory response, considered to be part of the normal wound healing process. The presence of a biomaterial typically exacerbates this response, occasionally resulting in foreign body giant cell formation and antigen release (when a biological component is present) at the site of implantation (Anderson et al., 2008). This immune response has been reviewed in depth in Chapters 2, 3, and 5 of this text but will be reviewed here to place subsequent comments in proper context. Briefly, interaction with bodily fluid leads to protein adsorption on the surface of the biomaterial, Vroman effect (Jung, 2003), and can initiate the coagulation cascade, complement system (which can polarize immune cells toward an inflammatory response), and the formation of a provisional matrix. These phenomena have been extensively investigated on different biomaterial surfaces and it is thought that they are correlated to the physicochemical surface properties of the biomaterial, thereby linking biomaterial properties with host immune cell responses (Anderson, 2001). Following matrix formation, antigen-presenting cells (APCs), including macrophages (MΦs) and dendritic cells (DCs), can be recruited to the implant site by chemokines released by the matrix as well as surrounding cells. Macrophages, in particular, persist at the implantation site, adhering to the implant surface and occasionally coalescing with neighboring macrophages to form a giant cell body, which attempts to engulf the material. Within this microenvironment, macrophages secrete a number of inflammatory mediators, including reactive oxygen species and degradative enzymes that can be detrimental to the structure and functionality of the implanted biomaterial (Brodbeck and Anderson, 2009). Incorporation of cells from an allogeneic or xenogeneic source only intensifies this immune response, with foreign cell-associated antigens prompting chronic inflammation, typically mediated by T-cells. DCs play a critical role in the initiation of this chronic adaptive response against tissue-engineered constructs delivering immunogenic cells, proteins, and other biologics.

DCs are widely considered the most efficient APCs. Their function in innate immunity includes recognition and clearance of foreign entities, including pathogens. More importantly, DCs initiate and control adaptive immunity through internalization, processing, and presentation of antigenic material to CD4$^+$ and CD8$^+$ T-cells via its major histocompatibility complex (MHC) pathways (Banchereau et al., 2000). In the context of biomaterial-based combination products, the DC has influence not only on the magnitude of the foreign body response but also on the direction and extent of adaptive immune responses to this non-self-entity. Herein, we discuss the responses of DCs to materials of varying chemistry, size, and topography, as well as the molecular devices that modulate DC behavior toward biomaterials. Figure 7.1 provides an

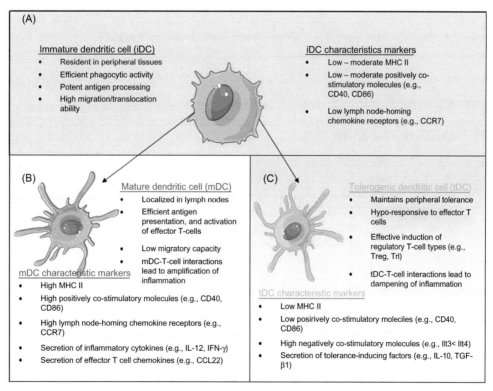

Figure 7.1 Major activation states of Mo-DCs: (A) immature, (B) mature, and (C) tolerogenic.

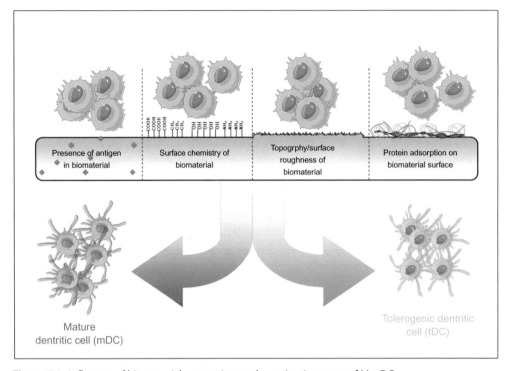

Figure 7.2 Influence of biomaterial properties on the activation state of Mo-DCs.

overview of the characteristics and roles of DCs in their primary maturation states, and Figure 7.2 summarizes current concepts in DC-biomaterial interactions.

DC IMMUNO-BIOLOGY

First described by Steinman et al. in 1973, DCs are often referred to as "professional" APCs due their unique ability to stimulate quiescent, naïve T-cells *in vitro* and *in vivo* (Banchereau et al., 2000; Ardavin et al., 2004). Steinman and coworkers described DCs as large, mononuclear cells (~10 μm) with elongated, stellate processes (or dendrites) extending in multiple directions from the cell body. Currently, DCs and subtypes are defined based on specific cell surface markers or clusters of differentiation (CD) and high expression levels of MHC class I and class II. Moreover, DCs are leukocytes distinguished based on their lack of CD3 (characteristic of T-cells), CD19 (B-cells), CD56 (NK-cells), CD14 (monocytes), CD15 (granulocytes), and CD34 (stem cells). Accordingly, DCs are termed lineage-negative (lin$^-$) DR$^+$ cells (Dopheide et al., 2012).

DC classes

DCs are further subtyped based on lineage origin (myeloid or plasmacytoid), anatomical location and immuno-phenotype. In humans, there are five major classes of DCs that have been characterized, namely: (i) peripheral blood DC, (ii) epithelial and interstitial DC, (iii) thymic DC, (iv) splenic DC, and (v) bone marrow DC (Summers et al., 2001).

Peripheral blood DCs are the main sources of DCs for immunotherapy, representing 0.5–1.5% of total peripheral blood mononuclear cells. There are subtypes of peripheral blood DCs classified based on their expression of CD11c and CD123 (Robinson et al., 1999). The $CD11c^+CD123^{low/+}$ DCs, often called conventional DC or myeloid DC (mDC), express CD13, CD33, CD45RO, and have impressive antigen uptake and allogeneic T-cell stimulatory capacities. Secretion of inflammatory cytokines, particularly interleukin-12 (IL-12), by this class of DC upon bacterial challenge has been demonstrated. Subclasses of this DC type express varying levels of CD16, blood DC antigen-1 (BDCA-1) and BDCA-3. Additionally, the peripheral blood DC is characterized by high expression of Toll-like receptor2 (TLR2) and TLR4 (MacDonald et al., 2002). The other major class of peripheral blood DCs is the plasmacytoid DC (pDC) originally named due to their morphological similarities to plasma cells. Immuno-phenotypically, pDCs lack myeloid markers (including CD13 and CD33) but express high levels of IL-3α, BDCA-2, BDCA-4, CD4, CD62L, and immunoglobulin (IgG)-λ-like transcript (Cao, 2009). pDCs are noted for their production of interferon-α (IFN-α) in response to CpG, certain viruses, and CD40L. TLR7 and TLR9 as well as C-type lectins—CD205 and CD209—are highly conserved on this distinct DC subset (Cao, 2009).

Langerhans cells (LCs) and interstitial DCs, found in peripheral tissues, comprise the *epithelial and interstitial DC* class. These cells are potent activators of naïve $CD4^+$ and $CD8^+$ T-cells and have high IL-12 secretory capacity. DCs found in the thymus have been coined "*thymic DCs*" and are reported to consist of three subpopulations— thymic pDCs, immature $CD11c^+$ DCs, and mature $CD11c^+$ DCs. Thymic pDCs are similar in immuno-phenotype to the aforementioned peripheral blood pDCs, while immature $CD11c^+$ DCs share common features with peripheral blood $CD11c^+$ DCs. Mature $CD11c^+$ DCs comprise less than 7% of thymic DCs and are noted for their expression of DC-lysosome-associated membrane protein (DC-LAMP), CCR7, and IL-12 production (Cao et al., 2007; Patterson et al., 2001). *Splenic DCs* are found in the B-cell-rich follicles, follicular mantle zone, and T-cell-rich areas of lymphoid tissues. Splenic DCs are primarily $CD11c^+$ with a small subpopulation of activated $CD86^+$ DCs found in T-cell zones. Cells with DC-like qualities were also identified in the bone marrow. These bone marrow DCs share common features with peripheral blood DCs and have been shown to be efficient APCs with capacity to induce primary immune responses in naïve $CD4^+$ and $CD8^+$ T-cells (McIlroy et al., 2001; Velasquez-Lopera et al., 2008; Van et al., 1984).

Additionally, *in vitro*–expanded DCs are categorized based on lineage origin, maturation, and functional state. The two major groups are *myeloid-derived DCs* and *lymphoid-derived DCs* (Fadilah and Cheong, 2007). A number of studies have demonstrated that human monocytes (and other myeloid precursor cells) in the presence of granulocyte macrophage colony-stimulating factor (GM-CSF) and IL-4 differentiate into monocyte-derived DCs (Mo-DCs) (Jacobs et al., 2008; Vandenabeele and Wu, 1999; Zheng et al., 2000). Others have used lymphoid progenitors, including T-cell precursors from the thymus (Ardavin et al., 1993) and CD19[+]-committed B-cell precursors (Bjorck and Kincade, 1998a,b), to generate DCs that are phenotypically similar to pDCs. The heterogeneity of lymphoid-derived DC is normally broad and dependent on the *in vitro* cocktail of factors used to induce DC development as well as the progenitor cell type. Generally, DCs are a heterogenous cell population, and this diversity may be necessary for the collective functionality of DCs to initiate adaptive immunity against plethora of invaders, including biomaterials. An overview of mechanisms by which DCs response to both foreign and self-antigens is presented below and will be followed by the role DCs play in the response to biomaterials.

DC receptors and adhesion to extracellular matrix proteins

Immature DCs (iDCs) function as the body's sentinels. They circulate throughout the peripheral blood and tissues and are able to "scavenge" pathogens, foreign materials, and apoptotic or necrotic cells (Banchereau et al., 2000). The mechanisms involved in this environmental sampling include (i) fluid-phase macropinocytosis, (ii) receptor-mediated endocytosis, and (iii) phagocytosis for larger particulate foreign bodies (Fadilah and Cheong, 2007). They are equipped with a wide array of endocytic and phagocytic surface receptors that recognize a host of molecules including proteins, lipids, sugars, glycoproteins, glycolipids, and oligonucleotides (Lewis et al., 2014). Notably, DC endocytic and phagocytic receptors for antigen uptake include C-type lectins (DEC205, CD206), Toll-like receptors (TLR4), Fcγ receptors, and integrins (αVβ5, CD11c) (Akira et al., 2006; Takeda et al., 2003; Lundberg et al., 2014). Interestingly, many of these receptors also direct intracellular signaling, adhesion, motility, and maturation of DCs.

The integrin family of cell-surface receptors is the primary receptor responsible for mediating adhesion to extracellular matrix proteins (Hynes, 2002). and integrins have been shown to modulate numerous cell functions such as viability, proliferation. and differentiation (Keselowsky et al., 2003, 2004, 2005, 2007; Tate et al., 2004; Lan et al., 2005). While it has been shown that DCs express multiple integrins, there are surprisingly few investigations into the effects of integrin binding to extracellular matrix proteins on DC maturation. Notably, Kohl et al. (2007) showed that Mo-DCs and CD34[+] stem cell–derived DCs employ α5β1 and α6β1 integrin, for initial adhesion to fibronectin and laminin adhesive substrates, respectively. Furthermore, Brand et al. (1998) have shown that β1 integrins were involved in adhesion-mediated maturation of human Mo-DCs. Similarly, Acharya et al. (2008) demonstrated that DC adhesion to various adhesive substrates as well as Arg-Gly-Asp (RGD) peptide surface density gradients (Acharya et al., 2010) through the αV integrins result in DC activation. Another report suggested that DCs cultured on adhesive protein substrates and simultaneously exposed to cyclic mechanical strain develop a semi-mature immuno-phenotype (Lewis et al., 2013). On the other hand, Lewis et al. (2012) reported that poly(D,L-lactic-co-glycolic acid) microspheres with surface immobilized ligands (DEC205 and CD11c antibodies and P-D2 peptide) are capable of improving DC internalization *in vitro* and *in vivo* without stimulating DC activation. Further, in a study by Bandyopadhyay et al. (2011), DEC205 antibody-tethered PLGA nanoparticles not only efficiently targeted DCs for uptake but also increased production of IL-10 in DCs. These studies elegantly demonstrate that DC receptor engagement is highly intertwined with DC adhesion, maturation state, and signaling.

Integrin binding to extracellular matrix ligands involves rapid association with the actin cytoskeleton and subsequent integrin clustering resulting in a mechanical coupling between the inside of the cell and its microenvironment. Integrin binding gives rise to adhesion complexes (focal adhesions) containing both structural (e.g., vinculin, talin) and signaling proteins (e.g., focal adhesion kinase (FAK), paxillin) and serves as sites for mechanical signal transduction (Romer et al., 2006; Keselowsky and Garcia, 2005). For example, FAK is a protein tyrosine kinase acting as an early modulator of the integrin signaling cascade and integrates both adhesive and soluble signals (van Nimwegen and van de Water, 2007). The Rho family of GTPases regulates actin cytoskeleton assembly and has been demonstrated to play a crucial role in diverse cellular processes such as membrane trafficking, transcriptional regulation, growth, differentiation, and apoptosis (Aspenstrom, 1999). Very few studies exist investigating the role of the cytoskeleton or focal adhesions in DCs. Swetman Andersen et al. (2006) demonstrated in DC dendrites the presence of microtubules and actin cytoskeleton co-localized with focal contacts proteins β1 integrin, actin, vinculin, paxillin, and talin. Madruga et al. (1999) demonstrated the co-localization of actin, FAK, paxillin, and tyrosine-phosphorylated proteins at the leading edge lamellipodia in motile DCs. Most importantly, the Shurin group recently demonstrated in DCs that the Rho GTPases RhoA, Rac1, and Cdc42 regulate endocytosis and antigen presentation (Tourkova et al., 2007; Shurin et al., 2005) demonstrating that mechanotransduction-related signals can regulate DC processes.

DC migration

DC migration is a key phenomenon intimately linked to localized antigen uptake. Prior to receptor engagement, iDCs secrete inflammatory cytokines including MIP-1α, MIP-1β, MCP-2, MCP-4, and stromal cell-derived factor-1 (SDF-1) and express receptors for the potent chemokine MIP-3α. These events promote recruitment of DCs as well as monocytes and neutrophils to the site of invasion. Following antigen uptake, DCs downregulate their expression of inflammatory cytokines and their receptors, while upregulating the chemokine receptor CCR7 which induces DC homing to lymphoid organs following CCR7 ligand (MIP-3β, CCL21) gradients (Cella et al., 1999; Saeki et al., 1999; Vulcano et al., 2001). Additionally, lymph node–bound DCs secrete the naïve and memory T-cell chemoattractants, CCL18 and CCL22, to help promote DC–T-cell interactions in the lymphoid tissue. mDCs and pDCs have different migratory capacities, routes and chemokine production profiles pointing to diverse roles of these two DC classes in the induction and regulation of adaptive immunity.

DC antigen presentation

Co-localization of both DCs and T-cells is critical for initiation of adaptive immunity. *Antigen presentation* is another mechanism which is important for the facilitation of DC–T-cell communication and activation. As DCs home to lymph nodes, MHC molecules, integral to the formation of immunological synapses with T-cells, are increasingly translocated to the cell surface membrane (via invagination processes) for presentation of antigens (Paglia and Colombo, 1999). Degraded antigen fragments are presented on the surface of DCs via different types of MHC molecules that provide signals via the T-cell receptor (TCR) complex to instigate T-cell selection, expansion, and activation. The antigen-presenting pathway is critical to the nature of the adaptive immune response. Most nucleated cells express MHC class I molecules (HLA-A, -B, and -C) on their surface, but, expression may vary with cell type (Svensson et al., 1997). MHC class II molecules (HLA-DP, -DQ, and -DR) are only expressed on professional APCs (DCs, B-cells, MΦs). Mature DCs, in particular, have high expression levels of both MHC class I and II complexes which allow for effective antigen presentation (Svensson et al., 1997). Endogenously derived (located within the cell cytosol) peptides are displayed primarily via class I MHCs. Peptides from endogenous sources are processed through a cytosolic pathway involving ubiquitination, proteasome degradation, transport via TAPs (transporters for antigen) and finally, insertion into MHC class I molecules for presentation. Peptide-MHC class I complexes interact with CD8$^+$ T-cells. Conversely, MHC class II complexes (expressed on APCs) are loaded primarily with epitopes from exogenous antigenic sources following endosomal degradation and form immunological synapses interacting with CD4$^+$ T-cells (Banchereau et al., 2000; Ardavin et al., 2004; Svensson et al., 1997). An alternative pathway of antigen presentation has been elucidated, where subsets of DCs efficiently present exogenously derived (located outside the cell) antigen fragments on MHC class I to CD8$^+$ T-cells. This phenomenon is referred to as "cross-presentation" and is thought to be important for the generation of normal and balanced immune responses to viruses and tumors (Cohn et al., 2013; Belz et al., 2002).

DC maturation

Increased expression of MHC molecules on the DC plasma membrane indicates a committed transformation of DC phenotype toward a "mature state." As DCs migrate from peripheral tissue, they undergo *DC maturation* which is triggered by the uptake of antigen, exposure to inflammatory cytokines (e.g., tumor necrosis factor (TNF), IL-1, and IL-6) or host molecules associated with inflammation or tissue injury (which are often referred to as "danger signals"; e.g., lipopolysaccharide (LPS), bacterial DNA, and CD40) (Akira et al., 2006). During this process, the primary role of the DC switches from that of antigen-capturing cell to T-cell stimulation. DC maturation is marked by a number of coordinated events including (i) upregulation of peptide–MHC class I and II complexes, (ii) increased expression of co-stimulatory molecules (e.g., CD40, CD80, and CD86), adhesion molecules (CD54, CD58), chemokine receptors (CCR1, CCR7), (iii) secretion of inflammatory cytokines (e.g., IL-12, IFN-γ), (iv) shift in lysosomal compartment type with increased expression of DC-LAMP. Morphologically, DCs lose their adhesive structures, undergo cytoskeleton reorganization which results in the development of cytoplasmic extensions or "veils" at this stage (Akira et al., 2006; Banchereau and Steinman, 1998). Finally, as mentioned above, DCs arriving to lymphoid tissue release chemokines to attract T- and B-cells from the vasculature to their vicinity, resulting in *DC–T-cell interaction* which induces the completion of DC maturation.

DC–T-cell interaction

T-cell priming by DCs occurs in the secondary lymphoid organs such as the spleen, lymph nodes, and gut-associated lymphoid tissue. DC–T-cell interactions typically results in either (i) induction of T-cell-mediated immunity against the presented antigen or (ii) induction of peripheral tolerance. The exact outcome is dependent on three signals: (i) ligation of peptide–MHC complexes to antigen-specific TCRs which constitutes the first signal; (ii) the second signal that is required for T-cell activation is the interaction between co-stimulatory molecules on the DC (e.g., CD80, CD86) and their receptors on the surfaces of T-cells (e.g., CD28, CD40); (iii) the third signal is the "polarizing" signal and can be either soluble or membrane-bound cytokines (e.g., IL-12) (Svensson et al., 1997; Banchereau and Steinman, 1998). Polarization refers to the differentiation of naïve T-cells to a distinct T-cell type. For instance, naïve CD4$^+$ T-cells can differentiate into T-helper cells (T_h cells) and regulatory T-cells (T_{reg} cells). The type of polarization is driven by the cytokine secretion profile of the interacting DC which is further dependent upon DC anatomic location and class as well as the type of maturation stimulus. For, example, mature monocyte-derived CD11c$^+$ DC-secreting IL-12p70 and in the presence of IFN-γ induce naïve CD4$^+$ T-cells to differentiate into T_{h1} IFN-γ-secreting, effector cells. The magnitude of the T-cell response may vary with (i) the surface density of peptide–MHC complexes, (ii) the affinity of the TCR for the corresponding peptide–MHC complex, (iii) DC activation state, and (iv) the type of maturation stimulus (de Jong et al., 2005; Kapsenberg, 2003). Finally, interaction with T-cells is thought to result in the termination of DCs via apoptotic mechanisms (Matsue et al., 1999).

Tolerogenic DCs

So far our discussion has centered on the role of DCs in the induction of inflammatory T-cell responses; however, it is important to recognize that DCs also initiate the suppressive networks that control peripheral tolerance. DCs are thought to play a critical role in the induction of peripheral tolerance through a number of mechanisms such as T-cell apoptosis, T-cell anergy, and T_{reg} induction. Classic immuno-biology describes the basis of T-cell anergy to be the lack of a second required signal in the interaction between APCs and naïve T-cells. The delivery of signal 1 (MHC class I– or class II–peptide complex to TCR) in the absence of signal 2, usually co-stimulatory molecules (CD80, CD86), or soluble cytokines (IL-12, TNF-α) (signal 3) results in an antigen-specific nonresponsive T-cell (Steinbrink et al., 1997). In addition to anergy, peripheral tolerance is maintained by induction of antigen-specific $CD4^+$ $CD25^+$ $FoxP3^+$ suppressor T-cells (T_{regs}) (Salomon et al., 2000). Depletion of this subset of T-cells has been shown to accelerate and induce autoimmunity in various animal models (Scalapino et al., 2006; Kohm et al., 2002; Nakahara et al., 2011). Researchers have shown that T_{regs} are thymic $CD4^+$ T-cells with relatively high affinity for "self" antigens which escape-negative selection, the developmental process in which self-reactive T-cells are clonally deleted (i.e., central tolerance) and develop into $FoxP3^+$ $CD25^+$ T-cells. Suppression of effector T-cells is accomplished by the ability of T_{regs} to impair antigen presentation by mature DCs. However, the crucial step in T_{reg}-mediated immunosuppression is generation of T_{regs} and this is initiated by DCs of definite phenotypes (Giannoukakis, 2013). Tolerogenic DCs are typically characterized by reduced levels of expression of stimulatory/costimulatory molecules (e.g., MHC class II, CD40, CD80, CD86), expression of inhibitory markers (e.g., IgG-like transcript 3) and tolerance-inducing factors (e.g., TGF-β1, IL-10, and indoleamine 2,3 deoxgenase) (Steinman et al., 2003).

DC RESPONSES TO BIOMATERIALS

DCs in the foreign body response

The response of MΦs to biomaterials has been extensively investigated for decades as detailed in other chapters of this textbook (See Chapters 2, 3, and 6). In contrast, studies on DC responses to biomaterials are sparse. A notable study by Vasilijic et al. (2005) delved into the phenotypical and functional changes of implant-infiltrated DCs and the potential role they may play in the foreign body response. Tissue injury associated with biomaterial implantation results in the release of chemotactic agents that recruit immune cells to the site of implantation, including monocytes (Takakura et al., 2000). Approximately 25% of recruited monocytes differentiate into DCs (Randolph et al., 1999). DC potency to stimulate adaptive immune responses has been well characterized, but an understanding of their role in the foreign body reaction to biomaterials is severely lacking. This study by Vasilijic et al. was the first and is currently still the only investigation of the role of the DC in acute and chronic inflammation, and wound healing around an implanted biomaterial (to the best of our knowledge). Briefly, polyvinyl sponges (two/animal) were implanted at dorsal sites of the skin in rats. Sponges were excised at different time periods, after implantation over the course of 14 days, and processed to isolate resident inflammatory immune cells. DCs were then purified from the immune cell population using a combination of isolation techniques including separation gradients, plastic adherence, and immuno-magnetic sorting. Their observations on total DC numbers in the sponge exudates indicate that DCs gradually infiltrated the biomaterial implant, reaching a maximum of day 10, after which their numbers decreased. The phenotypic characteristics of DCs were also investigated using immunohistochemical staining. DCs expressed common markers including MHC class II, CD11c, CD11b, and CD68. One remarkable observation from this study was that the number of DCs staining for His 24 or His 48 (putative pDC markers) was higher at the day 14 time point than that at day 6. Of further interest was the finding that DCs isolated at a later stage of inflammation (day 14 DCs) had a significantly lower capacity to stimulate proliferation of allogeneic T-cells, in comparison to DCs isolated from sponges at 6 days after implantation. This hyporesponsiveness to allogeneic T-cells correlated with not only a distinct change in the DC type (from mDC to pDC) with time, but also a downregulation of positively stimulatory markers CD80, CD86, and CD54. These findings indicated a switch in the phenotype and functionality of biomaterial-resident DCs from the early to late stages of inflammation. Increased amounts of IL-10 and TGF-β1 in culture supernatants and sponge exudate confirmed this functional change in DCs to that of a regulatory type. Conclusively, this study demonstrated that a significant number of DCs accumulate in biomaterials following subcutaneous implantation. Moreover, biomaterial-resident DCs acquire a tolerogenic phenotype as acute inflammation resolves, and these observations may be applied toward the suppression of chronic inflammation and prevention of unsolicited autoimmune responses (Vasilijic et al., 2005).

Adjuvant effects of biomaterials on DC maturation

Studies on DC responses to biomaterials primarily focus on the adjuvant effects of biomaterials in promoting immune responses to biomaterial–biological combination products used in tissue engineering. An adjuvant is a substance that can amplify immune responses to an accompanying antigen but alone does not evoke adaptive immune responses (Makela, 2000). It has been demonstrated that biomaterials act as adjuvants to boost adaptive immune responses to co-delivered antigen. Matzelle and Babensee (2004) established that the presence of the biomaterial resulted in an enhancement of the humoral immune response to co-delivered antigen using a simplified model system. Briefly, ovalbumin (OVA) was used as model antigen and co-delivered with biomaterial carrier vehicles commonly used in tissue engineering (e.g., microparticles (MPs), scaffolds) fabricated from the Food and Drug Administration (FDA)-approved polymer, poly(lactic-co-glycolic acid) (PLGA). OVA was pre-adsorbed onto the polymeric biomaterial carriers which were then inserted in C57BL/6 mice to determine the adjuvant nature of the biomaterials. Total anti-OVA IgG serum levels were used as the measure to compare the biomaterial vehicles against the well-known complete Freund's adjuvant (CFA; positive control). They found that OVA-adsorbed or co-delivered with carrier biomaterials including nonbiodegradable, polystyrene MPs and 75:25 PLGA MPs supported moderate humoral immune responses for an 18-week period. Moreover, the response was T_h2-driven as evidenced by the predominant IgG1 isotype antibody. This finding was further corroborated by the *in vivo* proliferation levels of fluorescently labeled, OVA-specific CD4$^+$ T-cells from transgenic OT-II mice in the presence of OVA delivered by biomaterial carriers, which were comparable to that of OVA combined with CFA. The common link between the biomaterial carriers, co-delivered antigen, and the observed adaptive immunity is the maturation of APCs, particularly DC maturation.

These experiments suggested that biomaterials (e.g., 75:25 PLGA; copolymer whose composition is 75% lactic acid and 25% glycolic acid) may promote the presentation of "danger signals" which elicit DC activation. As such, researchers have begun to take a closer look at the phenotype of DCs following biomaterial interaction. Yoshida and Babensee (2004) examined the phenotypic response of human Mo-DCs to treatment with 75:25 PLGA MPs or film in comparison to LPS-treated DC (for a positive control of matured DCs) and untreated iDCs (negative control). After 24 h exposure to the PLGA MPs and to a lesser extent PLGA films, they found DCs had elevated levels of expression of positively stimulatory molecules (CD40, CD80, CD83, and CD86), and MHC class II molecules (HLA-DQ and HLA-DR) compared to that of the iDC-negative control, but lower than that of LPS-matured DCs. Further, 75:25 PLGA MP-treated DCs display a "stellate" morphology with extended cellular processes, similar to that of mature DCs, and enhance proliferation of T-cells in an allogeneic mixed lymphocyte reaction (MLR). This report supports the claim that 75:25 PLGA can stimulate maturation of human Mo-DCs, and maturation may depend on the form of the biomaterial (Yoshida and Babensee, 2004). Yoshida and Babensee also confirmed that mDC responses to 75:25 PLGA films and MPs were independent of species, as comparable reactions to those described above with human Mo-DCS were observed using bone-marrow-derived DCs from C57BL/6 mice. Further, comparison of maturation states and cytokine secretion profiles of PLGA MP-treated DCs, PLGA film-exposed DC and untreated DCs suggest that DC activation may be contact-dependent (Yoshida and Babensee, 2006). Yoshida and coworkers also performed transmigration well studies to determine whether biomaterial-induced DC maturation was due to direct contact or mediated by soluble factors released from the material. This study established that direct contact with the biomaterial (75:25 PLGA) was required for biomaterial-induced DC maturation (Yoshida et al., 2007). Building on these reports, Park et al. (2015) comprehensively investigated the different pheno-typic changes in human Mo-DCs following exposure to a range of biomaterials com-monly used in combinatorial tissue engineering products. These biomaterials included films of alginate, agarose, chitosan, hyaluronic acid, and 75:25 PLGA. A complete array of immuno-phenotypic tests was performed on biomaterial-treated DCs includ-ing morphology, positively stimulatory molecule expression, MLR, NF-κB activity, and pro-inflammatory cytokine secretion assessments. Overall, differential effects of DC maturation were induced by different biomaterial films after 24 h exposure time period. More specifically, PLGA or chitosan films induced DC maturation, with higher levels of DC allo-stimulatory capacity, pro-inflammatory cytokine release, and expres-sion of CD80, CD86, CD83, HLA-DQ, and CD44 compared with iDCs. Alginate films evoked an increase in pro-inflammatory cytokine release as well as a decrease in CD44 expression. Whereas, hyaluronic acid films elicited suppressive effects on DC phenotype, with reduced expression of CD40, CD80, CD86, and HLA-DR observed, compared to iDCs.

It should be noted that other reports have described 50:50 PLGA (copoly-mer whose composition is 50% lactic acid and 50% glycolic acid) particles as being immune-inert systems that function only as vehicles (Waeckerle-Men and Groettrup, 2005). A study by Lewis et al. (2014) also supported the latter case, but differences in the PLGA compositions used are a likely explanation. The more hydrophobic nature of the 75:25 PLGA polymer compared to 50:50 PLGA may be a driving factor, as the more hydrophobic polymer will persist longer, and the composition and conformation of surface-adsorbed proteins are expected to be different. Interestingly, there are reports that the degradation products of PLGA into it constituent monomers, particularly lac-tic acid, can downregulate stimulatory molecules on DCs following exposure, which suggests that the time of DC exposure to this polymer may also be a factor (Gottfried et al., 2006; Kreutz et al., 2004).

Effect of biomaterial surface chemistry on DC phenotype

The finding that different biomaterials, and compositions, could prompt a variety of immuno-phenotypic changes in DCs compelled scientists to explore the relationship between biomaterial chemistry and DC maturation. To this extent, Shankar et al. inves-tigated how defined material surface chemistries modulated DC phenotype. DCs were cultured on self-assembled monolayers (SAM) surfaces of alkanethiols terminated with defined chemical groups, of either $-CH_3$, $-OH$, $-COOH$, and $-NH_2$, and assessed DC maturation based on cell morphology, allo-stimulatory capacity, and expres-sion of positive stimulatory molecules. DCs treated with $-OH$, $-COOH$, or $-NH_2$

SAMs showed moderate maturation, while DCs treated with $-CH_3$ SAMs were least mature based on the surface expression of markers. However, $-CH_3$ SAM-treated DCs treated elicited secretion of the highest levels of pro-inflammatory TNF-α and IL-6, despite being the least mature. Additionally, increased levels of apoptotic markers were observed for DCs and T-cells in contact with CH_3 SAMs. Various reports have shown that phagocytosis of apoptotic DCs has strong immunosuppressive effects on DCs; therefore, the increased number of apoptotic DCs on CH_3 SAMs may account for lower DC maturation. Finally, higher expression of cytotoxic T-lymphocyte-associated antigen receptor-4 (CTLA-4) on T-cells was shown, suggesting a mechanism of T-cell inhibition on CH_3 SAMs (Shankar et al., 2010a,b).

DC maturation responses to biomaterial surface roughness

Scientists have also sought to determine the correlation between biomaterial surface roughness and DC maturation. In a study by Kou et al., DCs were seeded on clinical dental titanium (Ti) surfaces with defined chemistries and surface roughness. More specifically, DCs were treated with Ti either pretreated (PT; smooth finish), grit-blasted and acid-etched (SLA), and hydrophilic SLA (modSLA). The roughness (R_a) of each of these surfaces was determined and found to be in the following increasing order: tissue culture polystyrene (control; TCPS) < PT (0.6 μm) < SLA = mod-SLA (3.97 μm). Surface energies of these Ti surfaces, measured in terms of water–air contact angle, were approximately 96°, 138.3°, and 0° for PT, SLA, and modSLA respectively. They found that DC maturation-associated markers were upregulated in a substrate-dependent manner. More specifically, DCs cultured on PT and SLA Ti surfaces showed significantly increased expression levels of CD86 in comparison to TCPS-seeded iDCs. The morphology of PT- and SLA-treated DCs, as determined by scanning electron microscopy, was demonstrated to be similar to that of LPS-matured DCs further suggesting that these substrates support DC maturation. Contrastingly, modSLA-treated DCs exhibited morphology close to that of iDCs. Additionally, PT surfaces stimulated increased secretion of IL-1ra from DCs in comparison to all other investigated substrates (SLA, modSLA). However, cytokine secretion of TNF-α, MIP-1α, and IL-10 was found to be statistically comparable for DCs treated on the different Ti surfaces. Given that SLA- and modSLA-treated substrates possess comparable surface roughness and microarchitecture, these results suggest that surface energy (and indirectly surface chemistry) is a more definitive factor in the polarization of DC maturation by biomaterial surfaces. Moreover, surface chemical composition analysis in conjunction with principal component analysis indicates that increasing surface carbon or surface nitrogen induces a mature DC phenotype, whereas increasing surface oxygen, or surface titanium promotes an immature DC phenotype (Kou et al., 2011, 2012).

Mechanisms involved in DC–biomaterial interactions

The mechanisms by which DCs recognize and respond to biomaterials are yet to be completely clarified. One hypothesis is that biomaterials activate DCs by triggering receptors and signaling cascades of the pathogen recognition receptors (PRRs), particularly the TLRs, C-type lectin receptors, and complement receptors (Babensee, 2008). Recently, Shokouhi et al. investigated the role of the TLR/MyD88 recognition and signaling cascade in DC responses to a number of physically and chemically diverse biomedical polymers. This group demonstrated that DCs from mice lacking TLRs (particularly TLR 2, TLR4, and TLR6) or MyD88 had reduced expression levels of activation markers (MHCII, CD40, CD80, and CD86) and inflammatory cytokines (IL-1β, IL-6, IL-10, IL-12p40, RANTES, and TNF-α), in comparison to wild-type controls. Further, DCs from murine wild-type systems were responsive to biomaterial as well as LPS stimulation and induced proliferation of antigen-specific T-cells. Taken altogether, these data suggest that engagement of PRRs such as TLRs can profoundly influence DC phenotype (Shokouhi et al., 2010). The ligands that bind and activate these receptors are termed "danger signals" and are constituted by proteins and carbohydrate moieties in the adsorbed protein layer on biomaterial surfaces following implantation (Kou and Babensee, 2011).

A number of reports have chronicled the recognition and responses of DCs to biomaterial-adsorbed protein layer dictated by the underlying surface chemistry (Shankar et al., 2010a,b; Kou et al., 2011, 2012). Moreover, a number of non-PRR receptors including Fc receptors and integrins have been implicated to play a role in the DC responses to biomaterial surfaces, in an adhesion-dependent manner. For instance, Acharya et al. demonstrated that different adsorbed, adhesive protein (fibronectin, laminin, collagen type I, vitronectin, fibrinogen, bovine serum albumin, and fetal bovine serum (control)) layers on biomaterials could influence DC morphology, co-stimulatory molecule expression, cytokine production, and allo-stimulatory capacity. They reported that adhesive substrates supported similar levels of DC adhesion and expression of positively stimulatory molecules. DC morphology and production of pro- and anti-inflammatory cytokines (IL-12p40 and IL-10, respectively) varied in an adhesive substrate-dependent manner. For example, DCs cultured on collagen and vitronectin substrates generated higher levels of IL-12p40, whereas DCs cultured on albumin and serum-coated tissue culture-treated substrates produce the higher levels of IL-10 compared to other substrates. Further, substrate-dependent modulation of DC IL-12p40 cytokine production correlated well with CD4$^+$ T-cell proliferation and Th1 type response in terms of IFN-γ producing T_h cells (Acharya et al., 2008). From this and other studies (Brand et al., 1998; Acharya et al., 2010, 2011), we can surmise that rationally designed biomaterials may direct the presentation, orientation, and conformation of the adsorbed layer of protein (following implantation) which may serve to influence DC phenotype and functionality. Biomaterial design represents a nonpharmacological tool, through which host immune responses can be modulated for applications in tissue engineering and immunotherapy.

CONCLUSION—DC ROLE IN HOST RESPONSES TO BIOMATERIALS

The advent and application of synthetic polymers at the end of the nineteenth century resulted in an explosion of implantable materials to correct or treat medical problems. For example, tissue engineering has recently emerged as a viable therapeutic method in regenerative medicine to regrow/replace damaged or diseased tissue. This strategy often employs biomaterial scaffolds in combination with relevant cells to recapitulate dysfunctional tissues and organs. However, once implanted, these constructs face a number of challenges, particularly the mammalian immune system. It is well known that innate immune cells including macrophages and DCs infiltrate the biomaterial implant site. However, the role of DCs in the body's response is still under investigation. This chapter presented a review of DC biology and DC responses to bulk biomaterials. DCs are positioned to play a key balancing role in opposing aspects including the suppression of chronic pro-inflammatory responses to the implant, and conversely, activation of pro-inflammatory T- and B-cells in the context of combinational products. There is promise that with careful material design, application-specific DC responses to biomaterial constructs may be dictated. It is anticipated that a more complete understanding of DC responses to biomaterial implantation will drive the development of novel strategies to circumvent host immunity and ultimately improve biomedical device integration and functionality.

REFERENCES

Acharya, A.P., Dolgova, N.V., Clare-Salzler, M.J., Keselowsky, B.G., 2008. Adhesive substrate-modulation of adaptive immune responses. Biomaterials 29, 4736–4750.

Acharya, A.P., Dolgova, N.V., Moore, N.M., Xia, C.Q., Clare-Salzler, M.J., Becker, M.L., et al., 2010. The modulation of dendritic cell integrin binding and activation by RGD-peptide density gradient substrates. Biomaterials 31, 7444–7454.

Acharya, A.P., Dolgova, N.V., Xia, C.Q., Clare-Salzler, M.J., Keselowsky, B.G., 2011. Adhesive substrates modulate the activation and stimulatory capacity of non–obese diabetic mouse-derived dendritic cells. Acta. Biomater. 7, 180–192.

Akira, S., Uematsu, S., Takeuchi, O., 2006. Pathogen recognition and innate immunity. Cell 124, 783–801.

Anderson, J.M., 2001. Biological responses to materials. Annu. Rev. Mater. Res. 31, 81–110.

Anderson, J.M., Rodriguez, A., Chang, D.T., 2008. Foreign body reaction to biomaterials. Semin. Immunol. 20, 86–100.

Ardavin, C., Wu, L., Li, C.L., Shortman, K., 1993. Thymic dendritic cells and T-cells develop simultaneously in the thymus from a common precursor population. Nature 362, 761–763.

Ardavin, C., Amigorena, S., Reis e Sousa, C., 2004. Dendritic cells: immunobiology and cancer immunotherapy. Immunity 20, 17–23.

Arinzeh, T.L., Peter, S.J., Archambault, M.P., van den Bos, C., Gordon, S., Kraus, K., et al., 2003. Allogeneic mesenchymal stem cells regenerate bone in a critical-sized canine segmental defect. J. Bone. Joint Surg. Am. 85A, 1927–1935.

Aspenstrom, P., 1999. The Rho GTPases have multiple effects on the actin cytoskeleton. Exp. Cell. Res. 246, 20–25.

Babensee, J.E., 2008. Interaction of dendritic cells with biomaterials. Semin. Immunol. 20, 101–108.

Banchereau, J., Steinman, R.M., 1998. Dendritic cells and the control of immunity. Nature 392, 245–252.

Banchereau, J., Briere, F., Caux, C., Davoust, J., Lebecque, S., Liu, Y.T., et al., 2000. Immunobiology of dendritic cells. Annu. Rev. Immunol. 18, 767.

Bandyopadhyay, A., Fine, R.L., Demento, S., Bockenstedt, L.K., Fahmy, T.M., 2011. The impact of nanoparticle ligand density on dendritic-cell targeted vaccines. Biomaterials 32, 3094–3105.

Belz, G.T., Carbone, F.R., Heath, W.R., 2002. Cross-presentation of antigens by dendritic cells. Crit. Rev. Immunol. 22, 439–448.

Bjorck, P., Kincade, P.W., 1998a. CD19(+) pro-B cells can develop into dendritic cells *in vitro*. J. Leukoc. Biol., 17.

Bjorck, P., Kincade, P.W., 1998b. Cutting edge: CD19(+) pro-B cells can give rise to dendritic cells *in vitro*. J. Immunol. 161, 5795–5799.

Brand, U., Bellinghausen, I., Enk, A.H., Jonuleit, H., Becker, D., Knop, J., et al., 1998. Influence of extracellular matrix proteins on the development of cultured human dendritic cells. Eur. J. Immunol. 28, 1673–1680.

Brodbeck, W.G., Anderson, J.M., 2009. Giant cell formation and function. Curr. Opin. Hematol. 16, 53–57.

Cao, W., 2009. Molecular characterization of human plasmacytoid dendritic cells. J. Clin. Immunol. 29, 257–264.

Cao, T., Ueno, H., Glaser, C., Fay, J.W., Palucka, A., Banchereau, J., 2007. Both Langerhans cells and interstitial DC cross-present melanoma antigens and efficiently activate antigen-specific CTL. Eur. J. Immunol. 37, 2657–2667.

Capo, J.T., Kokko, K.P., Rizzo, M., Adams, J.E., Shamian, B., Abernathie, B., et al., 2014. The use of skin substitutes in the treatment of the hand and upper extremity. Hand (New York, N.Y.) 9, 156–165.

Cella, M., Jarrossay, D., Facchetti, F., Alebardi, O., Nakajima, H., Lanzavecchia, A., et al., 1999. Plasmacytoid monocytes migrate to inflamed lymph nodes and produce large amounts of type I interferon. Nat. Med. 5, 919–923.

Cohn, L., Chatterjee, B., Esselborn, F., Smed-Soerensen, A., Nakamura, N., Chalouni, C., et al., 2013. Antigen delivery to early endosomes eliminates the superiority of human blood BDCA3(+) dendritic cells at cross presentation. J. Exp. Med. 210, 1049–1063.

Dopheide, J.F., Obst, V., Doppler, C., Radmacher, M.C., Scheer, M., Radsak, M.P., et al., 2012. Phenotypic characterisation of pro-inflammatory monocytes and dendritic cells in peripheral arterial disease. Thromb. Haemost. 108, 1198–1207.

Fadilah, S.A.W., Cheong, S.K., 2007. Dendritic cell immunobiology and potential roles in immunotherapy. Malays. J. Pathol. 29, 1–18.

Giannoukakis, N., 2013. Tolerogenic dendritic cells for type 1 diabetes. Immunotherapy 5, 569–571.

Gottfried, E., Kunz-Schughart, L.A., Ebner, S., Mueller-Klieser, W., Hoves, S., Andreesen, R., et al., 2006. Tumor-derived lactic acid modulates dendritic cell activation and antigen expression. Blood 107, 2013–2021.

Han, S.K., Kim, S.Y., Choi, R.J., Jeong, S.H., Kim, W.K., 2014. Comparison of tissue-engineered and artificial dermis grafts after removal of basal cell carcinoma on face—a pilot study. Dermatol. Surg. 40, 460–467.

Hynes, R.O., 2002. Integrins: bidirectional, allosteric signaling machines. Cell 110, 673–687.

Jacobs, B., Wuttke, M., Papewalis, C., Selssler, J., Schott, M., 2008. Dendritic cell subtypes and *in vitro* generation of dendritic cells. Horm. Metab. Res. 40, 99–107.

de Jong, E.C., Smits, H.H., Kapsenberg, M.L., 2005. Dendritic cell-mediated T cell polarization. Springer. Semin. Immunopathol. 26, 289–307.

Jung, S.Y., Lim, S.M., Albertorio, F., Kim, G., Gurau, M.C., Yang, R.D., 2003. The vroman effect: a molecular level description of fibrinogen displacement. J. Am. Chem. Society 125, 12782–12786.

Kapsenberg, M.L., 2003. Dendritic-cell control of pathogen-driven T-cell polarization. Nat. Rev. Immunol. 3, 984–993.

Keselowsky, B.G., Garcia, A.J., 2005. Quantitative methods for analysis of integrin binding and focal adhesion formation on biomaterial surfaces. Biomaterials 26, 413–418.

Keselowsky, B.G., Collard, D.M., Garcia, A.J., 2003. Surface chemistry modulates fibronectin conformation and directs integrin binding and specificity to control cell adhesion. J. Biomed. Mater. Res. A. 66A, 247–259.

Keselowsky, B.G., Collard, D.M., Garcia, A.J., 2004. Surface chemistry modulates focal adhesion composition and signaling through changes in integrin binding. Biomaterials 25, 5947–5954.

Keselowsky, B.G., Collard, D.M., Garcia, A.J., 2005. Integrin binding specificity regulates biomaterial surface chemistry effects on cell differentiation. Proc. Natl. Acad. Sci. USA. 102, 5953–5957.

Keselowsky, B., Wang, L., Schwartz, Z., Garcia, A., Boyan, B., 2007. Integrin alpha(5) controls osteoblastic proliferation and differentiation responses to titanium substrates presenting different roughness characteristics in a roughness independent manner. J. Biomed. Mater. Res. A. 80A, 700–710.

Kohl, K., Schnautz, S., Pesch, M., Klein, E., Aumailley, M., Bieber, T., et al., 2007. Subpopulations of human dendritic cells display a distinct phenotype and bind differentially to proteins of the extracellular matrix. Eur. J. Cell. Biol. 86, 719–730.

Kohm, A.P., Carpentier, P.A., Anger, H.A., Miller, S.D., 2002. Cutting edge: CD4(+)CD25(+) regulatory T cells suppress antigen-specific autoreactive immune responses and central nervous system inflammation during active experimental autoimmune encephalomyelitis. J. Immunol. 169, 4712–4716.

Kou, P.M., Babensee, J.E., 2011. Macrophage and dendritic cell phenotypic diversity in the context of biomaterials. J. Biomed. Mater. Res. A. 96A, 239–260.

Kou, P.M., Schwartz, Z., Boyan, B.D., Babensee, J.E., 2011. Dendritic cell responses to surface properties of clinical titanium surfaces. Acta. Biomater. 7, 1354–1363.

Kou, P.M., Pallassana, N., Bowden, R., Cunningham, B., Joy, A., Kohn, J., et al., 2012. Predicting biomaterial property–dendritic cell phenotype relationships from the multivariate analysis of responses to polymethacrylates. Biomaterials 33, 1699–1713.

Kreutz, M., Gottfried, E., Kunz-Ghart, L., Hoves, S., Andreesen, R., Muller-Klieser, W., 2004. Tumor-derived lactic acid modulates dendritic cell activation and differentiation. Blood 104, 147B.

Lan, M.A., Gersbach, C.A., Michael, K.E., Keselowsky, B.G., Garcia, A.J., 2005. Myoblast proliferation and differentiation on fibronectin-coated self assembled monolayers presenting different surface chemistries. Biomaterials 26, 4523–4531.

Langer, R., Vacanti, J.P., 1993. Tissue engineering. Science 260, 920–926.

Langer, R., Tirrell, D.A., 2004. Designing materials for biology and medicine. Nature 428, 487–492.

Lewis, J.S., Zaveri, T.D., Crooks, C.P., Keselowsky, B.G., 2012. Microparticle surface modifications targeting dendritic cells for non-activating applications. Biomaterials 33, 7221–7232.

Lewis, J.S., Dolgova, N.V., Chancellor, T.J., Acharya, A.P., Karpiak, J.V., Lele, T.P., et al., 2013. The effect of cyclic mechanical strain on activation of dendritic cells cultured on adhesive substrates. Biomaterials 34, 9063–9070.

Lewis, J.S., Roche, C., Zhang, Y., Brusko, T.M., Wasserfall, C.H., Atkinson, M., et al., 2014. Combinatorial delivery of immunosuppressive factors to dendritic cells using dual-sized microspheres. J. Mater. Chem. B 2, 2562–2574.

Lu, D., Mahmood, A., Qu, C., Hong, X., Kaplan, D., Chopp, M., 2007. Collagen scaffolds populated with human marrow stromal cells reduce lesion volume and improve functional outcome after traumatic brain injury. Neurosurgery 61, 596–602.

Lundberg, K., Rydnert, F., Greiff, L., Lindstedt, M., 2014. Human blood dendritic cell subsets exhibit discriminative pattern recognition receptor profiles. Immunology 142, 279–288.

MacDonald, K.P.A., Munster, D.J., Clark, G.J., Dzionek, A., Schmitz, J., Hart, D.N.J., 2002. Characterization of human blood dendritic cell subsets. Blood 100, 4512–4520.

Madruga, J., Koritschoner, N.P., Diebold, S.S., Kurz, S.M., Zenke, M., 1999. Polarised expression pattern of focal contact proteins in highly motile antigen presenting dendritic cells. J. Cell. Sci. 112, 1685–1696.

Makela, P.H., 2000. Vaccines, coming of age after 200 years. FEMS. Microbiol. Rev. 24, 9–20.

Matsue, H., Edelbaum, D., Hartmann, A.C., Morita, A., Bergstresser, P.R., Yagita, H., et al., 1999. Dendritic cells undergo rapid apoptosis *in vitro* during antigen-specific interaction with CD4(+) T cells. J. Immunol. 162, 5287–5298.

Matzelle, M.M., Babensee, J.E., 2004. Humoral immune responses to model antigen co-delivered with biomaterials used in tissue engineering. Biomaterials 25, 295–304.

Mauney, J.R., Nguyen, T., Gillen, K., Kirker-Head, C., Gimble, J.M., Kaplan, D.L., 2007. Engineering adipose-like tissue *in vitro* and *in vivo* utilizing human bone marrow and adipose-derived mesenchymal stem cells with silk fibroin 3D scaffolds. Biomaterials 28, 5280–5290.

McIlroy, D., Troadec, C., Grassi, F., Samri, A., Barrou, B., Autran, B., et al., 2001. Investigation of human spleen dendritic cell phenotype and distribution reveals evidence of *in vivo* activation in a subset of organ donors. Blood 97, 3470–3477.

Nakahara, M., Nagayama, Y., Ichikawa, T., Yu, L., Eisenbarth, G.S., Abiru, N., 2011. The effect of regulatory T-cell depletion on the spectrum of organ-specific autoimmune diseases in nonobese diabetic mice at different ages. Autoimmunity 44, 504–510.

van Nimwegen, M.J., van de Water, B., 2007. Focal adhesion kinase: a potential target in cancer therapy. Biochem. Pharmacol. 73, 597–609.

Paglia, P., Colombo, M.P., 1999. Presentation of tumor antigens—the role of dendritic cells. Minerva Biotecnologica 11, 261–270.

Park, J., Gerber, M.H., Babensee, J.E., 2015. Phenotype and polarization of autologous T cells by biomaterial-treated dendritic cells. J. Biomed. Mater. Res. A. 103, 170–184.

Patterson, S., Rae, A., Donaghy, H., 2001. Purification of dendritic cells from peripheral blood. Methods. Mol. Med. 64, 111–120.

Pei, M., He, F., Boyce, B., Kish, V., 2009. Repair of full-thickness femoral condyle cartilage defects using allogeneic synovial cell-engineered tissue constructs. Osteoarthr. Cartil. 17, 714–722.

Quint, C., Arief, M., Muto, A., Dardik, A., Niklason, L.E., 2012. Allogeneic human tissue-engineered blood vessel. J. Vasc. Surg. 55, 790–798.

Randolph, G.J., Inaba, K., Robbiani, D.F., Steinman, R.M., Muller, W.A., 1999. Differentiation of phagocytic monocytes into lymph node dendritic cells *in vivo*. Immunity 11, 753–761.

Robinson, S.P., Patterson, S., English, N., Davies, D., Knight, S.C., Reid, C.D.L., 1999. Human peripheral blood contains two distinct lineages of dendritic cells. Eur. J. Immunol. 29, 2769–2778.

Romer, L.H., Birukov, K.G., Garcia, J.G.N., 2006. Focal adhesions—paradigm for a signaling nexus. Circ. Res. 98, 606–616.

Saeki, H., Moore, A.M., Brown, M.J., Hwang, S.T., 1999. Cutting edge: secondary lymphoid-tissue chemokine (SLC) and CC chemokine receptor 7 (CCR7) participate in the emigration pathway of mature dendritic cells from the skin to regional lymph nodes. J. Immunol. 162, 2472–2475.

Sakiyama-Elbert, S.E., Hubbell, J.A., 2000. Controlled release of nerve growth factor from a heparin-containing fibrin-based cell ingrowth matrix. J. Control. Release 69, 149–158.

Salomon, B., Lenschow, D.J., Rhee, L., Ashourian, N., Singh, B., Sharpe, A., et al., 2000. B7/CD28 costimulation is essential for the homeostasis of the CD4(+)CD25(+) immunoregulatory T cells that control autoimmune diabetes. Immunity 12, 431–440.

Scalapino, K.J., Tang, Q., Bluestone, J.A., Bonyhadi, M.L., Daikh, D.I., 2006. Suppression of disease in New Zealand Black/New Zealand White lupus-prone mice by adoptive transfer of *ex vivo*, expanded regulatory T cells. J. Immunol. 177, 1451–1459.

Schense, J.C., Hubbell, J.A., 2000. Three-dimensional migration of neurites is mediated by adhesion site density and affinity. J. Biol. Chem. 275, 6813–6818.

Shankar, S.P., Chen, I.I., Keselowsky, B.G., Garcia, A.J., Babensee, J.E., 2010a. Profiles of carbohydrate ligands associated with adsorbed proteins on self-assembled monolayers of defined chemistries. J. Biomed. Mater. Res. A. 92A, 1329–1342.

Shankar, S.P., Petrie, T.A., Garcia, A.J., Babensee, J.E., 2010b. Dendritic cell responses to self-assembled monolayers of defined chemistries. J. Biomed. Mater. Res. A. 92A, 1487–1499.

Shokouhi, B., Coban, C., Hasirci, V., Aydin, E., Dhanasingh, A., Shi, N., et al., 2010. The role of multiple toll-like receptor signalling cascades on interactions between biomedical polymers and dendritic cells. Biomaterials 31, 5759–5771.

Shurin, G.V., Tourkova, I.L., Chatta, G.S., Schmidt, G., Wei, S., Djeu, J.Y., et al., 2005. Small rho GTPases regulate antigen presentation in dendritic cells. J. Immunol. 174, 3394–3400.

Steinbrink, K., Wolfl, M., Jonuleit, H., Knop, J., Enk, A.H., 1997. Induction of tolerance by IL-10-treated dendritic cells. J. Immunol. 159, 4772–4780.

Steinman, R.M., Hawiger, D., Nussenzweig, M.C., 2003. Tolerogenic dendritic cells. Annu. Rev. Immunol. 21, 685–711.

Summers, K.L., Hock, B.D., McKenzie, J.L., Hart, D.N.J., 2001. Phenotypic characterization of five dendritic cell subsets in human tonsils. Am. J. Pathol. 159, 285–295.

Svensson, M., Stockinger, B., Wick, M.J., 1997. Bone marrow-derived dendritic cells can process bacteria for MHC-I and MHC-II presentation to T cells. J. Immunol. 158, 4229–4236.

Swetman Andersen, C.A., Handley, M., Pollara, G., Ridley, A.J., Katz, D.R., Chain, B.M., 2006. beta1-Integrins determine the dendritic morphology which enhances DC-SIGN-mediated particle capture by dendritic cells. Int. Immunol. 18, 1295–1303.

Takakura, N., Watanabe, T., Suenobu, S., Yamada, Y., Noda, T., Ito, Y., et al., 2000. A role for hematopoietic stem cells in promoting angiogenesis. Cell 102, 199–209.

Takeda, K., Kaisho, T., Akira, S., 2003. Toll-like receptors. Annu. Rev. Immunol. 21, 335–376.

Tate, M.C., Garcia, A.J., Keselowsky, B.G., Schumm, M.A., Archer, D.R., LaPlaca, M.C., 2004. Specific beta(1) integrins mediate adhesion, migration, and differentiation of neural progenitors derived from the embryonic striatum. Mol. Cell. Neurosci. 27, 22–31.

Tourkova, I.L., Shurin, G.V., Wei, S., Shurin, M.R., 2007. Small Rho GTPases mediate tumor-induced inhibition of endocytic activity of dendritic cells. J. Immunol. 178, 7787–7793.

Van, D.E.R., Van Der, V.L.O.O., Jansen, J., Daha, M.R., Meijer, C.J.L.M., 1984. Analysis of lymphoid and dendritic cells in human lymph node tonsil and spleen a study using mono clonal and heterologous antibodies. Virchows Arch., B, Cell Pathol. 45, 169–186.

Vandenabeele, S., Wu, L., 1999. Dendritic cell origins: puzzles and paradoxes. Immunol. Cell. Biol. 77, 411–419.

Vasilijic, S., Savic, D., Vasilev, S., Vucevic, D., Gasic, S., Majstorovic, I., et al., 2005. Dendritic cells acquire tolerogenic properties at the site of sterile granulomatous inflammation. Cell. Immunol. 233, 148–157.

Velasquez-Lopera, M., Correa, L., Garcia, L., 2008. Human spleen contains different subsets of dendritic cells and regulatory T lymphocytes. Clin. Exp. Immunol. 154, 107–114.

Vulcano, M., Albanesi, C., Stoppacciaro, A., Bagnati, R., D'Amico, G., Struyf, S., et al., 2001. Dendritic cells as a major source of macrophage-derived chemokine/CCL22 in vitro and in vivo. Eur. J. Immunol. 31, 812–822.

Waeckerle-Men, Y., Groettrup, M., 2005. PLGA microspheres for improved antigen delivery to dendritic cells as cellular vaccines. Adv. Drug. Deliv. Rev. 57, 475–482.

www.clinicaltrials.gov and NCT01765244, 2014. Allogeneic tissue engineering (nanostructured artificial human cornea) in patients with corneal trophic ulcers in advanced stages, refractory to conventional (ophthalmic) treatment. 2014.

www.clinicaltrials.gov and NCT01242618, 2014. Tissue engineered nasal cartilage for reconstruction of the Alar Lobule.

www.clinicaltrials.gov and NCT01958502, 2014. Evaluation the treatment of nonunion of long bone fracture of lower extremities (femur and tibia) using mononuclear stem cells from the iliac wing within a 3-D tissue engineered scaffold. 2014.

Yoneno, K., Ohno, S., Tanimoto, K., Honda, K., Tanaka, N., Doi, T., et al., 2005. Multidifferentiation potential of mesenchymal stem cells in three-dimensional collagen gel cultures. J. Biomed. Mater. Res. A. 75A, 733–741.

Yoshida, M., Babensee, J.E., 2004. Poly(lactic-co-glycolic acid) enhances maturation of human monocyte-derived dendritic cells. J. Biomed. Mater. Res. A. 71A, 45–54.

Yoshida, M., Babensee, J.E., 2006. Differential effects of agarose and poly(lactic-co-glycolic acid) on dendritic cell maturation. J. Biomed. Mater. Res. A. 79A, 393–408.

Yoshida, M., Mata, J., Babensee, J.E., 2007. Effect of poly(lactic-co-glycolic acid) contact on maturation of murine bone marrow-derived dendritic cells. J. Biomed. Mater. Res. A. 80A, 7–12.

Zheng, Z.Y., Takahashi, M., Narita, M., Toba, K., Liu, A.C., Furukawa, T., et al., 2000. Generation of dendritic cells from adherent cells of cord blood by culture with granulocyte-macrophage colony-stimulating factor, interleukin-4, and tumor necrosis factor-alpha. J. Hematother. Stem. Cell. Res. 9, 453–464.

CHAPTER 8

The Acquired Immune System Response to Biomaterials, Including Both Naturally Occurring and Synthetic Biomaterials

Jonathan M. Fishman[1], Katherine Wiles[2] and Kathryn J. Wood[3]

[1]Honorary Clinical Lecturer University College London, UCL Institute of Child Health, London UK
[2]Department of Surgery, UCL Institute of Child Health, London, UK
[3]Transplantation Research Immunology Group, Nuffield Department of Surgical Sciences,
 University of Oxford John Radcliffe Hospital Headley Way, Headington, Oxford, UK

Contents

INTRODUCTION

Antigenicity versus immunogenicity

Antigenicity and immunogenicity are distinct aspects of the immune response that are both involved in the host response to biomaterials. "Antigenicity" describes the ability

Host Response to Biomaterials.
DOI: http://dx.doi.org/10.1016/B978-0-12-800196-7.00008-6

of a foreign material (antigen) to bind to, or interact with, the products of the final cell-mediated response such as B-cell or T-cell receptors. Antigenic determinants, or epitopes, are structural features on these antigens that interact with B-cell receptors, also known as antibodies or immunoglobulins. T-cell receptors recognize linear amino acid sequences within a protein antigen, also referred to as epitopes, when they combine with a major histocompatibility complex (MHC) molecule. An "immunogen," by contrast, initiates an immune response, first triggering the innate immune response and subsequently the adaptive (acquired) immune response, sensitizing the body to foreign antigens. Biomaterials, especially natural-derived allogenic, or xenogenic, materials, can act as immunogens. While all immunogenic materials are also antigenic, the reverse does not hold true. Thus, there are some molecules that are antigenic but not immunogenic by themselves. These include entities termed "haptens" such as metal ions. These play an important role in metal hypersensitivity postoperatively. Both antigenicity and immunogenicity, therefore, play a role in the host immune response to natural and synthetic biomaterials.

There are a myriad of factors that influence how immunogenic a foreign product is. Some of these criteria include the "foreignness" of the molecule, the type of molecule, and the composition of the molecule. Insoluble foreign materials are particularly immunogenic. In addition, proteins are generally more immunogenic than polysaccharides, lipids, and nucleic acids, respectively. The heterogeneity of a structure's complexity is also directly correlated with its immunogenicity. Since antigens must be phagocytosed and degraded before presentation to T-helper (Th) cells, the physical form of the foreign substance plays an integral role that influences, or dictates, the direction of the host immune response. For example, a denatured protein is usually more immunogenic than the same molecule in its native conformation. Additional factors that must be considered for the design and clinical application of biomaterial technology include the genetics of the recipient, the dosage to achieve optimal tolerance, the number of doses to be given, the route of administration, and the knock-on effects of adjuvants (Franz et al., 2011).

At a cellular level, antigenic determinants play a critical role in how the immune response is triggered through B- and T-cells. T-cells do not recognize antigens in a tertiary structure as mentioned above, but rather as peptide fragments. Internal linear, hydrophobic peptides are produced by antigen processing within an antigen presenting cell and are then bound to an MHC molecule. The MHC with its bound peptide may then be recognized by a T-cell receptor. It should be noted that some lipids and glycolipids can be presented by MHC-like molecules to T-cells. B-cells, on the other hand, can be triggered by the native tertiary conformation of the antigen in either soluble or membrane-bound form. The antigen must be accessible on the surface and therefore hydrophilic. No MHC is required as the B-cell receptor and secreted immunoglobulin can bind the soluble antigen. Large antigens may contain multiple B-cell epitopes with the potential to trigger the activation of multiple clones of B lymphocytes. An example thereof is collagen I whose three-dimensional helical conformation, centrally located amino acids, and terminal peptides have all been implicated as antigenic determinants. Collagen lacking in the terminal peptide has been produced and sold commercially; however, recent studies have demonstrated that interspecies antigenicity relies primarily on the centrally located amino acids (Lynn et al., 2004).

Developing strategies to either harness or suppress the adaptive immune response to foreign materials is a primary goal of clinical biomaterial usage. Lessons from transplantation, the most widely studied example of a foreign biomaterial, may help to inform the nascent investigations into the immunogenicity and antigenicity of natural, synthetic, and metallic biomaterials.

THE IMMUNE SYSTEM AND GRAFT REJECTION

Role of innate immune system in graft rejection

The innate immune system can be activated by microbial products, or endogenous proinflammatory ligands, the so-called damage associated molecular patterns, or DAMPs, that are released during mechanical, or ischemia/reperfusion injury (Murphy et al., 2011). These products are common to both transplant patients and to those undergoing surgery involving implantation of biomaterials. Some of the products associated with local tissue damage and ischemia include heat shock proteins, heparin sulfate, HMG box 1, and fibrinogen. These local mediators can all bind pattern recognition receptors found on cell types in the innate immune system. Furthermore, DAMPs, irrespective of whether they are nuclear or cytosolic proteins, lead to activation of the inflammasome. The inflammasome is a multiprotein complex that upregulates microRNA expression and secretes mediators which then upregulate cytokines such as IL-1, IL-6, TNF, and type I interferons (IFNs) (Wood et al., 2012; Wood and Goto, 2012; Carvalho-Gaspar et al., 2005). The innate immune system, although classically associated with acute phase rejection of transplants, also plays a role in the initiation of the adaptive immune system and the future development of graft tolerance. Even in the presence of almost complete depletion of T-cells, rejection still occurs due to monocyte, macrophage, and eosinophilic inflammation (Wu et al., 2006; Kirk et al., 2003). The complement system and the inflammatory response of phagocytes are therefore implicated in adaptive immune response-mediated graft rejection. Investigating the crosstalk between the innate and adaptive immune system may facilitate our understanding of the immune response toward biomaterials, so that their effects can be propagated or mitigated in order to achieve a favorable outcome.

Complement activation

Complement activation following implantation of biomaterials occurs in response to a number of current medical treatments, including but not limited to, insertion of catheters, prostheses, stents, and grafts. The complement cascade is a network of plasma proteins and cell surface receptors that recognize non-self-components and triggers one of the three pathways. An antigen–antibody complex triggers the classical pathway; carbohydrates trigger the lectin pathway; and foreign surfaces trigger the alternative pathway. Biomaterials, as one might expect, act primarily upon the alternative pathway. An important mediator of complement activation is the instant blood-mediated inflammatory reaction. The injury caused by surgical trauma leads to activation of the clotting cascade and endogenous upregulation of IgG and IgM, which then triggers complement, chondroitin sulfate, and tissue factor (Nilsson et al., 2010). Proteins such as albumin, gamma globulin, fibrinogen, fibronectin, vitronectin, and complement are adsorbed onto the surface of the biomaterial and activate complement (Anderson et al., 2008). Activation of complement leads to the conversion of C3 to C3a and C3b by the enzyme C3 convertase, C3bBb. The subsequent amplification loop generates the bulk of C3 activation. C3b can also bind covalently to cells, or other materials, triggering opsonization by macrophages and other phagocytic cells that express complement receptors. Further convertases then catalyze the conversion of C5 into C5a and C5b. C3a and C5a are potent anaphylatoxins, mediating acute inflammatory reactions. The final product of the complement pathway is the membrane attack complex comprising C5b–C59, which then punctures holes in the cell membrane thereby facilitating killing of foreign pathogens (Ricklin et al., 2010).

The effect of this very early immune response is to promote inflammatory (via complement as described above) and thrombotic (via chondroitin sulfate and tissue factor) reactions. The thrombotic pathway's products can bypass the early stages of the complement cascade in order to generate redundant complement activation (Ekdahl et al., 2011). Factor XIIa and Kallikrein, as well as thrombin and plasmin, can cleave complement components *in vitro* (Thoman et al., 1984). Furthermore, FXIa, FXa, and FIXa can bypass the convertases and directly generate C3a and C5a (Amara et al., 2010). C5a-mediated uptake of tissue factor induces coagulation of endothelial cells and neutrophils, highlighting the reciprocal effects of the thrombotic and inflammatory responses (Ikeda et al., 1997). How to modify this secondary effect on the innate immune response has yet to be determined, but given the unavoidability of tissue injury in surgical applications of biomaterials and the disastrous consequences of vessel occlusion postoperatively, the thrombotic pathway is a crucial area of further study.

Early studies suggest that the innate immune response affects the subsequent adaptive immune response. Peripheral synthesis of C3 is upregulated in transplant patients in proportion to the extent of cold time and the pathogenesis of tissue injury (Farrar et al., 2006). Initially elevated C3 expression has a negative effect on graft outcome 2–3 years postoperatively, suggesting that the initial reaction somehow modulates the adaptive immune system effect (Naesens et al., 2009). This adaptive response may be due to downstream products of the complement cascade. For example, sublytic, but lingering levels of the membrane attack complex, C5b–C9, lead to the production of pro-inflammatory cytokines, tissue necrosis factor (TNF), prostaglandins, intercellular adhesion molecule-1, tissue factor, and collagen (Qiu et al., 2012). Interestingly, these responses affect certain cell types more than others. Thus myocytes are preferentially affected following cardiovascular or intestinal injury, whereas tubular epithelial cells are typically preferentially affected following kidney failure (Thurman et al., 2006; Williams et al., 1999; Weisman et al., 1990). This selection seems to be due to complement "preference" toward these cell types. Suppressing this signature could overcome this vulnerability of myocytes and renal tubular epithelial cells.

Studies of the innate immune response to transplant grafts clearly suggest a relation between early injury and late distress (Sacks and Zhou, 2012). Donor production of complement is correlated with allograft kidney rejection in mice (Pratt et al., 2002). When CD55, an inhibitor of the complement cascade, was knocked out in a mouse heart transplant model, donor production of complement increased, leading to T-cell-mediated damage and rejection (Liu et al., 2005). Further studies have extended these findings to the human kidney, demonstrating complement-induced T-cell injury (Sacks and Zhou, 2012). The molecular mechanisms for this activation are beginning to be elucidated. C3a and C5a were demonstrated to be vital in the CD8+ T-cell-mediated rejection of a murine heart allograft model (Vieyra et al., 2011). C3a and C5a receptor signaling on CD4+ T-cells increases the level of the immune response against the foreign MHC (Li et al., 2004). C3a and C5a receptors also skew the differentiation of naive CD4+ T-cells toward Th1-type cells, which then mediate rejection through CD55 (Lalli et al., 2008; Strainic et al., 2008). CD55 therefore seems to play a dual role in complement activation and suppression. These transplant studies all highlight the importance of complement in the subsequent adaptive immune response to foreign materials. However, some biomaterials will not express antigens that can be recognized by T- or B-cells and therefore will have a different, or possibly no interplay, with the adaptive immune system. How important these differences will prove to be is currently unknown.

Chemotaxis and activation of phagocytes

Macrophages are the dominant infiltrating cells involved in the immune response toward foreign biomaterials (see the section "The Adaptive Host Immune Response to Biomaterials" and Chapters 2, 3, and 6). Macrophages respond to almost all biomaterials including metals, ceramics, cements, polymers, decellularized scaffolds, and collagen. Importantly, they remain within the biomaterial over its lifetime, mediating degradation, and resorption of the material via phagocytosis (Yahyouche et al., 2011; Valentin et al., 2009). Macrophages are initiators of the adaptive immune system, presenting antigen to primed T-cells and subsequently causing cell death in tandem with other elements of the immune system, including effector T-cells. However, macrophages are also essential for the recruitment and differentiation of cell types that will initiate the healing process (Xia and Triffitt, 2006). Macrophages are particularly important to understand as they are implicated in the development of constructive remodeling and immune tolerance toward biomaterials. Their activation and targeting in transplants may inform how the adaptive immune system responds to particular biomaterials.

Activation of the macrophage response occurs in response to a complex cascade of events. When host proteins from the extracellular matrix (ECM), or blood products, are adsorbed onto the foreign material's surface, they complex with the macrophage complement receptors (Xia and Triffitt, 2006). The complement anaphylatoxins C3a and C5a activate and recruit further macrophages, while target-bound C3 fragments facilitate the adherence of these responders to allografts (Li et al., 2012). Macrophages subsequently act as secreting cells, producing platelet-derived growth factor (PDGF), TNFα, IL-6, granulocyte and macrophage colony stimulating factor (G-CSF and M-CSF) to activate additional phagocytes (Anderson et al., 2008). M-CSF, in particular, is also produced via tubular epithelial cells in the kidney and by infiltrating leukocytes during acute rejection (Jose et al., 2003). Degranulating mast cells release histamine, which further recruits signaling factors (Zdolsek et al., 2007). Thus, there are convergent pathways by which macrophages are signaled.

Cytokines and other signaling molecules play an important role in the targeting of macrophages. The signaling factors that promote macrophage and monocyte transduction to their targets include transforming growth factor-β (TGFβ), PDGF, chemokine (C-X-C motif) ligand 4, leukotriene B4, nitric oxide, and IL-1. Some of these molecules have additional effects. Nitric oxide, for example, is also microbicidal and cytotoxic (Xia and Triffitt, 2006). While macrophages initially damage their targets, when subsequently recruited by cytokines IL-3 and IL-4, macrophages are also capable of inhibiting pro-inflammatory cytokines and contributing to wound repair (Gordon, 2003; Stein et al., 1992). Whether or not this switch is beneficial has yet to be determined. Some studies suggest that tissue response repair may be undesirable as occlusion of the native blood vessels may occur (as in the case of Budd–Chiari syndrome). The attachment of macrophages to natural versus synthetic biomaterials may have important effects. Integrins play a central role in the attachment of macrophages to allografts. However, macrophages may be undergoing apoptosis secondary to failed adhesion to foreign material such as metals, releasing toxic, and damaged waste products that further induce an immune response (Brodbeck et al., 2001). There is further evidence of both juxtacrine and paracrine signaling between macrophages and lymphocytes at the surface of biomaterials (Anderson et al., 2008). How to harness, or modulate, this response is beginning to be studied.

In chronic allograft necrosis, macrophage accumulation precedes and then correlates with long-term damage progression (Pilmore et al., 2000). Antibody induced or humoral activation of macrophages and monocytes is an important aspect of rejection. For example, the binding of IgG antibodies to FcγRIII receptors on natural killer cells can induce activation of monocyte cell function. Infiltrating leukocytes and the intrinsic parenchymal cells produce a host of factors including MCP-1, RANTES, MIP-1α, and MIF to implement this response (Fernández et al., 2002). Macrophages can also be activated classically through cell receptors. The antigen presenting cells (which include macrophages and dendritic cells) induce inflammation. These cells express pattern recognition receptors including Toll-like receptors (TLRs), scavenger receptors (SRs), and mannose receptors (MRs). TLRs recognize microbial products and trigger sentinel cell activation leading to downstream effects such as mast cell degranulation, recruitment of leukocytes via cytokines and chemokines, and the movement of inflammatory exudates (Xia and Triffitt, 2006). TLRs can also recognize and respond to DAMPs, including self-molecules such as nucleic acids from necrotic cells, ECM degradation products, and heat shock proteins. TLRs are an intriguing avenue of research into the immune response since in the transplant setting their activity has been shown to be inversely proportional to transplant tolerance (Iwasaki and Medzhitov, 2004). Animal models have demonstrated that animals deficient in MyD88 (an adaptor protein of TLRs) are more prone to the development of tolerance (Iwasaki and Medzhitov, 2004). Furthermore, after introducing TLR ligands into animals currently tolerating their grafts, rejection ensued (Chen et al., 2006; Thornley et al., 2006). How important the TLR pathway will be in biomaterials lacking in T-cells and MHCs has yet to be determined. Interestingly, studies of decellularized pulmonary valves (porcine and human) demonstrated that decellularization of the donor tissue decreases the subsequent monocyte response (Rieder et al., 2005).

Role of the acquired (adaptive) immune system in graft rejection

It has been evident since the earliest days of transplantation that the adaptive immune system plays a critical role in graft rejection. Understanding the mechanisms of the adaptive immune system in graft rejection may inform studies into the immune response toward biomaterials. This division of the adaptive immune response into the cell-mediated response and the antibody-mediated (or humoral response) is largely based on historical grounds but also provides a means to dichotomize the complicated machinations of the adaptive immune response. The cell-mediated response involves mostly T-cells and responds to any cell type with aberrant MHCs. Animal models have demonstrated that Th cells are both necessary and sufficient for allograft rejection, whereas regulatory T-cells (Tregs) are crucial for the development of immunological unresponsiveness and long-term tolerance (Murphy et al., 2011). Understanding the T-cell response to transplants will inform studies in biomaterials. The humoral response describes B-cells and antibodies that recognize antigens and pathogens circulating in the blood or lymphatics. In renal transplant failures, alloantibodies attack the peritubular and glomerular capillaries, while T-cells infiltrate tubules and the arterial endothelium, acting in tandem to destroy the graft (Colvin, 2007). There is considerable cross talk between these two facets of the adaptive immune response.

Humoral-mediated immunity

The humoral response to pathogens and antigens is mediated by B-cells, which recognize foreign substances in blood or lymph. Antigens bind to B-cells via the B-cell receptor expressed on the cell surface. Antigen recognition, together with cytokines produced by Th cells and the interaction between cell surface molecules such as C40 and CD154, results in co-stimulation of the responding B-cells, inducing them to proliferate and eventually differentiate into plasma cells whose primary product is secreted antibodies. B-cells also generate memory cells, which are instrumental in providing future immunity. Humoral-mediated immunity has been shown to be vital in both the rejection of allografts and the induction of tolerance.

Current thinking is that acute rejection is primarily T-cell-mediated except in the cases of hypersensitivity rejection, ABO incompatibility, transplants, and xenografts (Mauiyyedi et al., 2002). However, acute humoral rejection comprises at least 30% of acute rejection biopsies and is associated with a poor prognosis (Mauiyyedi et al., 2002). In late rejection, the humoral response may be even more important. Antibody-mediated microcirculation injury is the primary cause of late kidney transplant failure (Einecke et al., 2009). Indeed, most therapies target T-cell function: mycophenolic acid, T-cell antibodies, calcineurin inhibitors, rapamycin, and prednisolone. These drugs all increase graft survival by 88–95% at 1 year. However, acute rejection can still occur and chronic rejection is an all too familiar outcome following transplantation (Colvin and Smith, 2005). These findings suggest that the humoral immune response has an impact on long-term graft outcomes, and different approaches will be required to deal with the different pathways triggered. It is not clear what kind of humoral immune response exists toward biomaterials. ABO incompatibility may not be a problem; however, metals induce hypersensitivity and allografts and xenografts are being modified and used as biomaterials.

The understanding of antibody formation and pathology is well described in human allograft transplant models. Pretransplant donor-reactive antibodies correlate with acute rejection (Poggio et al., 2007). It has now been 20 years since Jeannet et al. (1970) showed that *de novo* specific antibodies are linked with poor transplant outcome. Furthermore, circulating post-transplant anti-donor alloreactive effector memory T (Tm) cells are also proportional to poor post-transplant outcomes (Bestard et al., 2008). There are several pathological stages of this antibody-mediated rejection that can be used for clinical diagnosis. Firstly, *de novo* generation of donor-reactive, or donor-specific antibodies, can be detected, but elicit no clinical response at least in the short term. When antibody reactivity and complement activation in the graft occur, C4d deposition in the peritubular and glomerular capillary endothelium may be found. Alloantibodies activate complement leading to tissue injury and coagulation (see the section "Complement Activation"). At this stage the graft is still functional, but pathological changes may begin to occur in conjunction with the presence of CD4+ T-cells. Macrophages are recruited and mediate phagocytosis and degradation of the foreign material (see the section "Chemotaxis and Activation of Phagocytes"). Finally, endothelial gene expression leads to arterial and basement membrane remodeling, giving rise to the lesions and endothelial dysfunction that is characteristic of transplant failure (Colvin and Smith, 2005). This graft dysfunction ultimately leads to failure.

How and where the humoral system is initially activated and whether and how it then leads to the cell-mediated immune response remains unclear. Some progress has, however, been made. Interestingly, humoral-mediated rejection has been demonstrated in patients with no prior exposure to antigen (Leech, 1998). It has been suggested that alloreactive Tm cells may be generated in these patients through cross-reactivity triggered by infection and/or homeostatic proliferation (Wu et al., 2004; Tough et al., 1996). In the presence of Tm cells, a mouse skin allograft was capable of inducing rejection of cardiac allografts that were being tolerated under the anti-CD154 monoclonal antibody protocol (Zhai et al., 2002). The importance of Tm cells may explain why even though there are many protocols capable of producing graft tolerance in mice, these protocols have failed in humans (Adams et al., 2003). As an alternative to pan-immunosuppression, it has been suggested that antigen-specific tolerance in Tm could be artificially activated (Brook et al., 2006). Kreuwel et al. (2002) demonstrated that tolerance to influenza hemaglutinin with CD8+ Tm could be generated either by soluble peptide or by cross-presentation of antigens by dendritic cells. How Tm cells will play a role in biomaterials is beginning to be elucidated (see the section "The Adaptive Host Immune Response to Biomaterials").

B-cell tolerance of transplants has been an area of increasing interest since the finding of B-cells with regulatory activity (Breg) (Wood et al., 2012). Rat models of long-term cardiac allograft tolerance induced by short-term immunosuppression suggest that tolerated allografts have a high number of B-cells and that the production thereof is regulated by the IgG alloantibody response (Le Texier et al., 2011). This could be because alloantibodies promote deviation of T-cells from a Th1 to a Th2 type, not activating *in vitro* donor endothelial cells but rather leading to cytoprotection. Suppressive Breg cells have even been generated *in vitro* from CD19+ B-cells (Rafei et al., 2009). These cells expressed MHC I and MHC II as well as IgM and IgD and secreted IL-10 similarly to native Breg cells. Interestingly, another study demonstrated that, in tolerant animals, an increase in B-cells was blocked at the IgM to IgG switch recombination. These B-cells were not IL-10 positive but rather expressed BANK-1 and Fcgr2b (Le Texier et al., 2011). These results suggest that there may be multiple populations of B-cells acting in allograft transplants, both positively and negatively. Indeed, targeted depletion of B-cells to prevent chronic rejection in humans has led to mixed results, perhaps due to the depletion of tolerant B-cells (Le Texier et al., 2011; Zarkhin et al., 2010). Further studies are necessary to elucidate how this switching occurs and if it can be harnessed for biomaterials.

Cell-mediated immunity

The cell–mediated response involves T-cell-mediated identification of infected or aberrant cells that are pathogenic, tumorigenic, or allogenically/xenogenically transplanted (Wood and Goto, 2012). T-cells are co-stimulated by antigen presenting cells displaying foreign alloantigens. For example, cytotoxic CD8+ T-cells are stimulated by antigen presenting cells expressing MHC I molecules and their bound peptides usually in the presence of "help" from CD4+ Th cells. When activated CD8+ T-cells encounter a target cell, they have the ability to release granules containing perforin and granzyme and secrete TNFα in order to mediate cell death (Anglicheau and Suthanthiran, 2008). By contrast, CD4+ Th cells recognize MHC II molecules and their bound peptides and are triggered to proliferate in the presence of co-stimulation. Th1 cells display delayed type hypersensitivity by releasing interleukins and other cytokines, which interact with B-cells to produce antibodies. These soluble mediators (in particular IL-1, IFNγ, and TNFα) interact with other cell types, such as natural killer cells, monocytes, eosinophils, and macrophages directing them to destroy foreign cells (Wood and Goto, 2012). An intriguing aspect of T-cell-mediated graft rejection is the difference between Th1 T-cells and Th2 T-cells (Badylak and Gilbert, 2008). Th1 cells release cytokines such as IL-2, IFNγ, and TNFβ, leading to macrophage activation, complement fixing antibody isotypes, and differentiation of CD8+ T-cells to the cytotoxic type (Abbas et al., 1996). In particular, this pathway is implicated in xenogenic transplant rejection (Chen et al., 1996). In contrast, the Th2-type pathway—and its interleukins IL-4, IL-5, IL-6, and IL-10—does not activate macrophages or complement fixing antibodies, but rather is implicated in both transplant acceptance and rejection (Allman et al., 2001; Piccotti et al., 1997).

After proliferating through many cell generations and in the presence of the appropriate microenvironment of cytokines, the Th cells can differentiate into effector cells, memory cells, or regulatory cells. There are at least three populations of Treg cells that are implicated in promoting graft tolerance: CD4+ Treg cells, CD8+ Treg cells, and CD4 − CD8− Treg cells (Wood et al., 2012). The population of CD25 + CD4+ T-cells gives rise to CD4+ Treg cells that, along with Breg cells and dendritic cells, can induce graft tolerance. Interestingly, at transplant, there are insufficient levels of CD4+ Treg cells in order to prevent initial rejection. However, pretreatment of mice with donor alloantigen generates a population of CD25 + CD4+ Treg cells capable of preventing skin allograft rejection (Karim et al., 2005). This bystander effect may prove to be a useful mechanism by which to induce graft tolerance. However, in practice, human allografts may actually induce Treg cells after prolonged exposure to alloantigen, which may explain why tolerance can develop (Tullius et al., 1997; Hamano et al., 1996). The second subpopulation of CD8+ Treg cells is produced via the CD8+ naive T-cell population and may be divided into two subtypes: CD8+ CD28− and CD8+ IL-10 producing cells. CD8+ CD28− Treg cells inhibit antigen presenting cell-mediated T-cell activation by direct cell contact-dependent mechanisms (Liu et al., 1999). When CD8+ Treg cells were given in combination with nongraft antigens, the Treg population facilitated cardiac allograft acceptance (Karim et al., 2005). This is another example of bystander activation in which third-party allografts may be suppressed. In this case, rejection was prevented as long as the Treg cells were exposed to the antigens before the adaptive transfer occurred. IL-10 producing CD8+ Treg cells have also been found in kidney transplant patients (Cai et al., 2004). Finally, CD4− CD8− Treg cells may also play a role in cell-mediated tolerance. In hematopoietic stem cell transplants, deficiency of this population is proportional to the extent of graft versus host disease. However, these cells are induced to express IFNγ, a mediator of rejection, by dendritic cells, which may undermine their utility (Hill et al., 2011). Modulating these populations could be of paramount importance in facilitating graft or biomaterial acceptance.

The key to harnessing tolerant cell populations may be through the use of cytokines. The role of cytokines in T-cell class switching in graft failure is highly complex. IFNγ plays an intriguing role in T-cell modulation (Wood and Sawitzki, 2006). It usually acts in an inflammatory capacity in the Th1-driven response mediating rejection, but through induced Tregs, IFNγ can control the immune response in other cells. Early production of IFNγ by Treg cells during an immune response directly inhibits activation and proliferation of immune effector cells. IFNγ, in this context, also creates a negative activation environment, influencing antigen presenting cells through nitric oxide, indoleamine 2,3 dioxygenase, and heme oxygenase expression (Refaeli et al., 2002). Mice deficient in Th1 cytokine IFNγ reject cardiac allografts rapidly (Konieczny et al., 1998). However, IFNγ is not both necessary and sufficient to cause allograft rejection. Both STAT4 and IL-17 seem to play a crucial role in Th1-mediated rejection. IL-17 producing CD4+ T-cells mediate accelerated allograft rejection with a very severe vascular inflammation and macrophage infiltration (Yuan et al., 2008). IL-2 may play a similarly important role during the initial T-cell response and subsequent control by Tregs in mediating tolerance (Malek and Bayer, 2004). T-bet, a Th1-specific transcription factor, plays a role in the development of the Th1 subtype. A mouse study has recently shown that Tbet −/− recipients developed accelerated allograft rejection when compared with controls (Yuan et al., 2008). The Th1 cytokines are not alone in their involvement in graft rejection. Th2 cytokines (IL-4, IL-5, IL-10, and IL-13) are primarily involved in promoting tolerance. In particular, the Th2 cytokine IL-10 has been found to inhibit primary T-cell responses (Rubtsov et al., 2008). However, Th2 cytokines are found in acute vascular rejection (Dallman, 1995). Understanding the complex interplay of cytokines is a crucial part of developing a therapeutic strategy to induce tolerance.

Ischemic reperfusion injury (see the section "Complement Activation") has an important role in the T-cell-mediated immune response. A study by Burne-Taney et al. (2006) demonstrated that ischemic preconditioning through splenectomy protects patients from future renal ischemic reperfusion injury. Low T-cell count is associated with a 10 times decrease in hepatic neutrophil release, a decrease in the level of necrosis, and a reduction of serum transaminase levels post-transplantation. Furthermore, CD4+, but not CD8+, T-cell population depletion inhibited this hepatic injury (Zwacka et al., 1997). A recent study into the visualization of the adaptive immune response and its role in graft rejection has helped to elucidate some of the underlying pathology (Celli et al., 2011). In a murine ear skin graft model, donor dermal dendritic cells initially migrated and were replaced by host mononuclear cells. The host cells captured donor antigen, went to the adjacent lymph node, and primed graft-reactive CD8+ T-cells. The CD8+ T-cells disseminated through the graft, and some were arrested. It is possible that host inflammatory mononuclear cells and dendritic cells within the graft may be a source for the initial antigen presenting cells ferrying antigen from the graft. These cells could then be activating alloreactive T-cells in the lymph node via an indirect pathway. Perhaps it is through this pathway that chronic graft rejection occurs. In such a scenario, T-cell tissue destruction would act in tandem with monocyte infiltration. However, this pathway would not be found in synthetic or metallic biomaterials and may help to explain some of their properties.

BIOMATERIALS AS SCAFFOLDS FOR TISSUE ENGINEERING

Biomaterials are traditionally defined as nonliving substances that are used in medical devices. This definition, however, is no longer sufficient (Campoccia et al., 2013). In the wake of decellularized scaffolds and cell-based therapies, a more appropriate definition may be any material intended to evaluate, treat, augment, or replace a tissue, organ, or bodily function (Nair and Laurencin, 2007). Fundamentally, however, one can agree upon the premise that biomaterials are substances that are designed to control or alter the biological environment inside the body. A biomaterial must, at minimum, have no sustained toxic response, a long shelf life, a degradation time proportional to healing time, and nontoxic clearance and metabolism. Additionally, in order to be used in surgical applications, a biomaterial must have appropriate tags for cell attachment, proliferation, migration, and differentiation as well as the delivery of growth factors where appropriate. Furthermore, a biomaterial's properties (porosity, tensile strength, compliance, and topography) must be in line with the tissue it endeavors to replace (Orlando et al., 2012; Nair and Laurencin, 2007). Ultimately, the immunogenicity of a biomaterial is integral to its successful implementation.

The first generation of biomaterials included bone cement, stainless steel, and poly-ethylene terephthalate. These materials were employed because they are mechanically stable and largely inert. However, these substances were quickly replaced by second-generation materials with specialized functions such as titanium (osseointegration), bioglass (tissue integration), biodegradable synthetic polymers (sutures), and natural polymers (dermal fillers) (Orlando et al., 2012). There are many subdivisions of bioma-terials based on their wide range of properties. Biomaterials may be injectable (hydro-gels, glues, self-assembled) or noninjectable (porous scaffolds, ECM mesh, ECM sheets, gels, sponges, sutures, microspheres, and nanofibers). Biomaterials may also be classed as small (staples, sutures, drug-delivery vehicles) or large (bone screws, bone plates, con-traception). Some biomaterials are adapted for use in soft/hard tissues (hip replace-ment, tooth replacements, outer ear reconstruction, etc.), whereas others interact directly with the vascular supply (heart valves, blood vessels, cardiopulmonary bypass, hemodialysis, plasmapheresis). The variable host responses to these biomaterials depend on many of the aforementioned properties, but in particular on the manufacturing process, rate of scaffold degradation (if at all), and the presence of cross-species antigen (Badylak and Gilbert, 2008). The main differences between natural-derived and syn-thetic biomaterials are highlighted in Table 8.1.

Table 8.1 Table outlining the major differences between naturally derived and synthetic biomaterials

Natural-derived	Synthetic
Composed of ECM components	Artificial materials (e.g., polyglycolic acid)
Hypo-immunogenic (if decellularized)	Increased likelihood of foreign body reaction following implantation
Improved biocompatibility	Biocompatibility somewhat dependent on implanted material
Tissue microarchitecture that resembles native tissue	Microarchitecture does not usually resemble native tissue
Enhanced bioactivity present if ECM constituents and growth factors preserved	Scaffold's bioactivity somewhat dependent on implanted material
Microvasculature maintained	Microvasculature rarely maintained
Less control over biodegradation characteristics	Biodegradation and porosity characteristics can be controlled to some extent
Less control over scaffold's biomechanical properties which depends on ECM components left behind	More control over material's biomechanical properties
Higher chance of microbial contamination during scaffold preparation and storage	Contamination less of a concern
Supply of ECM depends on availability of donor tissue	"Off-the-shelf" availability
Time required for tissue procurement and preparation (days to weeks)	Can be manufactured rapidly (hours to days)

Natural (decellularized) biomaterials

Natural biomaterials are still in their nascent stages of use. However, recent advances suggest that these biomaterials have a promising future. Natural biomaterials range from collagen to cell-based therapy to decellularized tissue scaffolds. Natural products have also found myriad uses as drug-delivery vehicles, surgical sutures, and whole tissue replacements. They are advantageous due to their biocompatibility; however, natural biomaterials are potentially immunogenic. Starting at the very smallest natural biomaterials, nanoparticles, there is still some concern as to their immunogenicity. Two studies describe antibody formation to C60 fullerene. In one study, the C60 antibodies had a cross-reactivity with C70 fullerene as well (Chen et al., 1998). In the other study, monoclonal antibodies to C60 were produced (Braden et al., 2000). Although these are the only studies currently suggesting the immunogenicity of something as simple as a carbon backbone, the results are worrying. Other studies have not replicated these results (Dobrovolskaia and McNeil, 2007). If an explanation for the discrepancy could be found, it might give insight into structures of drug-delivery vehicles. Given that increasing complexity and size correlate with a more robust immune response, natural biomaterials may be difficult to harness. Nevertheless, the processing of natural biomaterials has improved their outlook, and they have been successfully employed without immunosuppression, making them particularly advantageous over traditional allogenic transplants (Dobrovolskaia and McNeil, 2007).

Biomaterials have been extensively investigated as vehicles for cell-based approaches. Hematopoietic and mesenchymal stem cells (MSC) have been used in clinical pancreatic islet transplantation but have demonstrated little function (20–30% of what is expected) and face immediate destruction (Ryan et al., 2001). It appears that this response is primarily mediated by the innate immune system due to the instant blood-mediated inflammatory reaction when the islet cells contact the portal vein (Bennet et al., 1999). However, as discussed earlier, this blood-mediated reaction may also involve the adaptive immune response (see the section "Cell-Mediated Immunity"). These findings could be linked to islet transplantation and the site of implantation. Nevertheless, they highlight the possibility that certain forms of cell replacement therapy can elicit an immune response and cell transplants may exhibit a lower degree of "immune privilege" than solid organ transplants. On the other hand, embryonic stem cells have been shown to have decreased MHC expression and in their undifferentiated state do not stimulate T-cell expansion *in vitro* (Drukker et al., 2002). Furthermore under other conditions both mesenchymal and embryonic stem cells have been reported to suppress T-cell cytokine secretion and proliferation through the action of arginase I (Yachimovich-Cohen et al., 2010). Interestingly, however, differentiated embryonic stem cells elicit a very strong immune response and are rejected considerably quicker than their undifferentiated counterparts (Swijnenburg et al., 2005).

Robertson et al. (2007) found that ESC-derived TGFβ2 evoked immunological unresponsiveness and was expressed on differentiated cell types both *in vitro* and *in vivo*.

An intriguing model of the differences between transplants and biomaterials can be found in the study of islet pancreatic cell transplants. Islet pancreatic cell clusters generated *in vitro* are less susceptible to rejection by innate immune mechanisms than islet allografts. This observation ties in with the earlier hypothesis that biomaterials may not evoke as strong an innate immune response because they do not have leukocytes with antigen presenting cell capacity to mediate complement activation through the direct pathway (Boyd and Wood, 2010). Wu et al. demonstrated that implantation of differentiated embryonic stem cells into insulin expressing cells *in vivo* did elicit inflammatory cell infiltration of the graft site at 5 days postoperatively and that by 10 days after transplantation the cells had completely disappeared. The authors suggested that CD4+ T-cells could respond to MHC and minor histocompatibility complex mismatches to facilitate acute rejection of the implanted cells in tandem with CD8+ T-cells (Wu et al., 2001).

An alternative to using allogenic cells would be to utilize autologous-induced pluripotent stem cells (iPSCs). iPSCs are typically derived from the reprogramming, or reversion, of fully differentiated skin fibroblasts back into stem cells (Takahashi and Yamanaka, 2006). They are attractive for the following reasons: their abundance thereby offering a limitless supply of donor cells, potential widespread applications and lack of immunogenicity, although there is some controversy with respect to their immunogenicity (Araki et al., 2013; Guha et al., 2013; Zhao et al., 2011). In addition, autologous cells have the same genetic print as damaged, or diseased, cells and therefore without genetic correction may be limited in certain disease states where recipient cells display genetic anomalies. iPSCs also appear to have "memory" of their previous cell type, displaying aberrant features in culture (Kim et al., 2010). Furthermore, the introduction of expensive growth factors and cytokines raises concerns from a financial, safety (potentially tumorigenic), and immunological standpoint. Additional molecules may prove immunogenic in their own right. However, iPSCs remain a promising avenue for research since recent studies have demonstrated the reprogramming of cells into specific tissue types including alveolar epithelium (Ghaedi et al., 2014) and skeletal muscle (Tedesco et al., 2012). A novel way of processing iPSCs with high efficiency and a well-established safety profile, that does not require external agents and preserves cellular integrity, would provide unparalleled opportunity for this technology (Hou et al., 2013).

Natural biomaterials that have been used surgically as macrostructures include derivatives of collagen, fibrinogen, hyaluronic acid, glycosaminoglycans, hydroxyapatite, cellulose, chitosan, and silk fibroin (Campoccia et al., 2013). Other biomaterials include ECM scaffolds that can be used to replace heart valves, skin, the pericardium, and other anatomic structures (Badylak and Gilbert, 2008). Challenges to the use of natural biomaterials as scaffolds include restricted control over the physicochemical properties of the biomaterials themselves, the inability to moderate degradation rates, concerns over sterilization and purification, and the lasting presence of pathogens. Although natural biomaterials are biocompatible and undergo natural remodeling, they are also immunogenic. Xenogenic materials, in particular, exhibit antigens including the Gal epitope and DNA (Nair and Laurencin, 2007). However, allograft and xenograft natural biomaterials have been used as scaffolds in tissue engineering with some promising results (Fishman et al., 2011, 2012, 2013). Natural scaffolds are still far from achieving their full clinical potential, but considerable progress is being made (Birchall and Seifalian, 2014; Fulco et al., 2014; Gonfiotti et al., 2014; Sicari et al., 2014; Elliott et al., 2012; Olausson et al., 2012; Macchiarini et al., 2008).

The ideal scaffold should be bioactive, facilitate cell adhesion, be nonimmunogenic, nontoxic, and noncarcinogenic (Jungebluth et al., 2012). It should also be able to mimic the natural tissue microenvironment, maintain its biomechanical properties *in vivo*, as well as retain air and liquid seals where necessary. The biggest challenge associated with natural-derived scaffolds is overcoming their inherent immunogenicity. Decellularization of the natural biomaterial through the detergent-enzymatic method (DEM) has largely ameliorated this problem but often with a resultant loss of graft quality (Partington et al., 2013; Macchiarini et al., 2008). Less aggressive treatments, including freeze-thaw and chemical dehydration, have all been proposed to assist in the maintenance of the natural scaffold's biomechanical properties. However, studies have shown that the DEM is superior to chemicals, including formalin and acetone, in removing immunogenicity while avoiding as much degeneration as possible (Crapo et al., 2011). Through more than 17 cycles of detergent-enzymatic treatment of the tissue, studies have been able to demonstrate a complete removal of native DNA, protein, and MHC molecules (Conconi et al., 2005). Although this method is functional for tougher structures such as the trachea, for more sensitive structures such as the small bowel, only one cycle of DEM may be used. After four cycles, crypt and villous structure is completely eradicated (Totonelli et al., 2012b). Interestingly, Gillies et al. (2010) demonstrated the complete removal of DNA and intracellular proteins from rat tibialis anterior muscle using a nondetergent, nonproteolytic method consisting of only latrunculin B, hyper- and hypotonic solutions, and DNase (Gillies et al., 2010). While the method was similar to DEM in cell clearance, it better preserved the biomechanical properties of the scaffold. So far the DEM has proved the most useful in natural biomaterial processing. However, due to its harsh effects on the materials affected, a new form of decellularization protocol may be warranted.

In the few human autologous cell-seeded scaffold transplants that have taken place to date, studies have reported on the presence of a diminished immune response against the graft. Initial reports from airway tissue engineering follow-up studies commented on the presence of fungal infections within the first 6 weeks' post-transplant, suggesting that some local immunocompromise is occurring around the graft (Berg et al., 2013; Elliott et al., 2012; Macchiarini et al., 2008). Berg et al. (2013) reported in their posthumous findings that the trachea had a lymphocytic infiltrate in the submucosa in proximity to the graft. However, these studies should be considered in light of the observation that host responses to scaffolds differ based on source and processing. For example, *in vitro* studies of materials Graftjacket™ (human dermis, cryogenic processing) and Restore™ (porcine small intestinal submucosa, minimal processing) both elicited an immune response, but the latter was replaced by muscle and connective tissue, whereas Graftjacket fibrosed and underwent persistent low grade inflammation (Badylak and Gilbert, 2008; Valentin et al., 2006). In naturally occurring scaffolds, approximately 60% of the mass is degraded and resolved within 4 weeks and complete degradation often occurs by 3 months (Gilbert et al., 2007). However, this degradation may be an integral part of the healing process. Cross-linking that was initially thought to enhance durability in fact leads to a sustained host immune response (Badylak and Gilbert, 2008; Badylak et al., 2001). Separating out the innate (but resolving) immune response from the adaptive immune response (that can lead to graft failure) will be of paramount importance.

Synthetic biomaterials

Synthetic biomaterials have existed for millennia; the Ancient Egyptians employed linen sutures to bind wounds. However, the modern study of synthetic biomaterials dates back to the 1960s as new products were used in orthopedic and surgical settings. Synthetic biomaterials include polymers such as hydrogels, plastics, polysaccharides, and ceramics (Nilsson et al., 2010). Some of the advantageous properties of synthetic scaffolds are that they are biologically inert, have predictable properties, are uniform, mass-produced, and can be tailored. Furthermore, the most popular degradable synthetic scaffolds (polyglycolic acid (PGA), poly-L-lactide (PLLA), and the copolymer poly(lactic-co-glycolic acid)) are hydrolytically degraded due to their labile aliphatic ester links, rendering them the most diverse and versatile biomaterials available. The hydrolytic erosion permits the by-products to be removed naturally through the body's metabolism. Furthermore, by controlling the molecular weight and copolymerization of these synthetic scaffolds, the degradation rate can be partially controlled (Nair and Laurencin, 2007). Other scaffolds including polyurethane, bacterial poly-3-hydroxy-butyrate (PHB), polycaprolactone (PCL), polydiaxone, and polytrimethylene have also been employed. Polyurethanes and PHB are currently the most promising of these alternative materials.

PGA is a highly crystalline (45–55%), tensile synthetic scaffold with low solubility, a high melting point (>200°C), and the ability to form fibers. It has been used in resorbable sutures (due to its fiber-forming capability) and scaffold matrices (for tissue engineering applications). Nonwoven PGA has good degradability, cell viability, and initial mechanical properties and is being investigated as a bone internal fixation device

(Törmälä, 1992). The limitations of PGA usage include its rapid degradation rate, acidic degradation products, and low solubility. The rapid degradation rate is not necessarily a problem, but low solubility is correlated with eliciting an immune response. PGA is produced in minute amounts by *Staphylococcus epidermidis* and in larger amounts by *Bacillus anthracis*. It was demonstrated that PGA contributes to resistance of high salt concentrations by these pathogens (Kocianova et al., 2005). Therefore, using PGA may render a patient more prone to infection. Furthermore, acidic degradation products are dangerous in their own right. Cytology has demonstrated that in a PGA effusion posttransplant, lymphocytes were present. It has been suggested that the chronic inflammatory reaction to PGA may be induced to H_2O soluble oligomers released in the degradation process. However, there was no PGA-induced lymphocyte DNA synthesis. The PGA construct was thus immunologically inert but produced an inflammatory mononuclear cell migration and adhesion secondary to MHC II antigen and IL-2 receptor antigen (albeit smaller than that induced by mitogen or antigen-induced response) (Santavirta et al., 1990).

In human studies, PGA has been found to cause a sustained foreign body reaction (Athanasiou et al., 1996). However, a study comparing stainless steel screws and PGA in an orthopedic application found that there were no differences in immune response (Bucholz et al., 1994). A consensus has yet to be reached on the immune effects of PGA. Encouragingly, a tubular urethra made with PGA was seeded with autologous muscle and epithelial cells and implanted into five patients requiring urethral reconstruction. The grafts have been reported to survive for at least 6 years post-transplantation (Raya-Rivera et al., 2011).

PLLA is another crystalline (~37%) polymer with a high melting point (175°C), but, unlike PGA, it has a slow degradation time course, good tensile strength, low extension, and a high modulus (Middleton and Tipton, 2000). Therefore, it is particularly applicable to load-bearing situations such as occur in orthopedics. With a degradation time of 2–5.6 years *in vivo*, it may not be suitable for long-term orthopedic applications. PLLA has been used in dog meniscus reconstruction, but there were resulting clinical symptoms of inflammation from macrophage and lymphocytes infiltration (Klompmaker et al., 1991). A lower strength and faster degrading version of polylactide, poly-DL-lactide, is an amorphous polymer that has been used in drug delivery as it loses its mass in 12–16 months (Maurus and Kaeding, 2004). Unfortunately, PDLA and PLLA have the same problems with acidic degradation products as PGA, which limit their usage.

Poly(lactic-co)glycolide (PGLA) is used in meshes, suture reinforcement, skin replacement, dura mater substitutes, scaffolding substitutes, and drug delivery as microcapsules, microspheres, and nanospheres (Nair and Laurencin, 2007). It undergoes bulk erosion through ester bond hydrolysis with the rate of degradation proportional to the molecular weight, the shape, and the matrix structure. PGLA has good cell adhesive and proliferative properties, which is encouraging for tissue engineering applications. However, there are limits to its usage, particularly as a drug-delivery construct. Protein denaturation occurs within the vehicle as glycolic acid creates an acidic environment. Creating a surface-eroding polymer would eliminate this particular problem (Ueda and Tabata, 2003). As regards to the immunogenicity of PGLA, it has been used in a model of articular healing in rabbits and minimal inflammation was reported (Päivärinta et al., 1993). Furthermore, PGLA has been shown to increase bone-healing time in a model of rat tibia (Hollinger, 1983). Thus, PGLA is a versatile product that may find use in a variety of properties, but the toxicity and immunogenicity of its degradation products are limiting flaws.

Polyurethanes have been used in both pacemakers and vascular grafts. They are biocompatible with good mechanical properties. However, they do elicit an increase in chemokines, cytokines, and growth factors when studied in *in vitro* models (Schutte et al., 2009). A notable example of a polyurethane being used in clinical practice is the bioartificial polyhedral oligomeric silesquiaxone-poly(carbonate-urea) urethane (POSS-PCU) that has been employed in tissue engineering (Jungebluth et al., 2011). When implanted into a patient with an advanced tracheal tumor, the patient was asymptomatic and tumor-free at 5 months. The airway had patent anastomoses and a vascularized neo-mucosa. There was a local occurrence of fungal infection initially which suggests that the graft initiated some immunogenicity, probably through the innate immune response. However, at 5 months, epithelialization and wound repair had occurred and no evidence of infection was present. These results strongly suggest that this synthetic polymer is tolerated by the adaptive immune response. Long-term follow-up will be necessary to assess whether or not a chronic rejection pattern can occur. However, the drawback to POSS-PCU is that neovascularization and epithelialization were difficult to achieve on this synthetic scaffold (Totonelli et al., 2012a). Theoretically, however, this polymer is a promising resource for future use if it can be employed as a smart polymer that incorporates appropriate signaling molecules. Three-dimensional bioprinting of cells directly onto biomaterials may assist in the future to promote revascularization, recellularization, reepithelialization, as well as immune modulation of implanted biomaterials, either directly or through paracrine effects (Zopf et al., 2013).

Alternative synthetic scaffolds have been employed previously, but with less success and will be discussed here largely for completeness. Polydiaxone has been used in monofilament sutures (as multifilament sutures have been associated with infection and friction-induced injury). Polytrimethylene carbonate is another variable polymer that is used in its low weight form for drug delivery and in its high weight form for soft tissue engineering. PCL is a semicrystalline polymer that is cheap, slow to degrade, and highly permeable (Nair and Laurencin, 2007). It has therefore been used in the long-term delivery of drugs and vaccines and, most notably, contraceptive implants. That is not to say that PCL does not produce an immune response. When PCL was implanted into the nervous system, microglia were found to peak 3 days following implantation and persisted for 28 days. Astrocytes displayed a similar pattern of activation. However, 60 days postimplant, no scar or foreign body reaction was seen surrounding the scaffolds (Nisbet et al., 2009).

The bacterial polyester PHB has demonstrated good biocompatibility in studies to date. It elicits minimal acute inflammation, abscesses, and tissue necrosis (Artsis et al., 2010). PHB is tough and brittle but its piezoelectricity makes it an ideal candidate for orthopedic applications as it can undergo electrical stimulation to facilitate movement postoperatively (Pouton and Akhtar, 1996). PHB evokes a mild tissue response similar to that of PGA and PLA. However, the intermediate degradation product of PHB is biocompatible and not acidic unlike that of PGA and PLA (Artsis et al., 2010). Therefore, PHB may be an ideal candidate for future tissue engineering and biomaterial applications. Synthetic scaffolds have thus been used as biomaterials in a wide range of applications. In addition to identifying appropriate mechanical properties, studies have demonstrated that some biomaterials are more or less immunogenic than others. In particular, while PGA and its variants have found myriad uses as biomaterials, PHB may prove more effective for long-term applications where biocompatibility is of paramount importance. Polyurethanes with their proven biocompatibility *in vivo* should be further explored in *in vivo* applications of tissue engineering.

Of particular interest would be harnessing the immune responses to these biomaterials to generate a tolerant effect. Synthetic scaffolds can be coated in short peptides in order to facilitate binding of MSC to the scaffolds (Campoccia et al., 2013, Harris et al., 2004). Such MSC binding would be particularly beneficial in tissue engineering applications concerning these biomaterials. One example is the integrin-binding peptide present within fibronectin and laminin, which enables MSC adhesion. Interestingly, Tyr-Ile-Gly-Ser-Arg (YIGSR) is another laminin-derived short peptide that increases endothelial cell adhesion and proliferation but decreases platelet activation (Harris et al., 2004). What implications the use of these peptides could have on the triggering of the adaptive immune response to the foreign material is currently unknown. Modifying the coating on synthetic scaffolds to interplay with the adaptive immune response could provide an element of control over long-term graft survival.

Metals

Metals have been used in orthopedic and dental applications primarily to replace joints and teeth (see Chapter 12). For a synthetic or natural material to rival bone, it must possess the mechanical properties to mimic cortical bone-bearing properties, be a resorbable or degradable material in order to prevent fatigue fractures, and be osteo-inductive (Nilsson et al., 2010). Although the ideal material has yet to be found, metal has emerged as the most appropriate form at present. By contrast, ceramics, bioglass, and polymers may be resorbed but lack load-bearing capacity. Calcium phosphate is promising but the understanding and control of synthesis (the osteoinductive aspect of this material) have yet to be untangled (Bohner et al., 2012). Cobalt-chromium-molybdenum (CoCrMo) is an alloy that has often been used in hip arthroplasty (Golish and Anderson, 2012). Early reports of failure of CoCrMo on CoCrMo were reported in disk arthroplasty (spinal reconstruction) due to metallic wear debris and necrosis. By contrast, when CoCrMo is articulated with ultrahigh molecular weight polyethylene, the weight-bearing problems are alleviated. Nevertheless, recent orthopedic applications of metals have reverted to a metal-on-metal structure with questionable immune reaction improvement. Problems with metal-on-metal articulation include aseptic loosening, metal hypersensitivity, and ion toxicity.

Aseptic loosening is problematic for today's patients who need bone replacement solutions that can last tens of years. The perceived advantage for metal-on-metal bearings was that the volumetric wear would be less than metal-on-polyethylene pairings. However, metal-on-metal bearings release more particles than metal-on-polyethylene. This finding is due to the higher surface area of the former, leading to greater corrosion and subsequent release of small particles. A type IV hypersensitivity reaction results and the subsequent lymphocytic response then leads to aseptic osteolysis mediated by IL-2, IFNγ, and Receptor activator of nuclear factor kappa-B ligand (RANKL) (Jacobs and Hallab, 2006). In particular, RANKL can increase osteoclast formation and block osteoblast activity further impeding bone repair (Hallab et al., 2002). Galbraith et al. (2011) note how hard it is to distinguish a type IV hypersensitivity reaction from infection. For this reason, metal-on-metal bearings should probably be avoided in young patients who require orthopedic implants (Smith et al., 2012).

Metal hypersensitivity is a common allergic condition resulting from exposure to metal ions through skin contact, inhalation, or surgical exposure. In the latter, when aseptic loosening occurs, this often releases metal ions into the surrounding environment, triggering the response. Nickel and beryllium are the best-studied metals as the former plays a critical role in contact dermatitis. Studies have shown that αβ T-cells mediate this reaction. The metal ions function as haptens that bind the MHC II–peptide complex on metal-specific αβ T-cell receptors (Wang and Dai, 2013). Metal antigens do not simply help to mount the immune response but can also modulate antigen presenting cell activity. For example zinc binding increases antigen presenting cell activity. However, studies have demonstrated that gold blocks the antigen presenting cell by forming inert complexes. Further studies have demonstrated that the gold salts functionally inhibit cysteine residues on the T-cell receptor (Griem et al., 1996). One could conceivably coat metals in gold, but gold is toxic to the kidneys when metabolized and easily corrodes. How to mitigate or harness this metal-derived immune response is not yet well understood.

There are arguments for the use of heavy metals as biomaterials since many also have the added benefit of being bactericidal (in particular, silver, bismuth, zinc, and copper) (Campoccia et al., 2013). Incorporating bactericidal properties would be of considerable utility as foreign bodies are particularly prone to infection. In theory, one could incorporate one of these materials into the component structure of the biomaterial. Interestingly, Li et al. demonstrated that if an infection occurs, one can give IL-12 or MPC-1 which activated Th1 cells to secrete cytokines such as IFNγ to stimulate the bactericidal properties of macrophages. Unfortunately, in doing so, a local immune response is also elicited (Li et al., 2009). More work is required in this area, but metals may prove important in elucidating how bactericidal properties may be incorporated into biomaterials.

Finally, the immune response toward quantum nanoparticles (quantum dots) warrants brief discussion here (Zolnik et al., 2010). Nanoparticles that contain a metallic core (such as cadmium, zinc, or gold) can be engineered to either escape immune system recognition or specifically inhibit or enhance immune responses (Ye et al., 2012; Alkilany and Murphy, 2010; Hoshino et al., 2009). Three factors primarily affect the toxicity and biological behavior of quantum dots: modifying the core metalloid complex of the nanoparticle, surface modifications of the nanoparticle, and altering the external environmental conditions (Hoshino et al., 2011).

THE ADAPTIVE HOST IMMUNE RESPONSE TO BIOMATERIALS

Certain implanted biomaterials appear to exert an influence on the host immune response resulting in the generation of particular outcomes (favorable or unfavorable) with respect to overall biocompatibility, constructive tissue remodeling, tissue repair, neovascularization, and tissue regeneration. Thus, the recognition of the predominant phenotype of macrophages provides an indication of rejection, inflammation, or acceptance following implantation of biomaterials and their role in the context of certain implanted biomaterials has been borne out by previous studies (Brown et al., 2012a,b, 2009; Keane et al., 2012; Koch et al., 2012; Sicari et al., 2012; Porta et al., 2009; Valentin et al., 2009; Badylak and Gilbert, 2008; Badylak et al., 2008; Martinez et al., 2008).

M1-activated macrophages (also known as classically activated macrophages) express IL-12^{high}, IL-23^{high}, IL-10^{low}, and produce inflammatory cytokines such as IL-1β, IL-6, and TNFα which promote active inflammation, ECM destruction, and tissue injury. They are CCR7+ CD80+ CD86+ and are inducer and effector cells in Th1-type inflammatory and rejection responses. M2-activated macrophages on the other hand (also known as alternatively activated macrophages) express an IL-12^{low}, IL-23^{low}, and IL-10^{high} phenotype and are able to facilitate tissue repair, constructive

M1 (classical activation)

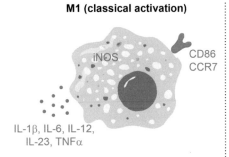

iNOS

CD86
CCR7

IL-1β, IL-6, IL-12,
IL-23, TNFα

M2 (alternative activation)

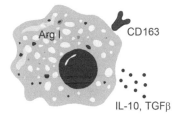

Arg I

CD163

IL-10, TGFβ

- Th1-like phenotype
- Pro-inflammatory
- ECM destruction/tissue injury
- Apoptosis

- Th2-like phenotype
- Anti-inflammatory
- Constructive remodelling
- Tissue regeneration
- Cell proliferation and chemotaxis
- Angiogenesis

Figure 8.1 M1 versus M2 macrophage response. (A) Classical pathway (M1) activation is associated with chronic inflammation, ECM destruction and apoptosis. (B) Alternative pathway (M2) activation is associated with anti-inflammatory effects, ECM construction, angiogenesis, and tissue regeneration. In reality a broad spectrum lies between the two extremes of polarization. iNOS = inducible nitric oxide synthase, Arg I = Arginase I. For a full review on the subject, see Gordon and Martinez (2010). Also see Chapter 6.

remodeling through ECM construction and angiogenesis. M2 macrophages are CD163+ CD206+ Arg I+ and predominantly induce a classical Th2 response that is anti-inflammatory and is hypothesized to be particularly beneficial for constructive tissue remodeling and tissue regeneration (Martinez et al., 2008) (Figure 8.1).

Previous evidence has demonstrated that decellularized biomaterials, in promoting the formation of M2 macrophages and retaining pertinent angiogenic growth factors (e.g., vascular endothelial growth factor, TGFβ, and basic fibroblast growth), may also be responsible for the pro-angiogenic effects seen which will be critical in ensuring viability of implanted biomaterials (Fishman et al., 2013; Takeda et al., 2011). In addition, unlike lymphocytes whose differentiation is relatively fixed upon differentiation, macrophages retain a degree of plasticity which enables them to switch relatively easily between M1 and M2 phenotypes in response to environmental cues (Arnold et al., 2007; Stout et al., 2005). The potential manipulation of macrophage effector mechanisms as a strategy for promoting site-appropriate and constructive remodeling as opposed to deleterious persistent inflammation and scar tissue formation is an area for future work (Brown et al., 2012a,b).

Similarly, polarization of T lymphocytes into Th1 and Th2 cells, each with differing profiles of cytokine expression, has been demonstrated to be associated with either graft acceptance (Th2 phenotype) or classical acute graft rejection (Th1 phenotype) (Badylak and Gilbert, 2008; Allman et al., 2001, 2002). It seems likely that the host immune response will vary depending on the source of material, processing methods, and site of implantation following implantation. Recent data also suggest that certain implanted biomaterials, particularly natural-derived biomaterials, may stimulate the production of Treg cells (Fishman et al., 2013; Haykal et al., 2013; Bollyky et al., 2009, 2011). The underlying mechanisms responsible for such findings remain elusive and are scope for future work. However, such mechanisms may in part explain why patients receiving tissue engineered implants using natural-derived scaffolds do not mount immune response against the grafts and therefore do not require immunosuppression to prevent rejection (Elliott et al., 2012; Olausson et al., 2012; Macchiarini et al., 2008). Thus, such scaffolds appear to be antigenic but not immunogenic (cross-reference to the section "Antigenicity Versus Immunogenicity").

GENERATION OF AN IMMUNOSUPPRESSION-FREE STATE

Use of immunosuppression prevents immune rejection but is associated with toxicity, unwanted systemic side effects and an increased risk of infection and malignancy. A major goal of transplantation and regenerative medicine, therefore, is organ/tissue replacement without the need for immunosuppressive drugs (clinical operational tolerance). To this end, two main approaches have been taken to reach this goal; induction of tolerance through modulation of the host immune system and/or a reduction in donor tissue antigenicity.

Modulation of host immunity

Central tolerance in transplantation is induced through the deletion of alloreactive T-cells in the thymus before they are exported into the periphery. *In utero* cell transplantation is one such approach that is being tried in order to achieve central tolerance (Fisher et al., 2013; Hayashi et al., 2002). The use of nonmyeloablative bone marrow transplantation leading to hematopoietic chimerism has been shown to induce central tolerance and long-term graft survival (Leventhal et al., 2012). The induction of peripheral tolerance targets peripheral T-cells typically using either costimulatory blockade (e.g., anti-CD154 and CTLA4-Ig), by transferring/inducing Treg cells, or by utilizing tolerogenic dendritic cells (Chandrasekharan et al., 2013; Issa and Wood, 2012; Leishman et al., 2011; Boyd and Fairchild, 2010; Long and Wood, 2009; Silk and Fairchild, 2009; Waldmann et al., 2008; Cobbold et al., 2006). Mechanisms of peripheral tolerance predominantly include clonal deletion, T-cell anergy, and regulation/suppression (Ashton-Chess et al., 2006).

The only strategy that has so far successfully achieved solid organ tolerance in human clinical trials is mixed chimerism (Leventhal et al., 2012). However, the risks of mixed chimerism tolerogenic protocols include the need for bone marrow transplantation, with the associated risks of graft rejection, graft versus host disease, toxicity of conditioning regimens and "engraftment syndrome," as well as the side effects of T-cell depletion, such as infection and loss of T-cell memory with newly engrafted T-cells (Ravindra et al., 2008).

Further progress might be made through a deeper understanding of the underlying mechanisms behind why some transplant patients develop spontaneous operational tolerance to allografts, usually secondary to noncompliance of immunosuppressive medications (Chandrasekharan et al., 2013). Thymic bioengineering and co-transplantation of vascularized thymic tissue, thereby allowing the deletion of T-cell clones responsible for allograft and xenograft rejection, is an alternative strategy for future tolerogenic approaches (Orlando, 2012; Yamada et al., 2005; Nikolic et al., 1999). Finally, the results of a multicenter phase I/II study to evaluate various types of immunomodulatory cells in living-donor kidney transplantation (The "*ONE Study*") are eagerly awaited and will develop protocols for the use of expanded recipient Treg cells, recipient Tr1 cells, donor regulatory macrophages, and donor tolerogenic dendritic cells (McMurchy et al., 2011) (Figure 8.2).

Reduction in donor tissue antigenicity and immunogenicity

A variety of different approaches have been taken to reduce tissue antigenicity in order to reduce the requirement for immunosuppression, including fixation with chemicals, cryopreservation, irradiation, and lyophilization (Fishman et al., 2011). While glutaraldehyde fixation and cryopreservation have been widely utilized for making tissues, such as heart valves and tracheal grafts, nonimmunogenic, this is only effective at

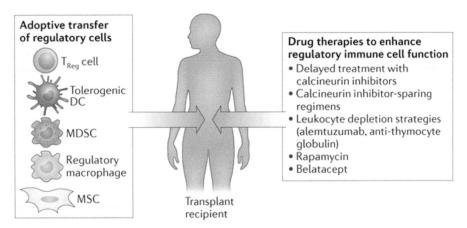

Figure 8.2 Clinical applications of therapies based on regulatory immune cells. Note: Myeloid-derived Suppressor Cells (MDSC). *Taken from Wood et al. (2012).*

reducing antigenicity in the short to medium term (Jacobs et al., 1999). Such pro-cesses typically involve the maintenance of cells within the graft, which is associated with rejection over time and structural deterioration and is generally believed to be responsible for the disappointing long-term results seen with such techniques (Bloch et al., 2011; Sotres-Vega et al., 2006; Hawkins et al., 2000). Due to the preservation and fixation process, grafts become nonviable bioprostheses, which is largely responsible for their lack of potential for remodeling, regeneration, and growth (Cebotari et al., 2006; Dohmen et al., 2006). Furthermore, cross-linking agents, such as glutaraldehyde, reduce cell permeation into scaffolds which may further hinder tissue remodeling and regen-erative potential (de Castro Bras et al., 2010).

Immunoisolation technology, having largely arisen out of the field of islet cell transplantation, has emerged as a way of preventing the recognition of non–self-anti-gens by the host immune system (Orlando, 2012; Pareta et al., 2012). By definition, the recipient cannot be considered immunologically "tolerant" and given the right cir-cumstances the immune system will still be able to mount an immune response against the antigens if encountered. The term immunological "ignorance" may be more appropriate in such circumstances. Despite encouraging results in preclinical studies, translation to humans has been hampered by significant morbidity and lack of efficacy, mainly due to inadequate immune isolation and cell death secondary to hypoxia. In this respect, decellularized ECM scaffolds may provide the optimal environment for encapsulated islets destined for transplantation.

An alternative approach to reduce donor tissue antigenicity comes from the field of xenotransplantation where pigs have been genetically engineered to remove the pig antigen α-gal, that is mainly responsible for hyperacute rejection in transplanting from pigs to humans, as well as pigs that express one or more complement regulatory proteins (Ekser et al., 2012; Yamada et al., 2005) (see Chapter 4). Although a reduction in host immune response has been demonstrated, it is probably not adequate to lower exog-enous immunosuppressive therapy sufficiently to permit clinical use, primarily due to an immune response directed against non-gal epitopes and further genetic modification of pigs will probably be necessary. Nevertheless, a host immune response against decellular-ized xenogenic tissues, if identified, could in theory be prevented further by harvesting of tissue for decellularization from transgenic α-gal knockout animals, or through treatment of harvested tissue with α-gal (Stapleton et al., 2011; Daly et al., 2009; Xu et al., 2009).

Interspecies blastocyst complementation, by injection of human iPSCs, offers the prospect of generating nonimmunogenic human organs for replacement through chi-merism (which has been recently demonstrated in pigs) (Matsunari et al., 2013; Usui et al., 2012; Kobayashi et al., 2010). However, this strategy may be limited by the pres-ence of highly immunogenic xenogenic vasculature, safety, and ethical concerns.

Tissue engineering, through the use of decellularized scaffolds, is a possible way of overcoming the above limitations since, hypothetically, decellularized scaffolds are capable of providing living tissue with remodeling, regeneration, and growth potential (see the section "Natural (Decellularized) Matrices"). The potential advantages of the decellularized scaffold approach, compared to previous approaches, lie in its similarity to native tissue, with the maintenance of tissue composition and microarchitecture, and the possibility of generating nonimmunogenic tissues. There is already a proof-of-principle that decellularized allogenic tissues fail to elicit a humoral-mediated immune response when transplanted into humans (Elliott et al., 2012; Kneib et al., 2012; Olausson et al., 2012; Macchiarini et al., 2008). There is also recent evidence from preclinical animal studies that decellularized scaffolds can also circumvent the cell-mediated immune response and modulate the host immune response toward a favorable phenotype (Fishman et al., 2012, 2013; Haykal et al., 2013; Ma et al., 2013; Zang et al., 2013; Bollyky et al., 2009, 2011; Scheibner et al., 2006).

FUTURE WORK AND CONCLUSIONS

Previous successes within the field of allotransplantation have enabled solid organ transplantation to proceed in the presence of immunosuppression. However, although successful in preventing immune rejection, lifelong immunosuppression (and the ever increasing array of immunosuppressive drugs that are being developed) carries notable risks including toxicity, systemic side effects, infection, and malignancy. Future research is geared toward developing a state of clinical operational tolerance, i.e., transplantation without the need for immunosuppression, or with only reduced requirements for immunosuppression ("prope" tolerance). In order to achieve this goal, various tolerogenic strategies are being deployed to induce acceptance of biomaterials without the need for immunosuppression. Part of this strategy may include redirecting the host immune response toward a more favorable phenotype (i.e., the promotion of M2 macrophages and Th2 lymphocytes), as well as the use of immunomodulatory cell types, including Treg cells, regulatory macrophages, and tolerogenic dendritic cells. The latter approach is being tested in the "ONE Study" which is currently under way, the results of which will have important implications concerning the immune response toward biomaterials (Juvet et al., 2014; Geissler and Hutchinson, 2013).

REFERENCES

Abbas, A.K., Murphy, K.M., Sher, A., 1996. Functional diversity of helper T lymphocytes. Nature 383, 787–793.

Adams, A.B., Pearson, T.C., Larsen, C.P., 2003. Heterologous immunity: an overlooked barrier to tolerance. Immunol. Rev. 196, 147–160.

Alkilany, A.M., Murphy, C.J., 2010. Toxicity and cellular uptake of gold nanoparticles: what we have learned so far? J. Nanopart. Res. 12, 2313–2333.

Allman, A.J., Mcpherson, T.B., Badylak, S.F., Merrill, L.C., Kallakury, B., Sheehan, C., et al., 2001. Xenogeneic extracellular matrix grafts elicit a TH2-restricted immune response. Transplantation 71, 1631–1640.

Allman, A.J., Mcpherson, T.B., Merrill, L.C., Badylak, S.F., Metzger, D.W., 2002. The Th2-restricted immune response to xenogeneic small intestinal submucosa does not influence systemic protective immunity to viral and bacterial pathogens. Tissue Eng. 8, 53–62.

Amara, U., Flierl, M.A., Rittirsch, D., Klos, A., Chen, H., Acker, B., et al., 2010. Molecular intercommunication between the complement and coagulation systems. J. Immunol. 185, 5628–5636.

Anderson, J.M., Rodriguez, A., Chang, D.T., 2008. Foreign body reaction to biomaterials. Semin. Immunol 20 (2), 86–100. PMCID: 2327202.

Anglicheau, D., Suthanthiran, M., 2008. Noninvasive prediction of organ graft rejection and outcome using gene expression patterns. Transplantation 86, 192.

Araki, R., Uda, M., Hoki, Y., Sunayama, M., Nakamura, M., Ando, S., et al., 2013. Negligible immunogenicity of terminally differentiated cells derived from induced pluripotent or embryonic stem cells. Nature 494, 100–104.

Arnold, L., Henry, A., Poron, F., Baba-Amer, Y., van Rooijen, N., Plonquet, A., et al., 2007. Inflammatory monocytes recruited after skeletal muscle injury switch into antiinflammatory macrophages to support myogenesis. J. Exp. Med. 204, 1057–1069.

Artsis, M., Bonartsev, A., Iordanskii, A., Bonartseva, G., Zaikov, G., 2010. Biodegradation and medical application of microbial poly (3-hydroxybutyrate). Mol. Cryst. Liq. Cryst. 523 21/[593]–49/[621].

Ashton-Chess, J., Brouard, S., Soulillou, J.P., 2006. Is clinical tolerance realistic in the next decade? Transpl. Int. 19, 539–548.

Athanasiou, K.A., Niederauer, G.G., Agrawal, C., 1996. Sterilization, toxicity, biocompatibility and clinical applications of polylactic acid/polyglycolic acid copolymers. Biomaterials 17, 93–102.

Badylak, S.F., Gilbert, T.W., 2008. Immune response to biologic scaffold materials. Semin. Immunol. 20, 109–116.

Badylak, S.F., Park, K., Peppas, N., Mccabe, G., Yoder, M., 2001. Marrow-derived cells populate scaffolds composed of xenogeneic extracellular matrix. Exp. Hematol. 29, 1310–1318.

Badylak, S.F., Valentin, J.E., Ravindra, A.K., Mccabe, G.P., Stewart-Akers, A.M., 2008. Macrophage phenotype as a determinant of biologic scaffold remodeling. Tissue Eng. Part A 14, 1835–1842.

Bennet, W., Sundberg, B., Groth, C.-G., Brendel, M.D., Brandhorst, D., Brandhorst, H., et al., 1999. Incompatibility between human blood and isolated islets of Langerhans: a finding with implications for clinical intraportal islet transplantation? Diabetes 48, 1907–1914.

Berg, M., Ejnell, H., Kovács, A., Nayakawde, N., Patil, P.B., Joshi, M., et al., 2013. Replacement of a tracheal stenosis with a tissue-engineered human trachea using autologous stem cells: a case report. Tissue Eng. Part A 20, 389–397.

Bestard, O., Nickel, P., Cruzado, J.M., Schoenemann, C., Boenisch, O., Sefrin, A., et al., 2008. Circulating alloreactive T cells correlate with graft function in longstanding renal transplant recipients. J. Am. Soc. Nephrol. 19, 1419–1429.

Birchall, M.A., Seifalian, A.M., 2014. Tissue engineering's green shoots of disruptive innovation. Lancet 384 (9940), 288–290.

Bloch, O., Golde, P., Dohmen, P.M., Posner, S., Konertz, W., Erdbrugger, W., 2011. Immune response in patients receiving a bioprosthetic heart valve: lack of response with decellularized valves. Tissue Eng. Part A 17, 2399–2405.

Bohner, M., Galea, L., Doebelin, N., 2012. Calcium phosphate bone graft substitutes: failures and hopes. J. Eur. Ceram. Soc. 32, 2663–2671.

Bollyky, P.L., Falk, B.A., Wu, R.P., Buckner, J.H., Wight, T.N., Nepom, G.T., 2009. Intact extracellular matrix and the maintenance of immune tolerance: high molecular weight hyaluronan promotes persistence of induced CD4+ CD25+ regulatory T cells. J. Leukoc. Biol. 86, 567–572.

Bollyky, P.L., Wu, R.P., Falk, B.A., Lord, J.D., Long, S.A., Preisinger, A., et al., 2011. ECM components guide IL-10 producing regulatory T-cell (TR1) induction from effector memory T-cell precursors. Proc. Natl. Acad. Sci. USA. 108, 7938–7943.

Boyd, A.S., Fairchild, P.J., 2010. Approaches for immunological tolerance induction to stem cell-derived cell replacement therapies. Expert Rev. Clin. Immunol. 6, 435–448.

Boyd, A.S., Wood, K.J., 2010. Characteristics of the early immune response following transplantation of mouse ES cell derived insulin-producing cell clusters. PLoS One 5, e10965.

Braden, B.C., Goldbaum, F.A., Chen, B.-X., Kirschner, A.N., Wilson, S.R., Erlanger, B.F., 2000. X-ray crystal structure of an anti-buckminsterfullerene antibody fab fragment: biomolecular recognition of C60. Proc. Natl. Acad. Sci. USA. 97, 12193–12197.

Brodbeck, W.G., Shive, M.S., Colton, E., Nakayama, Y., Matsuda, T., Anderson, J., 2001. Influence of biomaterial surface chemistry on the apoptosis of adherent cells. J. Biomed. Mater. Res. 55, 661–668.

Brook, M.O., Wood, K.J., Jones, N.D., 2006. The impact of memory T cells on rejection and the induction of tolerance. Transplantation 82, 1–9.

Brown, B.N., Valentin, J.E., Stewart-Akers, A.M., Mccabe, G.P., Badylak, S.F., 2009. Macrophage phenotype and remodeling outcomes in response to biologic scaffolds with and without a cellular component. Biomaterials 30, 1482–1491.

Brown, B.N., Londono, R., Tottey, S., Zhang, L., Kukla, K.A., Wolf, M.T., et al., 2012a. Macrophage phenotype as a predictor of constructive remodeling following the implantation of biologically derived surgical mesh materials. Acta Biomater. 8, 978–987.

Brown, B.N., Ratner, B.D., Goodman, S.B., Amar, S., Badylak, S.F., 2012b. Macrophage polarization: an opportunity for improved outcomes in biomaterials and regenerative medicine. Biomaterials 33, 3792–3802.

Bucholz, R.W., Henry, S., Henley, M.B., 1994. Fixation with bioabsorbable screws for the treatment of fractures of the ankle. J. Bone Joint Surg. 76, 319–324.

Burne-Taney, M.J., Liu, M., Baldwin, W.M., Racusen, L., Rabb, H., 2006. Decreased capacity of immune cells to cause tissue injury mediates kidney ischemic preconditioning. J. Immunol. 176, 7015–7020.

Cai, J., Lee, J., Jankowska-Gan, E., Derks, R., Pool, J., Mutis, T., et al., 2004. Minor H antigen HA-1-specific regulator and effector CD8+ T cells, and HA-1 microchimerism, in allograft tolerance. J. Exp. Med. 199, 1017–1023.

Campoccia, D., Montanaro, L., Arciola, C.R., 2013. A review of the biomaterials technologies for infection-resistant surfaces. Biomaterials 34, 8533–8554.

Carvalho-Gaspar, M., Billing, J.S., Spriewald, B.M., Wood, K.J., 2005. Chemokine gene expression during allograft rejection: comparison of two quantitative PCR techniques. J. Immunol. Methods 301, 41–52.

Cebotari, S., Lichtenberg, A., Tudorache, I., Hilfiker, A., Mertsching, H., Leyh, R., et al., 2006. Clinical application of tissue engineered human heart valves using autologous progenitor cells. Circulation 114, I132–I137.

Celli, S., Albert, M.L., Bousso, P., 2011. Visualizing the innate and adaptive immune responses underlying allograft rejection by two-photon microscopy. Nat. Med. 17, 744–749.

Chandrasekharan, D., Issa, F., Wood, K.J., 2013. Achieving operational tolerance in transplantation: how can lessons from the clinic inform research directions? Transpl. Int. 26, 576–589.

Chen, B.-X., Wilson, S., Das, M., Coughlin, D., Erlanger, B., 1998. Antigenicity of fullerenes: antibodies specific for fullerenes and their characteristics. Proc. Natl. Acad. Sci. USA. 95, 10809–10813.

Chen, L., Wang, T., Zhou, P., Ma, L., Yin, D., Shen, J., et al., 2006. TLR engagement prevents transplantation tolerance. Am. J. Transplant. 6, 2282–2291.

Chen, N., Gao, Q., Field, E.H., 1996. Prevention of Th1 responses is critical for tolerance 1. Transplantation 61, 1076–1083.

Cobbold, S.P., Adams, E., Graca, L., Daley, S., Yates, S., Paterson, A., et al., 2006. Immune privilege induced by regulatory T cells in transplantation tolerance. Immunol. Rev. 213, 239–255.

Colvin, R.B., 2007. Antibody-mediated renal allograft rejection: diagnosis and pathogenesis. J. Am. Soc. Nephrol. 18, 1046–1056.

Colvin, R.B., Smith, R.N., 2005. Antibody-mediated organ-allograft rejection. Nat. Rev. Immunol. 5, 807–817.

Conconi, M.T., Coppi, P.D., Liddo, R.D., Vigolo, S., Zanon, G.F., Parnigotto, P.P., et al., 2005. Tracheal matrices, obtained by a detergent-enzymatic method, support *in vitro* the adhesion of chondrocytes and tracheal epithelial cells. Transpl. Int. 18, 727–734.

Crapo, P.M., Gilbert, T.W., Badylak, S.F., 2011. An overview of tissue and whole organ decellularization processes. Biomaterials 32, 3233–3243.

Dallman, M.J., 1995. Cytokines and transplantation: Th1/Th2 regulation of the immune response to solid organ transplants in the adult. Curr. Opin. Immunol. 7, 632–638.

Daly, K.A., Stewart-Akers, A.M., Hara, H., Ezzelarab, M., Long, C., Cordero, K., et al., 2009. Effect of the alphaGal epitope on the response to small intestinal submucosa extracellular matrix in a nonhuman primate model. Tissue Eng. Part A 15, 3877–3888.

de Castro Bras, L.E., Proffitt, J.L., Bloor, S., Sibbons, P.D., 2010. Effect of crosslinking on the performance of a collagen-derived biomaterial as an implant for soft tissue repair: a rodent model. J. Biomed. Mater. Res. Part B Appl. Biomater. 95, 239–249.

Dobrovolskaia, M.A., Mcneil, S.E., 2007. Immunological properties of engineered nanomaterials. Nat. Nanotechnol. 2, 469–478.

Dohmen, P.M., da Costa, F., Holinski, S., Lopes, S.V., Yoshi, S., Reichert, L.H., et al., 2006. Is there a possibility for a glutaraldehyde-free porcine heart valve to grow? Eur. Surg. Res. 38, 54–61.

Drukker, M., Katz, G., Urbach, A., Schuldiner, M., Markel, G., Itskovitz-Eldor, J., et al., 2002. Characterization of the expression of MHC proteins in human embryonic stem cells. Proc. Natl. Acad. Sci. USA. 99, 9864–9869.

Einecke, G., Sis, B., Reeve, J., Mengel, M., Campbell, P., Hidalgo, L., et al., 2009. Antibody-mediated microcirculation injury is the major cause of late kidney transplant failure. Am. J. Transplant. 9, 2520–2531.

Ekdahl, K.N., Lambris, J.D., Elwing, H., Ricklin, D., Nilsson, P.H., Teramura, Y., et al., 2011. Innate immunity activation on biomaterial surfaces: a mechanistic model and coping strategies. Adv. Drug Deliv. Rev. 63, 1042–1050.

Ekser, B., Ezzelarab, M., Hara, H., van der Windt, D.J., Wijkstrom, M., Bottino, R., et al., 2012. Clinical xenotransplantation: the next medical revolution? Lancet 379, 672–683.

Elliott, M.J., De Coppi, P., Speggiorin, S., Roebuck, D., Butler, C.R., Samuel, E., et al., 2012. Stem-cell-based, tissue engineered tracheal replacement in a child: a 2-year follow-up study. Lancet 380, 994–1000.

Farrar, C.A., Zhou, W., Lin, T., Sacks, S.H., 2006. Local extravascular pool of C3 is a determinant of post-ischemic acute renal failure. FASEB J. 20, 217–226.

Fernández, N., Renedo, M., García-Rodríguez, C., Sánchez Crespo, M., 2002. Activation of monocytic cells through Fc gamma receptors induces the expression of macrophage-inflammatory protein (MIP)-1 alpha, MIP-1 beta, and RANTES. J. Immunol. 169, 3321–3328.

Fisher, J.E., Lillegard, J.B., Mckenzie, T.J., Rodysill, B.R., Wettstein, P.J., Nyberg, S.L., 2013. In utero transplanted human hepatocytes allow postnatal engraftment of human hepatocytes in pigs. Liver Transpl. 19, 328–335.

Fishman, J.M., De Coppi, P., Elliott, M.J., Atala, A., Birchall, M.A., Macchiarini, P., 2011. Airway tissue engineering. Expert Opin. Biol. Ther. 11, 1623–1635.

Fishman, J.M., Ansari, T., Sibbons, P., De Coppi, P., Birchall, M.A., 2012. Decellularized rabbit cricoarytenoid dorsalis muscle for laryngeal regeneration. Ann. Otol. Rhinol. Laryngol. 121, 129–138.

Fishman, J.M., Lowdell, M.W., Urbani, L., Ansari, T., Burns, A.J., Turmaine, M., et al., 2013. Immunomodulatory effect of a decellularized skeletal muscle scaffold in a discordant xenotransplantation model. Proc. Natl. Acad. Sci. USA. 110, 14360–14365.

Franz, S., Rammelt, S., Scharnweber, D., Simon, J.C., 2011. Immune responses to implants—a review of the implications for the design of immunomodulatory biomaterials. Biomaterials 32, 6692–6709.

Fulco, I., Miot, S., Haug, M.D., Barbero, A., Wixmerten, A., Feliciano, S., et al., 2014. Engineered autologous cartilage tissue for nasal reconstruction after tumour resection: an observational first-in-human trial. Lancet 384, 337–346.

Galbraith, J.G., Butler, J.S., Browne, T.-J., Mulcahy, D., Harty, J.A., 2011. Infection or metal hypersensitivity? The diagnostic challenge of failure in metal-on-metal bearings. Acta Orthop. Belg. 77, 145–151.

Geissler, E.K., Hutchinson, J.A., 2013. Cell therapy as a strategy to minimize maintenance immunosuppression in solid organ transplant recipients. Curr. Opin. Organ Transplant. 18, 408–415.

Ghaedi, M., Mendez, J.J., Bove, P.F., Sivarapatna, A., Raredon, M.S., Niklason, L.E., 2014. Alveolar epithelial differentiation of human induced pluripotent stem cells in a rotating bioreactor. Biomaterials 35, 699–710.

Gilbert, T.W., Stewart-Akers, A.M., Simmons-Byrd, A., Badylak, S.F., 2007. Degradation and remodeling of small intestinal submucosa in canine Achilles tendon repair. J. Bone Joint Surg 89, 621–630.

Gillies, A.R., Smith, L.R., Lieber, R.L., Varghese, S., 2010. Method for decellularizing skeletal muscle without detergents or proteolytic enzymes. Tissue Eng. Part C Methods 17, 383–389.

Golish, S.R., Anderson, P.A., 2012. Bearing surfaces for total disc arthroplasty: metal-on-metal versus metal-on-polyethylene and other biomaterials. Spine J. 12, 693–701.

Gonfiotti, A., Jaus, M.O., Barale, D., Baiguera, S., Comin, C., Lavorini, F., et al., 2014. The first tissue-engineered airway transplantation: 5-year follow-up results. Lancet 383, 238–244.

Gordon, S., 2003. Alternative activation of macrophages. Nat. Rev. Immunol. 3, 23–35.

Gordon, S., Martinez, F.O., 2010. Alternative activation of macrophages: mechanism and functions. Immunity 32, 593–604.

Griem, P., Panthel, K., Kalbacher, H., Gleichmann, E., 1996. Alteration of a model antigen by Au (III) leads to T cell sensitization to cryptic peptides. Eur. J. Immunol. 26, 279–287.

Guha, P., Morgan, J.W., Mostoslavsky, G., Rodrigues, N.P., Boyd, A.S., 2013. Lack of immune response to differentiated cells derived from syngeneic induced pluripotent stem cells. Cell Stem Cell 12, 407–412.

Hallab, N.J., Vermes, C., Messina, C., Roebuck, K.A., Glant, T.T., Jacobs, J.J., 2002. Concentration- and composition-dependent effects of metal ions on human MG-63 osteoblasts. J. Biomed. Mater. Res. 60, 420–433.

Hamano, K., Rawsthorne, M.-A., Bushell, A.R., Morris, P.J., Wood, K.J., 1996. Evidence that the continued presence of the organ graft and not peripheral donor microchimerism is essential for maintenance of tolerance to alloantigen *in vivo* in anti-CD4 treated recipients. Transplantation 62, 856–860.

Harris, L., Tosatti, S., Wieland, M., Textor, M., Richards, R., 2004. *Staphylococcus aureus* adhesion to titanium oxide surfaces coated with non-functionalized and peptide-functionalized poly(L-lysine)-grafted-poly(ethylene glycol) copolymers. Biomaterials 25, 4135–4148.

Hawkins, J.A., Breinholt, J.P., Lambert, L.M., Fuller, T.C., Profaizer, T., Mcgough, E.C., et al., 2000. Class I and class II anti-HLA antibodies after implantation of cryopreserved allograft material in pediatric patients. J. Thorac. Cardiovasc. Surg. 119, 324–330.

Hayashi, S., Peranteau, W.H., Shaaban, A.F., Flake, A.W., 2002. Complete allogeneic hematopoietic chimerism achieved by a combined strategy of *in utero* hematopoietic stem cell transplantation and postnatal donor lymphocyte infusion. Blood 100, 804–812.

Haykal, S., Zhou, Y., Marcus, P., Salna, M., Machuca, T., Hofer, S.O., et al., 2013. The effect of decellularization of tracheal allografts on leukocyte infiltration and of recellularization on regulatory T cell recruitment. Biomaterials 34, 5821–5832.

Hill, M., Thebault, P., Segovia, M., Louvet, C., Bériou, G., Tilly, G., et al., 2011. Cell therapy with autologous tolerogenic dendritic cells induces allograft tolerance through interferon-gamma and Epstein–Barr virus-induced gene 3. Am. J. Transplant. 11, 2036–2045.

Hollinger, J.O., 1983. Preliminary report on the osteogenic potential of a biodegradable copolymer of polyactide (PLA) and polyglycolide (PGA). J. Biomed. Mater. Res. 17, 71–82.

Hoshino, A., Hanada, S., Manabe, N., Nakayama, T., Yamamoto, K., 2009. Immune response induced by fluorescent nanocrystal quantum dots *in vitro* and *in vivo*. IEEE Trans. Nanobiosci 8, 51–57.

Hoshino, A., Hanada, S., Yamamoto, K., 2011. Toxicity of nanocrystal quantum dots: the relevance of surface modifications. Arch. Toxicol. 85, 707–720.

Hou, P., Li, Y., Zhang, X., Liu, C., Guan, J., Li, H., et al., 2013. Pluripotent stem cells induced from mouse somatic cells by small-molecule compounds. Science 341, 651–654.

Ikeda, K., Nagasawa, K., Horiuchi, T., Tsuru, T., Nishizaka, H., Niho, Y., 1997. C5a induces tissue factor activity on endothelial cells. Thromb. Haemost. 77, 394.

Issa, F., Wood, K.J., 2012. Translating tolerogenic therapies to the clinic—where do we stand? Front Immunol. 3, 254.

Iwasaki, A., Medzhitov, R., 2004. Toll-like receptor control of the adaptive immune responses. Nat. Immunol. 5, 987–995.

Jacobs, J.J., Hallab, N.J., 2006. Loosening and osteolysis associated with metal-on-metal bearings: a local effect of metal hypersensitivity? J. Bone Joint Surg. 88, 1171–1172.

Jacobs, J.P., Quintessenza, J.A., Andrews, T., Burke, R.P., Spektor, Z., Delius, R.E., et al., 1999. Tracheal allograft reconstruction: the total North American and worldwide pediatric experiences. Ann. Thorac. Surg. 68, 1043–1051. discussion 1052).

Jeannet, M., Pinn, V., Flax, M., Winn, H., Russell, P., 1970. Humoral antibodies in renal allotransplantation in man. N. Engl. J. Med. 282, 111–117.

Jose, M.D., Le Meur, Y., Atkins, R.C., Chadban, S.J., 2003. Blockade of macrophage colony-stimulating factor reduces macrophage proliferation and accumulation in renal allograft rejection. Am. J. Transplant. 3, 294–300.

Jungebluth, P., Alici, E., Baiguera, S., Le Blanc, K., Blomberg, P., Bozóky, B., et al., 2011. Tracheobronchial transplantation with a stem-cell-seeded bioartificial nanocomposite: a proof-of-concept study. Lancet 378, 1997–2004.

Jungebluth, P., Moll, G., Baiguera, S., Macchiarini, P., 2012. Tissue-engineered airway: a regenerative solution. Clin. Pharmacol. Ther. 91, 81–93.

Juvet, S.C., Whatcott, A.G., Bushell, A.R., Wood, K.J., 2014. Harnessing regulatory T cells for clinical use in transplantation: the end of the beginning. Am. J. Transplant. 14, 750–763.

Karim, M., Feng, G., Wood, K.J., Bushell, A.R., 2005. CD25+ CD4+ regulatory T cells generated by exposure to a model protein antigen prevent allograft rejection: antigen-specific reactivation *in vivo* is critical for bystander regulation. Blood 105, 4871–4877.

Keane, T.J., Londono, R., Turner, N.J., Badylak, S.F., 2012. Consequences of ineffective decellularization of biologic scaffolds on the host response. Biomaterials 33, 1771–1781.

Kim, K., Doi, A., Wen, B., Ng, K., Zhao, R., Cahan, P., et al., 2010. Epigenetic memory in induced pluripotent stem cells. Nature 467, 285–290.

Kirk, A.D., Hale, D.A., Mannon, R.B., Kleiner, D.E., Hoffmann, S.C., Kampen, R.L., et al., 2003. Results from a human renal allograft tolerance trial evaluating the humanized CD52-specific monoclonal antibody alemtuzumab (CAMPATH-1H). Transplantation 76, 120–129.

Klompmaker, J., Jansen, H., Veth, R., de Groot, J., Nijenhuis, A., Pennings, A., 1991. Porous polymer implant for repair of meniscal lesions: a preliminary study in dogs. Biomaterials 12, 810–816.

Kneib, C., von Glehn, C.Q., Costa, F.D., Costa, M.T., Susin, M.F., 2012. Evaluation of humoral immune response to donor HLA after implantation of cellularized versus decellularized human heart valve allografts. Tissue Antigens 80, 165–174.

Kobayashi, T., Yamaguchi, T., Hamanaka, S., Kato-Itoh, M., Yamazaki, Y., Ibata, M., et al., 2010. Generation of rat pancreas in mouse by interspecific blastocyst injection of pluripotent stem cells. Cell 142, 787–799.

Koch, H., Graneist, C., Emmrich, F., Till, H., Metzger, R., Aupperle, H., et al., 2012. Xenogenic esophagus scaffolds fixed with several agents: comparative *in vivo* study of rejection and inflammation. J. Biomed. Biotechnol. 2012, 948320.

Kocianova, S., Vuong, C., Yao, Y., Voyich, J.M., Fischer, E.R., Deleo, F.R., et al., 2005. Key role of poly-gamma-DL-glutamic acid in immune evasion and virulence of *Staphylococcus epidermidis*. J. Clin. Invest. 115, 688–694.

Konieczny, B.T., Dai, Z., Elwood, E.T., Saleem, S., Linsley, P.S., Baddoura, F.K., et al., 1998. IFN-gamma is critical for long-term allograft survival induced by blocking the CD28 and CD40 ligand T cell costimulation pathways. J. Immunol. 160, 2059–2064.

Kreuwel, H.T., Aung, S., Silao, C., Sherman, L.A., 2002. Memory CD8(+) T cells undergo peripheral tolerance. Immunity 17, 73–81.

Lalli, P.N., Strainic, M.G., Yang, M., Lin, F., Medof, M.E., Heeger, P.S., 2008. Locally produced C5a binds to T cell-expressed C5aR to enhance effector T-cell expansion by limiting antigen-induced apoptosis. Blood 112, 1759–1766.

Leech, S., 1998. Molecular mimicry in autoimmune disease. Arch. Dis. Child. 79, 448–451.

Leishman, A.J., Silk, K.M., Fairchild, P.J., 2011. Pharmacological manipulation of dendritic cells in the pursuit of transplantation tolerance. Curr. Opin. Organ Transplant. 16, 372–378.

Le Texier, L., Thebault, P., Lavault, A., Usal, C., Merieau, E., Quillard, T., et al., 2011. Long-term allograft tolerance is characterized by the accumulation of B cells exhibiting an inhibited profile. Am. J. Transplant. 11, 429–438.

Leventhal, J., Abecassis, M., Miller, J., Gallon, L., Ravindra, K., Tollerud, D.J., et al., 2012. Chimerism and tolerance without GVHD or engraftment syndrome in HLA-mismatched combined kidney and hematopoietic stem cell transplantation. Sci. Transl. Med. 4, 124ra28.

Li, B., Jiang, B., Boyce, B.M., Lindsey, B.A., 2009. Multilayer polypeptide nanoscale coatings incorporating IL-12 for the prevention of biomedical device-associated infections. Biomaterials 30, 2552–2558.

Li, K., Patel, H., Farrar, C.A., Hargreaves, R.E., Sacks, S.H., Zhou, W., 2004. Complement activation regulates the capacity of proximal tubular epithelial cell to stimulate alloreactive T cell response. J. Am. Soc. Nephrol. 15, 2414–2422.

Li, K., Fazekasova, H., Wang, N., Peng, Q., Sacks, S.H., Lombardi, G., et al., 2012. Functional modulation of human monocytes derived DCs by anaphylatoxins C3a and C5a. Immunobiology 217, 65–73.

Liu, J., Miwa, T., Hilliard, B., Chen, Y., Lambris, J.D., Wells, A.D., et al., 2005. The complement inhibitory protein DAF (CD55) suppresses T cell immunity *in vivo*. J. Exp. Med. 201, 567–577.

Liu, Z., Tugulea, S., Cortesini, R., Lederman, S., Suciu-Foca, N., 1999. Inhibition of CD40 signaling pathway in antigen presenting cells by T suppressor cells. Hum. Immunol. 60, 568–574.

Long, E., Wood, K.J., 2009. Regulatory T cells in transplantation: transferring mouse studies to the clinic. Transplantation 88, 1050–1056.

Lynn, A., Yannas, I., Bonfield, W., 2004. Antigenicity and immunogenicity of collagen. J. Biomed. Mater. Res. Part B Appl. Biomater. 71, 343–354.

Ma, R., Li, M., Luo, J., Yu, H., Sun, Y., Cheng, S., et al., 2013. Structural integrity, ECM components and immunogenicity of decellularized laryngeal scaffold with preserved cartilage. Biomaterials 34, 1790–1798.

Macchiarini, P., Jungebluth, P., Go, T., Asnaghi, M.A., Rees, L.E., Cogan, T.A., et al., 2008. Clinical transplantation of a tissue-engineered airway. Lancet 372, 2023–2030.

Malek, T.R., Bayer, A.L., 2004. Tolerance, not immunity, crucially depends on IL-2. Nat. Rev. Immunol. 4, 665–674.

Martinez, F.O., Sica, A., Mantovani, A., Locati, M., 2008. Macrophage activation and polarization. Front. Biosci. 13, 453–461.

Matsunari, H., Nagashima, H., Watanabe, M., Umeyama, K., Nakano, K., Nagaya, M., et al., 2013. Blastocyst complementation generates exogenic pancreas *in vivo* in apancreatic cloned pigs. Proc. Natl. Acad. Sci. USA. 110, 4557–4562.

Mauiyyedi, S., Crespo, M., Collins, A.B., Schneeberger, E.E., Pascual, M.A., Saidman, S.L., et al., 2002. Acute humoral rejection in kidney transplantation: II. Morphology, immunopathology, and pathologic classification. J. Am. Soc. Nephrol. 13, 779–787.

Maurus, P.B., Kaeding, C.C., 2004. Bioabsorbable implant material review. Oper. Tech. Sports Med. 12, 158–160.

Mcmurchy, A.N., Bushell, A., Levings, M.K., Wood, K.J., 2011. Moving to tolerance: clinical application of T regulatory cells. Semin. Immunol. 23, 304–313.

Middleton, J.C., Tipton, A.J., 2000. Synthetic biodegradable polymers as orthopedic devices. Biomaterials 21, 2335–2346.

Murphy, S.P., Porrett, P.M., Turka, L.A., 2011. Innate immunity in transplant tolerance and rejection. Immunol. Rev. 241, 39–48.

Naesens, M., Li, L., Ying, L., Sansanwal, P., Sigdel, T.K., Hsieh, S.-C., et al., 2009. Expression of complement components differs between kidney allografts from living and deceased donors. J. Am. Soc. Nephrol. 20, 1839–1851.

Nair, L.S., Laurencin, C.T., 2007. Biodegradable polymers as biomaterials. Prog. Polym. Sci. 32, 762–798.

Nikolic, B., Gardner, J.P., Scadden, D.T., Arn, J.S., Sachs, D.H., Sykes, M., 1999. Normal development in porcine thymus grafts and specific tolerance of human T cells to porcine donor MHC. J. Immunol. 162, 3402–3407.

Nilsson, B., Korsgren, O., Lambris, J.D., Ekdahl, K.N., 2010. Can cells and biomaterials in therapeutic medicine be shielded from innate immune recognition? Trends Immunol. 31, 32–38.

Nisbet, D.R., Rodda, A.E., Horne, M.K., Forsythe, J.S., Finkelstein, D.I., 2009. Neurite infiltration and cellular response to electrospun polycaprolactone scaffolds implanted into the brain. Biomaterials 30, 4573–4580.

Olausson, M., Patil, P.B., Kuna, V.K., Chougule, P., Hernandez, N., Methe, K., et al., 2012. Transplantation of an allogeneic vein bioengineered with autologous stem cells: a proof-of-concept study. Lancet 380, 230–237.

Orlando, G., 2012. Immunosuppression-free transplantation reconsidered from a regenerative medicine perspective. Expert Rev. Clin. Immunol. 8, 179–187.

Orlando, G., Wood, K.J., De Coppi, P., Baptista, P.M., Binder, K.W., Bitar, K.N., et al., 2012. Regenerative medicine as applied to general surgery. Ann. Surg. 255, 867–880.

Päivärinta, U., Böstman, O., Majola, A., Toivonen, T., Törmälä, P., Rokkanen, P., 1993. Intraosseous cellular response to biodegradable fracture fixation screws made of polyglycolide or polylactide. Arch. Orthop. Trauma Surg. 112, 71–74.

Pareta, R., Sanders, B., Babbar, P., Soker, T., Booth, C., Mcquilling, J., et al., 2012. Immunoisolation: where regenerative medicine meets solid organ transplantation. Expert Rev. Clin. Immunol. 8, 685–692.

Partington, L., Mordan, N.J., Mason, C., Knowles, J.C., Kim, H.W., Lowdell, M.W., et al., 2013. Biochemical changes caused by decellularization may compromise mechanical integrity of tracheal scaffolds. Acta Biomater. 9, 5251–5261.

Piccotti, J.R., Chan, S.Y., Vanbuskirk, A.M., Eichwald, E.J., Bishop, D.K., 1997. Are Th2 helper T lymphocytes beneficial, deleterious, or irrelevant in promoting allograft survival? Transplantation 63, 619–624.

Pilmore, H., Painter, D., Bishop, G., Mccaughan, G., Eris, J., 2000. Early up-regulation of macrophages and myofibroblasts: a new marker for development of chronic renal allograft rejection. Transplantation 69, 2658–2662.

Poggio, E.D., Augustine, J.J., Clemente, M., Danzig, J.M., Volokh, N., Zand, M.S., et al., 2007. Pretransplant cellular alloimmunity as assessed by a panel of reactive T cells assay correlates with acute renal graft rejection. Transplantation 83, 847–852.

Porta, C., Rimoldi, M., Raes, G., Brys, L., Ghezzi, P., Di Liberto, D., et al., 2009. Tolerance and M2 (alternative) macrophage polarization are related processes orchestrated by p50 nuclear factor kappaB. Proc. Natl. Acad. Sci. USA. 106, 14978–14983.

Pouton, C.W., Akhtar, S., 1996. Biosynthetic polyhydroxyalkanoates and their potential in drug delivery. Adv. Drug Deliv. Rev. 18, 133–162.

Pratt, J.R., Basheer, S.A., Sacks, S.H., 2002. Local synthesis of complement component C3 regulates acute renal transplant rejection. Nat. Med. 8, 582–587.

Qiu, W., Zhang, Y., Liu, X., Zhou, J., Li, Y., Zhou, Y., et al., 2012. Sublytic C5b-9 complexes induce proliferative changes of glomerular mesangial cells in rat Thy-1 nephritis through TRAF6-mediated PI3K-dependent Akt1 activation. J. Pathol. 226, 619–632.

Rafei, M., Hsieh, J., Zehntner, S., Li, M., Forner, K., Birman, E., et al., 2009. A granulocyte-macrophage colony-stimulating factor and interleukin-15 fusokine induces a regulatory B cell population with immune suppressive properties. Nat. Med. 15, 1038–1045.

Ravindra, K.V., Wu, S., Bozulic, L., Xu, H., Breidenbach, W.C., Ildstad, S.T., 2008. Composite tissue transplantation: a rapidly advancing field. Transplant. Proc. 40, 1237–1248.

Raya-Rivera, A., Esquiliano, D.R., Yoo, J.J., Lopez-Bayghen, E., Soker, S., Atala, A., 2011. Tissue-engineered autologous urethras for patients who need reconstruction: an observational study. Lancet 377, 1175–1182.

Refaeli, Y., Van Parijs, L., Alexander, S.I., Abbas, A.K., 2002. Interferon gamma is required for activation-induced death of T lymphocytes. J. Exp. Med. 196, 999–1005.

Ricklin, D., Hajishengallis, G., Yang, K., Lambris, J.D., 2010. Complement: a key system for immune surveillance and homeostasis. Nat. Immunol. 11, 785–797.

Rieder, E., Seebacher, G., Kasimir, M.-T., Eichmair, E., Winter, B., Dekan, B., et al., 2005. Tissue engineering of heart valves decellularized porcine and human valve scaffolds differ importantly in residual potential to attract monocytic cells. Circulation 111, 2792–2797.

Robertson, N.J., Brook, F.A., Gardner, R.L., Cobbold, S.P., Waldmann, H., Fairchild, P.J., 2007. Embryonic stem cell-derived tissues are immunogenic but their inherent immune privilege promotes the induction of tolerance. Proc. Natl. Acad. Sci. USA. 104, 20920–20925.

Rubtsov, Y.P., Rasmussen, J.P., Chi, E.Y., Fontenot, J., Castelli, L., Ye, X., et al., 2008. Regulatory T cell-derived interleukin-10 limits inflammation at environmental interfaces. Immunity 28, 546–558.

Ryan, E.A., Lakey, J.R., Rajotte, R.V., Korbutt, G.S., Kin, T., Imes, S., et al., 2001. Clinical outcomes and insulin secretion after islet transplantation with the Edmonton protocol. Diabetes 50, 710–719.

Sacks, S.H., Zhou, W., 2012. The role of complement in the early immune response to transplantation. Nat. Rev. Immunol. 12, 431–442.

Santavirta, S., Konttinen, Y.T., Saito, T., Gronblad, M., Partio, E., Kemppinen, P., et al., 1990. Immune response to polyglycolic acid implants. J. Bone Joint Surg. Br. Vol. 72, 597–600.

Scheibner, K.A., Lutz, M.A., Boodoo, S., Fenton, M.J., Powell, J.D., Horton, M.R., 2006. Hyaluronan fragments act as an endogenous danger signal by engaging TLR2. J. Immunol. 177, 1272–1281.

Schutte, R.J., Xie, L., Klitzman, B., Reichert, W.M., 2009. *In vivo* cytokine-associated responses to biomaterials. Biomaterials 30, 160–168.

Sicari, B.M., Johnson, S.A., Siu, B.F., Crapo, P.M., Daly, K.A., Jiang, H., et al., 2012. The effect of source animal age upon the *in vivo* remodeling characteristics of an extracellular matrix scaffold. Biomaterials 33, 5524–5533.

Sicari, B.M., Rubin, J.P., Dearth, C.L., Wolf, M.T., Ambrosio, F., Boninger, M., et al., 2014. An acellular biologic scaffold promotes skeletal muscle formation in mice and humans with volumetric muscle loss. Sci. Transl. Med. 6, 234ra58.

Silk, K.M., Fairchild, P.J., 2009. Harnessing dendritic cells for the induction of transplantation tolerance. Curr. Opin. Organ Transplant. 14, 344–350.

Smith, A.J., Dieppe, P., Vernon, K., Porter, M., Blom, A.W., 2012. Failure rates of stemmed metal-on-metal hip replacements: analysis of data from the national joint registry of England and wales. Lancet 379, 1199–1204.

Sotres-Vega, A., Villalba-Caloca, J., Jasso-Victoria, R., Olmos-Zuniga, J.R., Gaxiola-Gaxiola, M., Baltazares-Lipp, M., et al., 2006. Cryopreserved tracheal grafts: a review of the literature. J. Invest. Surg. 19, 125–135.

Stapleton, T.W., Ingram, J., Fisher, J., Ingham, E., 2011. Investigation of the regenerative capacity of an acellular porcine medial meniscus for tissue engineering applications. Tissue Eng. Part A 17, 231–242.

Stein, M., Keshav, S., Harris, N., Gordon, S., 1992. Interleukin 4 potently enhances murine macrophage mannose receptor activity: a marker of alternative immunologic macrophage activation. J. Exp. Med. 176, 287–292.

Stout, R.D., Jiang, C., Matta, B., Tietzel, I., Watkins, S.K., Suttles, J., 2005. Macrophages sequentially change their functional phenotype in response to changes in microenvironmental influences. J. Immunol. 175, 342–349.

Strainic, M.G., Liu, J., Huang, D., An, F., Lalli, P.N., Muqim, N., et al., 2008. Locally produced complement fragments C5a and C3a provide both costimulatory and survival signals to naive CD4+ T cells. Immunity 28, 425–435.

Swijnenburg, R.-J., Tanaka, M., Vogel, H., Baker, J., Kofidis, T., Gunawan, F., et al., 2005. Embryonic stem cell immunogenicity increases upon differentiation after transplantation into ischemic myocardium. Circulation 112, I-166–I-172.

Takahashi, K., Yamanaka, S., 2006. Induction of pluripotent stem cells from mouse embryonic and adult fibroblast cultures by defined factors. Cell 126, 663–676.

Takeda, Y., Costa, S., Delamarre, E., Roncal, C., Leite de Oliveira, R., Squadrito, M.L., et al., 2011. Macrophage skewing by Phd2 haplodeficiency prevents ischaemia by inducing arteriogenesis. Nature 479, 122–126.

Tedesco, F.S., Gerli, M.F., Perani, L., Benedetti, S., Ungaro, F., Cassano, M., et al., 2012. Transplantation of genetically corrected human iPSC-derived progenitors in mice with limb-girdle muscular dystrophy. Sci. Transl. Med. 4, 140ra89.

Thoman, M., Meuth, J., Morgan, E., Weigle, W., Hugli, T., 1984. C3d-K, a kallikrein cleavage fragment of iC3b is a potent inhibitor of cellular proliferation. J. Immunol. 133, 2629–2633.

Thornley, T.B., Brehm, M.A., Markees, T.G., Shultz, L.D., Mordes, J.P., Welsh, R.M., et al., 2006. TLR agonists abrogate costimulation blockade-induced prolongation of skin allografts. J. Immunol. 176, 1561–1570.

Thurman, J.M., Ljubanoviſá, D., Royer, P.A., Kraus, D.M., Molina, H., Barry, N.P., et al., 2006. Altered renal tubular expression of the complement inhibitor Crry permits complement activation after ischemia/reperfusion. J. Clin. Invest. 116, 357–368.

Törmälä, P., 1992. Biodegradable self-reinforced composite materials; manufacturing structure and mechanical properties. Clin. Mater. 10, 29–34.

Totonelli, G., Maghsoudlou, P., Fishman, J.M., Orlando, G., Ansari, T., Sibbons, P., et al., 2012a. Esophageal tissue engineering: a new approach for esophageal replacement. World J. Gastroenterol. WJG 18, 6900.

Totonelli, G., Maghsoudlou, P., Garriboli, M., Riegler, J., Orlando, G., Burns, A.J., et al., 2012b. A rat decellularized small bowel scaffold that preserves villus-crypt architecture for intestinal regeneration. Biomaterials 33, 3401–3410.

Tough, D.F., Borrow, P., Sprent, J., 1996. Induction of bystander T cell proliferation by viruses and type I interferon *in vivo*. Science 272, 1947–1950.

Tullius, S., Nieminen, M., Bechstein, W., Jonas, S., Steinmüller, T., Pratschke, J., et al., 1997. Chronically rejected rat kidney allografts induce donor-specific tolerance. Transplantation 64, 158–161.

Ueda, H., Tabata, Y., 2003. Polyhydroxyalkanonate derivatives in current clinical applications and trials. Adv. Drug Deliv. Rev. 55, 501–518.

Usui, J., Kobayashi, T., Yamaguchi, T., Knisely, A.S., Nishinakamura, R., Nakauchi, H., 2012. Generation of kidney from pluripotent stem cells via blastocyst complementation. Am. J. Pathol. 180, 2417–2426.

Valentin, J.E., Badylak, J.S., Mccabe, G.P., Badylak, S.F., 2006. Extracellular matrix bioscaffolds for orthopaedic applications. A comparative histologic study. J. Bone Joint Surg. 88, 2673–2686.

Valentin, J.E., Stewart-Akers, A.M., Gilbert, T.W., Badylak, S.F., 2009. Macrophage participation in the degradation and remodeling of extracellular matrix scaffolds. Tissue Eng. Part A 15, 1687–1694.

Vieyra, M., Leisman, S., Raedler, H., Kwan, W.-H., Yang, M., Strainic, M.G., et al., 2011. Complement regulates CD4 T-cell help to CD8 T cells required for murine allograft rejection. Am. J. Pathol. 179, 766–774.

Waldmann, H., Adams, E., Fairchild, P., Cobbold, S., 2008. Regulation and privilege in transplantation tolerance. J. Clin. Immunol. 28, 716–725.

Wang, Y., Dai, S., 2013. Structural basis of metal hypersensitivity. Immunol. Res. 55, 83–90.

Weisman, H.F., Bartow, T., Leppo, M.K., Marsh, H., Carson, G.R., Concino, M.F., et al., 1990. Soluble human complement receptor type 1: *in vivo* inhibitor of complement suppressing post-ischemic myocardial inflammation and necrosis. Science 249, 146–151.

Williams, D.F., 2008. On the mechanisms of biocompatibility. Biomaterials 29, 2941–2953.

Williams, J.P., Pechet, T.T., Weiser, M.R., Reid, R., Kobzik, L., Moore, F.D., et al., 1999. Intestinal reperfusion injury is mediated by IgM and complement. J. Appl. Physiol. 86, 938–942.

Wood, K.J., Goto, R., 2012. Mechanisms of rejection: current perspectives. Transplantation 93, 1–10.

Wood, K.J., Sawitzki, B., 2006. Interferon gamma: a crucial role in the function of induced regulatory T cells *in vivo*. Trends Immunol. 27, 183–187.

Wood, K.J., Bushell, A., Hester, J., 2012. Regulatory immune cells in transplantation. Nat. Rev. Immunol. 12, 417–430.

Wu, Q., Salomon, B., Chen, M., Wang, Y., Hoffman, L.M., Bluestone, J.A., et al., 2001. Reversal of spontaneous autoimmune insulitis in nonobese diabetic mice by soluble lymphotoxin receptor. J. Exp. Med. 193, 1327–1332.

Wu, T., Bond, G., Martin, D., Nalesnik, M.A., Demetris, A.J., Abu-Elmagd, K., 2006. Histopathologic characteristics of human intestine allograft acute rejection in patients pretreated with thymoglobulin or alemtuzumab. Am. J. Gastroenterol. 101, 1617–1624.

Wu, Z., Bensinger, S.J., Zhang, J., Chen, C., Yuan, X., Huang, X., et al., 2004. Homeostatic proliferation is a barrier to transplantation tolerance. Nat. Med. 10, 87–92.

Xia, Z., Triffitt, J.T., 2006. A review on macrophage responses to biomaterials. Biomed. Mater. 1, R1.

Xu, H., Wan, H., Zuo, W., Sun, W., Owens, R.T., Harper, J.R., et al., 2009. A porcine-derived acellular dermal scaffold that supports soft tissue regeneration: removal of terminal galactose-alpha-(1,3)-galactose and retention of matrix structure. Tissue Eng. Part A 15, 1807–1819.

Yachimovich-Cohen, N., Even-Ram, S., Shufaro, Y., Rachmilewitz, J., Reubinoff, B., 2010. Human embryonic stem cells suppress T cell responses via arginase I-dependent mechanism. J. Immunol. 184, 1300–1308.

Yahyouche, A., Zhidao, X., Czernuszka, J.T., Clover, A.J., 2011. Macrophage-mediated degradation of crosslinked collagen scaffolds. Acta Biomater. 7, 278–286.

Yamada, K., Yazawa, K., Shimizu, A., Iwanaga, T., Hisashi, Y., Nuhn, M., et al., 2005. Marked prolongation of porcine renal xenograft survival in baboons through the use of alpha1,3-galactosyltransferase gene-knockout donors and the cotransplantation of vascularized thymic tissue. Nat. Med. 11, 32–34.

Ye, L., Yong, K.T., Liu, L., Roy, I., Hu, R., Zhu, J., et al., 2012. A pilot study in non-human primates shows no adverse response to intravenous injection of quantum dots. Nat. Nanotechnol. 7, 453–458.

Yuan, X., Paez-Cortez, J., Schmitt-Knosalla, I., D'addio, F., Mfarrej, B., Donnarumma, M., et al., 2008. A novel role of CD4 Th17 cells in mediating cardiac allograft rejection and vasculopathy. J. Exp. Med. 205, 3133–3144.

Zang, M., Zhang, Q., Chang, E.I., Mathur, A.B., Yu, P., 2013. Decellularized tracheal matrix scaffold for tracheal tissue engineering: *in vivo* host response. Plast. Reconstr. Surg. 132, 549e–559e.

Zarkhin, V., Chalasani, G., Sarwal, M.M., 2010. The Yin and Yang of B cells in graft rejection and tolerance. Transplant. Rev. 24, 67–78.

Zdolsek, J., Eaton, J.W., Tang, L., 2007. Histamine release and fibrinogen adsorption mediate acute inflammatory responses to biomaterial implants in humans. J. Transl. Med. 5, 31–36.

Zhai, Y., Meng, L., Gao, F., Busuttil, R.W., Kupiec-Weglinski, J.W., 2002. Allograft rejection by primed/memory CD8+ T cells is CD154 blockade resistant: therapeutic implications for sensitized transplant recipients. J. Immunol. 169, 4667–4673.

Zhao, T., Zhang, Z.N., Rong, Z., Xu, Y., 2011. Immunogenicity of induced pluripotent stem cells. Nature 474, 212–215.

Zolnik, B.S., Gonzalez-Fernandez, A., Sadrieh, N., Dobrovolskaia, M.A., 2010. Nanoparticles and the immune system. Endocrinology 151, 458–465.

Zopf, D.A., Hollister, S.J., Nelson, M.E., Ohye, R.G., Green, G.E., 2013. Bioresorbable airway splint created with a three-dimensional printer. N. Engl. J. Med. 368, 2043–2045.

Zwacka, R.M., Zhang, Y., Halldorson, J., Schlossberg, H., Dudus, L., Engelhardt, J.F., 1997. CD4(+) T-lymphocytes mediate ischemia/reperfusion-induced inflammatory responses in mouse liver. J. Clin. Invest. 100, 279.

CHAPTER 9

Fibrotic Response to Biomaterials and all Associated Sequence of Fibrosis

Kim Jones
Department of Chemical Engineering and School of Biomedical Engineering, McMaster University, Hamilton, ON, Canada

Contents

Host Response to Biomaterials.
DOI: http://dx.doi.org/10.1016/B978-0-12-800196-7.00009-8
189

INTRODUCTION

One of the dirty little secrets of the biomaterials field is that virtually any implanted material will eventually cause scarring (fibrosis). When you get a sliver, the first, painful response is the classic hot, red inflammation. However, if you do not remove the sliver, over time, your body will accumulate collagen (scar tissue), essentially "walling off" the foreign body, even if it does not become infected. In this chapter, we will try to understand this protective mechanism.

While fibrosis is not always clinically problematic, it is important to recognize and try to address it during the design phase. We will present a number of examples in which fibrosis has been documented clinically and in research, and discuss the implications of this scar tissue formation.

In order to ultimately address fibrosis, we will need to understand the mechanism of action. Fibrosis is really just wound healing gone awry. Surgical implantation of a biomaterial, no matter how noninvasive, causes injury. If the material were not present, the body would go through classic wound healing, which would ultimately result (depending on the size of the injury) in regenerated tissue with only a small scar. After any injury, the body goes through inflammation, matrix formation, and matrix rearrangement. We must ask ourselves—at what stage does the biomaterial alter this response? In the other chapters in this textbook, evidence is presented that biomaterials are recognized, and a response generated, throughout their time in the body. So how do these early responses affect the long-term response—or do they? Thus, we will briefly discuss the wound healing response and the role biomaterials play in disrupting it.

There is a substantial literature examining pathological fibrosis. It is potentially useful to understand what happens in the body when disease states cause fibrosis. How do inflammatory stimuli affect or initiate fibrosis? What is the influence of the different cell type upon the fibrotic response? How do cytokines and chemokines affect the progression of fibrosis? In each section, we reflect upon the response to biomaterials and how it parallels and/or differs from the normal inflammatory response.

We examine the signals that initiate fibrosis. The initial injury due to implantation can initiate the fibrotic response. If infection is associated with the biomaterial, the degree of fibrosis will increase dramatically. Bacterial biofilms in particular cause adverse reactions. However, surface chemistry, mechanical properties, and topography have also been shown to influence the ultimate response.

There is some evidence from the factors which influence the body's response to biomaterials. Many of the cells associated with the innate immune response are involved in the fibrotic response. In particular, neutrophils, macrophages, foreign body giant cells (FBGCs), mast cells, and fibroblasts have all been implicated in sensing the biomaterial and in producing signals that alter fibrotic responses (for more details, see Chapters 2 and 4).

The question remains: how do we control fibrotic response? It seems that it is nearly impossible to create a truly "stealth" material; even if it superficially resembles the native tissue, there are enough differences that the body will respond. Nonetheless, a number of strategies have the potential to control fibrosis. Certainly, attempts have been made to alter fibrotic responses by altering surface chemistry (Valdes et al., 2011) and topography (Koschwanez et al., 2008). There is some potential to affect fibrotic responses, particularly in tissue engineering applications, by incorporating cells that have an effect on regeneration. Perhaps most promising is the ability to release drugs from biomaterials. A number of strategies have shown promise, including interfering with collagen assembly, altering inflammation, and altering macrophage phenotypes.

Biomaterials have proven themselves to be a very useful tool in medicine. In this chapter, we hope to convince you that research can move biomaterials from "good enough" to "perfect."

BIOMATERIALS AND THE WOUND HEALING PARADIGM

The surgical implantation of a biomaterial causes a wound, so it is worthwhile to explore how the biomaterial alters the default wound healing response. The basic stages of wound healing in response to biomaterials are acute inflammation, followed by granulation tissue formation and the foreign body reaction that includes fibrous tissue and contracture. In wound healing, the final step is remodeling and at least partial regeneration of the affected tissue, but this has not been observed in response to biomaterials.

Acute inflammation

Surgical implantation of biomaterials causes some degree of tissue injury (see Chapter 2). Fibrin deposition, the production of the provisional matrix, activation of the coagulation and complement cascades, and platelet release of growth factors, cytokines, and chemokines are all part of the acute response (Boateng et al., 2008; Markiewski et al., 2007). The proteins of the Vroman effect and of coagulation and complement cascades all interact directly with biomaterials as well, as do the platelets themselves, potentially exacerbating the acute inflammatory response (Gorbet and Sefton, 2004). The chemokines trigger migration and extravasation of neutrophils, monocytes, and fibrocytes (Schmid-Schönbein, 2006; McDonald et al., 2011). The neutrophils release cytokines that induce fibrosis (interleukin-1 (IL-1) and tumor necrosis factor α (TNFα)), while the monocytes release chemoattractants and mitogens for fibroblasts, such as fibroblast growth factor (FGF) and platelet-derived growth factor (PDGF) (Borthwick et al., 2013). Macrophages also release angiogenic molecules such as vascular endothelial growth factor (VEGF) (Jaipersad et al., 2014). Other chapters address how the biomaterials alter interactions with inflammatory cells, particularly macrophages (see Chapter 6). There is intriguing evidence that the macrophage phenotype might regulate the ultimate fibrotic response (Sindrilaru and Scharffetter-Kochanek, 2013).

In normal wound healing, the fibroblasts are activated by transforming growth factor β (TGFβ) to make pro-collagens, which are then enzymatically converted into collagen (Kendall and Feghali-Bostwick, 2014). Cells proliferate and matrix accumulates to fill the wound site and replace damaged tissue. Cell–cell and cell–matrix interactions are important here, depending on integrins, cadherins, selectins, and immunoglobulins. As the matrix matures, it is degraded by proteases including serum-derived plasmin, collagenase, and matrix metalloproteinases (MMPs) which allow cell migration (Giannandrea and Parks, 2014). These acute responses are all influenced by the presence of a biomaterial. This chapter focuses upon the long-term, chronic response to a biomaterial. Clinically, the body can extrude the material (as with some splinters), resorb it (e.g., degradable materials), integrate it (as would happen ideally in tissue engineering and does sometimes occur in response to surgical mesh materials (Badylak, 2014)), or encapsulate it. The latter, unfortunately, happens most frequently. Chronically, three things usually occur following biomaterial implantation: formation of granulation tissue, formation of an avascular fibrous capsule, and capsular contracture.

Granulation tissue and the foreign body reaction

Granulation tissue is vascularized tissue that forms as chronic inflammation evolves. The new capillaries make the tissue appear pink and granular, thus the name. Histologically, one can observe macrophages and proliferating fibroblasts within granulation tissue. This tissue can appear as early as 3–5 days after biomaterial implantation. In the early stages of granulation tissue production, proliferating fibroblasts produce primarily proteoglycans, while later they produce mostly type III collagen (Utsunomiya et al., 2005). In the presence of a persistent stimulus, granulation tissue, or chronic inflammation, can endure for the duration of the presence of the biomaterial. In some cases, wear debris or corrosion products are released throughout the lifetime of the implant. Hip implants are well known for producing such debris and causing concomitant damage (see Chapter 12). Degradable biomaterials have the potential to elicit such a response as well, depending on the mode of degradation (Galgut et al., 1991). In other cases, there is continuing injury due to biomaterial movement or mismatch of mechanical properties with the native tissue which serve as stimuli for granulation tissue formation.

In addition to granulation tissue, nondegradable and slowly degradable biomaterials generally elicit a foreign body response. This response has been described in Chapter 2.

Encapsulation by fibrous tissue and capsular contracture

Ultimately, nondegradable biomaterial implants become surrounded by a fibrous capsule. It is possible for implants to become fully integrated (such as macroporous polypropylene surgical meshes (Badylak, 2014), but this is the exception, not the rule. Most cells of the parenchyma are fully differentiated and thus do not easily divide to repopulate a wound site and regenerate it fully. In sites where cells normally multiply (such as skin), or when dividing cells are incorporated into tissue-engineered constructs, the potential exists for full integration/regeneration, yet that is still not usually what is observed.

In the absence of continuous stimuli, granulation tissue in a wound will remodel into scar tissue. The cellularity decreases due to apoptosis (Reinke and Sorg, 2012). MMPs help change the orientation and structure of the collagen fibrils, and the amounts of various types of collagen change with time (Kendall and Feghali-Bostwick, 2014). The dense parallel bundles of collagen do not have the strength of native tissue. Ultimately, myofibroblasts cause contracture of the wound margins. In normal wound healing, this contracture is beneficial; however, around biomaterials, as we shall see in the next section, contracture can be problematic.

Interestingly, there does not seem to be a strong correlation between the degree of protein deposition, coagulation, or acute inflammation induced by a biomaterial and the amount of fibrosis. Surface chemistry does play a small role, but it seems that the structure (e.g., size, shape, and mechanical properties) and surface topography (e.g., porosity and roughness) of biomaterials are more important in predicting degree of fibrosis (Lind et al., 2013). For example, implants with a smooth and nondegradable surface create a thicker fibrous capsule than rough or textured implants (Balderrama et al., 2009; Minami et al., 2006). More work needs to be done to understand the factors that contribute to the amount of fibrosis. Factors including anatomic site, blood supply, infection, and underlying pathological conditions are clearly very important.

Tissue remodeling as a consequence of biomaterial presence

The final step of successful wound healing is remodeling and regeneration so the wound site resembles the original tissue. It seems that the presence of the biomaterial interferes with this final step. It is not clear if the deviation from default wound healing is due to signals from the biomaterial, or if early effects on inflammation bias the response away from ultimate outcome. Nonetheless, the deviation from a normal tissue response is a particular concern in applications that require full, functional tissue regeneration around a biomaterial implant.

CLINICAL APPLICATIONS OF BIOMATERIALS AFFECTED BY FIBROSIS

There are as many instances where fibrosis will affect function as there are applications of biomaterials. Herein, we present some examples that highlight the clinical consequences of the fibrotic response.

Implanted sensors and drug delivery devices

It seems intuitive that devices that depend on rapid diffusion of a solute for their function would be affected by the formation of a fibrotic capsule. The most clinically mature probes and drug delivery devices have been developed to treat diabetes, so the tissue response to these devices will be the focus of the section, though any such implanted device will potentially face similar issues. We will discuss implanted glucose sensors, insulin pumps, microcapsules, and particles.

Most implanted sensors and drug delivery systems fail within 1–4 weeks of implantation (Gilligan et al., 2004), due in large part to the development of the fibrous capsule forming a diffusion barrier (Sharkawy et al., 1997, 1998a,b). The effects of this capsule can be seen as early as 1–3 days postimplantation (Mou et al., 2010), and this poses an obvious barrier for the implementation of this technology. When an implanted sensor must be so frequently replaced, the ostensible ease and convenience wanes compared to repeated pinprick blood tests. Thus far, all implanted sensors and devices suffer from these issues to some extent.

In particular, calibration and response time of sensors change as the body's response to the polymer changes the microenvironmental milieu. It is not altogether clear if the alterations are due to the additional diffusion barrier from the collagen layer or because there is less vascular exchange in the relatively acellular capsule. Nonetheless, the effect is significant enough that device manufacturers routinely include a calibration algorithm that compensates for time within the body (Mahmoudi et al., 2014).

Interestingly, in some cases, the calibration stays relatively consistent, but the response time of the sensor decays dramatically (Mou et al., 2010). One group modeled glucose sensor response times and discovered that in the cases of the thickest capsules, the response time could increase as much as threefold. A 200 μm thick capsular layer can increase the lag time in glucose detection from the blood from 5 to 20 min (Sharkawy et al., 1997). The supply of glucose at the sensor surface plummets to as low as 25% of that in normal tissue (Mou et al., 2010). This challenge to sensor responsiveness highlights the importance of engineering anti-fibrotic materials. The clinical implications to a diabetic individual of such significant time lags can be dangerous.

Indeed, there are a number of publications that describe efforts to address this very problem that include altering surface chemistry (Quinn et al., 1997), changing porosity (Ju et al., 2008), and release of bioactive agents (Frost and Meyerhoff, 2006; Ward et al., 2004; Hickey et al., 2002; Hetrick et al., 2007).

Measuring these effects is not straightforward. While diffusion measurements are fairly easily done *in vitro*, it is much more difficult to measure *in vivo*. Some researchers have extracted the fibrous capsule itself and treated it as a diffusion membrane *ex vivo* (Koschwanez and Reichert, 2007). More elegantly, microdialysis membranes can be subcutaneously implanted (Nandi and Lunte, 2009). In one study, calibration was affected, but the more serious problem was the delay in response time (Mou et al., 2010).

Presumably, similar issues will apply for other types of implanted sensors. Depending on the application, these changes in calibration and response time might by clinically acceptable. However, it is important to recognize the effect of the fibrous capsule, and, if possible, minimize it.

Implanted insulin pumps have been used clinically for some time. Early on, fibrous obstruction of the catheter that transported the insulin to the body was a common occurrence, which reduced the useful duration (and convenience) of the device. Twenty years ago, the 50% survival rate for patients with insulin pumps was as short as 27 months (Renard et al., 1995). While nearly half of the obstructions were due to a fibrin clot at the catheter tip, most of the rest were caused by fibrous tissue encapsulation around the catheter. In all cases, however, a fibrous capsule was present around the catheter, though it did not necessarily occlude the tip and prevent free flow of insulin. Again, this is a risky situation for the diabetic patient.

Similarly, permanent catheters are used in peritoneal dialysis to treat renal disease. Here, the catheter straddles applications between a "drug delivery" device and a permanently implanted biomaterial. Nonetheless, one of the serious side effects of peritoneal dialysis is peritonitis, which may lead to progressive peritoneal tissue fibrosis and inability for the peritoneum to act as an effective dialysis membrane. While this has been largely blamed on the dialysis solution, there is some evidence that the catheter itself is at least partly responsible for the failure of peritoneal dialysis clinically (Flessner et al., 2007, 2010).

One approach to treating diabetes (and many other conditions) has been to microencapsulate cells in a semipermeable polymer membrane. These microencapsulated cells are partly a drug delivery device and partly an early application of tissue engineering. In the case of diabetes, insulin-producing islets are encapsulated. The microcapsule membrane protects the implanted cells from the host immune system, as it allows the potential use of allogeneic (between different individuals) or even xenogeneic (between species) cell sources. Even if immune-matched cells can be used (e.g., induced pluripotent stem cells), type I diabetics have an autoimmune response that would otherwise kill the cells. The encapsulated cells produce insulin in a glucose-dependent manner. The insulin diffuses across the semipermeable microcapsule membrane. Similarly, oxygen, nutrients, and waste products will freely diffuse across the membrane, while preventing contact with cells of the immune system and (in some cases) antibodies. Microcapsules have been proposed for long-term release of many different compounds, often from cells that have been genetically altered to produce a protein drug continuously (Paredes JuÃ¡rez et al., 2014).

One barrier to the clinical success of this approach has been ongoing immune responses to antigens shed from the microcapsules, leading to a fibrous capsule forming around the microencapsulated cells and ultimate cell death (Clayton et al., 1993; Jones et al., 2004). There is evidence, however, that the response to the microcapsule material itself can also contribute to the loss of function of these implanted cells. One typical microencapsulation material, alginate–poly-L-lysine–alginate, typically does elicit a fibrous capsule. It has been shown that the purity of the naturally sourced material affects the magnitude of the fibrotic response (Paredes-Juarez et al., 2014). It has been very difficult to establish how much the presence of the fibrotic capsule contributes to device failure. Nonetheless, it likely is detrimental to optimum device function, requiring a larger implant volume than would be required under ideal circumstances.

Drug delivery approaches vary widely and include large devices that release drugs over very long periods. These devices would clearly be affected by long-term fibrosis in response to the polymer. In other cases, drug release is from smaller devices, including controlled release from microelectromechanical systems (MEMS) (Sutradhar and Sumi, 2014). The channels in MEMS devices are very small, so it would be easy to see how even modest fibrotic encapsulation could interfere with the success of this approach. Another very common drug delivery approach is the use of microparticles or nanoparticles. Often, the intent is to target these particles to specific cells, such as cancer cells (Jain et al., 2014). These small particles are usually taken up into the cells and therefore are unlikely to produce fibrosis. However, it should be noted that the majority of such particles (even those "targeted" to specific cell types) are phagocytosed by macrophages and do not reach their target (Kafshgari et al., 2014). In large enough quantities, there is a risk that such particles could produce a granulatomous or fibrotic response, as we will see in the next section.

Implanted biomaterials

Biomaterials have been implanted to supplement the structure and function of virtually every organ or tissue in the body. In many of these cases, a fibrotic response (to a degree) is acceptable clinically. The accumulation of extracellular matrix (ECM) is sometimes a desirable outcome by anchoring the implant and stabilizing it. Here, we will discuss some common applications of biomaterials: as filler materials, as surgical mesh materials, in cochlear implants, and in breast implants. The responses vary from chronic granulomatous tissue (foreign body reaction) to contracting fibrotic capsules.

Cosmetic surgery to buoy aging skin by inserting filler material is widespread: in 2009, over 10 million patients in the United States were implanted (American Society for Aesthetic Plastic Surgery, 2009). Many new compounds are available, yet some unwanted side effects occur with all fillers. The wide range of compounds includes degradable polymers, nondegradable gels, silicone oil, collagen, fat, and many others (Alijotas-Reig et al., 2013). These materials show a common histologic reaction in the long term. Near the filler particles are found T lymphocytes (mostly CD4+) and some B lymphocytes. Around the material are abundant macrophages with some eosinophils. The collagenization (fibrosis) can extend beyond the extent of the filler material and occasionally dystrophic calcification occurs (Alijotas-Reig et al., 2013).

In the case of nonpermanent (i.e., degradable biomaterial) fillers, the collagenization is actually a desirable outcome. Local fibrotic reactions in this application are clinically acceptable, as the filler material itself is not functional; it just needs to occupy a given volume. However, there are unacceptable side effects that have been documented in response to nearly every filler material. Immune-mediated delayed local reactions occur over a year postimplant for both permanent and nonpermanent fillers (Alijotas-Reig et al., 2013). In some instances, infection plays a role; however, chronic granulatomous reactions can occur even with no evidence of infection (Alijotas-Reig et al., 2013). Also observed have been systemic adverse reactions in which filler material migrates to distant sites causing panniculitis or axillary lymphadenitis (Alijotas-Reig et al., 2013). These documented clinical issues with particulate polymeric biomaterials do raise questions about the role of the host response when similar particles are used as drug delivery vehicles.

Surgical mesh materials have been used for many years in hernia repair, pelvic floor reconstruction, breast reconstruction, musculoskeletal and tendon repair, and urogenital tissue reconstruction (Badylak, 2014). They are also promising materials as scaffolds for tissue engineering. The surgical mesh materials are comprised of ECM derived from decellularized and processed allogeneic or xenogeneic tissue. When these tissues are thoroughly decellularized and processed in a way which does not chemically cross-link the ECM, they are constructively remodeled (Badylak, 2014). The materials must also contact the native tissue and experience anatomically appropriate mechanical loads. During remodeling, a rapid influx of neutrophils occurs, followed by macrophages. The scaffold material rapidly degrades while progenitor cells are recruited, resulting in new tissue formation that is at least partially functional and does not display chronic inflammation or fibrosis (Badylak, 2014).

Another commonly seen biomaterial application is the cochlear implant, with more than 324,000 recipients worldwide (NIH Publication No. 11-4798, 2012). The success in improving hearing and speech is very sensitive to acute and chronic damage due to the surgery itself and to the inflammatory reaction (host response) to the device. Clinically, there is evidence that fibrous encapsulation of the electrode, presumably due to a host response to the biomaterial, worsens hearing loss (Astolfi et al., 2014).

Perhaps the most commonly recognized example of fibrosis around a biomaterial is the breast implant. Over 1.5 million silicone breast implants are sold annually worldwide (Steiert et al., 2013). The association between breast implants and autoimmune disorders has been repudiated by well-designed epidemiological studies (Janowsky et al., 2000). This controversy has somewhat overshadowed the frequent complications associated with fibrosis. Among other causes of failure (rupture, leakage, and chronic inflammation) is capsule formation and contracture. The fibrous capsule forms as soon as 1–2 weeks postsurgery (Goldberg, 1997). Subsequently, as the wound tries to "close," the capsule contracts. Up to 80% of implant recipients experience capsular contracture, and it is thus the leading cause of revision surgery (Berry et al., 2010; Handel et al., 2006). On the plus side, a fibrous capsule helps maintain the correct positioning of the implant. However, capsular contracture can lead to pain, local tissue hardening, tightness, deformity, and distortion of the breast (Steiert et al., 2013).

In the capsule itself, myofibroblasts are the predominant cell type (27%), but also found are macrophages, polymorphonuclear leukocytes, lymphocytes, plasma cells, and mast cells (Hwang et al., 2010). From clinical observations, the mechanism leading to capsular contracture is not well understood. Textured implants in general have less capsular contracture than smooth implants (Wong et al., 2006). The incidence of infection is low but when present is an important cause of contracture. Bacteria can colonize the surface of breast implant and form a biofilm. Two-thirds of explanted contractures with high-grade capsular contraction had subclinical bacterial colonization. In contrast, there were no bacteria associated with explanted implants that had low-grade contracture (Schreml et al., 2007). Similarly, introducing bacteria with biomaterials in animal models increases the degree of contracture (Tamboto et al., 2010). Nevertheless, bacterial colonization is not the only contributing factor to capsular contracture. The formation of the fibrous capsule and its subsequent contraction are clinically problematic host responses in this instance.

Tissue-engineered constructs

In tissue engineering, biomaterials provide the structure (scaffold) that guides regeneration. The scaffold often contains cells that provide the biological function to the target tissue-engineered organ. In this context, the fibrotic response can be beneficial or detrimental.

Biomaterial scaffolds alone can facilitate healing. A wound of 1 cm would induce a great deal of scar tissue, but could be closed with minimal fibrosis where a scaffold is inserted to enhance cell migration into the wound site. When autologous cells are included in this strategy, wounds as large as 30 cm can be closed with minimal scarring (Atala, 2009).

The fibrotic response to biomaterials has actually been exploited to produce native scaffold materials. Here, the body is used as a bioreactor. The biomaterial is implanted (e.g., in the peritoneal cavity) and after several days, a fibrotic capsule forms. The capsule is removed and used as a scaffold for tissue engineering (Campbell et al., 2008). This strategy produces a scaffold that the body will at least perceive as "self," meaning that the tissue-engineered organ based on it is less likely to elicit its own foreign body response.

Most proposed scaffolds for tissue engineering are degradable polymers, whether naturally sourced or synthetic, and are thus likely to elicit a fibrotic response. The activity of the cells chosen will likely have a dramatic effect on the type of response. Researchers planning tissue engineering strategies must be cognizant of the consequences of a host response to the scaffold itself—and to the effect of the cells, implant site, and surgical injury. As with breast implants, a fibrotic response could have positive and negative consequences. Fibrotic tissue ingrowth would serve to anchor the construct and prevent further wounding due to micromovement. In some cases, this is interpreted as tissue integration. However, a scarring response that walls off the construct would be detrimental. Regeneration of new tissue might be thwarted if the host's response biases toward fibrosis rather than healing.

GENERAL MECHANISMS OF FIBROSIS

Fibrosis is a hallmark of numerous pathological conditions. These diseases, which cause up to 45% of deaths in the developed world (Wynn, 2008), are marked by an increase in the production and accumulation of ECM components, leading to a loss of tissue architecture and function. In many ways, this is the same progression that occurs in response to biomaterials, but these fields have been studied in far more depth, thus we can learn a great deal from the parallels and differences.

Generally, fibrosis is perceived as the last step in a continuum that begins with injury and inflammation. Anderson has a frequently reproduced diagram that shows the progression of responses to biomaterials over time, starting with influx of polymorphonuclear cells, then monocytes/macrophages, followed by neovascularization, development of FBGCs, then activation of fibroblasts, and finally fibrosis (see Chapter 2 for greater details). Though these events do generally occur sequentially, it is not clear if the early events actually cause the later events or if fibrosis could occur even without inflammatory signals.

Pathological fibrosis is generally accepted to be initiated by some sort of injury (Wynn, 2007). Damaged endothelial and/or epithelial cells release mediators of the coagulation cascade and a fibrin matrix forms (Chambers, 2008). Platelets interact with the fibrin and other ECM components, forming a blood clot, which (hopefully) causes hemostasis. Platelet degranulation affects epithelial/endothelial cells to promote vasodilation, MMP production, and cytokine and chemokine release (Barrientos et al., 2008). Local tissues also produce prostaglandins, which enhance vasodilation, vascular permeability, and leukocyte extravasation. The increased local permeability (along with other signals) induces leukocytes to migrate from the circulation to the site of damage.

The severity of acute inflammation depends on the extent of damage and resulting signaling molecules, the site of damage and the extent of provisional matrix formation. The initial extravasating cells are primarily neutrophils and mast cells. Mast cells release histamine from their granules, which recruits further phagocytes and causes vasodilation and increased vascular permeability (Overed-Sayer et al., 2013). Neutrophils outnumber mast cells and also release cell signaling and chemotactic molecules (Gifford and Chalmers, 2014). The life span of these cells is short, as degranulation is shortly followed by apoptosis. Monocytes and macrophages appear more gradually at the wound site. Much of the work in biomaterials has focused on macrophage–biomaterial interactions (Gardner et al., 2013). Both neutrophils and macrophages phagocytose tissue debris, dead cells, and foreign organisms or materials. Macrophages themselves release a wide variety of cytokines and chemokines that influence subsequent wound healing and fibrotic responses (Sindrilaru and Scharffetter-Kochanek, 2013). These include signals to endothelial/epithelial cells to initiate the formation of new blood vessels. Lymphocytes migrate into the site and their activation leads to release of several pro-fibrotic cytokines (Pellicoro et al., 2014).

The abundance of local pro-fibrotic mediators stimulates fibroblasts (and other cells) to differentiate into α-smooth muscle actin (SMA)-expressing myofibroblasts (Duffield, 2014). In the pathological fibrosis literature, this transition to myofibroblasts is often deemed the critical aspect of fibrogenesis. Myofibroblasts are primarily responsible for local ECM protein production.

If macrophages and other phagocytes cannot eliminate the initial stimulus (e.g., damaged tissue, foreign organisms, or foreign materials), activation of myofibroblasts persists and collagen-I-rich fibrous tissue is formed. As ECM production continues, immune cells undergo apoptosis (Reinke and Sorg, 2012), leaving an irreversible scar that impairs the function of the organ, tissue, or implant.

There are many molecular mediators of this process that are important in controlling the complex cell–cell and cell–microenvironment communication. Understanding these mediators will be critical in identifying possible targets to treat fibrosis. A simplified view of these events is shown in Figure 9.1.

INITIATION OF FIBROSIS

When we consider how to treat fibrosis, we can interfere with progression to fibrosis, which is very complex, or try to interfere with the initiation of fibrosis. Thus, understanding the variety of signals that can lead to fibrotic conditions is important and can help us recognize how host responses to biomaterials lead to fibrosis. Very minor shifts in tissue homeostasis can lead to fibrotic conditions. Often infection or injury

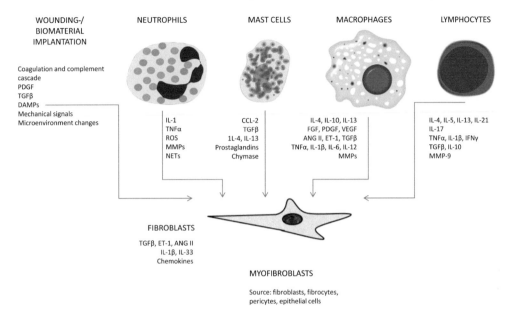

WOUNDING-/
BIOMATERIAL
IMPLANTATION

NEUTROPHILS   MAST CELLS   MACROPHAGES   LYMPHOCYTES

Coagulation and complement
cascade
PDGF
TGFβ
DAMPs
Mechanical signals
Microenvironment changes

IL-1   CCL-2   IL-4, IL-10, IL-13   IL-4, IL-5, IL-13, IL-21
TNFα   TGFβ   FGF, PDGF, VEGF   IL-17
ROS   1L-4, IL-13   ANG II, ET-1, TGFβ   TNFα, IL-1β, IFNγ
MMPs   Prostaglandins   TNFα, IL-1β, IL-6, IL-12   TGFβ, IL-10
NETs   Chymase   MMPs   MMP-9

FIBROBLASTS

TGFβ, ET-1, ANG II
IL-1β, IL-33
Chemokines

MYOFIBROBLASTS

Source: fibroblasts, fibrocytes,
pericytes, epithelial cells

Figure 9.1 Fibrosis in response to biomaterials is a complex process involving many cells and mediators.

leading to inflammation initiates pathological conditions, but it has been shown that severe injury is not a necessary prerequisite. Inflammatory cells are common in the pro-fibrotic environment but might not be required for the development of fibrotic conditions. For example, hemochromatosis often occurs in the absence of inflammatory cells, while still leading to liver cirrhosis (Lin and Adams, 1991). Similarly, lung fibrosis can be caused by over-expression of TGFβ1 without any apparent accompanying inflammation (Sime et al., 1997). The argument has been made that development of fibrosis does not depend on inflammation (Gauldie, 2002; Jones, 2008). In part, this might explain the standard prevalence of fibrosis due to biomaterials, even when the inflammatory responses to those materials differ significantly. Similarly, many of the anti-inflammatory strategies employed in biomaterials have been relatively ineffective in preventing long-term fibrosis.

So how is fibrosis initiated? Inflammatory cells often do produce pro-fibrotic signaling molecules and probably accelerate the development of fibrosis. Thus, the many modes of activation, particularly of macrophages, described in earlier chapters are likely contributors to the fibrosis associated with biomaterials. In addition, though, injury, infection, and the materials themselves can contribute to fibrotic development by producing pathogen-associated molecular patterns (PAMPs) and danger-associated molecular patterns (DAMPs) (Pearl et al., 2011; Yang and Jones, 2009). Hypoxia in the implant environment can also induce fibrosis. Given the trauma associated with biomaterial implantation and the time to develop a new vasculature, it is expected that cells surrounding a biomaterial would suffer from a paucity of oxygen (Bland et al., 2013). Associated with hypoxia and inflammation, shifts in redox homeostasis have also been shown to accelerate fibrosis. Of note, particularly when biomaterials create acidic degradation products (Pitt et al., 1981), pH can also change fibrotic progression. Finally, mechanical signals, such as those transferred due to mismatches in mechanical properties between biomaterial and tissue, can induce fibrosis (Lind et al., 2013). No doubt, this is not an exhaustive list, but it does highlight the many and overlapping ways that fibrosis can be induced in the presence of biomaterials. Many of the mechanisms of fibrosis development mentioned briefly in this section will be described in more detail later.

PAMPs and DAMPs due to biofilms, injury, and surface chemistry

Infection is a starting point of many pathological fibrotic conditions, particularly when the infection cannot be cleared (e.g., in cystic fibrosis: (Chmiel et al., 2014)). Similarly, bacterial biofilms that can easily form on biomaterial surfaces (and are very difficult to clear) have been shown to be associated with the most severe clinical fibrosis (Tamboto et al., 2010). In these cases, the adaptive immune system is undoubtedly involved, but additionally, the bacteria (or viruses or fungi) themselves produce a number of products called PAMPs that are recognized by pattern-recognition receptors (PRRs) on a wide variety of different cells (Greenfield, 2014). These PAMPs include bacterial DNA, double-stranded RNA, peptidoglycans, lipopolysaccharides, and flagellins (Prince et al., 2011). There is evidence that some biomaterial surfaces themselves are perceived as PAMPs (Yang and Jones, 2009).

Similarly, sterile tissue trauma can cause release of a number of molecules termed DAMPs that are recognized by PRRs (Manfredi et al., 2009). Biomaterial implantation itself causes tissue damage. In addition, when the biomaterial is not fully integrated, or when it has sharp edges or mismatched mechanical properties with the tissue, ongoing small-scale injury can occur, potentially releasing DAMPs (Malik et al., 2011; Rogers and Babensee, 2010). DAMPs and alarmins are released by damaged or dying epithelial cells that leak intracellular proteins. Examples include high-mobility box group 1 (HMGB-1), heat shock proteins (e.g., HSP60 and HSP90), IL–33, and IL–1α (Bellaye et al., 2014). IL-33 has been associated with fibrosis in chronic liver injury (Arshad et al., 2012), skin sclerosis, and pulmonary fibrosis (Yanaba et al., 2011). HMGB-1 has been shown to be associated with pulmonary fibrosis (Abe et al., 2011; Hamada et al., 2008). Similarly, Toll-like receptor (TLR—a PRR) expression in fibrotic patients is elevated, suggesting that their cells might be more "ready" to respond to DAMPs and PAMPs (Go et al., 2014).

PRRs are widely expressed on cells including neutrophils, macrophages, T-cells, B-cells, dendritic cells, eosinophils, epithelial cells, adipocytes, and fibroblasts (Jeong and Lee, 2011). Many of these cells, when activated, will release signaling molecules that induce fibrosis (discussed later in this chapter). Fibroblasts themselves express TLRs and IL-1R, which can directly drive differentiation to myofibroblasts (Farina et al., 2014).

Hypoxia

Typically, when biomaterials are implanted, they disrupt local tissue, and it takes time to redevelop the blood supply to the wounded tissue, thus producing a transient hypoxic, oxygen-deprived environment. In tissue engineering, this is a major design concern that is known to affect viability of cells within large constructs (Bland et al., 2013). Many researchers work on strategies to rapidly develop vasculature for large tissue-engineered constructs, given that an oxygen source is required within 200 μm of a metabolically active cell (Yuet et al., 1995). It is likely that, particularly in tissue engineering, hypoxia will at least temporarily affect local cells. In pathological conditions, the source of hypoxia could be from an initial injury that damages blood vessels and causes acute hypoxia (Lokmic et al., 2012). Also, inflammatory reactions cause an influx of cells that consume oxygen quickly, contributing to the hypoxic state (Ruthenborg et al., 2014).

No matter the cause of hypoxia, the result has many pro-fibrotic consequences. Hypoxia has been shown to induce macrophages to secrete VEGF, PDGF, FGF, TGFα and TGFβ, which are all involved in fibrotic tissue development (Murdoch et al., 2005). In fibrotic tissue, hypoxia can also induce epithelial to mesenchymal transition (EMT), which is a significant mechanism of myofibroblast differentiation (Lee and Nelson, 2012). Most of the consequences of hypoxia are mediated through the upregulation of hypoxia-inducible factor (HIF)-1. Elevated HIF-α helps macrophages survive and function (Cramer et al., 2003). It also might prevent excessive reactive oxygen species (ROS) generation and associated impaired resolution of healing (Kim et al., 2006). Among many other effects, HIF-1 induces transcription of pro-fibrotic factors including tissue inhibitor of metalloproteinases (TIMP)-1, plasminogen activator inhibitor (PAI)-1, and connective tissue growth factor (CTGF) (Murdoch et al., 2005). Elevated HIF-1 also induces glucose transporter-1, phosphoglycerate kinase 1, and VEGF (Li et al., 2007).

Shifts in redox homeostasis

There is some evidence that a pro-oxidant shift in redox homeostasis drives TGFβ-induced myofibroblast differentiation (Sampson et al., 2014). This redox shift on its own is not sufficient to cause fibrosis, but it is a contributing factor. In biomaterial implantation, a redox shift could be caused by frustrated phagocytosis. It has already been shown that neutrophils activated by a biomaterial surface release ROS in quantities high enough to damage the biomaterial (Patel et al., 2007). These same reactive oxygen intermediates could serve to cause a redox imbalance that drives fibrosis.

In pathological fibrosis, high expression of NADPH oxidase 4 (NOX4)-derived hydrogen peroxide (H_2O_2) and low levels of nitrous oxide (NO) and reactive oxygen scavengers alters the redox state. In cooperation with TGFβ1, this induces myofibroblast differentiation that then leads to excessive ECM production and wound contracture (Sampson et al., 2011). This interaction with TGFβ acts in a number of ways to accelerate myofibroblast differentiation. TGFβ itself acts on fibroblasts and fibrocytes to induce production of NOX4-induced H_2O_2 (Sampson et al., 2014). Angiotensin II (ANG II), PDGF, and hypoxia can also induce NOX4 activation in vascular smooth muscle cells and fibroblasts (Barnes and Gorin, 2011). The H_2O_2 and other reactive oxygen intermediates themselves can activate latent TGFβ by directly oxidizing the dissociation of latency-associated protein (LAP) (see details in the section on TGFβ), leading to a feedback loop (Jobling et al., 2006). Various antioxidants and NOX4 inhibitors have been shown to dedifferentiate myofibroblasts to a quiescent state (Sampson et al., 2011).

pH

High levels of lactic acid, potentially caused by inflammation, can activate TGFβ signaling and myofibroblast differentiation (Kottmann et al., 2012). Certainly, the inflammation due to biomaterials could contribute, but some biomaterials themselves alter the pH of their microenvironment as they degrade (Pitt et al., 1981). The classic example of this is poly(lactic-co-glycolic acid), which is widely used clinically. It has also been used as a tissue-engineered scaffold and to deliver drugs and vaccines.

In pathological fibrosis, increased lactic acid has been observed. For example, it is elevated in patients with idiopathic pulmonary fibrosis, which could be due to neutrophil activation (Kottmann et al., 2012; Hu et al., 2008). Generally, it is thought that the high metabolic demand from an influx of inflammatory cells causes higher lactic acid (Drent et al., 1996). If glycolytic metabolism is altered, that could also alter the pH. In any case, there is emerging evidence that these pH changes contribute to fibrosis.

Mechanical signals

Changes in mechanical signals from the surroundings can also contribute to fibrosis. Biomaterials can contribute to this change in a few ways. The materials themselves have mechanical properties that often do not match the surrounding tissue, which could transmit mechanical signals to surrounding cells (Lind et al., 2013). Similarly, how well-surrounding cells anchor to the biomaterial, determined both by chemical surface properties and topographical properties such as surface roughness and porosity, will affect mechanical signals received by surrounding cells (Koschwanez et al., 2008). Finally, the host response alters the mechanical properties of the surrounding tissue.

Changes in mechanical tension of the ECM get transmitted to the fibroblast cytoskeleton and cause RhoA/ROCK signaling (Jamieson et al., 1998). This causes fibroblasts to become activated to "protomyofibroblasts" which deposit new ECM components and secrete TGFβ (Kim et al., 2013). In turn, the TGFβ completes the myofibroblast differentiation. In addition, as myofibroblasts secrete more ECM, it increases the ECM stiffness (Wakatsuki et al., 2000). Integrins can then cause mechanical pulling of the LAP from ECM-bound TGFβ, causing its activation (Munger and Sheppard, 2011). These many ways of enhancing fibrosis highlight the difficulties inherent in preventing it.

CELLULAR CONTRIBUTORS TO FIBROSIS

In clinical fibrosis, relatively minor attention has been paid to the initiators of fibrosis, since these are more difficult to treat, particularly since the clinical symptoms of fibrotic disease do not appear until it has progressed significantly. In fact, early steps leading to fibrosis such as inflammation are necessary steps in wound healing. Instead, much more attention has been paid to reversing the final steps of fibrosis. In particular, researchers of pathological fibrosis focus on myofibroblast differentiation, since those cells are primarily responsible for collagen deposition and wound contraction. Dysregulated myofibroblasts are blamed for the clinical problems, and most antifibrotic strategies emphasize preventing or reversing myofibroblast differentiation. Nonetheless, it is worth exploring the effect of the wide variety of cell types that are involved in fibrosis. Only by understanding the full process of fibrosis can we hope to alter the progression. The cell types are described in the order that they typically appear at the site of biomaterial implantation.

Granulocytes (neutrophils, mast cells)

Neutrophils are among the first cells to arrive at the site of biomaterial implantation (Anderson et al., 2008). Because they have such a short life span, they are difficult to study and have not had as much attention paid to them as macrophages. They have PRRs on their surfaces and can release a number of molecules that mediate subsequent inflammatory reactions (Prince et al., 2011). There is even less information available about the role of basophils and eosinophils in fibrosis or biomaterial response, so they will not be mentioned further. However, eosinophils are a potential source of profibrotic cytokines, including TFGβ and IL-13 and the granules contain a number of proteins that contribute to inflammation, tissue damage, and remodeling (Acharya and Ackerman, 2014).

In pathological fibrosis, there is not a great deal of information on neutrophil effects. In hypersensitivity pneumonitis, depleting neutrophils reduce fibrosis, primarily because they reduce IL-17A production (Hasan et al., 2013). On the other hand, neutrophil depletion in bleomycin-induced lung fibrosis did not reduce fibrosis, despite altering the MMP-9/TIMP-1 balance (Manoury et al., 2007). Neutrophils have not been shown to have a direct effect on myofibroblasts. That being said, recent research has revealed a new and specific type of neutrophil cell death that might be involved in fibrosis. Neutrophil extracellular traps (NETs) are a result of neither necrosis nor apoptosis. They are induced by activated platelets and numerous other inflammatory stimuli. Their main components are DNA, granular antimicrobial proteins, chromatin, and proteases (Zawrotniak and Rapala-Kozik, 2013). Treatment of activated myofibroblasts with NETs increases CTGF expression, collagen production, and proliferation and migration (Chrysanthopoulou et al., 2014). So, continued inflammatory stimuli, such as those produced by ongoing injury or inflammatory degradation products, would be likely to enhance fibrosis.

Mast cells typically appear about the same time as neutrophils in response to biomaterial implantation. Mast cell precursors are recruited due to inflammatory chemotactic cues. These mast cells then mature and become activated at the wound site. There, they secrete vasodilators, chemokines (e.g., CC-chemokine ligand 2 (CCL2)), cytokines (notably TGFβ1, IL-4, and IL-13), and prostaglandins (Overed-Sayer et al., 2013; Avula et al., 2013). The cytokines they secrete have been shown to cause FBGC formation from macrophage fusion (McNally and Anderson, 1995; DeFife et al., 1997). There have been several studies in which mast cell action was blocked by using a tyrosine kinase inhibitor (Avula et al., 2013) or prevented by using mast cell deficient mice (Avula et al., 2014; Yang et al., 2014a; Klueh et al., 2010). Conflicting results have been reported in these models. In one study, there were no changes in FBGC formation or in thickness of fibrous capsules (Yang et al., 2014a). In other studies, however, mast cell deficient mice produced a thinner fibrous capsule and recruited fewer fibrocytes (Avula et al., 2014; Klueh et al., 2010). The role of mast cells in response to biomaterials is not altogether clear.

The role of mast cells in pathological fibrosis is becoming increasingly recognized. Mast cell depletion does delay tissue repair and remodeling but does not prevent it (Overed-Sayer et al., 2013). Mast cells tend to accumulate at the edges of wounds (Trautmann et al., 2000). They stimulate vascular permeability by secreting histamine, lipid mediators, and VEGF (Dvorak, 2005), and also can recruit other cell types (e.g., neutrophils via chymase: (Takato et al., 2011)). Most notably, mast cells can stimulate migration and proliferation of fibroblasts, partly due to release of keratinocyte growth factor, epidermal growth factor, PDGF, histamine, and tryptase (Levi-Schaffer and Piliponsky, 2003). Production of CCL2 attracts monocytes and fibrocytes (Oliveira and Lukacs, 2001), and of course, the TGFβ1 produced by mast cells is a key cytokine in fibrosis (Cho et al., 2015). It seems that mast cells contribute to the fibrotic process but are probably not necessary for fibrosis to proceed, particularly in the context of biomaterials.

Macrophages

The initial injury and inflammation due to biomaterial implantation recruits monocytes from the circulation (Zhang and Mosser, 2008; Janeway and Medzhitov, 2002). When they reach the implantation site, they differentiate into macrophages. There, macrophages phagocytose apoptotic neutrophils and produce growth factors and cytokines that can recruit fibroblasts and cause myofibroblast differentiation and resulting ECM production (Galli et al., 2011).

There has been a huge amount of research in the biomaterials field trying to understand the interaction between macrophages and biomaterials. These cells have been identified by the field as the primary actors in biomaterials-induced inflammation. Earlier chapters (e.g., Chapter 6) in this textbook address many of the questions of how macrophages and biomaterials interact, so this will be only very briefly mentioned here. We will focus on the role the macrophage plays in fibrosis. One key aspect we will explore in more detail is the effect of macrophage phenotype on fibrosis. There has been much recent research on which macrophage phenotypes are elicited by biomaterials, with conflicting results.

The role of macrophages in pathological fibrosis is becoming more prominent. Interestingly, wounds that have few macrophages heal with reduced scar formation. Particularly interesting is the observation that macrophages do not participate in neonatal scarless healing (Cowin et al., 1998). Macrophage depletion studies have, however, revealed a complex interplay of interactions in adult healing. Knockout mice have allowed selective, time-dependent macrophage knockouts. Early macrophage depletion does reduce scar formation, but also slows wound repair, showing that macrophages are required to coordinate early phases of adult wound healing (Goren et al., 2009; Mirza et al., 2009). Late macrophage depletion actually impairs clearance of fibrotic scars (Lucas et al., 2010). Macrophages participate in a number of ways to regenerate scar tissue. They release MMP-9 and MMP-13 that degrade the ECM (Skjøt-Arkil et al., 2010). Additionally, they can induce myofibroblast apoptosis and remove the apoptotic cells (Duffield et al., 2013). Finally, they can release IL-10, which has an anti-inflammatory function (Murray and Wynn, 2011). Thus, in adult wound healing, the macrophage plays different functions throughout the process.

The different functions macrophages have are controlled by the macrophage phenotype. As detailed elsewhere in the textbook, macrophages typically express as spectrum of phenotypes, as a correlate to Th1 and Th2 lymphocyte phenotypes. Classically activated or M1 macrophages are stimulated by interferon gamma (IFNγ) and lipopolysaccharide (Vogel et al., 2014). They produce TNFα, IL-1β, IL-6, and IL-12. They are microbicidal and play a role in cytotoxic host defense (Murray and Wynn, 2011). Alternatively activated or M2 macrophages are stimulated by IL-4 and IL-13 (Vogel et al., 2014). They produce IL-10, TGFβ1, VEGF, and PDGF (among others). These are typically thought to be involved in wound repair and immune suppression (Murray and Wynn, 2011).

Macrophage plasticity allows the cells to dynamically adapt during wound repair (Lech et al., 2012). Increasingly, macrophages are thought to exist on a range between M1 and M2, rather than being strictly divided into separate phenotypes. Additionally, many researchers further divide M2 macrophages into M2a which are pro-fibrotic and initiate type II inflammation, M2b which immunoregulate/immunosuppress, and M2c which participate in tissue repair and matrix remodeling (Martinez et al., 2008). Regulatory macrophages (Mreg) are yet another subset that are thought to participate in organ transplantation tolerance but are difficult to distinguish from M2c macrophages (Broichhausen et al., 2012). Recommendations for a uniform nomenclature have recently been published (Guilliams et al., 2014) and a more detailed description of the role of macrophages in the host response to biomaterials can be found in Chapters 2 and 6.

In diabetic ulcers, persistence of TNFα-producing M1-like macrophages amplifies tissue breakdown and impairs healing (Mirza and Koh, 2011). In contrast, overactivation of pro-fibrotic M2a-like macrophages promotes scar formation (Sindrilaru and Scharffetter-Kochanek, 2013). The role of M2c/Mreg-like cells has not yet been thoroughly researched but might help resolve fibrosis. Macrophages are not "bad" or "good," but dysregulation along the wound healing timeline is likely important in promoting or resolving fibrosis. There is evidence that macrophages alter their phenotype as a wound heals. At the start, they are highly inflammatory, releasing pro-inflammatory cytokines, ROS, and proteases, all of which is designed to quickly combat infection. Later, they phagocytose apoptotic cells and release anti-inflammatory growth factors and cytokines, at which point fibroblasts are recruited and differentiated into myofibroblasts (Sindrilaru et al., 2011; Daley et al., 2010). Ultimately, macrophages could be involved in ECM remodeling and scar resolution. Thus, any anti-fibrotic approach involving macrophages must take into account the different roles they play throughout the wound healing process.

Other monocyte-derived cells (dendritic cells, FBGCs, fibrocytes)

A number of other cells derive from a monocyte lineage and have a potential role to play in fibrosis. Dendritic cells certainly respond to biomaterials (see Chapter 7), but their role in fibrosis is less clear. Dendritic cells are resident mononuclear cells that survey the microenvironment for antigens. They are very responsive to DAMPs and PAMPs. When activated, they traffic via the lymphatics to local lymph nodes (Rahman and Aloman, 2013). If there are antigens (from delivered drugs, infection, or foreign cells), the dendritic cells would enhance the immune component of the response. Tissue dendritic cells can also produce pentraxin 3 which blocks P selectin on vascular endothelial cells, thus blocking further immune cell recruitment (Baruah et al., 2006). Dendritic cells can also produce MMPs that mediate ECM degradation (Kis-Toth et al., 2013).

Classically, biomaterial implantation induces the foreign body response of which FBGCs are a key component. As discussed in Chapter 2, these cells are formed at biomaterial surfaces as macrophages fuse during frustrated phagocytosis (McNally and Anderson, 2011; Anderson et al., 2008). It can be difficult to distinguish between adherent macrophages and FBGCs: they were found to produce MMP-9, TIMP-1, and TIMP-2 *in vitro* in response to biomaterials (Jones et al., 2008). These molecules are involved in ECM degradation and remodeling. FBGCs also release TGFβ, which is certainly involved in fibrosis (Hernandez-Pando et al., 2000). However, no direct link has been shown between FBGC development and fibrous capsule formation, though they do seem to appear concurrently (Kenneth Ward, 2008).

Fibrocytes are spindle-shaped mesenchymal progenitor cells that enter wound sites. They appear to differentiate from CD14+ peripheral blood monocytes (Keeley et al., 2010). They express markers of both hematopoietic cells and stromal cells (collagen I, collagen III, fibronectin, major histocompatibility complex II, CD11b, CD13, CD34, and CD45) (Keeley et al., 2010). Fibrocyte-like cells have been identified in the vicinity of biomaterial implants and can function as antigen-presenting cells or differentiate into myofibroblasts, laying down ECM. For example, CD45+/Col1+ fibrocytes appeared 4 days after implanting PLGA and peaked at 10 days postimplantation (Thevenot et al., 2011). The significance of these cells is not thoroughly understood in the context of biomaterials.

Fibrocytes have been shown to participate in normal and aberrant wound repair including hypertrophic scars, keloids, airway remodeling in asthma, interstitial pulmonary fibrosis, atherosclerosis, and many others (Bucala, 2012). Stimulation of CD14+ cells with pro-fibrotic cytokines, IL-4 and IL-13, and PDGF, as well as inflammatory cytokines cause differentiation into fibrocytes. Circulating fibrocytes are attracted to sites of injury primarily through the CC-chemokine receptor-2-mediated pathway (Sivakumar and Das, 2008).

Fibrocytes can play many roles, depending on their mode of activation. When stimulated by IL-1β or Th1 cytokines, fibrocytes respond by downregulating collagen expression, and increasing expression of IL-6, IL-8, CCL3, CCL4, and intercellular adhesion molecule 1, all of which promoted inflammatory cell recruitment and trafficking. However, IL-1β also upregulates IL-10, which is an anti-inflammatory cytokine (Shao et al., 2008). In response to serum (as in acute injury), antigen presentation and lipid metabolism are increased. Agonists of TLRs upregulate expression of major histocompatibility complexes I and II and costimulatory molecules CD80 and CD86, leading to antigen-presenting capabilities (Balmelli et al., 2007). Fibrocytes can also secrete TGFβ1 and PDGF, which act in a paracrine and autocrine fashion to increase fibrosis (Kao et al., 2011). They also participate in neoangiogenesis and inflammation by secreting high levels of MMPs, VEGF, hepatocyte growth factor, basic FGF, granulocyte macrophage colony-stimulating factor, IL-8, and IL-1β (Yeager et al., 2011). It is apparent that the potential functions of fibrocytes are extensive.

Lymphocytes

Lymphocytes have long been observed in the vicinity of implanted biomaterials, but their function has not been fully elucidated. As discussed elsewhere in this textbook, lymphocytes have the potential to interact directly with biomaterials through PRRs (Reynolds and Dong, 2013). They also interact with macrophages to enhance their activity. Of course, if there is an antigenic component introduced with the biomaterial, as an infection, or if the biomaterial is a combination product (e.g., delivering a protein or as a tissue-engineered scaffold with foreign cells), then lymphocytes will play a key role in guiding the overall response.

Helper T lymphocytes (CD4+) polarize into Th1 cells and Th2 cells and some other subsets (e.g., Th17), which each release a distinctive cytokine subset (see the next section for more details). The balance between the Th1 and Th2 cells appears to influence the extent of fibrotic response (Morishima and Ishii, 2010). For example, Balb/c mice, which lean to a Th2 response, display more fibrosis than C57BL/6 mice, which lean to a Th1 response, though there are organ-specific differences (Marques et al., 2014). In general, Th2 responses are thought to be more fibrogenic. For example, IL-13 (a Th2 cytokine) stimulates TGF-β and MMP-9 expression (Lee et al., 2001). Regulatory T (Treg) cells produce IL-10, and there is some evidence that they are anti-fibrotic (Katz et al., 2011). Cytotoxic T lymphocytes (CD8+) might be pro-fibrotic, but it is not entirely clear (Safadi et al., 2004). Similarly, the effects of natural killer cells and natural killer T cells are not certain (Wehr et al., 2013).

Fibroblasts and myofibroblasts

In the biomaterials literature, fibrous capsule formation has been primarily attributed to ECM secretion by fibroblasts. However, the pathological fibrosis literature describes the predominant ECM-secreting cells as myofibroblasts, cells that combine the ECM-producing capability of fibroblasts with the cytoskeletal and contractile properties of smooth muscle cells (Duffield et al., 2013; Kramann et al., 2013). In many cases, it can be difficult to distinguish "activated fibroblasts" from myofibroblasts (Orenstein, 2014).

Fibroblasts are the cells responsible for maintaining the homeostasis of the ECM. They both produce ECM and break it down, and in healthy tissue, the cells are relatively quiescent. After injury, however, the cells play a much more significant role. They are chemotactically attracted to the site of injury, where they are induced to proliferate and secrete ECM (Kendall and Feghali-Bostwick, 2014). Fibroblasts participate in inflammation, responding to TGFβ1, IL-1β, IL-6, IL-13, IL-33, prostaglandins, and leukotrienes (Kendall and Feghali-Bostwick, 2014). These stimuli can cause the fibroblasts to differentiate to myofibroblasts and increase matrix production. Fibroblasts can also themselves produce TGFβ1, IL-1β, IL-33, CXC and CC-chemokines, and ROS, which serve to recruit and activate macrophages (Kendall and Feghali-Bostwick, 2014). In angiogenesis, the ECM is critical in allowing endothelial cell migration, and fibroblasts also can produce VEGF (Kajihara et al., 2013). These autocrine and paracrine signals, together with many other molecules not described in detail here, can influence both fibrosis and myofibroblast differentiation.

Myofibroblasts combine an abundant production of ECM, usually associated with fibroblasts, with the contractile properties associated with smooth muscle cells. They are usually identified by the co-expression of α-SMA and collagen I (Yang et al., 2014b). They are resistant to apoptosis and have high constitutive expression of chemokines, cytokines, and cell surface receptors (Kramann et al., 2013). They have also been shown to display epigenetic changes (Mann and Mann, 2013). Myofibroblasts are not abundant in healthy tissue but can transiently be found in great numbers at wound sites. In normal wound healing, they are essential in restoring tissue integrity by producing ECM and contracting the wound bed (Hinz et al., 2012). Once the wound is largely healed, these cells apoptose. However, in many fibrotic conditions, these cells remain persistently active, producing excessive collagen and tissue contraction. The many pathways by which myofibroblasts appear then become deactivated are still being elucidated (Yang et al., 2014b).

The origin of myofibroblasts is still a subject of much debate. They can come from diverse tissues, though it appears that resident fibroblasts are the predominant source in most conditions (Mack and Yanagita, 2015). Epithelial cells can transform to myofibroblasts through EMT, though evidence in rodents suggests that this is at best a minor source of myofibroblasts (Kendall and Feghali-Bostwick, 2014). Similarly, endothelial cells are a rare potential source of myofibroblasts through a process termed endothelial to mesenchymal transition (EndoMT) (Lin et al., 2012). Vascular smooth muscle cells are very similar in phenotype to myofibroblasts, so there has been some speculation that they are related, but with little substantive evidence (Kendall and Feghali-Bostwick, 2014). Pericytes are cells that wrap around small blood vessel walls and control vascular permeability. These cells have been shown to be the main source of myofibroblasts in renal interstitial fibrosis (Duffield, 2014). Interestingly, both fibrocytes and monocytes appear to be able to differentiate into myofibroblasts under wounding conditions, suggesting that these cells act both directly and indirectly in stimulating fibrosis (Kendall and Feghali-Bostwick, 2014). Though they are not frequently discussed in the context of biomaterials, there is evidence that myofibroblasts do play a significant role. Indeed, it appears that the fibroblastic cells in a fibrous capsule have a monocytic origin (Mooney et al., 2014). The many signals that can induce myofibroblast differentiation will be discussed in more detail in the next section.

MOLECULAR MEDIATORS OF FIBROSIS

There are a huge number of signaling molecules involved in fibrosis, many with overlapping functions. Additionally, many of these molecules regulate wound healing differently at different stages of the process, making it difficult to dissect their purpose. Biomaterials have been shown to directly and indirectly cause release of most of these mediators. As an example, many of these factors were identified in a profile of gene expression during the fibrotic response to biomaterials in the peritoneal cavity (Le et al., 2010). Another study observed many changes in the temporal and spatial distribution of cytokines around an implant site (Higgins et al., 2009). Comprehensively reviewing these responses would be an enormous task and is beyond the scope of this chapter.

TGFβ: the hallmark of fibrosis

The prototypical pro-fibrotic cytokine is TGFβ. TGFβ has direct effects on fibroblast differentiation and ECM formation and indirect effects on many different cells types and mediators (Finnson et al., 2013). The different isoforms of TGFβ have somewhat different functions, with TGFβ1 having the major pro-fibrotic effect. The balance between TGFβ1 and TGFβ3 is important, as TGFβ1 promotes fibroproliferation by inducing TIMP-1 while TGFβ3 promotes non-fibrotic tissue repair (Ask et al., 2008). Many different cells are capable of producing TGFβ, but the primary source is from monocytes and macrophages (Lekkerkerker et al., 2012).

Part of the difficulty in understanding the function of TGFβ is that it is not secreted in its active form. It is secreted noncovalently bound to latency-associated peptide (LAP), which deactivate the cytokine (Lawrence, 2001). There are many enzymes that catalyze the dissociation of LAP, including cathepsins, plasmin, calpain, thrombospondin, integrin-αvβ6, and MMPs (Wynn, 2008). Integrins, pH, mechanical stresses, and ROS can also activate TGFβ (Munger and Sheppard, 2011). In its active form, it interacts with transmembrane receptors on a wide variety of cells. Downstream activation occurs via Smad 2/3 proteins or via a number of Smad-independent pathways including activation of mitogen–activated protein kinase and PI3 kinase/Akt pathways (Tsou et al., 2014). These latter pathways suggest that cell adhesion is likely to modulate TGFβ function. These control transcription of many target genes, including pro-collagen I and III (Roberts et al., 2003).

TGFβ attracts neutrophils, induces migration of fibroblasts, and promotes differentiation of myofibroblasts (Van Linthout et al., 2014). As mentioned previously, it can drive a pro-oxidant shift by inducing NOX4-derived hydrogen peroxide production (Sampson et al., 2011). It causes deposition of ECM and secretion of many paracrine and autocrine growth factors, including pro-fibrotic endothelin-1 (ET-1) and CTGF (Leask, 2009). Bone morphogenetic protein (BMP) 1 and BMP-7 oppose production and activation of TGFβ1 (Moustakas and Heldin, 2009). Smad knockout mice and TGFβ blockade have been used to try to understand its function in fibrosis (Borthwick et al., 2013). These studies have highlighted that fibrosis is not a simple phenomenon. While TGFβ is present in virtually all fibrotic conditions, blocking it (or its activation) has sometimes even resulted in increased fibrosis (Rozen-Zvi et al., 2013; Tsou et al., 2014).

Pro-fibrotic cytokines (ANG II, PDGF, CTGF, ET-1)

A number of cytokines have been identified specifically as pro-fibrotic. These proteins cooperate with TGFβ and each other to induce fibrosis (Leask, 2010). The renin–angiotensin–aldosterone system produces ANG II, which directly upregulates TGFβ1, stimulates fibroblast proliferation, and induces myofibroblast differentiation (Tomino, 2012; Rosenkranz, 2004; Yoshiji et al., 2007). Activated macrophages and fibroblasts both produce ANG II (Bataller et al., 2003). It can stimulate TGFβ1 production by inducing NOX activity and TGFβ1 signaling by increasing SMAD2 levels. It also stimulates CTGF and ET-1 production (Leask, 2010).

PDGF is a major mitogen of mesenchymal cells. It enhances migration into wound sites and proliferation of neutrophils, macrophages, fibroblasts, and smooth muscles cells (Heldin and Westermark, 1999). It stimulates fibroblasts to contract ECM and to differentiate into myofibroblasts. It appears to recruit pericytes, which might be a source of myofibroblasts. Blocking PDGF usually results in fewer myofibroblasts and decreased fibrosis (Nishioka et al., 2013).

CTGF/CCN2 is a matricellular protein that belongs to the ECM-associated signaling CCN family. It is involved in angiogenesis, cell migration, adhesion, proliferation, tissue wound repair, and ECM regulation (Tsou et al., 2014). It is induced by TGFβ, ANG II, ET-1, and IL-1β, and might also be a downstream mediator of these proteins (Jun and Lau, 2011). It is highly expressed in fibrotic conditions. It binds integrins, cell surface heparin sulfate proteoglycans, low-density lipoprotein receptor-related protein/α$_2$-macroglobulin receptor, and tyrosine kinase receptor TrkA. It also binds growth factors and ECM proteins including VEGF, TGFβ, BMPs, and fibronectin (Tsou et al., 2014). However, on its own, it is only weakly pro-fibrotic. As a cofactor with TGFβ, it maximally induces type I collagen synthesis and α-SMA RNA and protein expression. This downstream mediator of fibrosis seems to participate in a positive feedback loop with TGFβ and VEGF production (Jun and Lau, 2011).

ET-1 is a potent vasoconstrictor that also participates in angiogenesis, cell survival, EMT, and tumor-related activities (Levin, 1995). It is made primarily by endothelial cells, and also by epithelial cells, bone marrow mast cells, smooth muscle cells, fibroblasts, macrophages, polymorphonuclear leukocytes, and cardiomyocytes (Meyers and Sethna, 2013). Both ANG II and TGFβB can induce it, suggesting that its role is as a downstream mediator of fibrosis. It has been shown to induce ECM production and myofibroblast differentiation in fibroblasts (Tsou et al., 2014).

Other molecules involved in myofibroblast differentiation (lysophosphatidic acid, integrins)

Lysophosphatidic acid (LPA) is a phospholipid produced by the enzyme antaxin. There are six receptors (LPA1–6) (Budd and Qian, 2013). LPA1 acts through three families of G-proteins to drive cytoskeletal changes, serum response factor-mediated gene transcription, cell proliferation and migration, and collagen synthesis (Contos et al., 2000). Inhibiting LPA1 decreases CTGF and TGFβ expression, and causes fibroblast proliferation and myofibroblast accumulation (Sakai et al., 2013). LPA2 transactivates latent TGFβ. Mice deficient in LPA2 show decreased expression of fibronectin, αSMA, collagen, IL-6, and TGFβ (Huang et al., 2013).

Integrins modulate cell–cell and cell–matrix interactions, so would be expected to play some role in fibrosis. These heterodimeric transmembrane glycoproteins are involved in initiation, maintenance, and resolution of fibrosis. In particular, integrins αv have been shown to activate latent TGFβ1 and TGFβ3 by binding the Arg-Gly-Asp (RGD) motif on LAP (Tsou et al., 2014).

Th2 cytokines (IL-4, IL-13, IL-5, IL-21, and IL-10)

Although the function of lymphocytes in the vicinity of biomaterial implants has not been definitively established, it is likely that they play some role in controlling the cytokine milieu (Chang et al., 2009; Anderson and McNally, 2011). T helper cells polarize to produce specific sets of cytokines which then guide other cells to respond in different ways. Th2 cells produce a range of cytokines including IL-4, IL-13, IL-5, IL-21, and IL-10. In immunity, Th2 cells activate B-cells, mast cells, and eosinophils, stimulating the humoral immune system (Jiang and Dong, 2013). Th2 responses are thought to be generally pro-fibrotic, with the exception of IL-10, which is also produced by Treg cells and even Th1 cells.

Both IL-4 and IL-13 have been shown to be capable of initiating fibrosis, even in the absence of TGFβ. They can both drive differentiation of resident fibroblasts and recruited fibrocytes to myofibroblasts. They share the same IL-4Rα/Stat6 signaling pathway but do have distinct effects (Zurawski et al., 1993). IL-4 is a potent mediator of fibrosis and has been shown to stimulate production of type I and III collagen and fibronectin. In fibrosis, however, it seems that IL-13 is the dominant driver (Borthwick et al., 2013).

Both IL-4 and IL-13 alter the phenotype of macrophages to alternatively activated (M2), which is typically associated with fibrosis (Borthwick et al., 2013). Alternatively activated macrophages upregulate arginase, which controls L-proline production, which is required for collagen synthesis by activated myofibroblasts (Wynn and Barron, 2010). On the other hand, when macrophages cannot recognize IL-4 or IL-13 and in arginase-1 depleted mice, increased fibrosis results (Herbert et al., 2004; Pesce et al., 2009). This suggests that M2 macrophages are required for suppression or resolution of fibrosis and might compete with myofibroblasts for arginase-1.

The following examples highlight the importance of IL-13 in fibrosis. Blocking IL-13 in schistosomiasis led to an 85% decrease in collagen production, despite IL-4 levels being unchanged (Fallon et al., 2000). When IL-13 was over-expressed, it resulted in significant subepithelial airway fibrosis (Zhu et al., 1999), whereas IL-4 over-expression resulted only in inflammation but not fibrosis (Rankin et al., 1996). Treatment with anti-IL-13 antibody reduced collagen deposition in animals with fibrotic lungs (Blease et al., 2001). In addition to its ability to trigger fibrosis on its own,

IL-13 upregulates TGFβ signaling by increasing TGFβ production in macrophages and by causing LAP cleavage through MMP and cathepsin pathways (Lanone et al., 2002).

IL-5 and IL-21 do not contribute directly to development of fibrosis but promote production of Th2 cytokines. IL-5 is responsible for recruiting, differentiating, and activating eosinophils, which are important sources of pro-fibrotic growth factors and cytokines, including TGFβ and IL-13. Neutralizing IL-5 activity in some studies has decreased fibrosis (e.g., Cho et al., 2004), while others have found no effect (e.g., Hao et al., 2000). It seems that IL-5 and eosinophils do not directly cause fibrosis, but instead amplify production of other fibrotic mediators. Similarly, IL-21 acts by promoting Th2 cell migration and survival. It also increases IL-4 and IL-13 receptor expression on macrophages, potentiating pro-fibrotic macrophage responses (Pesce et al., 2006).

IL-10 balances the effects of other Th2 cytokines on fibrosis. This interesting anti-fibrotic cytokine has also been shown to be produced by Th1 cells and Treg cells, the latter of which also produce TGFβ (Mosser and Zhang, 2008). Mreg and monocytes also produce IL-10 (Mosser and Edwards, 2008). IL-10 is immunosuppressive, inhibiting activation and effector functions of T cells, monocytes, and macrophages. It can limit and terminate inflammation (Moore et al., 2001). It also causes direct inhibition of collagen synthesis and secretion from fibroblasts (Wangoo et al., 1997). IL-10 might not act entirely on its own; there is evidence that it acts cooperatively with other Th1 cytokines to reduce collagen production (Hoffmann et al., 2000).

Th17 cytokines (IL-17A)

Th17 cells are a subset of CD4+ T lymphocytes that are thought mostly to mediate autoimmunity but might also serve a purpose in fibrosis (Borthwick et al., 2013). They primarily produce IL-17 but also produce IL-13. In order to stimulate Th17 cells to form, they need to be exposed to TGFβ, IL-6, and IL-21 in mice; in humans, the latter two cytokines can be replaced with IL-23 or IL-1β. Stability and expansion of Th17 cells requires IL-23 (Wilson et al., 2007). The function of IL-17 is primarily inflammatory. It acts on myeloid cells, epithelial cells, and mesenchymal cells to induce cytokines and chemokines that increase granulopoiesis and recruitment of leukocytes (mostly neutrophils) to the site of inflammation (Ouyang et al., 2008; Dong, 2008). In some fibrotic diseases and models, IL-17 is increased. Neutralizing antibodies to IL-17 have been shown to reduce granuloma formation (Borthwick et al., 2013). The effect on fibrosis is likely indirect.

Th1 and inflammatory cytokines (IFNγ, IL-1β, and TNFα)

Generally, Th1 responses are thought to be anti-fibrotic. Th1 cells stimulate cell-based immune responses by activating cytotoxic T lymphocytes (CD8+ cells) and increasing macrophage phagocytosis and killing. The cells are stimulated by IL-12 and produce IFNγ (among other cytokines), which in turn induces macrophages to produce

IL-12 (Jiang and Dong, 2013). IFNγ is a potent anti-fibrotic. In liver fibrosis, it inhibits activation and proliferation of hepatic stellate cells and ECM deposition (Baroni et al., 1996). It indirectly mitigates fibrosis by stopping the TGFβ1 signaling pathway by inhibiting the Smad3 phosphorylation pathway (Ulloa et al., 1999). It also has direct anti-fibrotic actions by inhibiting fibroblast proliferation and TGFβ1-induced expression of genes encoding pro-collagen I and III and collagen synthesis in activated myofibroblasts (Gurujeyalakshmi and Giri, 1995). IFNγ inhibits Th2 cytokine-induced differentiation of fibrocytes into myofibroblasts (Shao et al., 2008). It also stimulates macrophages to produce IL-12, which itself has been shown to reduce fibrosis (Szekanecz and Koch, 2007). However, treatment with IFNγ has led to conflicting results, suggesting that it does not have a straightforward anti-fibrotic effect (Borthwick et al., 2013).

Classically activated macrophages (M1) are activated by IFNγ and IL-12. They then secrete TNFα and IL-1β, inflammatory cytokines that are themselves involved in fibrosis. IL-1β levels are high in several fibrotic conditions. It can drive EMT and myofibroblast differentiation in a TGFβ1-dependent manner. Both IL-1β and TNFα increase TGFβ1 production and have been implicated in EMT and EndoMT (Borthwick et al., 2013).

Morphogen pathways (Wnt, hedgehog, and Notch)

A number of developmental signaling molecules including Wnt, Notch, and hedgehog ligands have been shown to be involved in myofibroblast differentiation (Beyer and Distler, 2013). As fibrotic disease progresses, chronic activation of fibroblasts becomes increasingly independent of inflammatory stimuli and becomes self-perpetuating (Varga and Abraham, 2007). In many ways, this is similar to cancer, so researchers started examining many of the morphogen pathways identified in uncontrolled proliferation in cancers. These evolutionarily conserved pathways control normal organ development and adult homeostasis. In cell renewal and tissue regeneration, these pathways become upregulated.

Wnt signals through a variety of pathways, but only canonical Wnt signaling has been related to fibrotic diseases (Beyer and Distler, 2013). Here, soluble Wnt ligands bind to the family of frizzled membrane receptors and low–density lipoprotein-related protein membrane co-receptors. Together, they recruit dishevelled to the plasma membrane, which then destabilizes the intracellular β-catenin destruction complex. The resulting increased β-catenin translocates to the nucleus and interacts with the family of T cell factor/lymphoid enhancer-binding factor-1 transcription factors, activating transcription (Nusse and Varmus, 2012).

Activation of the Wnt pathway has been shown to promote fibrosis in the lung, kidneys, liver, and other organ systems, and in experimental models of fibrosis

(Akhmetshina et al., 2012) and has been shown in response to biomaterial implants (e.g., Thorfve et al., 2014). Wnt ligands can be released by a variety of different cells including fibroblasts and adipocytes (Wei et al., 2011). Experimentally, canonical Wnt signaling induces pathological activation of fibroblasts and release of ECM proteins (Wei et al., 2012). Also, TGFβ reduces expression of a Wnt inhibitor, and Wnt signaling might also stimulate the TGFβ pathway, augmenting fibrosis (Akhmetshina et al., 2012). Because there are 19 overlapping Wnt ligands and 10 receptors, it has been a difficult pathway to target, but recently a number of Wnt-targeted drugs have emerged and shown some promise (e.g., Chen et al., 2009; Huang et al., 2009).

The hedgehog pathway is another involved in fibrosis. It has three ligands: desert hedgehog (Dhh), Indian hedgehog (Ihh), and sonic hedgehog (Shh). These ligands bind to the patched (Ptch) receptor which is a negative regulator of smoothened (Smo) (Beyer and Distler, 2013). Overexpression of Shh elevates gene transcription, fibroblast activation, and collagen release (Horn et al., 2012a). Increased sonic hedgehog expression has been associated with better wound healing in response to biomaterials (Fitzpatrick et al., 2012). Pathologically activated hedgehog signaling has been observed in skin and liver fibrosis. Its blockade can prevent development of disease, though side effects of this treatment are difficult to overcome (Horn et al., 2012b; Choi et al., 2011).

The Notch signaling pathway is involved in cell differentiation and tissue homeostasis and there is evidence that it is also involved in fibrosis. While there is no direct evidence of its involvement in biomaterial responses, altering Notch signaling through drug delivery has been used as a strategy to increase angiogenesis in response to biomaterials (Cao et al., 2009). Membrane-bound Notch ligands can have interactions with other cells (*trans*), usually activating the canonical Notch signaling cascade or can interact with the same, ligand-bearing cell (*cis*), which is mostly inhibitory. There are five Notch ligands and four receptors (Beyer and Distler, 2013). *In vitro*, increased Notch signaling causes fibroblasts to differentiate into myofibroblasts and increase collagen release (Dees et al., 2011). Inhibition of the Notch pathway has been shown to decrease fibrosis, but the side effects are potentially serious (Kavian et al., 2010).

Matrix degrading enzymes (MMPs and TIMPs)

MMPs degrade many ECM proteins. Given that fibrosis is an imbalance between matrix production and degradation, the enzymes that degrade the ECM would be expected to be important and have been shown to be involved in many pathological conditions (Amălinei et al., 2010). MMPs are a 25-member family of extracellular endopeptidases that are either secreted or membrane bound (Giannandrea and Parks, 2014). Traditionally, they were thought to only be involved in turnover and degradation of ECM substrates. Now, however, they have also been shown to be involved in immunity and repair (Gill and Parks, 2008; Manicone and McGuire, 2008). For example, they participate in cell migration, leukocyte activation, antimicrobial defense, and chemokine processing among many activities (Ra and Parks, 2007). They have also been shown in a number of papers to change in response to biomaterial implantation (e.g., Jones et al., 2008; Moretti et al., 2012). Many non-ECM substrates have been identified for MMPs. There are diverse roles for the different MMPs: while some do inhibit fibrosis, others actually promote it (Giannandrea and Parks, 2014). To help keep tight control on the activity of MMPs, there are four tissue inhibitors of metalloproteinases—TIMP-1, TIMP-2, TIMP-3, and TIMP-4 (Hemmann et al., 2007). MMPs are active in every stage of wound healing: initial injury and repair, onset and resolution of inflammation, activation and deactivation of myofibroblasts, and deposition and breakdown of ECM (Martins et al., 2013). They probably play different roles depending on the tissue and dissecting their function is not straightforward. They can also act by activating or deactivating cytokines and cell signaling molecules, adding further complexity (Van Lint and Libert, 2007). MMPs have proven to be a difficult target in combating fibrosis.

Chemokines

The role of chemokines in fibrosis is not well understood. Certainly, they are involved early in wound healing in recruiting inflammatory cells and might play an important role in fibrogenesis. Macrophages that have responded or adhered to a biomaterial have been shown to produce chemokines such as CCL2, CCL4, CCL13, and CCL22 (Rhodes et al., 1997; Jones et al., 2007). These probably act to recruit more macrophages to the implant site. In pulmonary fibrosis, CXC chemokines have been shown to be pro-fibrotic, as neutralization of macrophage inflammatory protein 2 effectively suppressed fibrosis (Keane et al., 1999).

Epigenetic factors

There are certainly genetic variations in vulnerability to fibrosis (Marques et al., 2014), but genetics are not the whole story. Epigenetics describes functional changes in genome activity while the genetic sequence remains unchanged. These can be due to changes in DNA methylation, histone modification, and microRNAs (miRNAs), all of which work in close cooperation to regulate gene expression (Weigel et al., 2014).

DNA methylation regulates gene expression and genomic stability. Methylation changes during development and differentiation and is tightly controlled. Permanent changes in the myofibroblast growth program are associated with changes in DNA methylation. Furthermore, many genes involved in fibrosis show altered methylation patterns and expression changes in enzymes of the methylation machinery (Jones, 2012; Mann and Mann, 2013).

miRNAs are a class of short noncoding RNAs that help regulate gene expression posttranscriptionally. They have been shown to contribute to the development of fibrosis in the heart, lung, kidney, liver, and skin (Jiang et al., 2010). Many genes that are pro- and anti-fibrotic are regulated by miRNAs (Bowen et al., 2013).

Histone modifications help determine constitutive and inducible gene expression. A histone methyltransferase has been shown to regulate genes associated with myofibroblast differentiation (Perugorria et al., 2012). There is one report of microgrooves in a biomaterial causing epigenetic changes via biophysical cues (Downing et al., 2013).

ENGINEERING ANTI-FIBROTIC RESPONSES TO BIOMATERIALS

Altering fibrotic responses to biomaterials is not a straightforward task. Very little progress has been made in preventing the formation of a fibrous capsule around biomaterial implants over the long term (Yang et al., 2014b). This is perhaps not surprising, given that there are virtually no successful approaches to dealing with pathological fibrosis, despite the fact that fibrotic diseases account for up to 45% of deaths in developed countries (Wynn, 2008). In the United States, there are very few approved anti-fibrotic treatments; these include direct injection of collagenase and the "anti-fibrotic" drug is Pirfenidone, which has an unknown mechanism but probably inhibits TGFβ (King et al., 2014). There have been number of clinical trials, including ones for a drug that reduces TGFβ synthesis (Hawinkels and Ten Dijke, 2011), a recombinant human IFNγ (unsuccessful: (Pockros et al., 2007)), an endothelin agonist (unsuccessful: (Coyle and Metersky, 2013)), and kinase inhibitors (Richeldi et al., 2014). Clearly, fibrosis is caused by a complex and multifactorial series of events that are difficult to modify.

In the biomaterials field, we have two significant advantages. First, we have the opportunity to intervene from the moment of implantation (or even before), meaning we can try to prevent the initiation of pro-fibrotic signals. In pathological fibrosis, usually the disease has progressed considerably before clinical symptoms appear and treatment can begin. Second, we can use the biomaterial itself as a means to deliver anti-fibrotic agents. This local, targeted delivery has the potential to be more successful and have fewer side effects than the approaches taken in treating fibrotic diseases (Love and Jones, 2009). It is also likely that the timing of delivery of different agents through the wound healing/biomaterial response process will be important, which some new methods of drug delivery have the potential to address. Having said that, many drug delivery approaches from biomaterials have failed in the long term, since after time, the drug becomes depleted. Once the drug stops acting, the default fibrotic response to the biomaterial resumes (Bhardwaj et al., 2007). Thus, approaches that permanently alter the phenotype or progression of fibrosis would be preferable over those that have a temporary effect.

The previous description of the cells and molecules involved in fibrosis highlights the wide variety of possible anti-fibrotic targets. Using knockout animals provides illuminating results but is obviously only an experimental approach. Many other tactics have been suggested in the fibrosis literature, including enzymes, cytokines, small

Table 9.1 Fibrotic pathways and inhibiting compounds (Love and Jones, 2009)

Fibrotic pathway/target	Inhibiting compound(s)
Inflammation/ immunosuppression	Glucocorticoids, retinoids, colchicine, azathioprine, cyclophosphamide, thalidomide, pentoxifylline, theophylline
Collagen synthesis	Prolyl-4-hydroxylase inhibitors (e.g., HOE0 077 or phenanthrolinones)
TGFβ	Decorin, pirfenidone, relaxin, BMP-7, hepatocyte growth factor, SMAD7
CTGF	Antisense oligonuceotides, cAMP, TNFα
ET-1	Bosentan
ANG II	ARBs, ACE inhibitors
Rho GTPases	Y-27362, fasudil
MMP-2 and MMP-9	Bay 12-9566
TIMP-1	Monoclonal antibodies specific for TIMP-1
B-cell antagonists	Rituximab

molecule inhibitors, or agonists revealed by drug discovery trials, neutralizing antibodies, DNA-binding drugs, antisense RNA, siRNA, and genetic engineering approaches. The targets vary from specific cell types to cytokines, chemokines and growth factors, and signaling cascades, just to name a few. A list of potentially fibrosis-inhibiting compounds is provided in Table 9.1. It is impossible to identify every possible anti-fibrotic approach here; instead, the major targets will be highlighted.

Most of the effort in producing drug-releasing biomaterials that reduce fibrosis has been from researchers in implanted glucose sensors that rapidly biofoul and lose their glucose sensitivity (Koh et al., 2011), but there has also been work in glaucoma (Shao et al., 2011; Löbler et al., 2011), microencapsulation (Dang et al., 2013), and drug-eluting stents (Forte et al., 2014). Table 9.2 summarizes the approaches that have been taken to minimize fibrosis caused by biomaterials.

Minimizing fibrosis-initiating signals

Many anti-fibrotic efforts in the biomaterials field have concentrated on preventing the initial signals that precipitate fibrosis. Essentially, researchers have tried to create "stealth" materials that resemble the body and will not be recognized as foreign. Early efforts just tried to prevent protein adsorption; subsequent efforts have become much more sophisticated. DAMPs are released upon wounding and surgical implantation (Rogers and Babensee, 2010). Minimizing surgical damage and preventing DAMPs from adhering to the biomaterial surface will help with this. Similarly, some material surfaces appear to resemble PAMPs (Yang and Jones, 2009); ensuring materials are not recognized by PRRs will help. Others have worked on mimicking membrane chemistry on biomaterial surfaces and mimicking mechanical properties of local tissue, with some (but limited) success (Jin et al., 2010; Grainger, 2013). Interestingly, altering

Table 9.2 Drug-release strategies from biomaterials to reduce local fibrosis

Drug	Mode of action	References
None	Hydrogel materials; "invisible" surfaces; use of native ECM	Yang et al. (2011), Grainger (2013), Jin et al. (2010), Badylak (2014), Faulk et al. (2014)
None	Fluctuating properties to "clean" surface	Gant et al. (2009, 2010), Ding et al. (2000), Vaddiraju et al. (2012)
None	Mechanically altered microenvironment with microstructures	Pinney et al. (2014)
Dexamethasone	Anti-inflammatory steroid	Astolfi et al. (2014), Hickey et al. (2002), Patil et al. (2007), Ju et al. (2008), Bohl et al. (2012), Bünger et al. (2005), Dang et al. (2013)
VEGF	Angiogenesis induction	Ju et al. (2008), Patil et al. (2007)
Paclitaxel; triamcinolone	Anti-proliferative; anti-inflammatory	Löbler et al. (2011)
Diazeniumdiolate	Nitric oxide release	Hetrick et al. (2007)
Heparin	Anti-coagulant and unknown mode of action	Vaithilingam et al. (2014), Saito and Tabata (2012) Lee et al. (2011)
Cromolyn	Mast cell inhibitor	Thevenot et al. (2011)
Tranilast	TGFβ2 agonist	Spitzer et al. (2012)
SB431543	TGFβ inhibitor	Baker et al. (2014)
1,4-DPCA	Prolyl-4-hydroxylase inhibitor—inhibits collagen assembly	Love and Jones (2013)

surface topography (e.g., increasing porosity or surface roughness) does have some effect on fibrosis. There are so many ways that the body can recognize foreign materials that it seems unlikely that engineering the materials alone can completely overcome the fibrotic response. However, in some applications, reduction in fibrosis might be sufficient for device function.

Inhibiting inflammation, pro-fibrotic factors, and signaling cascades

Since inflammation has often been identified as the initiator of the fibrotic pathway, abrogating the inflammatory response to biomaterials might reduce later fibrosis. Inflammatory cells produce many pro-fibrotic molecules that mediate fibrotic capsule formation. Glucocorticoids (e.g., dexamethasone) are promising treatment agents because they are potently anti-inflammatory, are nonirritating, and suppress cell proliferation, though they do have undesirable side effects. Indeed, dexamethasone has been released from biomaterials to try to reduce fibrotic responses (Hickey et al., 2002; Astolfi et al., 2014) along with other approaches including NO release (Koh et al., 2011).

Glucocorticoids also modulate the phenotype of infiltrating macrophages and lympho-cytes, which, as we have seen, has the potential to alter the fibrotic response (Peek et al., 2005; Mosser and Edwards, 2008). Other general immunosuppressive drugs include col-chicine, azathioprine, cyclophosphamide, prednisone, thalidomide, pentoxifylline, and the-ophylline. Blocking the action of a range of inflammatory cytokines and growth factors (e.g., IL-1β, IL-5, IL-6, and IL-13) might also prove useful, or even delivering anti-fibrotic cytokines such as IL-10, IFNγ, or IL-12 (Hinz and Gabbiani, 2010). Preventing the accu-mulation of inflammatory cells near biomaterials by blocking CC and CXC chemokines is another interesting approach. For example, inhibiting CXCL12 blocks fibrocyte migra-tion and differentiation and decreases fibrosis (Garibaldi et al., 2013). In fibrotic disease models, many of these approaches have been attempted, with some success.

Blockade of pro-fibrotic factors has been attempted, most notably with TGFβ. Blockade of endothelin, ANG II, CTGF, and PDGF have also been attempted in fibrotic models with varying degrees of success (Leask, 2009, 2010). Again, timing and site of implantation are important factors to consider. There has been a lot of work in the fibrosis field in developing drugs that block Wnt, Notch, and hedgehog pathways (Beyer and Distler, 2013), which also has some potential for success in the biomaterials field. Similarly blocking the signaling of pathogen-associated receptors such as TLRs might help. There has also been some work targeting the gene transcription mecha-nism downstream of Rho, which is downstream of many of the pro-fibrotic molecules (Sampson et al., 2014).

Targeting specific cell responses

Many different cells respond to biomaterial implantation and can potentially be targeted to minimize fibrosis. Macrophages are key cells that might control down-stream fibrotic effects. As mentioned above, several different cytokines, growth factors, and chemokines likely affect the number and activation of macrophages in the implant location. Additionally, approaches can be made to intentionally alter the macrophages to express a noninflammatory phenotype, perhaps by releasing cytokines such as IL-4, IL-13, or IL-10. One interesting molecule is serum amyloid P (pentraxin 2), which has been shown to inhibit pro-fibrotic macrophage generation, promote immunoregula-tory macrophages, inhibit monocyte to fibrocyte differentiation, and regulate neutro-phil function (Cox et al., 2014). Pentraxin 2 also controls monocyte differentiation and activation, promoting Mreg/M2c-like macrophages and blocking collagen deposition (Duffield and Lupher, 2010).

Mast cells have been targeted in a biomaterials context by releasing the tyrosine kinase inhibitor mastinib, which did result in some reduction in fibrosis in response to a biomaterial (Avula et al., 2013). However, it was not certain if the drug was acting primarily on mast cells or on other pro-fibrotic pathways.

Much work has been done to try to interfere with or reverse myofibroblast dif-ferentiation (Hinz and Gabbiani, 2010; Sivakumar and Das, 2008; Yang et al., 2014b).

Arguably, many of the cytokines and growth factors listed above are essential. In addition, blocking LPA or integrin function could prevent myofibroblast differentiation (Pyne et al., 2013). Myofibroblasts are the number one target in pathological fibrosis.

Regulating ECM production and catabolism

Fibrosis is essentially an imbalance between ECM production and catabolism. Altering these two processes seems like a natural approach for inhibiting fibrous capsule formation. Inhibiting enzymes involved in collagen synthesis seems a straightforward approach. Alternatively, myofibroblasts could be targeted with pro-apoptotic drugs. One enzyme that has attracted the attention of fibrosis researchers is prolyl-4-hydroxylase, since hydroxyproline is important in maintaining the triple helix structure of collagen. When released from PLGA, it significantly reduced fibrosis (Love and Jones, 2013). As previously mentioned, the MMPs degrade components of the ECM, though their mode of action is extensive. MMP-1 in particular catabolizes collagen, so upregulating MMP-1 and downregulating TIMP-1 might reduce fibrotic tissue formation. In contrast, MMP-2, MMP-9, and MMP-12 promote fibrosis by inducing EMT and increasing vascular permeability for immune cells. Some researchers have inhibited these compounds to reduce immune cell infiltration and myofibroblast formation. Timing and location of injury are very important in targeting MMP activity.

Other approaches

Many other approaches have been attempted to reduce fibrosis, including systemic approaches such as altering diet. Redox balances have been altered by inhibiting NOX4 (Sampson et al., 2011). Also, scavenging of ROS or release of antioxidants has been shown to help de-differentiate myofibroblasts to quiescent fibroblasts (Sampson et al., 2014). Enhanced nitrous oxide synthase (NOS) activity can be achieved by releasing the NOS substrate, L-arginine. Also NO donors can be released, and soluble guanylate cyclase can be activated/enhanced and phosphodiesterase can be inhibited (Sampson et al., 2014). These changes alter signaling and redox levels. Even altering heat shock protein activity might alter fibrotic responses. There are numerous approaches to altering fibrosis; the list here is not comprehensive. Nonetheless, there is promise in many of these approaches that can be applied to biomaterials.

CONCLUSIONS

Fibrosis around implanted biomaterials is ubiquitous and has deleterious effects on many clinical applications including sensors, drug delivery devices, soft tissue implants, and, potentially, tissue-engineered constructs. Despite a great deal of work in the field to alter these responses via surface modification, fibrous capsule formation seems inevitable. The sequence of events that occurs in response to biomaterial implantation is similar to that encountered in wound healing, with the exception being that remodeling and resolution do not occur. We thus looked to the fibrosis field to understand what the cellular and molecular mechanisms of pathological fibrosis were. While many cells including macrophages do play a role in fibrosis, the major player is the myofibroblast. Many cytokines (most notably TGFβ), growth factors, chemokines, signaling pathways, and enzymes control the complex progression of fibrosis and present targets for its treatment. In the biomaterials field, we have the opportunity to use our devices not only for their intended original function, but also to deliver anti-fibrotic drugs. These new approaches have the potential to turn fibrotic responses to biomaterials into truly biocompatible, regenerative responses.

REFERENCES

Abe, S., Hayashi, H., Seo, Y., Matsuda, K., Kamio, K., Saito, Y., et al., 2011. Reduction in serum high mobility group box-1 level by polymyxin B-immobilized fiber column in patients with idiopathic pulmonary fibrosis with acute exacerbation. Blood. Purif. 32 (4), 310–316.

Acharya, K.R., Ackerman, S.J., 2014. Eosinophil granule proteins: form and function. J. Biol. Chem. 289 (25), 17406–17415.

Akhmetshina, A., Palumbo, K., Dees, C., Bergmann, C., Venalis, P., Zerr, P., et al., 2012. Activation of canonical Wnt signalling is required for TGF-β-mediated fibrosis. Nat. Commun. 3, 735.

Alijotas-Reig, J., Fernández-Figueras, M.T., Puig, L., 2013. Late-onset inflammatory adverse reactions related to soft tissue filler injections. Clin. Rev. Allergy. Immunol. 45 (1), 97–108.

Amălinei, C., Draga Căruntu, I., Eliza Giuşcă, S., Anca Bălan, R., 2010. Matrix metalloproteinases involvement in pathologic conditions. Rom J. Morphol. Embryol. 51 (2), 215–228.

American Society for Aesthetic Plastic Surgery., 2009. Cosmetic Surgery National Data Bank Statistics. Available from: <http://www.surgery.org/sites/default/files/2009stats.pdf>.

Anderson, J.M., McNally, A.K., 2011. Biocompatibility of implants: lymphocyte/macrophage interactions. Semin. Immunopathol. 33 (3), 221–233.

Anderson, J.M., Rodriguez, A., Chang, D.T., 2008. Foreign body reaction to biomaterials. Semin. Immunol. 20 (2), 86–100.

Arshad, M.I., Piquet-Pellorce, C., Samson, M., 2012. IL-33 and HMGB1 alarmins: sensors of cellular death and their involvement in liver pathology. Liver Int. 32 (8), 1200–1210.

Ask, K., Bonniaud, P., Maass, K., Eickelberg, O., Margetts, P.J., Warburton, D., et al., 2008. Progressive pulmonary fibrosis is mediated by TGF-beta isoform 1 but not TGF-beta3. Int. J. Biochem. Cell. Biol. 40 (3), 484–495.

Astolfi, L., Guaran, V., Marchetti, N., Olivetto, E., Simoni, E., Cavazzini, A., et al., 2014. Cochlear implants and drug delivery: in vitro evaluation of dexamethasone release. J. Biomed. Mater. Res. B. Appl. Biomater. 102 (2), 267–273.

Atala, A., 2009. Engineering organs. Curr. Opin. Biotechnol 20 (5), 575–592.

Avula, M.N., Rao, A.N., McGill, L.D., Grainger, D.W., Solzbacher, F., 2013. Modulation of the foreign body response to implanted sensor models through device-based delivery of the tyrosine kinase inhibitor, masitinib. Biomaterials 34 (38), 9737–9746.

Avula, M.N., Rao, A.N., McGill, L.D., Grainger, D.W., Solzbacher, F., 2014. Foreign body response to subcutaneous biomaterial implants in a mast cell-deficient Kit(w-Sh) murine model. Acta. Biomater. 10 (5), 1856–1863.

Badylak, S.F., 2014. Decellularized allogeneic and xenogeneic tissue as a bioscaffold for regenerative medicine: factors that influence the host response. Ann. Biomed. Eng. 42 (7), 1517–1527.

Baker, D.W., Tsai, Y.-T., Weng, H., Tang, L., 2014. Alternative strategies to manipulate fibrocyte involvement in the fibrotic tissue response: pharmacokinetic inhibition and the feasibility of directed-adipogenic differentiation. Acta. Biomater. 10 (7), 3108–3116.

Balderrama, C.M.S., Rojas, J.M., Ribas-Filho, O.M., Gregori Czeczko, N., Alexandre Dietz, U., Giacometti Sakamoto, D., et al., 2009. Healing reaction to mammary prostheses covered by textured silicone and silicone foam in rats. Acta. Cir. Bras. 24 (5), 367–376.

Balmelli, C., Alves, M.P., Steiner, E., Zingg, D., Peduto, N., Ruggli, N., et al., 2007. Responsiveness of fibrocytes to toll-like receptor danger signals. Immunobiology 212 (9-10), 693–699.

Barnes, J L, Gorin, Y, 2011. Myofibroblast differentiation during fibrosis: role of NAD(P)H oxidases. Kidney. Int 79 (9), 944–956. International Society of Nephrology.

Baroni, G.S., D'Ambrosio, L., Curto, P., Casini, A., Mancini, R., Jezequel, A.M., et al., 1996. Interferon gamma decreases hepatic stellate cell activation and extracellular matrix deposition in rat liver fibrosis. Hepatology (Baltimore, MD) 23 (5), 1189–1199.

Barrientos, S., Stojadinovic, O., Golinko, M.S., Brem, H., Tomic-Canic, M., 2008. Growth factors and cytokines in wound healing. Wound Repair Regen. 16 (5), 585–601.

Baruah, P., Dumitriu, I.E., Peri, G., Russo, V., Mantovani, A., Manfredi, A.A., et al., 2006. The tissue pentraxin PTX3 limits C1q-mediated complement activation and phagocytosis of apoptotic cells by dendritic cells. J. Leukoc. Biol. 80 (1), 87–95.

Bataller, R., Schwabe, R.F., Choi, Y.H., Yang, L., Paik, Y.H., Lindquist, J., et al., 2003. NADPH oxidase signal transduces angiotensin II in hepatic stellate cells and is critical in hepatic fibrosis. J. Clin. Invest. 112 (9), 1383–1394.

Bellaye, P.-S., Burgy, O., Causse, S., Garrido, C., Bonniaud, P., 2014. Heat shock proteins in fibrosis and wound healing: good or evil? Pharmacol. Ther. 143 (2), 119–132.

Berry, M.G., Cucchiara, V., Davies, D.M., 2010. Breast augmentation: part II—adverse capsular contracture. J. Plast. Reconstr. Aesthet. Surg. : JPRAS 63 (12), 2098–2107.

Beyer, C., Distler, J.H.W., 2013. Curr. Rheumatol. Rep. 15 (1), 299.

Bhardwaj, U., Sura, R., Papadimitrakopoulos, F., Burgess, D.J., 2007. Controlling acute inflammation with fast releasing dexamethasone-PLGA microsphere/PVA hydrogel composites for implantable devices. J. Diabetes Sci. Technol. 1 (1), 8–17.

Bland, E., Dréau, D., Burg, K.J.L., 2013. Overcoming hypoxia to improve tissue-engineering approaches to regenerative medicine. J. Tissue Eng. Regen. Med. 7 (7), 505–514.

Blease, K., Jakubzick, C., Westwick, J., Lukacs, N., Kunkel, S.L., Hogaboam, C.M., 2001. Therapeutic effect of IL-13 immunoneutralization during chronic experimental fungal asthma. J. Immunol (Baltimore, Md. : 1950) 166 (8), 5219–5224.

Boateng, J.S., Matthews, K.H., Stevens, H.N.E., Eccleston, G.M., 2008. Wound healing dressings and drug delivery systems: a review. J. Pharm. Sci. 97 (8), 2892–2923.

Bohl, A., Rohm, H.W., Ceschi, P., Paasche, G., Hahn, A., Barcikowski, S., et al., 2012. Development of a specially tailored local drug delivery system for the prevention of fibrosis after insertion of cochlear implants into the inner ear. J. Mater. Sci. Mater. Med. 23 (9), 2151–2162.

Borthwick, L.A., Wynn, T.A., Fisher, A.J., 2013. Cytokine mediated tissue fibrosis. Biochim. Biophys. Acta. 1832 (7), 1049–1060.

Bowen, T., Jenkins, R.H., Fraser, D.J., 2013. MicroRNAs, transforming growth factor beta-1, and tissue fibrosis. J. Pathol. 229 (2), 274–285.

Broichhausen, C., Riquelme, P., Geissler, E.K., Hutchinson, J.A., 2012. Regulatory macrophages as therapeutic targets and therapeutic agents in solid organ transplantation. Curr. Opin. Organ Transplant. 17 (4), 332–342.

Bucala, R., 2012. Review series—inflammation & fibrosis. Fibrocytes and fibrosis. QJM 105 (6), 505–508.

Budd, D.C., Qian, Y., 2013. Development of lysophosphatidic acid pathway modulators as therapies for fibrosis. Future Med.l Chem. 5 (16), 1935–1952.

Bünger, C.M., Tiefenbach, B., Jahnke, A., Gerlach, C., Freier, T., Schmitz, K.P., et al., 2005. Deletion of the tissue response against alginate-Pll capsules by temporary release of co-encapsulated steroids. Biomaterials 26 (15), 2353–2360.

Campbell, G.R., Turnbull, G., Xiang, L., Haines, M., Armstrong, S., Rolfe, B.E., et al., 2008. The peritoneal cavity as a bioreactor for tissue engineering visceral organs: bladder, uterus and vas deferens. J. Tissue Eng. Regen. Med. 2 (1), 50–60.

Cao, L., Arany, P.R., Wang, Y.-S., Mooney, D.J., 2009. Promoting angiogenesis via manipulation of VEGF responsiveness with notch signaling. Biomaterials 30 (25), 4085–4093.

Chambers, R.C., 2008. Procoagulant signalling mechanisms in lung inflammation and fibrosis: novel opportunities for pharmacological intervention? Br. J. Pharmacol. 153 (March), S367–S378.

Chang, D.T., Colton, E., Matsuda, T., Anderson, J.M., 2009. Lymphocyte adhesion and interactions with biomaterial adherent macrophages and foreign body giant cells. J. Biomed. Mater. Res. A. 91 (4), 1210–1220.

Chen, B., Dodge, M.E., Tang, W., Lu, J., Ma, Z., Fan, C.-W., et al., 2009. Small molecule-mediated disruption of Wnt-dependent signaling in tissue regeneration and cancer. Nat. Chem. Biol. 5 (2), 100–107.

Chmiel, J.F., Aksamit, T.R., Chotirmall, S.H., Dasenbrook, E.C., Elborn, J.S., LiPuma, J.J., et al., 2014. Antibiotic management of lung infections in cystic fibrosis: part I. The microbiome, MRSA, gram-negative bacteria, and multiple infections. Ann. Am. Thorac. Soc. 11 (7), 1120–1129.

Cho, J.Y., Miller, M, Baek, K.J., Han, J.W., Nayar, J., Young Lee, S., et al., 2004. Inhibition of airway remodeling in IL-5-deficient mice. J. Clin. Invest. 113 (4), 551–560.

Cho, S.H., Lee, S.H., Kato, A., Takabayashi, T., Kulka, M., Shin, S.C., et al., 2015. Cross-talk between human mast cells and bronchial epithelial cells in PAI-1 production via TGF-β1. Am. J. Respir. Cell Mol. Biol. 52 (1), 88–95.

Choi, S.S., Omenetti, A., Syn, W.-K., Mae Diehl, A., 2011. The role of hedgehog signaling in fibrogenic liver repair. Int. J. Biochem. Cell. Biol. 43 (2), 238–244.

Chrysanthopoulou, A., Mitroulis, I., Apostolidou, E., Arelaki, S., Mikroulis, D., Konstantinidis, T., et al., 2014. Neutrophil extracellular traps promote differentiation and function of fibroblasts. J. Pathol. 233 (3), 294–307.

Clayton, H.A., James, R.F., London, N.J., 1993. Islet microencapsulation: a review. Acta. Diabetol. 30 (4), 181–189.

Contos, J.J.A., Ishii, I., Chun, J., 2000. Lysophosphatidic acid receptors. Mol. Pharmacol. 58 (6), 1188–1196.

Cowin, A.J., Brosnan, M.P., Holmes, T.M., Ferguson, M.W., 1998. Endogenous inflammatory response to dermal wound healing in the fetal and adult mouse. Dev. Dyn. 212 (3), 385–393.

Cox, N, Pilling, D, Gomer, R.H., 2014. Serum amyloid P: a systemic regulator of the innate immune response. J. Leukoc. Biol. 96 (5), 739–743.

Coyle, T.B., Metersky, M.L., 2013. The effect of the endothelin-1 receptor antagonist, bosentan, on patients with poorly controlled asthma: a 17-week, double-blind, placebo-controlled crossover pilot study. J. Asthma 50 (4), 433–437.

Cramer, T., Yamanishi, Y., Clausen, B.E., Förster, I., Pawlinski, R., Mackman, N., et al., 2003. HIF-1alpha is essential for myeloid cell-mediated inflammation. Cell 112 (5), 645–657.

Daley, J.M., Brancato, S.K., Thomay, A.A., Reichner, J.S., Albina, J.E., 2010. The phenotype of murine wound macrophages. J. Leukoc. Biol. 87 (1), 59–67.

Dang, T.T., Thai, A.V., Cohen, J., Slosberg, J.E., Siniakowicz, K., Doloff, J.C., et al., 2013. Enhanced function of immuno-isolated islets in diabetes therapy by co-encapsulation with an anti-inflammatory drug. Biomaterials 34 (23), 5792–5801.

DeFife, K.M., Jenney, C.R., McNally, A.K., Colton, E., Anderson, J.M., 1997. Interleukin-13 induces human monocyte/macrophage fusion and macrophage mannose receptor expression. J. Immunol. (Baltimore, Md. : 1950) 158 (7), 3385–3390.

Dees, C., Tomcik, M., Zerr, P., Akhmetshina, A., Horn, A., Palumbo, K., et al., 2011. Notch signalling regulates fibroblast activation and collagen release in systemic sclerosis. Ann. Rheum. Dis. 70 (7), 1304–1310.

Ding, X.-B., Sun, Z.-H., Zhang, W.-C., Peng, Y.-X., Wan, G.-X., Jiang, Y.-Y., 2000. Adsorption/desorption of protein on magnetic particles covered by thermosensitive polymers. J. Appl. Polym. Sci. 77 (13), 2915–2920.

Dong, C., 2008. Regulation and pro-inflammatory function of interleukin-17 family cytokines. Immunol. Rev. 226 (December), 80–86.

Downing, T.L., Soto, J., Morez, C., Houssin, T., Fritz, A., Yuan, F., et al., 2013. Biophysical regulation of epigenetic state and cell reprogramming. Nat. Mater. 12 (12), 1154–1162.

Drent, M., Cobben, N.A., Henderson, R.F., Wouters, E.F., van Dieijen-Visser, M., 1996. Usefulness of lactate dehydrogenase and its isoenzymes as indicators of lung damage or inflammation. Eur. Respir. J. 9 (8), 1736–1742.

Duffield, J.S., 2014. Cellular and molecular mechanisms in kidney Fibrosis. J. Clin. Invest. 124 (6), 2299–2306.

Duffield, J.S., Lupher, M.L., 2010. PRM-151 (recombinant human serum amyloid P/pentraxin 2) for the treatment of fibrosis. Drug. News. Perspect. 23 (5), 305–315.

Duffield, J.S., Lupher, M., Thannickal, V.J., Wynn, T.A., 2013. Host responses in tissue repair and fibrosis. Annu. Rev. Pathol. 8 (January), 241–276.

Dvorak, A.M., 2005. Mast cell-derived mediators of enhanced microvascular permeability, vascular permeability factor/vascular endothelial growth factor, histamine, and serotonin, cause leakage of macromolecules through a new endothelial cell permeability organelle, the vesic. Chem. Immunol. Allergy. 85 (January), 185–204.

Fallon, P.G., Richardson, E.J., McKenzie, G.J., McKenzie, A.N., 2000. Schistosome infection of transgenic mice defines distinct and contrasting pathogenic roles for IL-4 and IL-13: IL-13 is a profibrotic agent. J. Immunol. (Baltimore, Md. : 1950) 164 (5), 2585–2591.

Farina, A., Cirone, M., York, M., Lenna, S., Padilla, C., McLaughlin, S., et al., 2014. Epstein–Barr virus infection induces aberrant TLR activation pathway and fibroblast–myofibroblast conversion in scleroderma. J. Invest. Dermatol. 134 (4), 954–964.

Faulk, D.M., Londono, R., Wolf, M.T., Ranallo, C.A., Carruthers, C.A., Wildemann, J.D., et al., 2014. ECM hydrogel coating mitigates the chronic inflammatory response to polypropylene mesh. Biomaterials 35 (30), 8585–8595.

Finnson, K.W., Arany, P.R., Philip, A., 2013. Transforming growth factor beta signaling in cutaneous wound healing: lessons learned from animal studies. Adv. Wound Care 2 (5), 225–237.

Fitzpatrick, L.E., Lisovsky, A., Sefton, M.V., 2012. The expression of sonic hedgehog in diabetic wounds following treatment with poly(Methacrylic Acid-Co-Methyl Methacrylate) beads. Biomaterials 33 (21), 5297–5307.

Flessner, M.F., Credit, K., Henderson, K., Vanpelt, H.M., Potter, R., He, Z., et al., 2007. Peritoneal changes after exposure to sterile solutions by catheter. J. Am. Soc. Nephrol. 18 (8), 2294–2302.

Flessner, M.F., Credit, K., Richardson, K., Potter, R., Li, X., He, Z., et al., 2010. Peritoneal inflammation after twenty-week exposure to dialysis solution: effect of solution versus catheter-foreign body reaction. Perit. Dial. Int. 30 (3), 284–293.

Forte, A., Rinaldi, B., Berrino, L., Rossi, F., Galderisi, U., Cipollaro, M., 2014. Novel potential targets for prevention of arterial restenosis: insights from the pre-clinical research. Clin. Sci. (London, England : 1979) 127 (11), 615–634.

Frost, M., Meyerhoff, M.E., 2006. *In vivo* chemical sensors: tackling biocompatibility. Anal. Chem. 78 (21), 7370–7377. American Chemical Society.

Galgut, P., Pitrola, R., Waite, I., Doyle, C., Smith, R., 1991. Histological evaluation of biodegradable and non-degradable membranes placed transcutaneously in rats. J. Clin. Periodontol. 18 (8), 581–586.

Galli, S.J., Borregaard, N., Wynn, T.A., 2011. Phenotypic and functional plasticity of cells of innate immunity: macrophages, mast cells and neutrophils. Nat. Immunol. 12 (11), 1035–1044.

Gant, R.M., Hou, Y., Grunlan, M.A., Coté, G.L., 2009. Development of a self-cleaning sensor membrane for implantable biosensors. J. Biomed. Mater. Res. A. 90 (3), 695–701.

Gant, R.M., Abraham, A.A., Hou, Y., Cummins, B.M., Grunlan, M.A., Coté, G.L., 2010. Design of a self-cleaning thermoresponsive nanocomposite hydrogel membrane for implantable biosensors. Acta. Biomaterialia 6 (8), 2903–2910.

Gardner, A.B., Lee, S.K.C., Woods, E.C., Acharya, A.P., 2013. Biomaterials-based modulation of the immune system. BioMed Res. Int. 2013 (January), 732182.

Garibaldi, B.T., D'Alessio, F.R., Mock, J.R., Files, D.C., Chau, E., Eto, Y., et al., 2013. Regulatory T cells reduce acute lung injury fibroproliferation by decreasing fibrocyte recruitment. Am. J. Respir. Cell. Mol. Biol. 48 (1), 35–43.

Gauldie, J., 2002. Pro: inflammatory mechanisms are a minor component of the pathogenesis of idiopathic pulmonary fibrosis. Am. J. Respir. Crit. Care Med. 165 (9), 1205–1206.

Giannandrea, M., Parks, W.C., 2014. Diverse functions of matrix metalloproteinases during fibrosis. Dis. Model Mech. 7 (2), 193–203.

Gifford, A.M., Chalmers, J.D., 2014. The role of neutrophils in cystic fibrosis. Curr. Opin. Hematol. 21 (1), 16–22.

Gill, S.E., Parks, W.C., 2008. Metalloproteinases and their inhibitors: regulators of wound healing. Int. J. Biochem. Cell. Biol. 40 (6-7), 1334–1347.

Gilligan, B.C., Shults, M., Rhodes, R.K., Jacobs, P.G., Brauker, J.H., Pintar, T.J., et al., 2004. Feasibility of continuous long-term glucose monitoring from a subcutaneous glucose sensor in humans. Diabetes. Technol. Ther. 6 (3), 378–386. Mary Ann Liebert, Inc.

Go, H., Koh, J., Sung Kim, H., Kyung Jeon, Y., Hyun Chung, D., 2014. Expression of toll-like receptor 2 and 4 is increased in the respiratory epithelial cells of chronic idiopathic interstitial pneumonia patients. Respir. Med. 108 (5), 783–792.

Goldberg, E.P., 1997. Silicone breast implant safety: physical, chemical, and biologic problems. Plast. Reconstr. Surg. 99 (1), 258–261.

Gorbet, M.B., Sefton, M.V., 2004. Biomaterial-associated thrombosis: roles of coagulation factors, complement, platelets and leukocytes. Biomaterials 25 (26), 5681–5703.

Goren, I., Allmann, N., Yogev, N., Schürmann, C., Linke, A., Holdener, M., et al., 2009. A transgenic mouse model of inducible macrophage depletion: effects of diphtheria toxin-driven lysozyme m-specific cell lineage ablation on wound inflammatory, angiogenic, and contractive processes. Am. J. Pathol. 175 (1), 132–147.

Grainger, D.W., 2013. All charged up about implanted biomaterials. Nat. Biotechnol. 31 (6), 507–509.

Greenfield, E.M., 2014. Do genetic susceptibility, toll-like receptors, and pathogen-associated molecular patterns modulate the effects of wear? Clin. Orthop. Relat. Res. July.

Guilliams, M., Ginhoux, F., Jakubzick, C., Naik, S.H., Onai, N., Schraml, B.U., et al., 2014. Dendritic cells, monocytes and macrophages: a unified nomenclature based on ontogeny. Nat. Rev. Immunol. 14 (8), 571–578.

Gurujeyalakshmi, G., Giri, S.N., 1995. Molecular mechanisms of antifibrotic effect of interferon gamma in bleomycin-mouse model of lung fibrosis: downregulation of TGF-beta and procollagen I and III gene expression. Exp. Lung Res. 21 (5), 791–808.

Hamada, N., Maeyama, T., Kawaguchi, T., Yoshimi, M., Fukumoto, J., Yamada, M., et al., 2008. The role of high mobility group box1 in pulmonary fibrosis. Am. J. Respir. Cell. Mol. Biol. 39 (4), 440–447.

Handel, N., Cordray, T., Gutierrez, J., Jensen, J.A., 2006. A long-term study of outcomes, complications, and patient satisfaction with breast implants. Plast. Reconstr. Surg. 117 (3), 757–767. discussion 768–72.

Hao, H., Cohen, D.A., Jennings, C.D., Bryson, J.S., Kaplan, A.M., 2000. Bleomycin-induced pulmonary fibrosis is independent of eosinophils. J. Leukoc. Biol. 68 (4), 515–521.

Hasan, S.A., Eksteen, B., Reid, D., Paine, H.V., Alansary, A., Johannson, K., et al., 2013. Role of IL-17A and neutrophils in fibrosis in experimental hypersensitivity pneumonitis. J. Allergy. Clin. Immunol. 131 (6), 1663–1673.

Hawinkels, L.J.A.C., Ten Dijke, P., 2011. Exploring anti-TGF-β therapies in cancer and fibrosis. Growth Factors (Chur, Switzerland) 29 (4), 140–152.

Heldin, C.H., Westermark, B., 1999. Mechanism of action and in vivo role of platelet-derived growth factor. Physiol. Rev. 79 (4), 1283–1316.

Hemmann, S., Graf, J., Roderfeld, M., Roeb, E., 2007. Expression of MMPs and TIMPs in liver fibrosis - a systematic review with special emphasis on anti-fibrotic strategies. J. Hepatol. 46 (5), 955–975.

Herbert, D.R., Hölscher, C., Mohrs, M., Arendse, B., Schwegmann, A., Radwanska, M., et al., 2004. Alternative macrophage activation is essential for survival during schistosomiasis and downmodulates T helper 1 responses and immunopathology. Immunity 20 (5), 623–635.

Hernandez-Pando, R., Bornstein, Q.L., Aguilar Leon, D., Orozco, E.H., Madrigal, V.K., Martinez Cordero, E., 2000. Inflammatory cytokine production by immunological and foreign body multinucleated giant cells. Immunology 100 (3), 352–358.

Hetrick, E.M., Prichard, H.L., Klitzman, B., Schoenfisch, M.H., 2007. Reduced foreign body response at nitric oxide-releasing subcutaneous implants. Biomaterials 28 (31), 4571–4580.

Hickey, T., Kreutzer, D., Burgess, D.J., Moussy, F., 2002. Dexamethasone/PLGA microspheres for continuous delivery of an anti-inflammatory drug for implantable medical devices. Biomaterials 23 (7), 1649–1656.

Higgins, D.M., Basaraba, R.J., Hohnbaum, A.C., Lee, E.J., Grainger, D.W., Gonzalez-Juarrero, M., 2009. Localized immunosuppressive environment in the foreign body response to implanted biomaterials. Am. J. Pathol. 175 (1), 161–170.

Hinz, B, Gabbiani, G, 2010. Fibrosis: recent advances in myofibroblast biology and new therapeutic perspectives. F1000 Biol. Rep. 2, 78.

Hinz, B., Phan, S.H., Thannickal, V.J., Prunotto, M., Desmoulière, A., Varga, J., et al., 2012. Recent developments in myofibroblast biology: paradigms for connective tissue remodeling. Am. J. Pathol. 180 (4), 1340–1355.

Hoffmann, K.F., Cheever, A.W., Wynn, T.A., 2000. IL-10 and the dangers of immune polarization: excessive Type 1 and Type 2 cytokine responses induce distinct forms of lethal immunopathology in murine schistosomiasis. J. Immunol. (Baltimore, Md. : 1950) 164 (12), 6406–6416.

Horn, A., Kireva, T., Palumbo-Zerr, K., Dees, C., Tomcik, M., Cordazzo, C., et al., 2012a. Inhibition of hedgehog signalling prevents experimental fibrosis and induces regression of established fibrosis. Ann. Rheum. Dis. 71 (5), 785–789.

Horn, A., Palumbo, K., Cordazzo, C., Dees, C., Akhmetshina, A., Tomcik, M., et al., 2012b. Hedgehog signaling controls fibroblast activation and tissue fibrosis in systemic sclerosis. Arthritis. Rheum. 64 (8), 2724–2733.

Hu, J.Z., Rommereim, D.N., Minard, K.R., Woodstock, A., Harrer, B.J., Wind, R.A., et al., 2008. Metabolomics in lung inflammation:a high-resolution (1)h NMR study of mice exposedto silica dust. Toxicol. Mech. Methods 18 (5), 385–398. Informa UK Ltd UK.

Huang, S.-M.A., Mishina, Y.M., Liu, S., Cheung, A., Stegmeier, F., Michaud, G.A., et al., 2009. Tankyrase inhibition stabilizes axin and antagonizes wnt signalling. Nature 461 (7264), 614–620.

Huang, L.S., Fu, P., Patel, P., Harijith, A., Sun, T., Zhao, Y., et al., 2013. Lysophosphatidic acid receptor-2 deficiency confers protection against bleomycin-induced lung injury and fibrosis in mice. Am. J. Respir. Cell. Mol. Biol 49 (6), 912–922.

Hwang, K., Sim, H.B., Huan, F., Joong Kim, D., 2010. Myofibroblasts and capsular tissue tension in breast capsular contracture. Aesthetic. Plast. Surg. 34 (6), 716–721.

Jain, V., Shikha Jain, Mahajan, S.C., 2014. Nanomedicines based drug delivery systems for anti-cancer targeting and treatment. Curr. Drug. Deliv Epub ahead (August).

Jaipersad, A.S., Lip, G.Y.H., Silverman, S., Shantsila, E., 2014. The role of monocytes in angiogenesis and atherosclerosis. J. Am. Coll. Cardiol. 63 (1), 1–11.

Jamieson, S., Going, J.J., D'Arcy, R., George, W.D., 1998. Expression of gap junction proteins connexin 26 and connexin 43 in normal human breast and in breast tumours. J. Pathol. 184 (1), 37–43.

Janeway, C.A., Medzhitov, R., 2002. Innate immune recognition. Annu. Rev. Immunol. 20 (January), 197–216.

Janowsky, E.C., Kupper, L.L., Hulka, B.S., 2000. Meta-analyses of the relation between silicone breast implants and the risk of connective-tissue diseases. N. Engl. J. Med. 342 (11), 781–790.

Jeong, E., Young Lee, J., 2011. Intrinsic and extrinsic regulation of innate immune receptors. Yonsei. Med. J. 52 (3), 379–392.

Jiang, S., Dong, C., 2013. A complex issue on CD4(+) T-cell subsets. Immunol. Rev. 252 (1), 5–11.

Jiang, X., Tsitsiou, E., Herrick, S.E., Lindsay, M.A., 2010. MicroRNAs and the regulation of fibrosis. FEBS J. 277 (9), 2015–2021.

Jin, Z., Feng, W., Zhu, S., Sheardown, H., Brash, J.L., 2010. Protein-resistant materials via surface-initiated atom transfer radical polymerization of 2-methacryloyloxyethyl phosphorylcholine. J. Biomater. Sci. Polym. Ed 21 (10), 1331–1344.

Jobling, M.F., Mott, J.D., Finnegan, M.T., Jurukovski, V., Erickson, A.C., Walian, P.J., et al., 2006. Isoform-specific activation of latent transforming growth factor beta (LTGF-Beta) by reactive oxygen species. Radiat. Res. 166 (6), 839–848.

Jones, J.A., Chang, D.T., Meyerson, H., Colton, E., Kwon, I.L.K, Matsuda, T., et al., 2007. Proteomic analysis and quantification of cytokines and chemokines from biomaterial surface-adherent macrophages and foreign body giant cells. J. Biomed. Mater. Res. A 83 (3), 585–596.

Jones, J.A., McNally, A.K., Chang, D.T., Abigail Qin, L., Meyerson, H., Colton, E., et al., 2008. Matrix metalloproteinases and their inhibitors in the foreign body reaction on biomaterials. J. Biomed. Mater. Res. A 84 (1), 158–166.

Jones, K.S., 2008. Effects of biomaterial-induced inflammation on fibrosis and rejection. SSemin. Immunol. 20 (2), 130–136.

Jones, P.A., 2012. Functions of DNA methylation: Islands, start sites, gene bodies and beyond. Nat. Rev. Genet. 13 (7), 484–492.

Jones, K.S., Sefton, M.V., Gorczynski, R.M., 2004. In vivo recognition by the host adaptive immune system of microencapsulated xenogeneic cells. Transplantation 78 (10), 1454–1462.

Ju, Y.M., Yu, B., Koob, T.J., Moussy, Y., Moussy, F., 2008. A novel porous collagen scaffold around an implantable biosensor for improving biocompatibility. I. In vitro/in vivo stability of the scaffold and in vitro sensitivity of the glucose sensor with scaffold. J. Biomed. Mater. Res. A. 87 (1), 136–146.

Jun, J.I., Lau, L.F., 2011. Taking aim at the extracellular matrix: CCN proteins as emerging therapeutic targets. Nat. Rev. Drug. Discov. 10 (12), 945–963.

Kafshgari, M.H., Harding, F.J., Voelcker, N.H., 2014. Insights into cellular uptake of nanoparticles. Curr. Drug. Deliv Epub ahead (August).

Kajihara, I., Jinnin, M., Honda, N., Makino, K., Makino, T., Masuguchi, S., et al., 2013. Scleroderma dermal fibroblasts overexpress vascular endothelial growth factor due to autocrine transforming growth factor β signaling. Mod. Rheumatol. 23 (3), 516–524.

Kao, H.-K., Chen, B., Murphy, G.F., Li, Q., Orgill, D.P., Guo, L., 2011. Peripheral blood fibrocytes: enhancement of wound healing by cell proliferation, re-epithelialization, contraction, and angiogenesis. Ann. Surg. 254 (6), 1066–1074.

Katz, S.C., Ryan, K., Ahmed, N., Plitas, G., Chaudhry, U.I., Kingham, T.P., et al., 2011. Obstructive jaundice expands intrahepatic regulatory T cells, which impair liver T lymphocyte function but modulate liver cholestasis and fibrosis. J. Immunol. (Baltimore, Md. : 1950) 187 (3), 1150–1156.

Kavian, N., Servettaz, A., Mongaret, C., Wang, A., Nicco, C., Chéreau, C., et al., 2010. Targeting ADAM-17/notch signaling abrogates the development of systemic sclerosis in a murine model. Arthritis. Rheum. 62 (11), 3477–3487.

Keane, M.P., Belperio, J.A., Moore, T.A., Moore, B.B., Arenberg, D.A., Smith, R.E., et al., 1999. Neutralization of the CXC chemokine, macrophage inflammatory protein-2, attenuates bleomycin-induced pulmonary fibrosis. J. Immunol. (Baltimore, Md. : 1950) 162 (9), 5511–5518.

Keeley, E.C., Mehrad, B., Strieter, R.M., 2010. Fibrocytes: bringing new insights into mechanisms of inflammation and fibrosis. Int. J. Biochem. Cell. Biol. 42 (4), 535–542.

Kendall, R.T., Feghali-Bostwick, C.A., 2014. Fibroblasts in fibrosis: novel roles and mediators. Front. Pharmacol. 5 (May), 123.

Kenneth Ward, W., 2008. A review of the foreign-body response to subcutaneously-implanted devices: the role of macrophages and cytokines in biofouling and fibrosis. J. Diabetes Sci. Technol. 2 (5), 768–777.

Kim, J-w, Tchernyshyov, I., Semenza, G.L., Dang, C.V., 2006. HIF-1-mediated expression of pyruvate dehydrogenase kinase: a metabolic switch required for cellular adaptation to hypoxia. Cell. Metab. 3 (3), 177–185.

Kim, M., Shin, D.W., Shin, H., Noh, M., Shin, J.H., 2013. Tensile stimuli increase nerve growth factor in human dermal fibroblasts independent of tension-induced TGFβ production. Exp. Dermatol. 22 (1), 72–74.

King, T.E., Bradford, W.Z., Castro-Bernardini, S., Fagan, E.A., Glaspole, I., Glassberg, M.K., et al., 2014. A phase 3 trial of pirfenidone in patients with idiopathic pulmonary fibrosis. N. Engl. J. Med. 370 (22), 2083–2092.

Kis-Toth, K., Bacskai, I., Gogolak, P., Mazlo, A., Szatmari, I., Rajnavolgyi, E., 2013. Monocyte-derived dendritic cell subpopulations use different types of matrix metalloproteinases inhibited by GM6001. Immunobiology 218 (11), 1361–1369.

Klueh, U., Kaur, M., Qiao, Y., Kreutzer, D.L., 2010. Critical role of tissue mast cells in controlling long-term glucose sensor function in vivo. Biomaterials 31 (16), 4540–4551.

Koh, A., Nichols, S.P., Schoenfisch, M.H., 2011. Glucose sensor membranes for mitigating the foreign body response. J. Diabetes Sci. Technol. 5 (5), 1052–1059.

Koschwanez, H.E., Reichert, W.M., 2007. In vitro, in vivo and post explantation testing of glucose-detecting biosensors: current methods and recommendations. Biomaterials 28 (25), 3687–3703.

Koschwanez, H.E., Yap, F.Y., Klitzman, B., Reichert, W.M., 2008. In vitro and in vivo characterization of porous poly-L-lactic acid coatings for subcutaneously implanted glucose sensors. J. Biomed. Mater. Res. A 87 (3), 792–807.

Kottmann, R., Matthew, A.A., Kulkarni, K.A., Smolnycki, E., Lyda, T., Dahanayake, R., et al., 2012. Lactic acid is elevated in idiopathic pulmonary fibrosis and induces myofibroblast differentiation via pH-dependent activation of transforming growth factor-β. Am. J. Respir. Crit. Care. Med. 186 (8), 740–751.

Kramann, R., DiRocco, D.P., Humphreys, B.D., 2013. Understanding the origin, activation and regulation of matrix-producing myofibroblasts for treatment of fibrotic disease. J. Pathol. 231 (3), 273–289.

Lanone, S., Zheng, T., Zhu, Z., Liu, W., Geun Lee, C., Ma, B., et al., 2002. Overlapping and enzyme-specific contributions of matrix metalloproteinases-9 and -12 in IL-13-induced inflammation and remodeling. J. Clin. Invest. 110 (4), 463–474.

Lawrence, D.A., 2001. Latent-TGF-beta: an overview. Mol. Cell. Biochem. 219 (1-2), 163–170.

Le, S.J., Gongora, M., Zhang, B., Grimmond, S., Campbell, G.R., Campbell, J.H., et al., 2010. Gene expression profile of the fibrotic response in the peritoneal cavity. Differentiation. 79 (4-5), 232–243.

Leask, A, 2009. Signaling in fibrosis: targeting the TGF beta, endothelin-1 and CCN2 axis in scleroderma. Front. Biosci. (Elite ed.) 1 (January), 115–122.

Leask, A, 2010. Potential therapeutic targets for cardiac fibrosis: TGFbeta, angiotensin, endothelin, CCN2, and PDGF, partners in fibroblast activation. Circ. Res. 106 (11), 1675–1680.

Lech, M., Gröbmayr, R., Weidenbusch, M., Anders, H.-J., 2012. Tissues use resident dendritic cells and macrophages to maintain homeostasis and to regain homeostasis upon tissue injury: the immunoregulatory role of changing tissue environments. Mediators. Inflamm. 2012 (January), 951390.

Lee, C.G., Homer, R.J., Zhu, Z., Lanone, S., Wang, X., Koteliansky, V., et al., 2001. Interleukin-13 induces tissue fibrosis by selectively stimulating and activating transforming growth factor beta(1). J. Exp. Med. 194 (6), 809–821.

Lee, J.-H., Lee, H., Joung, Y.K., Jung, K.H., Choi, J.-H., Lee, D.-H., et al., 2011. The use of low molecular weight heparin-pluronic nanogels to impede liver fibrosis by inhibition the TGF-β/Smad signaling pathway. Biomaterials 32 (5), 1438–1445.

Lee, K., Nelson, C.M., 2012. New insights into the regulation of epithelial-mesenchymal transition and tissue fibrosis. Int. Rev. Cell. Mol. Biol. 294 (January), 171–221.

Lekkerkerker, A.N., Aarbiou, J., van Es, T., Janssen, R.A.J., 2012. Cellular players in lung fibrosis. Curr. Pharm. Des. 18 (27), 4093–4102.

Levi-Schaffer, F., Piliponsky, A.M., 2003. Tryptase, a novel link between allergic inflammation and fibrosis. Trends. Immunol. 24 (4), 158–161.

Levin, E.R., 1995. Endothelins. N. Engl. J. Med. 333 (6), 356–363.

Li, J., Chen, J., Kirsner, R., 2007. Pathophysiology of acute wound healing. Clin. Dermatol. 25 (1), 9–18.

Lin, E., Adams, P.C., 1991. Biochemical liver profile in hemochromatosis. A survey of 100 patients. J. Clin. Gastroenterol. 13 (3), 316–320.

Lin, F., Wang, N., Zhang, T.-C., 2012. The role of endothelial-mesenchymal transition in development and pathological process. IUBMB. Life. 64 (9), 717–723.

Lind, G., Eriksson Linsmeier, C., Schouenborg, J., 2013. The density difference between tissue and neural probes is a key factor for glial scarring. Sci. Rep. 3 (January), 2942.

Löbler, M., Sternberg, K., Stachs, O., Allemann, R., Grabow, N., Roock, A., et al., 2011. Polymers and drugs suitable for the development of a drug delivery drainage system in glaucoma surgery. J. Biomed. Mater. Res. B. Appl. Biomater. 97 (2), 388–395.

Lokmic, Z., Musyoka, J., Hewitson, T.D., Darby, I.A., 2012. Hypoxia and hypoxia signaling in tissue repair and fibrosis. Int. Rev. Cell. Mol. Biol. 296 (January), 139–185.

Love, R.J., Jones, K.S., 2009. Biomaterials, fibrosis, and the use of drug delivery systems in future antifibrotic strategies. Crit. Rev. Biomed. Eng. 37 (3), 259–281.

Love, R.J., Jones, K.S., 2013. Transient inhibition of connective tissue infiltration and collagen deposition into porous poly(lactic-co-glycolic acid) discs. J. Biomed. Mater. Res. A. 101 (12), 3599–3606.

Lucas, T., Waisman, A., Ranjan, R., Roes, J., Krieg, T., Müller, W., et al., 2010. Differential roles of macrophages in diverse phases of skin repair. J. Immunol. (Baltimore, Md. : 1950) 184 (7) 3964–77.

Mack, M., Yanagita, M., 2015. Origin of Origin of myofibroblasts and cellular events triggering fibrosis. Kidney. Int 87 (2), 297–307. Nature Publishing Group.

Mahmoudi, Z., Jensen, M.H., Johansen, M.D., Christensen, T.F., Tarnow, L, Christensen, J.S., et al., 2014. Accuracy evaluation of a new real-time continuous glucose monitoring algorithm in hypoglycemia. Diabetes. Technol. Ther. 16 (10), 667–678.

Malik, A.F., Hoque, R., Ouyang, X., Ghani, A., Hong, E., khan, K, et al., 2011. Inflammasome components Asc and caspase-1 mediate biomaterial-induced inflammation and foreign body response. Proc. Natl. Acad. Sci. U.S.A. 108 (50), 20095–20100.

Manfredi, A.A., Capobianco, A., Bianchi, M.E., Rovere-Querini, P., 2009. Regulation of dendritic- and T-cell fate by injury-associated endogenous signals. Crit. Rev. Immunol. 29 (1), 69–86.

Manicone, A.M., McGuire, J.K., 2008. Matrix metalloproteinases as modulators of inflammation. Semin. Cell. Dev. Biol. 19 (1), 34–41.

Mann, J., Mann, D.A., 2013. Epigenetic regulation of wound healing and fibrosis. Curr. Opin. Rheumatol. 25 (1), 101–107.

Manoury, B, Nétran, S, Guénon, I, Lagente, V, Boichot, E., 2007. Influence of early neutrophil depletion on MMPs/TIMP-1 balance in bleomycin-induced lung fibrosis. Int. Immunopharmacol. 7 (7), 900–911.

Markiewski, M.M., Nilsson, B, Ekdahl, K.N., Mollnes, T.E., Lambris, J.D., 2007. Complement and coagulation: strangers or partners in crime? Trends. Immunol. 28 (4), 184–192.

Marques, S.M., Castro, P.R., Campos, P.P., Viana, C.T.R., Parreiras, P.M., Ferreira, M.A.N., et al., 2014. Genetic strain differences in the development of peritoneal fibroproliferative processes in mice. Wound Repair Regen. 22 (3), 381–389.

Martinez, F.O., Sica, A., Mantovani, A., Locati, M., 2008. Macrophage activation and polarization. Front. Biosci. 13 (January), 453–461.

Martins, V.L., Caley, M., O'Toole, E.A., 2013. Matrix metalloproteinases and epidermal wound repair. Cell. Tissue Res. 351 (2), 255–268.

McDonald, J.R., Finck, B.K., McIntosh, L.M., Wilson, S.E., 2011. Anti-inflammatory approaches that target the chemokine network. Recent Pat. Inflamm. Allergy Drug Discov. 5 (1), 1–16.

McNally, A.K., Anderson, J.M., 1995. Interleukin-4 induces foreign body giant cells from human monocytes/macrophages. Differential lymphokine regulation of macrophage fusion leads to morphological variants of multinucleated giant cells. Am. J. Pathol. 147 (5), 1487–1499.

McNally, A.K., Anderson, J.M., 2011. Macrophage fusion and multinucleated giant cells of inflammation. Adv. Exp. Med. Biol. 713 (January), 97–111.

Meyers, K.E.C., Sethna, C., 2013. Endothelin antagonists in hypertension and kidney disease. Pediatr. Nephrol. (Berlin, Germany) 28 (5), 711–720.

Minami, E., Koh, I.H.J., Ferreira, J.C.R., Waitzberg, A.F.L., Chifferi, V., et al., 2006. The composition and behavior of capsules around smooth and textured breast implants in pigs. Plast. Reconstr. Surg. 118 (4), 874–884.

Mirza, R., Koh, T.J., 2011. Dysregulation of monocyte/macrophage phenotype in wounds of diabetic mice. Cytokine 56 (2), 256–264.

Mirza, R., DiPietro, L.A., Koh, T.J., 2009. Selective and specific macrophage ablation is detrimental to wound healing in mice. Am. J. Pathol. 175 (6), 2454–2462.

Mooney, J.E., Summers, K.M., Gongora, M., Grimmond, S.M., Campbell, J.H., Hume, D.A., et al., 2014. Transcriptional switching in macrophages associated with the peritoneal foreign body response. Immunol. Cell. Biol. 92 (6), 518–526.

Moore, K.W., de Waal Malefyt, R., Coffman, R.L., O'Garra, A., 2001. Interleukin-10 and the interleukin-10 receptor. Annu. Rev. Immunol. 19 (January), 683–765.

Moretti, A.I.S., Souza Pinto, F.J.P., Cury, V., Jurado, M.C., Marcondes, W., Velasco, I.T., et al., 2012. Nitric oxide modulates metalloproteinase-2, collagen deposition and adhesion rate after polypropylene mesh implantation in the intra-abdominal wall. Acta. Biomater. 8 (1), 108–115.

Morishima, Y., Ishii, Y., 2010. Targeting Th2 cytokines in fibrotic diseases. Curr. Opin. Investig. Drugs (London, England : 2000) 11 (11), 1229–1238.

Mosser, D.M., Edwards, J.P., 2008a. Exploring the full spectrum of macrophage activation. Nat. Rev. Immunol. 8 (12), 958–969.

Mosser, D M, Zhang, X, 2008b. Interleukin-10: new perspectives on an old cytokine. Immunol. Rev. 226 (December), 205–218.

Mou, X., Lennartz, M.R., Loegering, D.J., Stenken, J.A., 2010. Long-term calibration considerations during subcutaneous microdialysis sampling in mobile rats. Biomaterials 31 (16), 4530–4539.

Moustakas, A., Heldin, C.-H., 2009. The regulation of TGFbeta signal transduction. Development (Cambridge, England) 136 (22), 3699–3714.

Munger, J.S., Sheppard, D., 2011. Cross talk among TGF-β signaling pathways, integrins, and the extracellular matrix. Cold Spring Harb. Perspect. Biol. 3 (11), a005017.

Murdoch, C., Muthana, M., Lewis, C.E., 2005. Hypoxia regulates macrophage functions in inflammation. J. Immunol. (Baltimore, Md. : 1950) 175 (10), 6257–6263.

Murray, P.J., Wynn, T.A., 2011. Protective and pathogenic functions of macrophage subsets. Nat. Rev. Immunol. 11 (11), 723–737.

Nandi, P., Lunte, S.M., 2009. Recent trends in microdialysis sampling integrated with conventional and microanalytical systems for monitoring biological events: a review. Anal. Chim. Acta. 651 (1), 1–14.

NIH Publication No. 11-4798, 2012. Cochlear implants. National Institute on Deafness and Other Communication Disorders. Available from: < http://www.nidcd.nih.gov/health/hearing/pages/coch.aspx>.

Nishioka, Y., Azuma, M., Kishi, M., Aono, Y., 2013. Targeting platelet-derived growth factor as a therapeutic approach in pulmonary fibrosis. J. Med. Invest.: JMI 60 (3-4), 175–183.

Nusse, R., Varmus, H., 2012. Three decades of Wnts: a personal perspective on how a scientific field developed. EMBO. J. 31 (12), 2670–2684.

Oliveira, S.H., Lukacs, N.W., 2001. Stem cell factor and igE-stimulated murine mast cells produce chemokines (CCL2, CCL17, CCL22) and express chemokine receptors. Inflamm. Res. 50 (3), 168–174.

Orenstein, J.M., 2014. The "myofibroblast" that is omnipresent in pathology and key to the EMT concepts does not actually exist, since normal fibroblasts contain stress fibril organelles (SMA bundles with dense bodies) variably detected by TEM and IHC: conclusions by a diagnost. Ultrastruct. Pathol. August, 1–12.

Ouyang, W., Kolls, J.K., Zheng, Y., 2008. The biological functions of T helper 17 cell effector cytokines in inflammation. Immunity 28 (4), 454–467.

Overed-Sayer, C., Rapley, L., Mustelin, T., Clarke, D.L., 2013. Are mast cells instrumental for fibrotic diseases? Front. Pharmacol 4 (January), 174.

Paredes JuÃ¡rez, G.A., Spasojevic, M., Faas, M.M., de Vos, P., 2014a. Immunological and technical considerations in application of alginate-based microencapsulation systems. Front. Bioeng. Biotechnol. 2 (August) Frontiers Media SA: 26.

Paredes-Juarez, G., de Haan, B, Faas, M., de Vos, P., 2014b. A technology platform to test the efficacy of purification of alginate. Materials 7 (3), 2087–2103. Multidisciplinary Digital Publishing Institute.

Patel, J.D., Krupka, T., Anderson, J.M., 2007. iNOS-mediated generation of reactive oxygen and nitrogen species by biomaterial-adherent neutrophils. J. Biomed. Mater. Res. A. 80 (2), 381–390.

Patil, S.D., Papadmitrakopoulos, F., Burgess, D.J., 2007. Concurrent delivery of dexamethasone and VEGF for localized inflammation control and angiogenesis. J. Control. Release 117 (1), 68–79.

Pearl, J.I., Ma, T., Irani, A.R., Huang, Z., Robinson, W.H., Smith, R.L., et al., 2011. Role of the Toll-like receptor pathway in the recognition of orthopedic implant wear-debris particles. Biomaterials 32 (24), 5535–5542.

Peek, E.J., Richards, D.F., Faith, A., Lavender, P., Lee, T.H., Corrigan, C.J., et al., 2005. Interleukin-10-secreting "regulatory" T cells induced by glucocorticoids and beta2-agonists. Am. J. Respir. Cell. Mol. Biol. 33 (1), 105–111.

Pellicoro, A., Ramachandran, P., Iredale, J.P., Fallowfield, J.A., 2014. Liver fibrosis and repair: immune regulation of wound healing in a solid organ. Nat. Rev. Immunol. 14 (3), 181–194.

Perugorria, M.J., Wilson, C.L., Zeybel, M., Walsh, M., Amin, S., Robinson, S., et al., 2012. Histone methyltransferase ASH1 orchestrates fibrogenic gene transcription during myofibroblast transdifferentiation. Hepatology (Baltimore, Md.) 56 (3), 1129–1139.

Pesce, J., Kaviratne, M., Ramalingam, T.R., Thompson, R.W., Urban, J.F., Cheever, A.W., et al., 2006. The IL-21 receptor augments Th2 effector function and alternative macrophage activation. J. Clin. Invest. 116 (7), 2044–2055.

Pesce, J.T., Ramalingam, T.R., Mentink-Kane, M.M., Wilson, M.S., El Kasmi, K.C., Smith, A.M., et al., 2009. Arginase-1-expressing macrophages suppress Th2 cytokine-driven inflammation and fibrosis. PLoS. Pathog. 5 (4), e1000371.

Pinney, J.R., Du, Perla Ayala, K.T., Fang, Q., Sievers, R.E., Chew, P., Delrosario, L., et al., 2014. Discrete microstructural cues for the attenuation of fibrosis following myocardial infarction. Biomaterials 35 (31), 8820–8828.

Pitt, C.G., Gratzl, M.M., Kimmel, G.L., Surles, J., Schindler, A., 1981. Aliphatic polyesters II. The degrada-tion of poly (DL-lactide), poly (epsilon-caprolactone), and their copolymers *in vivo*. Biomaterials 2 (4), 215–220.

Pockros, P.J., Jeffers, L., Afdhal, N., Goodman, Z.D., Nelson, D., Gish, R.G., et al., 2007. Final results of a double-blind, placebo-controlled trial of the antifibrotic efficacy of interferon-gamma1b in chronic hepatitis C patients with advanced fibrosis or cirrhosis. Hepatology (Baltimore, Md.) 45 (3), 569–578.

Prince, L.R., Whyte, M.K., Sabroe, I., Parker, L.C., 2011. The role of TLRs in neutrophil activation. Current Opinion in Pharmacology 11 (4), 397–403.

Pyne, N.J., Dubois, G., Pyne, S., 2013. Role of sphingosine 1-phosphate and lysophosphatidic acid in fibro-sis. Biochim. Biophys. Acta. 1831 (1), 228–238.

Quinn, C.A.P., Connor, R.E., Heller, A., 1997. Biocompatible, glucose-permeable hydrogel for *in situ* coat-ing of implantable biosensors. Biomaterials 18 (24), 1665–1670.

Ra, H.-J., Parks, W.C., 2007. Control of matrix metalloproteinase catalytic activity. Matrix Biol. 26 (8), 587–596.

Rahman, A.H., Aloman, C., 2013. Dendritic cells and liver fibrosis. Biochim. Biophys. Acta. 1832 (7), 998–1004.

Rankin, J.A., Picarella, D.E., Geba, G.P., Temann, U.A., Prasad, B., DiCosmo, B., et al., 1996. Phenotypic and physiologic characterization of transgenic mice expressing interleukin 4 in the lung: lymphocytic and eosinophilic inflammation without airway hyperreactivity. Proc. Natl. Acad. Sci. U.S.A. 93 (15), 7821–7825.

Reinke, J.M., Sorg, H., 2012. Wound repair and regeneration. Eur. Surg. Res. 49 (1), 35–43. Karger Publishers.

Renard, E., Baldet, P., Picot, M.C., Jacques-Apostol, D., Lauton, D., Costalat, G., et al., 1995. Catheter com-plications associated with implantable systems for peritoneal insulin delivery. An analysis of frequency, predisposing factors, and obstructing materials. Diabetes. Care. 18 (3), 00–306.

Reynolds, J.M., Dong, C., 2013. Toll-like receptor regulation of effector T lymphocyte function. Trends. Immunol. 34 (10), 511–519.

Rhodes, N.P., Hunt, J.A., Williams, D.F., 1997. Macrophage subpopulation differentiation by stimulation with biomaterials. J. Biomed. Mater. Res. 37 (4), 481–488.

Richeldi, L., du Bois, R.M., Raghu, G., Azuma, A., Brown, K.K., Costabel, U., et al., 2014. Efficacy and safety of nintedanib in idiopathic pulmonary fibrosis. N. Engl. J. Med. 370 (22), 2071–2082.

Roberts, A.B., Russo, A., Felici, A., Flanders, K.C., 2003. Smad3: a key player in pathogenetic mechanisms dependent on TGF-beta. Ann. N.Y. Acad. Sci. 995 (May), 1–10.

Rogers, T H, Babensee, J E, 2010. Altered adherent leukocyte profile on biomaterials in Toll-like receptor 4 deficient mice. Biomaterials 31 (4), 594–601.

Rosenkranz, S., 2004. TGF-beta1 and angiotensin networking in cardiac remodeling. Cardiovasc. Res. 63 (3), 423–432.

Rozen-Zvi, B., Hayashida, T., Hubchak, S.C., Hanna, C., Platanias, L.C., William Schnaper, H., 2013. TGF-β/Smad3 activates mammalian target of rapamycin complex-1 to promote collagen production by increasing HIF-1α expression. Am. J. Physiol. Renal. Physiol. 305 (4), F485–F494.

Ruthenborg, R.J., Ban, J.-J., Wazir, A., Takeda, N., Kim, J.-W., 2014. Regulation of wound healing and fibrosis by hypoxia and hypoxia-inducible factor-1. Mol. Cells 37 (9), 637–643.

Safadi, R., Ohta, M., Alvarez, C.E., Isabel Fiel, M., Bansal, M., Mehal, W.Z., et al., 2004. Immune stimulation of hepatic fibrogenesis by CD8 cells and attenuation by transgenic interleukin-10 from hepatocytes. Gastroenterology 127 (3), 870–882.

Saito, T., Tabata, Y., 2012. Preparation of gelatin hydrogels incorporating low-molecular-weight heparin for anti-fibrotic therapy. Acta. Biomater. 8 (2), 646–652.

Sakai, N., Chun, J., Duffield, J.S., Wada, T., Luster, A.D., Tager, A.M., 2013. LPA1-induced cytoskeleton reorganization drives fibrosis through CTGF-dependent fibroblast proliferation. FASEB J. 27 (5), 1830–1846.

Sampson, N., Berger, P., Zenzmaier, C., 2014. Redox signaling as a therapeutic target to inhibit myofibro-blast activation in degenerative fibrotic disease. BioMed Res. Int. 2014 (January), 131737.

Sampson, N., Koziel, R., Zenzmaier, C., Bubendorf, L., Plas, E., Jansen-Dürr, P., et al., 2011. ROS signal-ing by NOX4 drives fibroblast-to-myofibroblast differentiation in the diseased prostatic stroma. Mol. Endocrinol. (Baltimore, Md.) 25 (3), 503–515. Endocrine Society Chevy Chase, MD.

Schmid-Schönbein, G.W., 2006. Analysis of inflammation. Annu. Rev. Biomed. Eng. 8 (January), 93–131.

Schreml, S., Heine, N., Eisenmann-Klein, M., Prantles, L., 2007. Bacterial colonization is of major relevance for high-grade capsular contracture after augmentation mammaplasty. Ann. Plast. Surg. 59 (2), 126–130.

Shao, D.D., Suresh, R.,Vakil,V., Gomer, R.H., Pilling, D., 2008. Pivotal Advance:Th-1 cytokines inhibit, and Th-2 cytokines promote fibrocyte differentiation. J. Leukoc. Biol. 83 (6), 1323–1333.

Shao,T., Li, X., Ge, J., 2011.Target drug delivery system as a new scarring modulation after glaucoma filtration surgery. Diagn. Pathol. 6 (January), 64.

Sharkawy, A.A., Klitzman, B.,Truskey, G.A., Reichert,W.M., 1997. Engineering the tissue which encapsulates subcutaneous implants. I. Diffusion properties. J. Biomed. Mater. Res. 37 (3), 401–412.

Sharkawy, A.A., Klitzman, B.,Truskey, G.A., Reichert,W.M., 1998a. Engineering the tissue which encapsulates subcutaneous implants. II. Plasma-tissue exchange properties. J. Biomed. Mater. Res. 40 (4), 586–597.

Sharkawy, A.A., Klitzman, B.,Truskey, G.A., Reichert,W.M., 1998b. Engineering the tissue which encapsulates subcutaneous implants. III. Effective tissue response times. J. Biomed. Mater. Res. 40 (4), 598–605.

Sime, P.J., Xing, Z., Graham, F.L., Csaky, K.G., Gauldie, J., 1997. Adenovector-mediated gene transfer of active transforming growth factor-beta1 induces prolonged severe fibrosis in rat lung. J. Clin. Invest. 100 (4), 768–776.

Sindrilaru, A., Scharffetter-Kochanek, K., 2013. Disclosure of the culprits: macrophages–versatile regulators of wound healing. Adv. Wound Care 2 (7), 357–368.

Sindrilaru, A., Peters, T.,Wieschalka, S., Baican, C., Baican, A., Peter, H., et al., 2011. An unrestrained proinflammatory M1 macrophage population induced by iron impairs wound healing in humans and mice. J. Clin. Invest. 121 (3), 985–997.

Sivakumar, P., Das, A.M., 2008. Fibrosis, chronic inflammation and new pathways for drug discovery. Inflamm. Res. 57 (9), 410–418.

Skjøt-Arkil, H., Barascuk, N., Register, T., Karsdal, M.A., 2010. Macrophage-mediated proteolytic remodeling of the extracellular matrix in atherosclerosis results in neoepitopes: a potential new class of biochemical markers. Assay. Drug. Dev. Technol 8 (5), 542–552.

Spitzer, M.S., Sat, M., Schramm, C, Schnichels, S, Schultheiss, M, yoerueek, E, et al., 2012. Biocompatibility and antifibrotic effect of UV-cross-linked hyaluronate as a release-system for tranilast after trabeculectomy in a rabbit model--a pilot study. Curr. Eye. Res. 37 (6), 463–470.

Steiert, A.E., Boyce, M., Sorg, H., 2013. Capsular contracture by silicone breast implants: possible causes, biocompatibility, and prophylactic strategies. Med. Devices (Auckland, N.Z.) 6 (January), 211–218. Dove Press.

Sutradhar, K.B., Datta Sumi, C., 2014. Implantable microchip: the futuristic controlled drug delivery system. Drug. Deliv Epub ahead (April).

Szekanecz, Z, Koch, A E, 2007. Macrophages and their products in rheumatoid arthritis. Current Opinion in Rheumatology 19 (3), 289–295.

Takato, H.,Yasui, M., Ichikawa,Y., Waseda,Y., Inuzuka, K., Nishizawa,Y., et al., 2011. he specific chymase inhibitor TY-51469 suppresses the accumulation of neutrophils in the lung and reduces silica-induced pulmonary fibrosis in mice. Exp. Lung. Res. 37 (2), 101–108.

Tamboto, H.,Vickery, K., Deva, A.K., 2010. Subclinical (biofilm) infection causes capsular contracture in a porcine model following augmentation mammaplasty. Plast. Reconstr. Surg. 126 (3), 835–842.

Thevenot, P.T., Baker, D.W., Weng, H., Sun, M.-W., Tang, L., 2011. The pivotal role of fibrocytes and mast cells in mediating fibrotic reactions to biomaterials. Biomaterials 32 (33), 8394–8403.

Thorfve, A., Bergstrand, A., Ekström, K., Lindahl, A., Thomsen, P., Larsson, A., et al., 2014. Gene expression profiling of peri-implant healing of PLGA-Li+ implants suggests an activated wnt signaling pathway in vivo. PLoS. One. 9 (7), e102597.

Tomino,Y, 2012. Mechanisms and interventions in peritoneal fibrosis. Clin. Exp. Nephrol. 16 (1), 109–114.

Trautmann, A., Toksoy, A., Engelhardt, E., Bröcker, E.B., Gillitzer, R., 2000. Mast cell involvement in normal human skin wound healing: expression of monocyte chemoattractant protein-1 is correlated with recruitment of mast cells which synthesize interleukin-4 in vivo. J. Pathol. 190 (1), 100–106.

Tsou, P-S, Haak, A J, Khanna, D, Neubig, R R, 2014. Cellular mechanisms of tissue fibrosis. 8. Current and future drug targets in fibrosis: focus on Rho GTPase-regulated gene transcription. Am. J. Physiol. Cell. Physiol. 307 (1), C2–C13.

Ulloa, L., Doody, J., Massagué, J., 1999. Inhibition of transforming growth factor-beta/SMAD signalling by the interferon-gamma/STAT pathway. Nature 397 (6721), 710–713.

Utsunomiya, H., Tilakaratne, W.M., Oshiro, K., Maruyama, S., Suzuki, M., Ida-Yonemochi, H., et al., 2005. Extracellular matrix remodeling in oral submucous fibrosis: its stage-specific modes revealed by immunohistochemistry and *in situ* hybridization. J. Oral Pathol. Med. 34 (8), 498–507.

Vaddiraju, S., Wang, Y., Qiang, L., Burgess, D.J., Papadimitrakopoulos, F., 2012. Microsphere erosion in outer hydrogel membranes creating macroscopic porosity to counter biofouling-induced sensor degradation. Anal. Chem. 84 (20), 8837–8845.

Vaithilingam, V., Kollarikova, G., Qi, M., Larsson, R., Lacik, I., Formo, K., et al., 2014. Beneficial effects of coating alginate microcapsules with macromolecular heparin conjugates—*in vitro* and *in vivo* study. Tissue Eng. Part A. 20 (1-2), 324–334.

Valdes, T.I., Ciridon, W., Ratner, B.D., Bryers, J.D., 2011. Modulation of fibroblast inflammatory response by surface modification of a perfluorinated ionomer. Biointerphases 6 (2), 43–53.

Van Lint, P., Libert, C., 2007. Chemokine and cytokine processing by matrix metalloproteinases and its effect on leukocyte migration and inflammation. J. Leukoc. Biol. 82 (6), 1375–1381.

Van. Linthout, S, Miteva, K., Tschöpe, C., 2014. Crosstalk between fibroblasts and inflammatory cells. Cardiovasc. Res. 102 (2), 258–269.

Varga, J., Abraham, D., 2007. Systemic sclerosis: a prototypic multisystem fibrotic disorder. J. Clin. Invest. 117 (3), 557–567.

Vogel, D.Y.S., Glim, J.E., Stavenuiter, A.W.D., Breur, M., Heijnen, P., Amor, S., et al., 2014. Human macrophage polarization *in vitro*: maturation and activation methods compared. Immunobiology 219 (9), 695–703.

Wakatsuki, T., Kolodney, M.S., Zahalak, G.I., Elson, E.L., 2000. Cell mechanics studied by a reconstituted model tissue. Biophys. J. 79 (5), 2353–2368.

Wangoo, A., Laban, C., Cook, H.T., Glenville, B., Shaw, R.J., 1997. Interleukin-10- and corticosteroid-induced reduction in type I procollagen in a human *ex vivo* scar culture. Int. J. Exp. Pathol. 78 (1), 33–41.

Ward, W., Kenneth, M.D., Wood, H.M., Casey, M.J., Quinn, Federiuk, I.F., 2004. The effect of local subcutaneous delivery of vascular endothelial growth factor on the function of a chronically implanted amperometric glucose sensor. Diabetes. Technol. Ther. 6 (2), 137–145. Mary Ann Liebert, Inc.

Wehr, A., Baeck, C., Heymann, F., Maria Niemietz, P., Hammerich, L., Martin, C., et al., 2013. Chemokine receptor CXCR6-dependent hepatic NK T Cell accumulation promotes inflammation and liver fibrosis. J. Immunol. (Baltimore, Md. : 1950) 190 (10), 5226–5236.

Wei, J., Melichian, D., Komura, K., Hinchcliff, M., Lam, A.P., Lafyatis, R., et al., 2011. Canonical Wnt signaling induces skin fibrosis and subcutaneous lipoatrophy: a novel mouse model for scleroderma? Arthritis. Rheum. 63 (6), 1707–1717.

Wei, J., Fang, F., Lam, A.P., Sargent, J.L., Hamburg, E., Hinchcliff, M.E., et al., 2012. Wnt/β-catenin signaling is hyperactivated in systemic sclerosis and induces Smad-dependent fibrotic responses in mesenchymal cells. Arthritis. Rheum. 64 (8), 2734–2745.

Weigel, C., Schmezer, P., Plass, C., Popanda, O., 2014. Epigenetics in radiation-induced fibrosis. Oncogene July. [Epub ahead of print].

Wilson, N.J., Boniface, K., Chan, J.R., McKenzie, B.S., Blumenschein, W.M., Mattson, J.D., et al., 2007. Development, cytokine profile and function of human interleukin 17-producing helper T cells. Nat. Immunol. 8 (9), 950–957.

Wong, C.-H, Samuel, M., Tan, B.-K., Song, C., 2006. Capsular contracture in subglandular breast augmentation with textured versus smooth breast implants: a systematic review. Plast. Reconstr. Surg 118 (5), 1224–1236.

Wynn, T.A., 2007. Common and unique mechanisms regulate fibrosis in various fibroproliferative diseases. J. Clin. Invest. 117 (3), 524–529.

Wynn, T.A., 2008. Cellular and molecular mechanisms of fibrosis. J. Pathol. 214 (2), 199–210.

Wynn, T.A., Barron, L., 2010. Macrophages: master regulators of inflammation and fibrosis. Semin. Liver. Dis. 30 (3), 245–257.

Yanaba, K., Yoshizaki, A., Asano, Y., Kadono, T., Sato, S., 2011. Serum IL-33 levels are raised in patients with systemic sclerosis: association with extent of skin sclerosis and severity of pulmonary fibrosis. Clin. Rheumatol. 30 (6), 825–830.

Yang, D., Jones, K.S., 2009. Effect of alginate on innate immune activation of macrophages. Effect of alginate on innate immune activation of macrophages. J. Biomed. Mater. Res. Part A 90 (2), 411–418.

Yang, W., Xue, H., Carr, L.R., Wang, J., Jiang, S., 2011. Zwitterionic poly(carboxybetaine) hydrogels for glucose biosensors in complex media. Biosens. Bioelectron. 26 (5), 2454–2459.

Yang, J., Jao, B., McNally, A.K., Anderson, J.M., 2014a. *In vivo* quantitative and qualitative assessment of foreign body giant cell formation on biomaterials in mice deficient in natural killer lymphocyte subsets, mast cells, or the interleukin-4 receptorα and in severe combined immunodeficient mice. J. Biomed. Mater. Res. Part A 102 (6), 2017–2023.

Yang, X., Chen, B., Liu, T., Chen, X., 2014a. Reversal of myofibroblast differentiation: a review. Reversal of myofibroblast differentiation: a review. Eur. J. Pharmacol. 734 (July), 83–90.

Yeager, M.E., Frid, M.G., Stenmark, K.R., 2011. Progenitor cells in pulmonary vascular remodeling. Pulm. Circ. 1 (1), 3–16.

Yoshiji, H., Kuriyama, S., Fukui, H., 2007. Blockade of renin–angiotensin system in antifibrotic therapy. J. Gastroenterol. Hepatol. 22 (1), S93–S95.

Yuet, P.K., Harris, T.J., Goosen, M.F., 1995. Mathematical modelling of immobilized animal cell growth. Artif. Cells. Blood. Substit. Immobil. Biotechnol. 23 (1), 109–133.

Zawrotniak, M., Rapala-Kozik, M., 2013. Neutrophil extracellular traps (NETs)—formation and implications. Acta. Biochim. Pol. 60 (3), 277–284.

Zhang, X., Mosser, D.M., 2008. Macrophage activation by endogenous danger signals. J. Pathol. 214 (2), 161–178.

Zhu, Z., Homer, R.J., Wang, Z., Chen, Q., Geba, G.P., Wang, J., et al., 1999. Pulmonary expression of interleukin-13 causes inflammation, mucus hypersecretion, subepithelial fibrosis, physiologic abnormalities, and eotaxin production. J. Clin. Invest. 103 (6), 779–788.

Zurawski, S.M., Vega, F., Huyghe, B., Zurawski, G., 1993. Receptors for interleukin-13 and interleukin-4 are complex and share a novel component that functions in signal transduction. EMBO J. 12 (7), 2663–2670.

CHAPTER 10

Human Anti-Gal and Anti-Non-Gal Immune Response to Porcine Tissue Implants

Uri Galili

Department of Surgery, University of Massachusetts Medical School, Worcester, MA, USA (email:uri.galili@rcn.com)

Contents

INTRODUCTION

Tissues and organs of porcine origin have been the focus of extensive research in two disciplines: (i) Xenotransplantation of porcine organs, tissues, or cells in order to solve the problem of insufficient supply of human allografts for transplantation. (ii) Tissue engineering in which extracellular matrix (ECM), decellularized tissues and organs, and cross-linked tissues have been studied for use as implants that provide a biological scaffold for tissue remodeling and regeneration. The term xenograft refers here to a graft containing live cells, whereas the term implant describes a processed graft

Host Response to Biomaterials.
DOI: http://dx.doi.org/10.1016/B978-0-12-800196-7.00010-4

239

containing dead cells or lacking cells and containing ECM as a result of decellularization (i.e., a naturally occurring "biomaterial"). The choice of the pig as a donor species for xenografts and implants is based on similarity in size of organs and on availability of the donor species.

Analysis of various mechanistic aspects of the immune response to implants in several experimental animal models has been covered in previous comprehensive reviews such as that of Badylak and Gilbert (2008). The present chapter focuses primarily on the immune response to porcine implants in humans and is based primarily on studies evaluating the immune response in patients receiving xenografts or porcine implants in the last two decades. Studies in monkeys which contribute to the understanding of the primate immune response to pig implants are discussed as well. Observations in recipients of porcine implants have led to several conclusions on the principles of the human immune response to porcine implants. The human immune system is not "indifferent" to the introduction of porcine implants and it mounts an extensive immune response against porcine ECM. As argued below, since implants contain dead cells or no cells, antibodies and macrophages are a significant components of the anti-implant detrimental immune response. The two major types of antibodies active in human recipients against porcine implants are: (i) the anti-Gal antibody and (ii) anti-non-gal antibodies. This chapter discusses these antibodies, the porcine antigens they recognize and the mechanisms by which they affect porcine implants. This chapter further suggests methods for overcoming the detrimental effects of these anti-implant antibodies.

IMMUNE MECHANISMS THAT AFFECT TISSUE IMPLANTS

The immune response against implants differs from that against xenografts or allografts containing live cells in that cytotoxic T cells have no functional relevance in implant recipients since implants contain dead cells (as in tissues cross-linked by glutaraldehyde) or no cells (as in decellularized ECM bioscaffold implants). In the absence of cytotoxic T cell activity, the immune mechanisms affecting implants are mediated by effector cells of the innate immune system such as macrophages (see Chapters 3 and 6) and by antibodies which are produced against the implant antigens with the assistance of helper T cells (See Chapter 8). The antibodies generated against porcine xenografts or implants have similar specificities and when they bind to antigens they activate the complement system, as in most antigen/antibody interactions. However, the activated complement cascade can cause direct lysis of live cells by "boring" holes in the cell membrane in xenografts, whereas complement activation does not affect the "intactness" of the ECM or of dead cells that are chemically cross-linked. Activation of the complement system by anti-implant antibodies has at least two outcomes: (i) The newly generated complement cleavage peptides C3a and C5a are among the most effective physiologic chemotactic factors (chemoattractants) and they induce recruitment of neutrophils and of macrophages into the implant (Klos et al., 2013). (ii) Neutrophils and macrophages have cell surface receptors (C3bR, also known as CR1 and CD35) for C3b complement molecules that are deposited on the ECM or on cross-linked cells of the implant as a result of the antibodies binding to the implant (van Lookeren Campagne et al., 2007). Macrophages and neutrophils further bind to the ECM glycoproteins and proteoglycans coated with antibodies by the interaction between the Fcγ receptors (FcγR) on these cells and the Fc portion of antibodies immunocomplexed to the implant (Ravetch and Bolland, 2001; Selvaraj et al., 2004). Both the C3b/C3bR and Fc/FcγR interaction stimulate neutrophils and macrophages to release their proteases which cause degradation of the implant and to phagocytoze the fragmented implant.

Another mechanism which may be detrimental to the constructive remodeling process is prevention of the interaction between stem cells and the ECM because of masking of ECM molecules by bound anti-implant antibodies. Stem cells recruited into implants by macrophages are "instructed" to differentiate into specialized mature cells by interaction with various components of the ECM (Yano et al., 2006; Lolmede et al., 2009; Mantovani et al., 2013; Atala, 2009; Badylak et al., 2012; Crapo et al., 2011). Such interaction generates signals that instruct the stem cells to differentiate into cells that restore structure and function of the target tissue. Extensive binding of antibodies to the implanted ECM may mask the ECM molecules and prevent the interaction with stem cells. Such prevention of interaction is suggested by the observed inhibition of stem cells adhesion to ECM with antibodies to ECM or to cell surface molecules on stem cells (Williams et al., 1991; Shakibaei, 1998; Jung et al., 2005). Inhibition of stem cell/ECM interaction may prevent stem cell differentiation into the cells that are required for repopulating the ECM and converting the implant into the functionally remodeled tissue. Therefore, the immune response against the implant may result in partial or complete failure of the porcine implant to convert into an autologous tissue with the desired structure and biological function.

The ultimate outcome of implant conversion into functional tissue depends on multiple factors including intensity of the anti-implant immune response, the extent of recruitment of macrophages and of stem cells into the implant at various time points, and the efficacy of the "cues" provided by the ECM to the stem cells. In the absence of the appropriate cues for differentiation of stem cells, it is probable that the implant will convert into a connective tissue since fibrosis is the default mechanism of the body for repair of external as well as internal injuries.

THE ANTI-GAL ANTIBODY AND THE α-GAL EPITOPE
Characteristics of the anti-Gal antibody

All humans produce a natural antibody that readily binds to a carbohydrate antigen that is abundant in many porcine implants. This natural antibody, called anti-Gal, is the most abundant antibody in humans, comprising approximately 1% of circulating immunoglobulins (Galili et al., 1984; Galili, 1993) and the carbohydrate antigen-binding anti-Gal is called the α-gal epitope (also called α-galactosyl and Galα1-3Gal epitope) (Galili, 1993; Galili et al., 1985). Anti-Gal is found in human serum as several isotypes (classes) including IgG, IgM, and IgA and in various body secretions as IgG and IgA (Hamadeh et al., 1995; Parker et al., 1999; Yu et al., 1999). The most abundant anti-Gal IgG subclass is IgG2 followed by IgG3, IgG1, and the least amount of the antibody is found as IgG4 (Parker et al., 1999; Yu et al., 1999). In a small proportion of the population anti-Gal may be present also as an IgE isotype which can mediate allergic reactions (Chung et al., 2008; Commins et al., 2009; Morisset et al., 2012). The α-gal epitope which is the ligand for anti-Gal has the structure Galα1-3Galβ1-4GlcNAc-R and is abundant on glycolipids and glycoproteins of nonprimate mammals, including pigs (Figure 10.1) (Galili et al., 1987, 1988b). Anti-Gal IgG crosses the placenta and is found in newborn blood in titers comparable to those in the maternal blood (Galili et al., 1984). Its production is initiated at approximately 6 months and it is continuously produced throughout life as an immune response against carbohydrate antigens with structures similar to the α-gal epitopes that are presented on bacteria of the normal human gastrointestinal flora (Galili et al., 1988a).

As many as 1% of human B cells are capable of producing anti-Gal (Galili et al., 1993). Most of these B cells (designated anti-Gal B cells) are quiescent and only those along the gastrointestinal tract continuously produce this natural antibody. However, as detailed below, the introduction of xenogeneic implants presenting α-gal epitopes into humans (Konakci et al., 2005; Stone et al., 2007b) and monkeys (Galili et al., 1997; Stone et al., 1998, 2007a) results in activation of the quiescent anti-Gal B cells by glycoproteins carrying α-gal epitopes that are released from the implant. This results in increase in anti-Gal IgG activity by approximately 100-fold, within about 2 weeks. Analysis of the immunoglobulin genes in human anti-Gal B cells indicated that these B cells are a polyclonal population; however, the immunoglobulin heavy chain genes in most clones cluster in the VH3 family (Wang et al., 1995).

Distribution of the α-gal epitope and anti-Gal antibody in mammals

The α-gal epitope is a carbohydrate antigen that is found only in mammals and is absent from other vertebrates (Galili, 1993; Galili et al., 1987, 1988b). Its amount on nucleated cells varies in different tissues and different mammals, and ranges between 1×10^6 and 30×10^6 epitopes/cell (Galili et al., 1988b). Since red cells are usually smaller than nucleated cells, they carry less α-gal epitopes, in the range of 1×10^4–2×10^6 epitopes/cell (Ogawa and Galili, 2006). The α-gal epitope is carried on the cell membrane both on glycolipids and glycoproteins (Figure 10.1) and is synthesized by a glycosylation enzyme called α1,3galactosyltransferase (α1,3GT) (Galili et al., 1988b; Basu and Basu, 1973; Betteridge and Watkins, 1983; Blake and Goldstein, 1981; Blanken

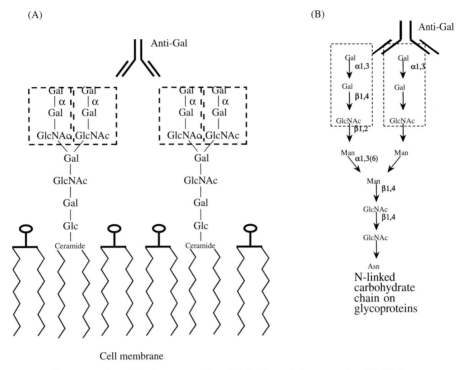

Figure 10.1 Structure of α-gal epitopes on glycolipids (A) and glycoproteins (B). (A) A representative α-gal glycolipid in which the carbohydrate chain with 10 units and two branches (ceramide decahexoside) is capped by α-gal epitopes (marked with dashed rectangles). The carbohydrate chain is linked to a ceramide that is anchored among phospholipids in the outer leaflet of the cell membrane. The glycolipid may have 1–8 branches each capped with an α-gal epitope. (B) A representative carbohydrate chain linked to a protein via an asparagine (N) in amino acid sequences Asn-X-Ser/Thr. The two branches of the carbohydrate chain are capped with α-gal epitopes (marked with dashed rectangles). Each carbohydrate chain may have 2–4 branches. α-Gal epitopes on both glycolipids and glycoproteins bind the natural anti-Gal antibody.

and van den Eijnden, 1985). The α-gal epitope displays a unique distribution pattern in mammals. It is expressed on cells of marsupials such as kangaroo and opossum and on cells of nonprimate placental mammals like mouse, rat, rabbit, bat, pig, cow, horse, cat, dog, and dolphin (Galili et al., 1987, 1988b) (Table 10.1). In addition, the α-gal epitope is found on cells of two distinct groups of primates, prosimians (e.g., lemurs) and New World monkeys (i.e., monkeys of South America). The α-gal epitope is completely absent, however, in Old World monkeys (monkeys of Asia and Africa), apes (chimpanzee, gorilla, orangutan, and gibbon) and in humans (Galili et al., 1987, 1988b) (Table 10.1). Because of the absence of α-gal epitopes in humans, apes, and Old World

Table 10.1 Distribution of the α-gal epitope and the natural anti-Gal antibody in mammals

	Mammalian group	α-Gal epitope (Galα1-3Galβ1-4GlcNAc-R)	Natural anti-Gal antibody
1.	Nonprimate mammals	+	−
2.	Lemurs (prosimians)	+	−
3.	New World monkeys (NWM)	+	−
4.	Old World monkeys (OWM)	−	+
5.	Apes	−	+
6.	Humans	−	+

monkeys, they are not immunotolerant to the α-gal epitope and all produce large amounts of the natural anti-Gal antibody against it (Galili et al., 1987). In pigs, as in other nonprimate mammals, the α-gal epitope is present on multiple cell surface glycoproteins and glycolipids. Thus, immunostaining of Western blots of porcine kidney, liver, lung, and thyroid cell membranes with the human natural anti-Gal antibody results in a smear pattern of staining, rather than distinct bands, since the bands of multiple glycoproteins carrying α-gal epitopes overlap each other (Tanemura et al., 2000a; Thall et al., 1991). In addition, the α-gal epitope is common on secreted porcine glycoproteins (e.g., thyroglobulin, fibrinogen, and immunoglobulin) (Spiro and Bhoyroo, 1984; Thall and Galili, 1990), as well as on ECM glycoproteins and proteoglycans (see below).

Since the α-gal epitope is abundant in both marsupials and placental mammals and since it is absent in nonmammalian vertebrates (fish, amphibians, reptiles, and birds) (Galili et al., 1987, 1988b), it is most probable that the α1,3GT gene and its product, the α-gal epitope, appeared in mammalian evolution at least 140 million years ago (i.e., before marsupials and placental mammals diverged from a common ancestor). Indeed α1,3GT activity could be demonstrated in cells of nonprimate mammals (Galili et al., 1988b; Thall et al., 1991). The activity of α1,3GT in cells of New World monkeys further implies that the α1,3GT gene was inactivated in ancestral Old World monkeys and apes after they diverged from ancestral New World monkeys (Galili, 1993; Galili et al., 1988b). Analysis of the α1,3GT gene in various primate species demonstrated the presence of this gene as a pseudogene in Old World monkeys, apes, and humans (Galili and Swanson, 1991; Galili and Andrews, 1995; Larsen et al., 1990; Joziasse et al., 1991; Koike et al., 2002, 2007; Lantéri et al., 2002), all of which have an inactive α1,3GT gene. This inactivation is the result of few single base deletions that generate premature stop codons which truncate the enzyme molecule and thus inactivate it. Based on the sequence of the α1,3GT pseudogene in Old World primates and humans, it seems that the inactivation of the α1,3GT gene in ancestral Old World primates occurred 20–28 million years ago (Galili and Swanson, 1991; Galili and Andrews, 1995; Joziasse et al., 1991; Koike et al., 2007). This evolutionary event could be associated with a major catastrophic epidemiological event which affected only ancestral Old World primates (Galili and Andrews, 1995). New World monkeys (evolving in South America) and lemurs (prosimians evolving in Madagascar) have not been subjected to this selective pressure since they have evolved in geographic areas that are separated from the Old World land mass by oceanic barriers. This evolutionary event could be mediated by a pathogen endemic to the Old World which was detrimental to primates and which expressed α-gal epitopes, or a pathogen that used the α-gal epitope on cells as a receptor (Galili et al., 1988b; Galili and Andrews, 1995). Following inactivation of the α1,3GT gene, ancestral Old World primates ceased to synthesize α-gal epitopes and thus could produce the anti-Gal antibody which was likely to provide immune protection against such a putative pathogen expressing α-gal epitopes (Galili et al., 1987; Galili and Andrews, 1995; Galili, 2013c).

Expression of α-gal epitopes on ECM glycoproteins and proteoglycans

The extensive tissue engineering research into the use of porcine ECM as implants for induction of tissue remodeling raises the question of whether glycoproteins and proteoglycans of porcine ECM carry α-gal epitopes. Presence of α-gal epitopes on ECM is likely to result in anti-Gal binding to these glycoproteins and proteoglycans. Binding of antibodies to the ECM may accelerate macrophage-mediated degradation of the ECM as well as mask the ECM thereby preventing the interaction with stem cells. Fibrosis of a connective tissue ECM implant may occur either as part of the remodeling process or as the default regeneration mechanism in the body following an anti-implant immune response. However, remodeling and functional regeneration of an implant into a tissue that also includes cells other than fibroblasts requires stem cell/ECM interaction. This interaction is needed for "instructing" stem cells to differentiate into the various specialized cells (other than fibroblasts) that repopulate and regenerate the tissue (Yano et al., 2006; Lolmede et al., 2009; Mantovani et al., 2013; Atala, 2009; Badylak et al., 2012; Crapo et al., 2011; Zhang et al., 2009; Guilak et al., 2009; Chen, 2010; Hidalgo-Bastida and Cartmell, 2010; Decaris and Leach, 2011). If an ECM implant expresses multiple α-gal epitopes, binding of the natural anti-Gal antibody to these epitopes on ECM may mask portions of various ECM molecules and thus may interfere with the stem cell/ECM interaction.

ECM in most and possibly all pig tissues is likely to include glycoproteins and proteoglycans that carry α-gal epitopes. Most of the α-gal epitopes of the ECM are present on N-linked carbohydrate chains. Evaluation of the predicted number of N-linked carbohydrate chains on ECM glycoproteins (i.e., amino acid sequences of Asn-X-Ser/Thr) indicates that they have multiple such carbohydrate chains which may carry α-gal epitopes. Pig laminin has 14 N-linked carbohydrate chains/molecule, fibronectin—9, decorin—3, thrombospondin—12, elastin—5, and tenascin—9 (based on GeneBank information). The proteoglycan aggrecan also has 14 N-linked carbohydrate chains/molecule. As indicated above, the α-gal epitope is synthesized in mammalian cells (including pig cells) by the glycosylation enzyme α1,3GT which transfers galactose from the sugar donor UDP-Gal to N-acetyllactosamine (Galβ1-4GlcNAc-R) to synthesize the α-gal epitope (Galili et al., 1988b; Basu and Basu, 1973; Betteridge and Watkins, 1983; Blake and Goldstein, 1981; Blanken and van den Eijnden, 1985). This glycosylation enzyme is active in the trans-Golgi compartment where it competes with other glycosyltransferases, such as sialyltransferase, for capping the N-acetyllactosamine residues with terminal α-galactosyl units or with sialic acid, respectively (Smith et al., 1990). The ultimate number of α-gal epitopes versus that of sialic acid terminal units on the carbohydrate chains of cell surface or secreted glycoconjugates is the result of the activity of α1,3GT relative to other competing glycosyltransferases.

Various porcine ECM glycoproteins and proteoglycans express multiple α-gal epitopes. This is indicated by the binding of anti-Gal to porcine kidney and lung laminin, heparan sulfate proteoglycans, and fibronectin, in co-localization studies in confocal microscopy immunostaining, ELISA, and Western blot analyses (Maruyama et al., 1999a, 2000). In contrast, no binding of anti-Gal was observed with ECM proteins from human origin (Maruyama et al., 1999a, 2000). Porcine ligament and cartilage, both poor in cells and rich ECM, were also found to contain high concentrations of α-gal epitopes ($>1 \times 10^{11}$ epitopes/mg tissue) (Stone et al., 1998, 2007b). α-Gal epitopes were found to be abundant also on ECM molecules of other mammalian species. Mouse laminin expresses approximately 50 α-gal epitopes/molecule (Thall and Galili, 1990), and α-gal epitopes were found on purified bovine laminin, Type IV collagen, and collagen α-1 extracted from bovine glomerular basement membrane, lens, and muscle (Mohan and Spiro, 1986; Takahashi et al., 2014).

It is of note that porcine small intestinal submucosa (SIS) ECM also expresses α-gal epitopes; however, their concentration in SIS is much lower than that in cartilage or tendon, primarily because SIS is comprised mostly of collagen which lacks carbohydrate chains (McPherson et al., 2000; Raeder et al., 2002; Daly et al., 2009). However, as discussed below, the presence of these epitopes on SIS does not seem to affect its remodeling in monkeys (Daly et al., 2009). Accordingly, SIS was found to function successfully as a remodeled ECM implant in hernia repair in multiple patients (Hiles et al., 2009).

Anti-Gal response in recipients of porcine implants

The detrimental effects of anti-Gal on porcine ECM and on other porcine biomaterial implants carrying α-gal epitopes may be further exacerbated by elicited anti-Gal antibody produced *de novo* in high titers as a result of the immune response against these α-gal epitopes. As indicated above, anti-Gal B cells comprise approximately 1% of B cells in humans (Galili et al., 1993). The natural anti-Gal antibody is produced by a small proportion of anti-Gal B cells, those residing along the gastrointestinal tract, whereas the majority of anti-Gal B cells are quiescent and are found in the circulation and probably in the lymph nodes and spleen (Galili et al., 1993). Introduction of implants carrying α-gal epitopes into humans results in rapid activation of the quiescent anti-Gal B cells which produce the anti-Gal antibody. This extensive anti-Gal antibody response against the α-gal epitopes of porcine origin was first demonstrated in diabetic patients that were immunosuppressed and transplanted with an allogeneic kidney together with pig fetal pancreatic islet cells (Groth et al., 1994; Galili et al., 1995). For this purpose, fetal islet cells were isolated from fetal pig pancreas and cultured *in vitro* to form clusters of islet cells (Groth et al., 1994). These pig islet cell clusters were administered at a volume corresponding to 2–6 mL packed cells either in the subcapsular space of a transplanted allogeneic kidney graft or infused into the portal vein of diabetic recipients of an allogeneic kidney. The patients were treated by immunosuppression regimens potent enough to prevent immune rejection of the kidney allograft. Despite this immunosuppression, the patients displayed an increase of 20–80-folds in anti-Gal titer within the period of 25–50 days post-transplantation (Galili et al., 1995). The increase in anti-Gal activity was mostly in the IgG isotype and to a much lesser extent of IgM and IgA isotypes. This production of elicited anti-Gal in xenograft recipients suggests that the immunosuppressive protocols that are used for prevention of allograft immune rejection do not prevent the activation of anti-Gal B cells by α-gal epitopes introduced into humans by porcine tissues or by other mammalian xenografts.

The extensive ability of mammalian α-gal epitopes to activate anti-Gal B cells and elicit an elevated anti-Gal immune response was further demonstrated in patients with impaired liver function, who were treated by temporary extracorporeal perfusion of their blood through a pig liver (Yu et al., 1999; Cotterell et al., 1995). The elevated anti-Gal activity in these patients implies that the release of xenoglycoproteins from the pig liver, perfused for only several hours, was sufficient to induce the activation of the many quiescent anti-Gal B cells for the increased production of the anti-Gal antibody. Another example for the elicited anti-Gal response in humans is of an ovarian carcinoma patient undergoing an experimental gene therapy treatment in which the patient received several intraperitoneal infusions of a mouse "packaging" cell line containing replication defective virus with the transgene studied. Anti-Gal activity in the blood was determined by ELISA with synthetic α-gal epitopes linked to bovine serum albumin (α-gal BSA) as solid-phase Ag. Within 14 days post-infusion, anti-Gal IgG titer increased by 100-fold as a result of both increase in concentration of anti-Gal and in the affinity of the antibody due to the affinity maturation process in the anti-Gal B cells activated by the α-gal epitopes expressed on the infused mouse cells (Galili et al., 2001). Most (~90%) of the increase in anti-Gal was of the IgG2 subclass and the rest of IgG3. No significant changes in anti-Gal activity were observed in IgM or IgA isotypes following the intraperitoneal infusion of mouse fibroblasts (Galili et al., 2001). A similar rapid and extensive elicited anti-Gal antibody production was observed in baboons immunized with synthetic α-gal epitopes linked to BSA (Maruyama et al., 1999a,b, 2000).

Analysis of anti-Gal antibody response against α-gal epitopes on xenografts could be performed in knockout mice for the α1,3GT gene (GT-KO mice). These mice have disrupted α1,3GT genes and thus cannot synthesize the α-gal epitope (Thall et al., 1995; Tearle et al., 1996). In the absence of α-gal epitopes, these mice lose the immune tolerance to it and can produce the anti-Gal antibody when immunized with pig glycoproteins carrying α-gal epitopes. Studies in these mice indicated that the α-gal epitope can activate anti-Gal B cells, but like other carbohydrate antigens of the complex type, it cannot activate T cells (Tanemura et al., 2000b; Galili, 2012). However, the T cell help required for activation of anti-Gal B cells by α-gal epitopes on xenografts is provided by helper T cells. These helper T cells are activated by the multiple peptides in pig proteins that are immunogenic in mice, as well as in humans (Galili, 2012).

An extensive immune response resulting in elevation of anti-Gal antibody activity was also observed in recipients of porcine implants expressing α-gal epitopes and cross-linked by glutaraldehyde. Glutaraldehyde cross-linking of the amino groups of lysine and of N-terminus amino acids of proteins does not alter the structure and immunogenicity of α-gal epitopes. The human immune response against α-gal epitopes in glutaraldehyde cross-linked porcine implants could be closely monitored for prolonged periods in patients with torn anterior cruciate ligament (ACL) that were implanted with pig patellar tendon carrying bone plugs at both ends (Stone et al., 2007a,b). These harvested pig tendons were engineered for elimination of α-gal epitopes by incubation for 12 h with recombinant α-galactosidase (Stone et al., 2007b). This enzyme cleaves the terminal α-galactosyl unit (Zhu et al., 1995, 1996), thereby destroying the α-gal epitope and preventing the binding of human anti-Gal antibody (Stone et al., 2007b). Such processing does not eliminate, however, α-gal epitopes from red cells and from nucleated cells within the cavities of the cancellous bone in the bone plugs since the enzyme cannot reach the cells encased in these cavities. The pig tendon underwent further processing by washes for removal of the enzyme, mild cross-linking by 12 h incubation in 0.1% glutaraldehyde, washes for removal of the glutaraldehyde and blocking the glutaraldehyde groups remaining reactive, by glycine. The torn autologous ACL was replaced by the tendon implant that was placed across the knee joint within femoral and tibial tunnels using a ligament guide and fixed in the tunnels with titanium screws (Stone et al., 2007b).

Patients receiving the tendon implant demonstrated elicited anti-Gal IgG production already 2 weeks after implantation. This anti-Gal response, which peaked in the period of 2 weeks to 2 months postimplantation, declined after 6 months and displayed further decline to almost the preimplantation level after 12 months (Stone et al., 2007b). The elevated anti-Gal IgG antibody titers were the result of the immune response to α-gal epitopes on cells and cell fragments released from the bone plug cavities as part of the bone remodeling process and the fusion to the femur and tibia. The elevated production of anti-Gal continued as long as pig cell fragments carrying α-gal epitopes were released from the remodeling bone plugs. However, once pig cells were completely eliminated, the production of anti-Gal reverted to the physiologic production in response to antigens of the gastrointestinal flora. No significant changes in activity of anti-Gal IgM were observed in these recipients of the engineered pig tendon (Stone et al., 2007b). These observations strongly suggest that the production of elicited high affinity anti-Gal IgG antibody by the human immune system continues as long as α-gal epitopes of the implant are present within the recipient.

An increase in anti-Gal antibody production in response to α-gal epitopes on glutaraldehyde cross-linked porcine implants was also observed in patients receiving porcine heart valve for replacing the impaired heart valve (Konakci et al., 2005). Accordingly, α-gal epitopes could be demonstrated in porcine heart valves (Kasimir et al., 2005; Naso et al., 2013). This elicited anti-Gal response in porcine valve recipients occurs despite the extensive cross-linking of these heart valves by glutaraldehyde, implying that α-gal epitopes on various glycoproteins released from the implant can activate quiescent anti-Gal B cells for the production of anti-Gal in increased titers. The information on the detrimental effects of natural and elicited anti-Gal antibodies on ECM implants expressing α-gal epitopes is very limited because many studies on xenogeneic ECM implants have been performed in experimental animal models other than monkeys. Since standard mammalian experimental models such as mouse, rat, guinea pig, rabbit, and dog, like all other nonprimate mammals, they synthesize α-gal epitopes, are immunotolerant to it, and thus cannot produce the anti-Gal antibody. Presently, the only available experimental mammalian models lacking α-gal epitopes and thus are capable of producing anti-Gal are Old World monkeys (Galili et al., 1987; Teranishi et al., 2002), GT-KO mice (Thall et al., 1995; Tearle et al., 1996), and GT-KO pigs (Lai et al., 2002; Phelps et al., 2003; Takahagi et al., 2005). Based on the limited information obtained in these models and in humans, it seems that the extent of detrimental effects of anti-Gal on porcine ECM implants depends on α-gal epitope concentration in the implant and on the type of cells expected to repopulate the implant in the course of remodeling.

SIS is an example for an ECM that does not seem to be affected by natural and elicited anti-Gal antibodies. SIS is comprised mostly of a mesh of collagen fibers with very few other proteins. Since the most common amino acid motif in collagen is glycine-proline-X and glycine-X-hydroxyproline and there are very few glycosylation sequences, collagen has very few carbohydrate chains and thus a very low concentration of α-gal epitopes. Other glycoproteins and proteoglycans are present in very low concentration in SIS. One example is fibronectin which comprises less than 0.1% of SIS dry weight (McPherson and Stephen, 1998). Because of the low α-gal epitope concentration in SIS, serum anti-Gal binding to these epitopes is below the level capable of activating serum complement (McPherson et al., 2000). In accord with the low concentration of α-gal epitope, no significant differences in remodeling and regeneration of SIS expressing or lacking α-gal epitopes were reported in murine or primate recipients of SIS despite the activity of natural and elicited anti-Gal antibody in the recipients (Raeder et al., 2002; Daly et al., 2009). Moreover, SIS was reported to function successfully as a remodeled ECM implant in hernia repair in a large number of patients (Hiles et al., 2009). In contrast, implantation of porcine cartilage ECM into monkeys was found to elicit an extensive anti-Gal response and an extensive inflammatory response that destroys the cartilage implant within 2 months (Galili et al., 1997; Stone et al., 1998). This cartilage contains relatively few dead fibrochondrocytes and is mostly comprised of ECM that carries an abundance of α-gal epitopes which induce an extensive elicited anti-Gal antibody response (Stone et al., 1997, 1998). The studies of porcine meniscus cartilage implants in cynomolgus monkey further demonstrated an extensive recruitment of macrophages and T cells into the implant and degradation of the cartilage ECM (Stone et al., 1998). Elimination of α-gal epitopes by treatment of the meniscus cartilage with recombinant α-galactosidase prior to implantation of the cartilage resulted in approximately 95% decrease in the inflammatory response against the cartilage when the implants were histologically evaluated 2 months postimplantation (Stone et al., 1998). This suggests that a large proportion of the immune response against this porcine ECM was mediated by anti-Gal interacting with the α-gal epitopes within the ECM. The detrimental effect of anti-Gal on ECM expressing high concentration of α-gal epitopes was further observed indirectly, in pigs infused with elicited baboon anti-Gal antibody. Such administration of anti-Gal resulted in the induction of inflammatory lesions in the ECM of kidney and lung similar to lesions induced in laboratory animals by anti-laminin and anti-heparan sulfate proteoglycans antibodies (Maruyama et al., 1999a, 2000).

Overall the presence of high concentrations of α-gal epitopes within porcine implants seems to be detrimental to the remodeling of the implant into a live functional tissue by several mechanisms including: (i) Anti-Gal/α-gal epitope interaction activates the complement system to induce rapid recruitment of macrophages into the implant. Binding of these macrophages via FcγR to the Fc portion of anti-Gal on ECM of the implant and via C3bR (CR1) to C3b deposits on the ECM results in accelerated degradation of the ECM.

Slow macrophage-mediated degradation of the ECM implant was found to be beneficial to remodeling since released small peptides display chemoattractant potential for several cell types *in vitro* and *in vivo*, including endothelial cells and multipotential progenitor cells that participate in remodeling of the ECM (Li et al., 2004; Yang et al., 2010; Badylak et al., 2001). However, binding of large amounts of anti-Gal to multiple α-gal epitopes on the ECM is likely to result in degradation of the ECM that is too fast for enabling appropriate remodeling of the implant. (ii) The α-gal epitopes on implant elicit production of large amounts of high affinity anti-Gal IgG antibody that exacerbates the degradation of the ECM. (iii) Binding of anti-Gal to α-gal epitopes on the ECM is likely to mask ECM molecules thereby preventing the interaction of stem cells with the ECM. This interaction is required for instructing the stem cells to differentiate into specialized cells, other than fibroblasts, that are required for regeneration of the target tissue. It is possible that in ECM of tissues aimed to differentiate into connective tissue (e.g., SIS), such masking may not have a detrimental effect since fibrosis is the default mechanism of tissue regeneration and thus, it may occur whether or not the ECM is masked. However, ECM with more complex components than SIS may display an impaired "instructive" ability for differentiation of stem cells into specialized cells, if significant amounts of anti-Gal antibodies are bound to the multiple α-gal epitopes on the ECM glycoproteins and proteoglycans.

Avoiding the anti-Gal barrier to porcine implants

Currently, it is impossible to prevent the production of anti-Gal in humans without complete "shutoff" of immunoglobulins production (Galili et al., 1995). Therefore, prevention of the interaction between anti-Gal and α-gal epitopes on porcine ECM requires the use of implants that lack α-gal epitopes. Three methods have been studied for achieving this goal: (i) Enzymatic treatment of porcine implants with α-galactosidase. (ii) The generation of knockout pigs for the α1,3GT gene. (iii) Decellularization of implants.

Destruction of α-gal epitopes by α-galactosidase

The enzyme α-galactosidase is naturally found in green coffee beans and in several other plants and mammals (including humans). α-Galactosidase cleaves the terminal α-galactosyl from the α-gal epitopes on these glycolipids (Galα1-3Galβ1-4GlcNAc-R) and converts it to an *N*-acetyllactosamine residue (Galβ1-4GlcNAc-R). Based on this enzymatic activity, it was hypothesized that incubation of implants in a solution of α-galactosidase may result in penetration of the enzyme into the tissue and destruction of the α-gal epitopes within the tissue (Stone et al., 2007b, 1998). The recombinant α-galactosidase encoded by a coffee beans gene was produced in an yeast expression system for studying the enzymatic destruction of α-gal epitopes in porcine implants (Zhu et al., 1995, 1996). Porcine meniscus cartilage was estimated to have approximately 1×10^{12} α-gal epitopes/mg tissue (Stone et al., 1998). Overnight incubation of porcine meniscus cartilage in a solution of recombinant α-galactosidase results in complete elimination of α-gal epitopes from the cartilage, as indicated by the complete lack of binding of a monoclonal anti-Gal antibody to the treated cartilage (Stone et al., 1998). Moreover, treated pig cartilage implanted into cynomolgus monkey elicited no production of anti-Gal IgG above the preimplantation level, whereas untreated cartilage induced extensive production of elicited anti-Gal within 2 weeks postimplantation (Stone et al., 1998). In the absence of α-gal epitopes, the inflammatory response in the monkey recipients against the cartilage implants was greatly attenuated. This was indicated by the 95% decrease in the infiltrating mononuclear cells (macrophages and T cells) observed within the implants that were retrieved 2 months postimplantation (Stone et al., 1998).

Another orthopedic implant studied for enzymatic elimination of α-gal epitopes has been porcine patellar tendon used for replacement of torn ACL in patients. By using the ELISA Inhibition Assay with the monoclonal anti-Gal antibody M86 for measuring α-gal epitope expression (Galili et al., 1998), the porcine tendon was estimated to have approximately 1×10^{11} α-gal epitopes/mg tissue (Stone et al., 2007b). As with porcine cartilage, 12 h incubation of porcine tendon in a solution of recombinant α-galactosidase results in diffusion of the enzyme throughout the tendon and complete destruction of the α-gal epitopes (Stone et al., 2007b). This removal of α-gal epitopes prevents anti-Gal-mediated destruction of the tendon implant. However, this processing was not sufficient for prevention of implant degradation at a rate that is slow enough to enable gradual repopulation of the destroyed implant tissue with fibroblasts of the recipient. These fibroblasts have to align with the porcine collagen fibers scaffold and secrete their autologous collagen and other ECM components. As discussed below in the section of anti-non-gal antibodies, the additional slowing of the degradation process was achieved by "fine-tuning" of glutaraldehyde cross-linking process.

The use of recombinant α-galactosidase for elimination of α-gal epitopes from porcine implants was further demonstrated with porcine heart valves (Park et al., 2009), which like other porcine tissues express an abundance of α-gal epitopes (Kasimir et al., 2005; Naso et al., 2013). In the absence of α-gal epitopes on the valve, binding of anti-Gal will be prevented. This may decrease the extent of macrophage binding to the surface of the valve, thereby this enzymatic treatment may delay the calcification process on the valve surface and thus may delay impairment of the implant biomechanical activity.

GT-KO pigs as a source of implants lacking α-gal epitopes

The most convenient source for porcine implants devoid of α-gal epitopes is GT-KO pigs. These pigs have been generated to provide xenografts that lack α-gal epitopes in order to prevent anti-Gal-mediated hyperacute rejection of organs such as heart and kidney transplanted into humans (Lai et al., 2002; Phelps et al., 2003; Takahagi et al., 2005). In the presence of α-gal epitopes, such pig organs undergo hyperacute rejection in monkeys within 30 min to several hours as a result of anti-Gal binding to these epitopes on endothelial cells and lysis of these cells followed by the collapse of the vascular bed within the xenograft (Collins et al., 1994; Xu et al., 1998; Simon et al., 1998).

The use of GT-KO pigs as a source for porcine implants lacking α-gal epitopes has been explored with pig valves. GT-KO pig heart valves were found to be less immunogenic in monkey recipients than wild-type pig heart valves (McGregor et al., 2013). It is assumed that binding of the serum anti-Gal to the α-gal epitopes on the wild-type pig valve results in subsequent binding of macrophages to the implanted valves via Fc/FcγR interaction with anti-Gal. The resulting stimulation of the macrophages to secrete the content of their vesicles induces the calcification process, in addition to the chemical processes between glutaraldehyde and free calcium ions in the blood. It is further assumed that in the absence of anti-Gal to the implant, calcification would be much slower, thus prolonging the biomechanic activity of the valve implant (McGregor et al., 2013; Manji et al., 2014). A similar prevention of anti-Gal response was observed with SIS from GT-KO pigs implanted in monkeys (Daly et al., 2009).

Decellularization of implants

Decellularization of ECM implants was reported to result in elimination of α-gal epitopes from ECM implants. Among such studies, elimination was reported with porcine heart valves (Kasimir et al., 2005; Naso et al., 2013) and with porcine cornea (Gonzalez-Andrades et al., 2011) by using solutions with various detergent strength. It is important to determine the presence of residual α-gal epitopes by methods that are more sensitive than direct immunostaining (Stone et al., 2007b, 1998; Naso et al., 2013) since if these epitopes are not close enough to enable antibody or lectin bridging, it is possible that interaction via only one combining site may not be strong enough to prevent detachment of antibody or lectin during washes of the specimen. In addition, as discussed above, if the ECM implant is planned to be repopulated with cells other than fibroblasts, the presence of various ECM proteins and proteoglycans might be important for directing stem cell differentiation. If decellularizing detergent solutions remove essential ECM components, the stem cells may not receive the required information to differentiate into the appropriate repopulating cells, and the remodeling of the implant may result in fibrosis.

PRODUCTION OF ANTI-NON-GAL ANTIBODIES IN HUMANS

Most homologous porcine proteins are immunogenic in humans

Mammalian species differ from each other in the amino acid sequence of most homologous proteins. The extent of sequence differences is proportional to the evolutionary distance between the various species. These sequence differences are the result of random mutations accumulated in various lineages and referred to as the evolutionary molecular clock (Sarich and Wilson, 1967; Wilson, 1985). The rate of mutations in introns or in pseudogenes is estimated to be approximately 0.5% of the bases per million years (Britten, 1986). Whereas some of the mutations are lethal since they destroy the function of an essential protein, many of the mutations in exons are tolerated since they do not alter significantly functions of proteins. In most proteins, regions that are not essential for the protein function (e.g., tethers of cell surface receptors) mutate at rates that are much higher than regions with biological function such as ligand-binding regions of receptors or catalytic domains. Thus, with the exception of highly conserved proteins such as collagen and histones, the majority of proteins in species of different lineages have multiple amino acid sequence differences which confer immunogenicity to such proteins when administered into another species. Thus, the further two species are from each other on an evolutionary scale, the more immunogenic their proteins are to each other. Porcine implants in humans are likely to elicit a much stronger anti-protein antibody response than ape implants. Accordingly, studies on anti-albumin antibody production demonstrated a direct relationship between the distance on an evolutionary scale of the albumin donor species from the species immunized with the assayed albumin and the intensity of the anti-albumin antibody response in the immunized species (Sarich and Wilson, 1967; Wilson, 1985). Since most pig proteins differ in their amino acid sequence from homologous proteins in humans, it is probable that the immune system in human recipients of pig implants will produce antibodies against the majority of proteins in the porcine implant (with the possible exception of collagen and histones). These anti-protein antibodies, called "anti-non-gal antibodies," may play an important role in the immune response against porcine implants in humans.

Anti-non-gal antibody response to pig implants

Production of anti-non-gal antibodies in monkey recipients of implants was first studied in cynomolgus monkeys implanted in the suprapatellar pouch with porcine meniscus and articular cartilage (Stone et al., 1998). Most of these implants which contained no live cells were pretreated with α-galactosidase in order to eliminate α-gal epitopes. Accordingly, monkeys implanted with α-galactosidase-treated cartilage produced only natural, and no elicited anti-Gal antibody, whereas those implanted with untreated porcine cartilage displayed increase of at least 100-fold in anti-Gal titers within 2 weeks postimplantation (Galili et al., 1997). Production of anti-non-gal antibodies (anti-cartilage antibodies in Stone et al., 1998) was determined by ELISA with porcine cartilage homogenate as solid-phase antigen, using monkey sera depleted of anti-Gal. Extensive production of anti-non-gal antibodies was observed both in monkeys implanted with cartilage expressing or lacking α-gal epitopes, 3–4 weeks postimplantation (Stone et al., 1998). A distinct difference in kinetics of anti-Gal and anti-non-gal antibody production was observed in monkeys implanted with porcine cartilage expressing α-gal epitopes. Whereas anti-Gal production reached its highest level within 2 weeks postimplantation (Galili et al., 1997), anti-non-gal antibody activity reached the highest level 3–5 weeks postimplantation (Stone et al., 1998). As discussed below, the slow anti-non-gal antibody response may be exploited for overcoming detrimental effects of this antibody.

Production of anti-non-gal antibodies against pig implants in humans could be closely monitored by ELISA in the clinical trial mentioned above in which torn ACL was replaced with glutaraldehyde cross-linked pig patellar tendon pretreated with recombinant α-galactosidase (Stone et al., 2007b). In these studies, pig tendon homogenate served as solid-phase antigen and the sera of the implanted patients were depleted of anti-Gal. As previously observed in monkey recipients of cartilage implants, anti–non-gal antibody response developed slower than anti-Gal response in these patients. Ultimately, an extensive anti–non-gal antibody response was observed in all recipients of the pig tendon implant. This antibody response peaked 2–6 months post-implantation, continued to be produced for at least 1 year and returned to the preimplantation background level after about 2 years (Stone et al., 2007b).

Specificity analysis of anti–non-gal antibodies was performed by Western blot of solubilized pig tendon proteins immunostained with sera of the implanted patients. The sera were depleted of anti-Gal prior to analysis in order to prevent binding of this antibody to α-gal epitopes of the glycoproteins. No anti–non-gal antibodies were found in the preimplantation sera. However, extensive production of these antibodies which demonstrated a very wide range of specificities against a large number of por-cine proteins was observed in sera obtained few months postimplantation (Stone et al., 2007b). No binding of these anti–non-gal antibodies was observed in Western blots with human tendon proteins immunostained with postimplantation sera. This finding implies that the immune response against the multiple pig tendon proteins did not cause any breakdown in the physiologic immune tolerance to human antigens. It is of interest to further note that many of the anti–non-gal antibodies produced in the implanted patients also bound in the Western blot to multiple antigens in pig kidney homogenate, probably because of the presence of the same proteins in different types of pig cells.

During the 2-year monitoring of patients implanted with the processed pig tendon, the implants maintained their biomechanical function while a gradual "ligamentiza-tion" process occurred within them. In that process, macrophages were recruited into the implant. It is possible that part of that recruitment was mediated by anti–non-gal antibodies which interacted with the pig proteins within the implant and activated the complement system, thereby generating macrophage chemotactic factors. These mac-rophages bound to the implant ECM via Fc/FcγR and C3b/C3bR interactions and mediated gradual degradation of the pig ECM. The recipient's fibroblasts infiltrating the implant via the *de novo* vascularization aligned with the porcine collagen fibers bioscaffold and secreted their autologous ECM. This ligamentization process gradually converts the implant into an autologous remodeled ACL (Stone et al., 2007b).

The complete conversion of the porcine tendon into human ACL seems to take about 24 months. This is based on the observation that the level of anti–non-gal anti-bodies in the implanted patients reversed after about 24 months to the preimplantation background level of antibody binding in the ELISA wells. The extensive production of anti–non-gal antibodies for at least 1 year further implies that the human immune sys-tem continuously produces anti–non-gal antibodies against pig proteins as long as these proteins are present within the implanted tissue. However, once the implanted pig proteins are fully degraded and eliminated (possibly as a result of uptake by macrophages), the immune system ceases to produce anti–non-gal antibodies since there is no further antigenic stimulation by pig proteins.

Production of anti–non-gal antibodies was also observed within few weeks postimplantation in human recipients of SIS implants (Ansaloni et al., 2007). SIS is comprised mostly of porcine collagen, which is of low immunogenicity in humans, as indicated by the wide use of such collagen in cosmetic procedures. In view of the well-documented very effective functional remodeling of the SIS (Hiles et al., 2009), it is probable that the mild immune response against this ECM enables the effective remodeling of SIS implants into connective tissue without their inflammatory rejection. The anti-SIS antibody activity was found to disappear within 6 months postimplantation (Ansaloni et al., 2007). This suggests that, similar to the elimination of anti–non-gal antibodies in recipients of porcine tendon, the gradual degradation of the implanted SIS and its conversion into autologous connective tissue eliminated the antigenic stimulation that induced the production of such antibodies in SIS recipients.

Significance of the extent of cross-linking in regeneration of connective tissue implants

The rate of immune-mediated degradation of the porcine tendon implant in recipients with torn ACL was slowed enough to enable ligamentization by a combination of α-galactosidase treatment and mild cross-linking with 0.1% glutaraldehyde for 12 h (Stone et al., 2007b). Subsequently, the unbound glutaraldehyde was washed away and the remaining reactive glutaraldehyde groups were blocked by incubation with 0.1 M glycine. The optimal cross-linking conditions were determined empirically with porcine tendon treated at various concentration of glutaraldehyde prior to implantation in monkeys (Stone et al., 2007a). Milder cross-linking (i.e., <0.1% glutaraldehyde for 12 h) resulted in subsequent extensive infiltration of macrophages. This extensive infiltration was followed by degradation of the implant at a pace that was too fast for enabling the appropriate angiogenesis and alignment of fibroblasts with the porcine bioscaffold of collagen fibers. In contrast, a higher concentration of glutaraldehyde results in cross-linking which is extensive enough to prevent subsequent infiltration of macrophages and fibroblasts.

Pig heart valves serve as an example for extensive cross-linking which prevents remodeling. The pig heart valves are usually cross-linked for many days in glutaraldehyde at a concentration of at least 0.25%. Histological inspection of such implants, which are explanted because of impaired function, usually demonstrates a calcification process on the surface of the valve. However, penetration of cells into the implant is greatly inhibited because of the extensive cross-linking (Purinya et al., 1994; Dittrich et al., 2000). Thus, incubation of the porcine tendon for 12 h in glutaraldehyde at a concentration higher than 0.1% or for a longer period may result in a similar formation of cross-linking glutaraldehyde covalent bonds at a density that too high for enabling the appropriate infiltration of macrophages. In the absence of infiltrating macrophages, no angiogenesis can occur and no fibroblasts can infiltrate the implant and remodel the pig tissue into a human ACL. The gradual breaking of porcine collagen fibers caused by the pulling forces, bending, and impingement on the bone is likely to gradually impair the function of the implant, ultimately resulting in its tear. Conversely, a too low concentration of glutaraldehyde (e.g., 0.01%) results in an insufficient density of covalent cross-linking bonds. Such a density is too low for slowing macrophage infiltration, resulting in premature destruction of the implant bioscaffold, before the infiltration and appropriate alignment of fibroblasts with the porcine collagen bioscaffold can occur. Since the density of various porcine ECM implants and the physiologic forces applied on implants differ from one type of implant to the other, the optimal cross-linking conditions may have to be determined for each type of implant.

The studies on porcine tendon implants for the remodeling into human ACL suggest that if the regenerating tissue is comprised primarily of fibroblasts, a combination of α-gal epitopes elimination (or use of GT-KO pig as source of the biomaterial implant) and "fine-tuning" of the porcine tissue cross-linking may ultimately result in gradual degradation of the implant at an optimal rate that enables its regeneration by infiltrating fibroblasts while maintaining its biomechanical function. These studies further suggest that monitoring anti–non-gal antibodies production in the serum by methods similar to those described above for recipients of pig tendon implant will provide useful information on whether the implant has fully remodeled and converted into human tissue. Cross-linking by agents such as glutaraldehyde may be useful in the remodeling of various types of connective tissue. However, it is likely that this processing may not be effective in the regeneration of tissues other than connective tissue, since stem cells require "cues" from ECM molecules for differentiation into cells other than fibroblasts. As indicated above, glutaraldehyde cross-links the amino groups of lysines and those of the amino acids at the amino terminus of proteins. Such cross-linking is likely to alter the structure of ECM molecules and thus may prevent the appropriate interaction with stem cells. As discussed below, providing the appropriate ECM cues to stem cells may therefore require accelerated recruitment of stem cells into the implant prior to the formation of anti–non-gal antibodies at detrimental levels.

Rapid stem cell recruitment for avoiding effects of anti-non-gal antibodies

As indicated above, the physiologic default mechanism for repair and regeneration of external and internal injuries is the process of fibrosis in which fibroblasts recruited into the injury site form dense connective tissue. Because of this mechanism, healing of injuries, such as large wounds in the skin, extensive ischemia in the myocardium, and severed nerves in spinal cord injuries, usually results in fibrosis and irreversible scars are formed before constructive remodeling and appropriate regeneration can occur. Thus, in considering methods for overcoming anti-non-gal-mediated immune rejection of an implant, the objectives for remodeling of tissues containing specialized cells other than fibroblasts differ from those for remodeling of connective tissue. The remodeling of a bioscaffold for connective tissue, such as SIS or pig ligament, can be achieved by migration of fibroblasts to the bioscaffold or by fibrosis as the default repair mechanism in case the implant undergoes rapid destruction. In contrast, remodeling of biomaterial implants requiring more specialized cells, such as ECM patches of urinary bladder wall or of myocardium, may be viewed as "complex type" remodeling processes. These patches are expected to undergo constructive remodeling into tissues comprised of specialized cells such as transitional epithelium (urothelium) and smooth muscle in the urinary bladder wall, or cardiomyocytes in myocardial regeneration. Multiple studies have indicated that the success of the complex type remodeling of tissues is determined by the ability of the ECM implants to instruct stem cells reaching the implant to differentiate into specialized cells that repopulate it (Atala, 2009; Badylak et al., 2012). Since antibodies against ECM molecules or those against stem cell receptors for ECM ligands can inhibit adhesion of stem cells to ECM, it is reasonable to assume that by masking the ECM, anti-non-gal antibodies can prevent the interaction of stem cell with ECM molecules (Guilak et al., 2009; Chen, 2010; Hidalgo-Bastida and Cartmell, 2010; Decaris and Leach, 2011). Similarly, it is probable that rapid degradation of the ECM can be mediated by binding of anti-non-gal antibodies to it. Adhesion of recruited macrophages to these ECM complexed antibodies will also result in ECM degradation and prevention of stem cells from receiving the appropriate cues. Under such circumstances it is likely that the default fibrosis will occur instead of the desired constructive remodeling of the implant.

Presently, effective suppression of anti-non-gal antibody response against porcine implants may be feasible only by complete "shutting off" the immune system by excessive administration of immunosuppressive drugs. Since this is not a practical solution, an alternative approach which may be considered is the accelerated recruitment of stem cells into the implant. As indicated above, production of anti-non-gal antibodies may take several weeks postimplantation. Therefore, it is hypothesized that shortly after implantation, there is a "window" of time during which stem cells may be effectively guided by the ECM to differentiate, prior to the formation of anti-non-gal antibodies at detrimental titers. Thus, constructive remodeling of implants prior to the formation of anti-non-gal antibodies may be achieved by induction of rapid recruitment of stem cells into the implant. A suggested method for inducing rapid recruitment may be by administration of α-gal nanoparticles within the implant (Galili, 2013a,b). No studies have been performed as yet for evaluating the efficacy of α-gal nanoparticles in inducing regeneration of implants. However, the ability of α-gal nanoparticles to accelerate wound healing and burn healing and to prevent scar formation in GT-KO mouse (Wigglesworth et al., 2011; Galili et al., 2010) and GT-KO pig experimental models (Hurwitz et al., 2012) raises the possibility that α-gal nanoparticles may also induce rapid recruitment of stem cells into implants shortly after implantation. Characteristics of α-gal nanoparticles and experimental observations supporting the hypothesis that these nanoparticles may be beneficial in overcoming the detrimental effects of anti-non-gal antibodies for achieving constructive remodeling of porcine implants are described below.

Structure and activity of α-gal nanoparticles

α-Gal nanoparticles are nanoparticles that present on their surface many α-gal epitopes, thereby they enable the harnessing of the therapeutic potential of the natural anti-Gal antibody. One type of α-gal nanoparticles which has been studied in recent years is submicroscopic α-gal liposomes comprised of glycolipids with one to several α-gal epitopes (α-gal glycolipids), phospholipids, and cholesterol (Wigglesworth et al., 2011; Galili et al., 2010; Hurwitz et al., 2012) (Figure 10.2). These three components of α-gal nanoparticles are extracted from rabbit red cell membranes by incubation in chloroform and methanol (Galili et al., 2007). Rabbit red cells are the richest known source of α-gal glycolipids in mammals (Eto et al., 1968; Stellner et al., 1973; Dabrowski et al., 1984; Egge et al., 1985) and thus, membranes of these red cells serve as a convenient source for α-gal glycolipids. The chloroform:methanol extracts are filtered to remove particulate materials, dried and sonicated in saline into submicroscopic nanoparticles designated α-gal nanoparticles (size range of ~10–300 nm). These nanoparticles are sterilized by filtration through a 0.2 μm filter. The α-gal nanoparticles were found to present as many as about 10^{15} α-gal epitopes/mg nanoparticles (Wigglesworth et al., 2011).

Because of their abundant expression of α-gal epitopes, α-gal nanoparticles administered into injury sites readily bind the natural anti-Gal antibody and thus have important effects on macrophages that orchestrate healing of various injuries (Galili, 2013a,b). Studies in GT-KO mice and pigs (Galili, 2013b; Wigglesworth et al., 2011; Galili et al., 2010; Hurwitz et al., 2012) indicated that several consecutive processes occur as a result of anti-Gal binding to α-gal epitopes on these nanoparticles (Figure 10.2): (i) *In vivo* binding of the natural anti-Gal antibody to administered α-gal nanoparticles activates the complement system similar to complement activation observed when porcine xenografts expressing α-gal epitopes are transplanted into monkeys (Collins et al., 1994; Xu et al., 1998; Simon et al., 1998). (ii) The chemotactic factors (chemoattractant) C5a and C3a generated as complement cleavage peptides (because of complement activation) induce rapid recruitment of macrophages to the site of α-gal nanoparticles. This recruitment can be observed *in vivo* within 24 h from administration of α-gal nanoparticles into GT-KO mice and is completely inhibited in the presence of cobra venom factor which inactivates the complement

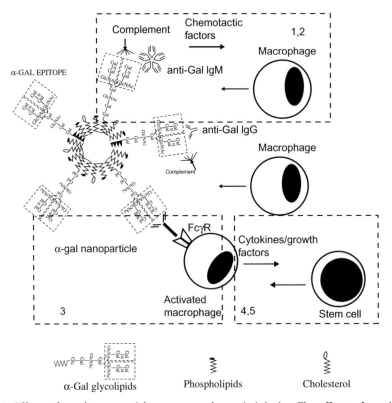

Figure 10.2 *Effects of α-gal nanoparticles on macrophages in injuries* . The effects of α-gal nanoparticles may be divided into several stages as illustrated in the various dashed line rectangles: 1. Interaction of the natural anti-Gal antibody with α-gal nanoparticles applied to injuries activates the local complement system, resulting in the generation of complement cleavage chemotactic peptides. 2. The chemotactic peptides induce extravasation of monocytes and their differentiation into macrophages that rapidly migrate toward the α-gal nanoparticles within the injured site. 3. The recruited macrophages interact via their cell surface FcγR with the Fc "tails" of anti-Gal immunocomplexed to the α-gal nanoparticles. 4. This Fc/FcγR interaction activates the macrophage to produce and secrete "pro-healing" cytokines/growth factors. It is hypothesized that some of these cytokines/growth factors secreted by the activated macrophages are capable of recruiting stem cells. The components of α-gal nanoparticles (α-gal glycolipids, phospholipids, and cholesterol) are illustrated at the bottom of the figure.

system (Wigglesworth et al., 2011). (iii) The recruited macrophages interact via their FcγR with the Fc portion of anti-Gal coating the α-gal nanoparticles. This interaction could be visualized by electron microscopy as multiple nanoparticles adhering to the surface of macrophages (Galili, 2013b). (iv) This Fc/FcγR interaction activates the macrophages to secrete a wide range of cytokines and growth factors such as fibroblast growth factor, IL1, platelet-derived growth factor, and colony-stimulating factor detected by quantitative real-time polymerase chain reaction studies of macrophages recruited *in vivo* by α-gal nanoparticles (Wigglesworth et al., 2011). *In vitro* analysis of macrophages-binding anti-Gal-coated α-gal nanoparticles via Fc/FcγR interaction indicated that as a result of activation by this interaction, the macrophages markedly increase their secretion of vascular endothelial growth factor (VEGF) (Wigglesworth et al., 2011). This high secretion of VEGF by the activated macrophages results in extensive vascularization of the granulation tissue in wounds treated with α-gal nanoparticles at a level that is much higher than that in untreated wounds (Hurwitz et al., 2012). Ultimately, the cytokines/growth factors secreted by these activated macrophages display a "pro-healing" effect on injuries, decreasing healing time by 40–60% (Wigglesworth et al., 2011; Galili et al., 2010; Hurwitz et al., 2012). Moreover, the accelerated healing of wounds treated with α-gal nanoparticles avoided the fibrosis and scar formation in wounds. The accelerated vascularization and possibly the rapid recruitment of stem cells by the pro-healing cytokines/growth factors resulted in restoration of the normal histology of the injured skin prior to the onset of the fibrosis process and scar formation (Wigglesworth et al., 2011).

Recruitment of stem cells by activated macrophages within injury sites has been observed in some experimental models such heart regeneration (Lolmede et al., 2009; Arenas-Herrera et al., 2013). Taken together, these reports on macrophage-mediated progenitor/stem cell recruitment and the recruiting and activating effects of α-gal nanoparticles on macrophages raise the possibility that administration of these nanoparticles within porcine implants may accelerate the remodeling process by rapid recruitment of macrophages followed by recruitment of stem cells prior to detrimental interaction of anti-non-gal antibodies with the implant.

α-Gal nanoparticles may be introduced into decellularized porcine implants by diffusion into the implant soaked in a nanoparticles suspension. If the implant is of a decellularized organ (e.g., kidney), α-gal nanoparticles may be introduced by perfusion of the implant with an α-gal nanoparticles suspension, after the perfusion performed with detergent solutions for the decellularization process and subsequent washes (Crapo et al., 2011, p. 114). It is hypothesized that anti-Gal and complement molecules which are present throughout the body in humans will diffuse into decellularized implants, bind to α-gal nanoparticles, activate the complement system, and generate complement cleavage chemotactic factors that will rapidly recruit many macrophages into the implant. Interaction of these macrophages with anti-Gal-coated α-gal nanoparticles is likely to further activate these cells to secrete many cytokines/growth factors that promote vascularization, recruit stem cells, and generate a microenvironment that is conducive to recruited stem cells. Because of the fast kinetics of these processes, the recruited stem cells may reach the implanted ECM before the generation of anti-non-gal antibodies at detrimental titers. This, in turn, may enable the stem cells to interact with the intact ECM prior to its degradation or its masking by the anti-non-gal antibodies, thus enabling the appropriate differentiation of the stem cells into mature cells that restore the structure and function of the tissue from which the ECM implant is derived. It is further hypothesized that in order to maximize the success of such an accelerated remodeling process, the anti-Gal/α-gal epitope interaction should be confined to the introduced α-gal nanoparticles, i.e., the implant should be devoid of α-gal epitopes in order to prevent anti-Gal binding to the implant itself. Future studies with various porcine implants in GT-KO mice, GT-KO pigs, or monkeys will enable the evaluation of α-gal nanoparticles efficacy in inducing constructive remodeling of implants and avoiding the fibrosis process.

CONCLUSIONS

The immune-mediated rejection of porcine implants in humans is primarily the result of antibody activity against the implant. The two main types of antibodies that constitute the human immune response against porcine implants are anti-Gal and anti–non-gal antibodies. Production of these antibodies cannot be prevented by currently used immunosuppression protocols without complete suppression of the immune system. Anti-Gal is a natural antibody constituting about 1% of the immunoglobulins and it interacts specifically with α-gal epitopes which are abundantly expressed on porcine tissues and implants. These α-gal epitopes further activate the multiple quiescent anti-Gal B cells, resulting in elevated production of anti-Gal antibodies. These elicited anti-Gal antibodies continue to be produced as long as the implant is not eliminated and they exacerbate the destruction of implants. The effects of anti-Gal/α-gal epitope interaction can be avoided either by elimination of α-gal epitopes from the implant with α-galactosidase or by using implants prepared from tissues of GT-KO pigs which lack α-gal epitopes.

Anti–non-gal antibodies are produced against the multiple pig proteins that are immunogenic in humans because of amino acid sequence differences between homologous proteins in humans and pigs. These antibodies are produced by the human immune system as long as the porcine implant proteins are present in the recipient. Production of anti–non-gal antibodies is slower than that of elicited anti-Gal antibodies and may peak 3–5 weeks postimplantation. Acceleration of the constructive remodeling process in implants may help in avoiding anti–non-gal antibody effects. It is hypothesized, but not proven as yet that such accelerated remodeling may be induced by administration of α-gal nanoparticles within porcine implants.

REFERENCES

Ansaloni, L., Cambrini, P., Catena, F., Di Saverio, S., Gagliardi, S., Gazzotti, F., et al., 2007. Immune response to small intestinal submucosa (surgisis) implant in humans: preliminary observations. J. Invest. Surg. 20, 237–241.

Arenas-Herrera, J.E., Ko, I.K., Atala, A., Yoo, J.J. 2013, Decellularization for whole organ bioengineering. Biomed. Mater. 8, 1–9.

Atala, A., 2009. Engineering organs. Curr. Opin. Biotechnol. 20, 575–593.

Badylak, S.F., Gilbert, T.W., 2008. Immune response to biologic scaffold materials. Semin. Immunol. 20, 109–116.

Badylak, S.F., Park, K., Peppas, N., McCabe, G., Yoder, M., 2001. Marrow-derived cells populate scaffolds composed of xenogeneic extracellular matrix. Exp. Hematol. 29, 1310–1318.

Badylak, S.F., Weiss, D.J., Caplan, A., Macchiarini, P., 2012. Engineered whole organs and complex tissues. Lancet 379, 943–952.

Basu, M., Basu, S., 1973. Enzymatic synthesis of blood group related pentaglycosyl ceramide by an α-galac tosyltransferase. J. Biol. Chem. 248, 1700–1706.

Betteridge, A., Watkins, W.M., 1983. Two α-3-D galactosyltransferases in rabbit stomach mucosa with different acceptor substrate specificities. Eur. J. Biochem. 132, 29–35.

Blake, D.D., Goldstein, I.J., 1981. An α-D-galactosyltransferase in Ehrlich ascites tumor cells: Biosynthesis and characterization of a trisaccharide (α-D-galacto(1-3)-N-acetyllactosamine). J. Biol. Chem. 256, 5387–5393.

Blanken, W.M., van den Eijnden, D.H., 1985. Biosynthesis of terminal Galα1-3Galß1-4GlcNAc-R oligosaccharide sequence on glycoconjugates: purification and acceptor specificity of a UDP-Gal: N-acetyllactosamine α1,3galactosyltransferase. J. Biol. Chem. 260, 12927–12934.

Britten, R.J., 1986. Rates of DNA sequence evolution differ between taxonomic groups. Science 231, 1393–1399.

Chen, X.D., 2010. Extracellular matrix provides an optimal niche for the maintenance and propagation of mesenchymal stem cells. Birth Defects Res. 90, 45–54.

Chung, C.H., Mirakhur, B., Chan, E., Le, Q.T., Berlin, J., Morse, M., et al., 2008. Cetuximab-induced anaphylaxis and IgE specific for galactose-α-1,3-galactose. N. Engl. J. Med. 358, 1109–1117.

Collins, B.H., Cotterell, A.H., McCurry, K.R., Alvarado, C.G., Magee, J.C., Parker, W., et al., 1994. Cardiac xenografts between primate species provide evidence of the α-galactosyl determinant in hyperacute rejection. J. Immunol. 154, 5500–5510.

Commins, S.P., Satinover, S.M., Hosen, J., Mozena, J., Borish, L., Lewis, B.D., et al., 2009. Delayed anaphylaxis, angioedema, or urticaria after consumption of red meat in patients with IgE antibodies specific for galactose-α-1,3-galactose. J. Allergy. Clin. Immunol. 123, 426–433.

Cotterell, A.H., Collins, B.H., Parker, W., Harland, R.C., Platt, J.L., 1995. The humoral immune response in humans following cross-perfusion of porcine organs. Transplantation 60, 861–868.

Crapo, P.M., Gilbert, T.W., Badylak, S.F., 2011. An overview of tissue and whole organ decellularization processes. Biomaterials 32, 3233–3243.

Dabrowski, U., Hanfland, P., Egge, H., Kuhn, S., Dabrowski, J., 1984. Immunochemistry of I/i-active oligo- and polyglycosylceramides from rabbit erythrocyte membranes. Determination of branching patterns of a ceramide pentadecasaccharide by 1H nuclear magnetic resonance. J. Biol. Chem. 259, 7648–7651.

Daly, K.A., Stewart-Akers, A.M., Hara, H., Ezzelarab, M., Long, C., Cordero, K., et al., 2009. Effect of the α-Gal epitope on the response to small intestinal submucosa extracellular matrix in a nonhuman primate model. Tissue. Eng. Part. A. 15, 3877–3888.

Decaris, M.L., Leach, J.K., 2011. Design of experiments approach to engineer cell-secreted matrices for directing osteogenic differentiation. Ann. Biomed. Eng. 39, 1174–1185.

Dittrich, S., Alexi-Meskishvili, V.V., Yankah, A.C., Dähnert, I., Meyer, R., Hetzer, R., et al., 2000. Comparison of porcine xenografts and homografts for pulmonary valve replacement in children. Ann. Thorac. Surg. 70, 717–722.

Egge, H., Kordowicz, M., Peter-Katalinic, J., Hanfland, P., 1985. Immunochemistry of I/i-active oligo- and polyglycosylceramides from rabbit erythrocyte membranes. J. Biol. Chem. 260, 4927–4935.

Eto, T., Iichikawa, Y., Nishimura, K., Ando, S., Yamakawa, T., 1968. Chemistry of lipids of the posthemolytic residue or stroma of erythrocytes. XVI. Occurrence of ceramide pentasaccharide in the membrane of erythrocytes and reticulocytes in rabbit. J. Biochem. (Tokyo) 64, 205–213.

Galili, U., 1993. Evolution and pathophysiology of the human natural anti-Gal antibody. Springer. Semin. Immunopathol. 15, 155–171.

Galili, U., 2012. Induced anti-non gal antibodies in human xenograft recipients. Transplantation 93, 11–16.

Galili, U., 2013a. Anti-Gal: An abundant human natural antibody of multiple pathogeneses and clinical benefits. Immunology 140, 1–11.

Galili, U., 2013b. Anti-Gal macrophage recruitment and activation by α-gal nanoparticles accelerate regeneration and can improve biomaterials efficacy in tissue engineering. Open Tissue Eng. Regen. Med. J. 6, 1–11.

Galili, U., 2013c. α1,3Galactosyltransferase knockout pigs produce the natural anti-Gal antibody and simulate the evolutionary appearance of this antibody in primates. Xenotransplantation 20, 267–276.

Galili, U., Swanson, K., 1991. Gene sequences suggest inactivation of α1-3 galactosyltransferase in catarrhines after the divergence of apes from monkeys. Proc. Natl. Acad. Sci. USA 88, 7401–7404.

Galili, U., Andrews, P., 1995. Suppression of α-galactosyl epitopes synthesis and production of the natural anti-Gal antibody: A major evolutionary event in ancestral Old World primates. J. Human Evol. 29, 433–442.

Galili, U., Rachmilewitz, E.A., Peleg, A., Flechner, I., 1984. A unique natural human IgG antibody with anti-α-galactosyl specificity. J. Exp. Med. 160, 1519–1531.

Galili, U., Macher, B.A., Buehler, J., Shohet, S.B., 1985. Human natural anti-α-galactosyl IgG. II. The specific recognition of α(1-3)-linked galactose residues. J. Exp. Med. 162, 573–582.

Galili, U., Clark, M.R., Shohet, S.B., Buehler, J., Macher, B.A., 1987. Evolutionary relationship between the anti-Gal antibody and the Galα1→3Gal epitope in primates. Proc. Natl. Acad. Sci. USA 84, 1369–1373.

Galili, U., Mandrell, R.E., Hamadeh, R.M., Shohet, S.B., Griffis, J.M., 1988a. Interaction between human natural anti-α-galactosyl immunoglobulin G and bacteria of the human flora. Infect. Immun. 56, 1730–1737.

Galili, U., Shohet, S.B., Kobrin, E., Stults, C.L.M., Macher, B.A., 1988b. Man, apes, and Old World monkeys differ from other mammals in the expression of α-galactosyl epitopes on nucleated cells. J. Biol. Chem. 263, 17755–17762.

Galili, U., Anaraki, F., Thall, A., Hill-Black, C., Radic, M., 1993. One percent of circulating B lymphocytes are capable of producing the natural anti-Gal antibody. Blood 82, 2485–2493.

Galili, U., Tibell, A., Samuelsson, B., Rydberg, B., Groth, C.G., 1995. Increased anti-Gal activity in diabetic patients transplanted with fetal porcine islet cell clusters. Transplantation 59, 1549–1556.

Galili, U., LaTemple, D.C., Walgenbach, A.W., Stone, K.R., 1997. Porcine and bovine cartilage transplants in cynomolgus monkey: II. Changes in anti-Gal response during chronic rejection. Transplantation 63, 646–651.

Galili, U., LaTemple, D.C., Radic, M.Z., 1998. A sensitive assay for measuring α-gal epitope expression on cells by a monoclonal anti-Gal antibody. Transplantation 65, 1129–1132.

Galili, U., Chen, Z.C., Tanemura, M., Seregina, T., Link, C.J., 2001. Induced antibody response in xenograft recipients. GRAFT 4, 32–35.

Galili, U., Wigglesworth, K., Abdel-Motal, U.M., 2007. Intratumoral injection of α-gal glycolipids induces xenograft-like destruction and conversion of lesions into endogenous vaccines. J. Immunol. 178, 4676–4687.

Galili, U., Wigglesworth, K., Abdel-Motal, U.M., 2010. Accelerated healing of skin burns by anti-Gal/α-gal liposomes interaction. BURNS 36, 239–251.

Gonzalez-Andrades, M., de la Cruz Cardona, J., Ionescu, A.M., Campos, A., del Mar Perez, M., Alaminos, M., 2011. Generation of bioengineered corneas with decellularized xenografts and human keratocytes. Invest. Ophthalmol. Vis. Sci. 52, 215–222.

Groth, C.G., Korsgren, O., Tibell, A., Tollemar, J., Möller, E., Bolinder, J., et al., 1994. Transplantation of porcine fetal pancreas to diabetic patients. Lancet 344, 1402–1404.

Guilak, F., Cohen, D.M., Estes, B.T., Gimble, J.M., Liedtke, W., Chen, C.S., 2009. Control of stem cell fate by physical interactions with the extracellular matrix. Cell. Stem. Cell. 5, 17–26.

Hamadeh, R.M., Galili, U., Zhou, P., Griffis, J.M., 1995. Human secretions contain IgA, IgG and IgM anti-Gal (anti-α-galactosyl) antibodies. Clin. Diagnos Lab Immunol. 2, 125–131.

Hidalgo-Bastida, L.A., Cartmell, S.H., 2010. Mesenchymal stem cells, osteoblasts and extracellular matrix proteins: enhancing cell adhesion and differentiation for bone tissue engineering. Tissue. Eng. Part. B. Rev. 16, 405–412.

Hiles, M., Record Ritchie, R.D., Altizer, A.M., 2009. Are biologic grafts effective for hernia repair? A systematic review of the literature. Surg. Innov. 16, 26–37.

Hurwitz, Z., Ignotz, R., Lalikos, J., Galili, U., 2012. Accelerated porcine wound healing with α-Gal nanoparticles. Plast. Reconst. Surgery. 129, 242–251.

Joziasse, D.H., Shaper, J.H., Jabs, E.W., Shaper, N.L., 1991. Characterization of an α1-3-galactosyltransferase homologue on human chromosome 12 that is organized as a processed pseudogene. J. Biol. Chem. 266, 6991–6998.

Jung, Y., Wang, J., Havens, A., Sun, Y., Wang, J., Jin, T., et al., 2005. Cell-to-cell contact is critical for the survival of hematopoietic progenitor cells on osteoblasts. Cytokine 32, 155–171.

Kasimir, M.T., Rieder, E., Seebacher, G., Wolner, E., Weigel, G., Simon, P., 2005. Presence and elimination of the xenoantigen gal (α1, 3) gal in tissue-engineered heart valves. Tissue Eng. 11, 1274–1280.

Klos, A., Wende, E., Wareham, K.J., Monk, P.N., 2013. International Union of Pharmacology. LXXXVII. Complement peptide C5a, C4a, and C3a receptors. Pharmacol. Rev. 65, 500–543.

Koike, C., Fung, J.J., Geller, D.A., Kannagi, R., Libert, T., Luppi, P., et al., 2002. Molecular basis of evolutionary loss of the α1,3-galactosyltransferase gene in higher primates. J. Biol. Chem. 277, 10114–10120.

Koike, C., Uddin, M., Wildman, D.E., Gray, E.A., Trucco, M., Starzl, T.E., et al., 2007. Functionally important glycosyltransferase gain and loss during catarrhine primate emergence. Proc. Natl. Acad. Sci. USA 104, 559–564.

Konakci, K.Z., Bohle, B., Blumer, R., Hoetzenecker, W., Roth, G., Moser, B., et al., 2005. α-Gal on bioprosthesis: xenograft immune response in cardiac surgery. Eur. J. Clin. Invest. 35, 17–23.

Lai, L., Kolber-Simonds, D., Park, K.W., Cheong, H.T., Greenstein, J.L., Im, G.S., et al., 2002. Production of α-1,3-galactosyltransferase knockout pigs by nuclear transfer cloning. Science 295, 1089–1092.

Lantéri, M., Giordanengo, V., Vidal, F., Gaudray, P., Lefebvre, J.-C., 2002. A complete α1,3-galactosyltransferase gene is present in the human genome and partially transcribed. Glycobiology 12, 785–792.

Larsen, R.D., Rivera-Marrero, C.A., Ernst, L.K., Cummings, R.D., Lowe, J.B., 1990. Frameshift and nonsense mutations in a human genomic sequence homologous to a murine UDP-Galß-D-Gal(1,4)-D-GlcNAcα(1,3) galactosyltransferase cDNA. J. Biol. Chem. 265, 7055–7061.

Li, F., Li, W., Johnson, S., Ingram, D., Yoder, M., Badylak, S., 2004. Low-molecular-weight peptides derived from extracellular matrix as chemoattractants for primary endothelial cells. Endothelium 11, 199–206.

Lolmede, K., Campana, L., Vezzoli, M., Bosurgi, L., Tonlorenzi, R., Clementi, E., et al., 2009. Inflammatory and alternatively activated human macrophages attract vessel-associated stem cells, relying on separate HMGB1- and MMP-9-dependent pathways. J. Leukoc. Biol. 85, 779–787.

Manji, R.A., Ekser, B., Menkis, A.H., Cooper, D.K., 2014. Bioprosthetic heart valves of the future. Xenotransplantation 21, 1–10.

Mantovani, A., Biswas, S.K., Galdiero, M.R., Sica, A., Locati, M., 2013. Macrophage plasticity and polarization in tissue repair and remodelling. J. Pathol. 229, 176–185.

Maruyama, S., Cantu, E., DeMartino, C., Wang, C.Y., Chen, J., Al-Mohanna, F., et al., 1999a. Interaction of baboon anti-α-galactosyl antibody with pig tissues. Am. J. Pathol. 155, 1635–1649.

Maruyama, S., Cantu, E., Pernis, B., Galili, U., Godman, G., Stern, D.M., et al., 1999b. α-Galactosyl antibody redistributes α-galactosyl at the surface of pig blood and endothelial cells. Transpl. Immunol. 7, 101–106.

Maruyama, S., Cantu, E., Galili, U., D'Agati, V., Godman, G., Stern, D.M., et al., 2000. α-Galactosyl epitopes on glycoproteins of porcine renal extracellular matrix. Kidney Int. 57, 655–663.

McGregor, C.G., Kogelberg, H., Vlasin, M., Byrne, G.W., 2013. Gal-knockout bioprostheses exhibit less immune stimulation compared to standard biological heart valves. J. Heart Valve Dis. 22, 383–390.

McPherson, T.B., S., F. Badylak., Spring 1998. Characterization of fibronectin derived from porcine small intestinal submucosa. Tiss. Eng. 4, 75–83.

McPherson, T.B., Liang, H., Record, D., Badylak, S.F., 2000. Galα(1,3)Gal epitope in porcine small intestinal submucosa. Tissue Eng. 6, 233–239.

Mohan, P.S., Spiro, R.G., 1986. Macromolecular organization of basement membranes. Characterization and comparison of glomerular basement membrane and lens capsule components by immunochemical and lectin affinity procedures. J. Biol. Chem. 261, 4328–4336.

Morisset, M., Richard, C., Astier, C., Jacquenet, S., Croizier, A., Beaudouin, E., et al., 2012. Anaphylaxis to pork kidney is related to IgE antibodies specific for galactose-α-1,3-galactose. Allergy 67, 699–704.

Naso, F., Gandaglia, A., Bottio, T., Tarzia, V., Nottle, M.B., d'Apice, A.J., et al., 2013. First quantification of alpha-Gal epitope in current glutaraldehyde-fixed heart valve bioprostheses. Xenotransplantation 20, 252–256.

Ogawa, H., Galili, U., 2006. Profiling terminal N-acetyllactoamines of glycans on mammalian cells by an immuno-enzymatic assay. Glycoconj. J. 23, 663–674.

Park, S., Kim, W.H., Choi, S.Y., Kim, Y.J., 2009. Removal of α-Gal epitopes from porcine aortic valve and pericardium using recombinant human α-galactosidase A. J. Korean. Med. Sci. 24, 1126–1131.

Parker, W., Lin, S.S., Yu, P.B., Sood, A., Nakamura, Y.C., Song, A., et al., 1999. Naturally occurring anti-α-galactosyl antibodies: relationship to xenoreactive anti-α-galactosyl antibodies. Glycobiology 9, 865–873.

Phelps, C.J., Koike, C., Vaught, T.D., Boone, J., Wells, K.D., Chen, S.H., et al., 2003. Production of α1,3-galactosyltransferase-deficient pigs. Science 299, 411–414.

Purinya, B., Kasyanov, V., Volkolakov, J., Latsis, R., Tetere, G., 1994. Biomechanical and structural properties of the explanted bioprosthetic valve leaflets. J. Biomech. 27, 1–11.

Raeder, R.H., Badylak, S.F., Sheehan, C., Kallakury, B., Metzger, D.W., 2002. Natural anti-galactose α1,3 galactose antibodies delay, but do not prevent the acceptance of extracellular matrix xenografts. Transpl. Immunol. 10, 15–24.

Ravetch, J.V., Bolland, S., 2001. IgG Fc receptors. Annu. Rev. Immunol. 19, 275–290.

Sarich, V.M., Wilson, A.C., 1967. Rates of albumin evolution in primates. Proc. Natl. Acad. Sci. USA 58, 142–148.

Selvaraj, P., Fifadara, N., Nagarajan, S., Cimino, A., Wang, G., 2004. Functional regulation of human neutrophil Fc gamma receptors. Immunol. Res. 29, 219–230.

Shakibaei, M., 1998. Inhibition of chondrogenesis by integrin antibody in vitro. Exp. Cell. Res. 240, 95–106.

Simon, P.M., Neethling, F.A., Taniguchi, S., Goode, P.L., Zopf, D., Hancock, W.W., et al., 1998. Intravenous infusion of Galα1-3Gal oligosaccharides in baboon delays hyperacute rejection of porcine heart xenografts. Transplantation 56, 346–353.

Smith, D.F., Larsen, R.D., Mattox, S., Lowe, J.B., Cummings, R.D., 1990. Transfer and expression of a murine UDP-Gal:β-D-Gal-α1,3-galactosyltransferase gene in transfected Chinese hamster ovary cells. Competition reactions between the α1,3-galactosyltransferase and the endogenous α2,3-sialyltransferase. J. Biol. Chem. 265, 6225–6234.

Spiro, R.G., Bhoyroo, V.D., 1984. Occurrence of α-D-galactosyl residues in the thyroglobulin from several species. Localization in the saccharide chains of the complex carbohydrate units. J. Biol. Chem. 259, 9858–9866.

Stellner, K., Saito, H., Hakomori, S., 1973. Determination of aminosugar linkage in glycolipids by methylation. Aminosugar linkage of ceramide pentasaccharides of rabbit erythrocytes and of Forssman antigen. Arch. Biochem. Biophys. 133, 464–472.

Stone, K.R., Walgenbach, A.W., Abrams, T., Nelson, J., Gellett, N., Galili, U., 1997. Porcine and bovine cartilage transplants in cynomolgus monkey: I. A model for chronic xenograft rejection. Transplantation 63, 640–645.

Stone, K.R., Ayala, G., Goldstein, J., Hurst, R., Walgenbach, A., Galili, U., 1998. Porcine cartilage transplants in the cynomolgus monkey. III. Transplantation of α-galactosidase-treated porcine cartilage. Transplantation 65, 1577.

Stone, K.R., Walgenbach, A.W., Turek, T.J., Somers, D.L., Wicomb, W., Galili, U., 2007a. Anterior cruciate ligament reconstruction with a porcine xenograft: a serologic, histologic, and biomechanical study in primates. Arthroscopy 23, 411–419.

Stone, K.R., Abdel-Motal, U.M., Walgenbach, A.W., Turek, T.J., Galili, U., 2007b. Replacement of human anterior cruciate ligaments with pig ligaments: a model for anti-non-gal antibody response in long-term xenotransplantation. Transplantation 83, 211–219.

Takahagi, Y., Fujimura, T., Miyagawa, S., Nagashima, H., Shigehisa, T., Shirakura, R., et al., 2005. Production of α1,3-galactosyltransferase gene knockout pigs expressing both human decay-accelerating factor and N-acetylglucosaminyltransferase III. Mol. Reprod. Dev. 71, 331–338.

Takahashi, H.1., Chinuki, Y., Tanaka, A., Morita, E., 2014. Laminin γ-1 and collagen α-1 (VI) chain are galactose-α-1,3-galactose-bound allergens in beef. Allergy 69, 199–207.

Tanemura, M., Maruyama, S., Galili, U., 2000a. Differential expression of α-gal epitopes (Galα1-3Galß1-4GlcNAc-R) on pig and mouse organs. Transplantation 69, 187–190.

Tanemura, M., Yin, D., Chong, A.S., Galili, U., 2000b. Differential immune response to α-gal epitopes on xenografts and allografts: implications for accommodation in xenotransplantation. J. Clin. Invest. 105, 301–310.

Tearle, R.G., Tange, M.J., Zannettino, Z.L., Katerelos, M., Shinkel, T.A., Van Denderen, B.J., et al., 1996. The α-1,3-galactosyltransferase knockout mouse. Implications for xenotransplantation. Transplantation 61, 13–19.

Teranishi, K., Manez, R., Awwad, M., Cooper, D.K., 2002. Anti-Gal α1-3Gal IgM and IgG antibody levels in sera of humans and old world non-human primates. Xenotransplantation 9, 48–154.

Thall, A., Galili, U., 1990. Distribution of Gal α1-3Galβ1-4GlcNAc residues on secreted mammalian glycoproteins (thyroglobulin, fibrinogen, and immunoglobulin G) as measured by a sensitive solid-phase radioimmunoassay. Biochemistry 29, 3959–3965.

Thall, A., Etienne-Decerf, J., Winand, R.J., Galili, U., 1991. The α-galactosyl epitope on mammalian thyroid cells. Acta Endocrinol. 124, 692–699.

Thall, A.D., Maly, P., Lowe, J.B., 1995. Oocyte Gal α1,3Gal epitopes implicated in sperm adhesion to the zona pellucida glycoprotein ZP3 are not required for fertilization in the mouse. J. Biol. Chem. 270, 21437–21440.

van Lookeren Campagne, M., Wiesmann, C., Brown, E.J., 2007. Macrophage complement receptors and pathogen clearance. Cell. Microbiol. 9, 2095–2102.

Wang, L., Radic, M.Z., Galili, U., 1995. Human anti-Gal heavy chain genes: preferential use of VH3 and the presence of somatic mutations. J. Immunol. 155, 1276–1285.

Wigglesworth, K.M., Racki, W.J., Mishra, R., Szomolanyi-Tsuda, E., Greiner, D.L., Galili, U., 2011. Rapid recruitment and activation of macrophages by anti-Gal/α-gal liposome interaction accelerates wound healing. J. Immunol. 186, 4422–4432.

Williams, D.A., Rios, M., Stephens, C., Patel, V.P., 1991. Fibronectin and VLA-4 in haematopoietic stem cell–microenvironment interactions. Nature 352, 438–441.

Wilson, A.C., 1985. The molecular basis of evolution. Sci. Am. 253, 164–173.

Xu, Y., Lorf, T., Sablinski, T., Gianello, P., Bailin, M., Monroy, R., et al., 1998. Removal of anti-porcine natural antibodies from human and nonhuman primate plasma *in vitro* and *in vivo* by a Galα1-3Galβ1-4Glc-R immunoaffinity column. Transplantation 65, 172–179.

Yang, B., Zhou, L., Sun, Z., Yang, R., Chen, Y., Dai, Y., 2010. *In vitro* evaluation of the bioactive factors preserved in porcine small intestinal submucosa through cellular biological approaches. J. Biomed. Mater. Res. A. 93, 1100–1109.

Yano, T., Miura, T., Whittaker, P., Miki, T., Sakamoto, J., Nakamura, Y., et al., 2006. Macrophage colony-stimulating factor treatment after myocardial infarction attenuates left ventricular dysfunction by accelerating infarct repair. J. Am. Coll. Cardiol. (47), 626–634.

Yu, P.B., Parker, W., Everett, M.L., Fox, I.J., Platt, J.L., 1999. Immunochemical properties of anti-Gal alpha 1-3Gal antibodies after sensitization with xenogeneic tissues. J. Clin. Immunol. 19, 116–126.

Zhang, Y., He, Y., Bharadwaj, S., Hammam, N., Carnagey, K., Myers, R., et al., 2009. Tissue-specific extracellular matrix coatings for the promotion of cell proliferation and maintenance of cell phenotype. Biomaterials 30, 4021–4028.

Zhu, A., Monahan, C., Zhang, Z., Hurst, R., Leng, L., Goldstein, J., 1995. High-level expression and purification of coffee bean alpha-galactosidase produced in the yeast *Pichia pastoris*. Arch. Biochem. Biophys. 324, 65–70.

Zhu, A., Leng, L., Monahan, C., Zhang, Z., Hurst, R., Lenny, L., et al., 1996. Characterization of recombinant alpha-galactosidase for use in seroconversion from blood group B to O of human erythrocytes. Arch. Biochem. Biophys. 327, 324–329.

CHAPTER 11

Aging and the Host Response to Implanted Biomaterials

Archana N. Rao[1,√], Mahender N. Avula[2,#] and David W. Grainger[1,2]
[1]Department of Pharmaceutics and Pharmaceutical Chemistry; [√]Early Development Analytics Department, Alcon Laboratories, Inc., Norcross, GA, USA
[2]Department of Bioengineering, University of Utah, UT, USA; [#]Research and Development, Catheter Connections, Inc., Salt Lake City, UT, USA

Contents

INTRODUCTION

Aging is a natural physiological process characterized by graded reductions in functional abilities of various organs, organ systems, and physiological networks, resulting in compromised homeostasis, defense and repair functions, with associated increased risks of disease and death (Boccardi and Paolisso, 2014). The global human population is aging (i.e., that population of age >60 years) and estimated to triple to two billion from its current 605 million by 2050 (WHO, 2012). Advancements in modern medicine,

Host Response to Biomaterials.
DOI: http://dx.doi.org/10.1016/B978-0-12-800196-7.00011-6

its increased global availability, and improvements in quality of life have resulted in an increased number of people living to be over 80 years of age. Concomitantly, implantation of pacemakers, continuous glucose sensors, cardiovascular and ocular devices, artificial replacement hip, knee and other orthopedic implants, and many other biomaterials have increased to maintain the well-being and quality of life of this expanding geriatric patient class (Avula and Grainger, 2013). New clinical considerations have arisen in assessing device performance in this increasing population, with new risks and adverse events associated specifically with aging and patient fragility (Report to Congress, 2012). With increased life expectancy, and the increased need for improved medical devices compatible with weaker/aging human physiologies, an understanding of the effects of age on medical device implant performance *in vivo* is important. Rational criteria of implants designed specifically for geriatric populations might become apparent with such analysis. Musculoskeletal implants addressing structural aspects of bone repair in the context of osteoporosis are examples of such a need.

Medical device use in general has witnessed exponential growth in clinical applications over the past five decades (Simchi et al., 2011). Scope and fields of use for implanted medical devices (IMDs) have increased multiple-fold with the advent of new technologies, innovation, and improved understanding of human physiology and its underlying problems. Increasing rates of medical device adoption can be attributed to various factors including aging median populations worldwide, innovations in design and function that increase performance and reliability, rising standards of living among patients in developing nations, and noted improvements in patient quality of life offered by the devices (Raymond Brood, 2012). Given these factors, the global medical device market is expected to continue growing, reaching approximately $434 billion by 2017 with an annual growth rate of approximately 7.1% between 2012 and 2017 (http:// www.reportsnreports.com/reports/142514-the-outlook-for-medical-devices-worldwide. html). New IMDs continue to offer improved treatment alternatives for cardiovascular, orthopedic, oncologic, and many other diseases, specifically applications where deterioration of the body with age cannot be avoided (Kramer et al., 2012). Millions of people in the United States alone depend on some kind of implantable medical device for chronic use. Despite improvements in safety and efficacy of these devices, much is yet to be understood about human factors affecting device performance *in vivo*, especially with respect to aging. Age-specific implants are certainly under design consideration; that host reactions to implants might also be age-specific is therefore a compelling question.

The human body has several key regulatory mechanisms to maintain physiological homeostasis. Inflammation, infection control, tissue turnover, cell apoptosis and autophagy, wound healing, foreign body reactions (FBR), complement activation, and coagulation are among the tightly controlled regulatory mechanisms that work continually, individually, or in combination to maintain homeostasis. These networks respond ubiquitously to medical implants, producing a complex, intricate, and dynamic cross talk between inflammatory, immune, and coagulation cascades over both space and time to orchestrate wound healing in the presence of a foreign body/IMD. The process of aging is generally characterized by functional decline from both a histological and biochemical perspective, especially in tissues and organ systems under chronic oxidative stress. Diminishing capacity to respond to injury or stress parallels declining functionality (Rossi et al., 2008). Age progression and associated attenuation in physiological repair and homeostatic cascade intensities and durations change the host immune and inflammatory competence. These changes are largely associated with cumulative damage and mutations resulting from free radical exposure and dysregulation of host redox balancing mechanisms. Overall, this maintenance "slowdown" manifests as compromised wound healing, which also logically affects the host FBR to IMDs. While such changes appear logical given the "natural" anecdotal consequences of aging, the precise mechanisms underlying host response in geriatric patients and how the host implant–tissue relationship is altered are largely unexplored.

This chapter seeks to outline various components of host physiological aging and how it might relate to host response to implants in order to understand the impact of aging-related physiological changes on IMD performance and adverse events. Given the current complexity in understanding the FBR as described in Chapter 2, one might predict that analysis of the complex acute and chronic regulatory mechanisms within the human body that elicit FBR activities, namely inflammation, immunity, repair, defense, and healing, in the context of aging is particularly difficult. The current paucity of age-specific data specific to correlating patient aging to function and performance of IMDs, and their respective failure modes, in their various clinical contexts makes such correlations even more difficult.

THE HOST FBR

As detailed extensively in Chapters 2 and 3, the human body responds to foreign materials through a sequence of physiological events that begin as normal wound healing but ultimately result in various combinations of implant destruction/degradation, clearance, integration, or complete foreign body isolation from the surrounding environment (Anderson et al., 2008).

The host FBR to materials including IMDs is mediated by several different, coordinated, and spatially proximal events that act individually or in concert (Anderson, 2001). These reactions are conceptualized in Figure 11.1.

Each host reactionary cascade to an IMD has age-dependent intensities and compromises that are poorly understood in general and particularly in the context of the FBR. As the FBR begins as an acute wound healing process that is continuously interrupted by chronically unresolved inflammatory processes, the FBR is often characterized conceptually as a chronically aborted wound healing process with abnormal host

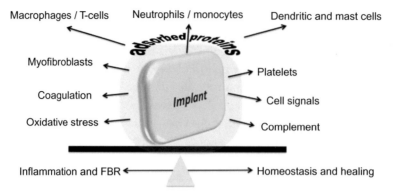

Figure 11.1 The diversity of host responses to an implant. *(Adapted from Gorbet and Sefton, 2004, with permission.)*

accommodation. Normal wound healing is highly dynamic, involving complex interactions of extracellular matrix (ECM) molecules, soluble mediators, various resident cells, and infiltrating leukocyte subtypes in the wound site (Eming et al., 2007). To achieve tissue integrity and homeostasis, wound healing occurs in three phases: inflammation, tissue formation, and remodeling (Martin and Leibovich, 2005; Singer and Clark, 1999). Chronic inflammation, a hallmark of the nonhealing wound, also predisposes tissue to cancer development in select tissues such as skin (Eming et al., 2007). Age-related molecular changes cause dysfunction and impaired repair capacity that involves the normal wound healing process. A variety of age-induced effects on certain aspects of wound healing have been reported, and these will be discussed in the following sections as a basis for understanding how these effects might analogously impact the FBR in aged patients.

HOST INFLAMMATORY RESPONSE

The inflammatory response manifests primarily as acute (minutes-to-days) and chronic (weeks-to-months) responses based on the duration and intensity of inflammatory stimuli and its mitigation *in situ*. Generally, the acute inflammatory response to biomaterials resolves quickly, usually within a week, depending on the extent of injury at the implant site and the type of biomaterial in the IMD. Chronic inflammation is less uniform histologically, resulting from constant and variable inflammatory stimuli from the implant's presence, mechanical irritation as implant–tissue micro-motion, or degradation components produced by the implant. The chronic inflammatory response to biomaterials is usually confined to the implant site and can range from weeks to months to years (Anderson, 1988). In fact, the host response can be expected to persist for as long as the biomaterial remains in the individual. Multiple cell types, both resident within and recruited to the tissue around the implant site, as well as diverse molecular mediators, are involved in propagating, sustaining, and resolving the inflammatory response.

The predominant cell type presents in the inflammatory response varies with the age of the injury. Neutrophils (polymorphonuclear leukocytes, PMNs) characterize the acute inflammatory response. In general, neutrophils dominate during the first several days following injury and then are replaced by infiltrating blood-derived monocytes/macrophages as the predominant cell type. Neutrophils are short-lived cells that attack pathogens and foreign materials at the wound site and disintegrate after 24–48 h of wound formation. Neutrophils are often accompanied by host mast cells in acute inflammatory phases. Mast cell activation results in degranulation, with histamine release and fibrinogen adsorption known to mediate acute inflammatory responses to implanted biomaterials (Tang et al., 1998). The extent of release of cytokines interleukin-4 (IL-4) and IL-13 from mast cells in degranulation processes plays a significant role in subsequent development and degree of the FBR (Zdolsek et al., 2007). Biomaterial-mediated inflammatory responses may be modulated by histamine-mediated phagocyte recruitment and phagocyte adhesion to implant surfaces facilitated by adsorbed host fibrinogen, among many other possible host proteins (Anderson and Patel, 2013). Monocytes arriving at the implantation site following earlier PMNs undergo phenotypic changes, differentiating into macrophages. Monocyte infiltration depends on chemotactic cues from tissue injury as well as inflammatory signals secreted by PMNs. That this recruitment depends on the implanted biomaterial characteristics and tissue site is arguable: it appears to be relatively ubiquitous. Chronic inflammation is characterized by the presence of precursor monocytes, macrophages, and lymphocytes adhered to the biomaterial in addition to the proliferation of blood vessels associated with both macrophage and endothelial cell actions, and abundant connective tissue produced by late arriving myofibroblasts.

The progression of events in host inflammation and eventual FBR requires the extravasation and migration of monocytes/macrophages to the implant site. The guided movement of monocytes/macrophages to the implant occurs in response to evolving presence of multiple cytokines, chemokines, and other chemoattractants produced at the implant site upon injury, resulting acute hemostasis, and associated immediate acute inflammatory cell responses. Following blood–material interactions associated with acute wounding (surgery and implant placement naturally always produces wounding, even if minimally invasive as discussed in Chapter 2), platelets in the resulting clot release chemoattractants such as transforming growth factor (TGF-β), platelet-derived growth factor (PDGF), CXCL4 (platelet factor, PF4), leukotriene (LTB4), and IL-1. These agents can direct blood monocytes and tissue-resident macrophages to the wound site (Broughton et al., 2006). Interaction of implant-adsorbed proteins with adhesion receptors present on inflammatory cell populations constitutes the major cellular recognition system for implantable synthetic materials and medical devices (Hu et al., 2001). Adsorbed wound-site proteins such as albumin, fibrinogen, complement, fibronectin, vitronectin, globulins, and many others are implicated in modulating host inflammatory cell interactions and are thus linked to subsequent inflammatory and wound healing responses (Jenney and Anderson, 2000). Understanding protein adsorption *in vivo* is complicated by the number and different types of proteins present, and that their adsorptive interactions with biomaterials surfaces vary with time, often independent of their relative mass fractions present in biological milieu (i.e., the so-called Vroman effect, Bamford et al., 1992) and Chapter 5. That these proteins likely change their compositional fractions and resulting wound-site reactivities further confounds interpretations of their involvement in the aged FBR response. Most Vroman effects with biomaterials have been studied in the context of blood coagulation. Little is known about the alterations in the Vroman response or protein alterations of the FBR as a function of age.

Recruitment of macrophages to the implant site further propagates chemoattractant signals. Macrophage activation *in situ* prompts production of PDGF, tumor necrosis factor (TNF-α), granulocyte colony-stimulating factor (G-CSF), and granulocyte macrophage colony-stimulating factor (GM-CSF) attracting more macrophages to the wound site (Broughton et al., 2006). Monocyte chemotactic protein (CCL2 or MCP-1) is known to surround implanted polyethylene materials (Hu et al., 2001). An array of other inflammatory mediators including IL-1, IL-6, IL-10, IL-12, IL-18, TGF-β, IL-8, and macrophage inflammatory protein (MIP)-1α/β are also produced by monocytes/macrophages (Rot and von Andrian, 2004; Fujiwara and Kobayashi, 2005). Macrophages are also capable of secreting growth and angiogenic factors important in the regulation of fibro-proliferation and angiogenesis (Singer and Clark, 1999). Alternatively, activated macrophages over-express certain ECM proteins, such as fibronectin, and are involved in tissue remodeling during wound healing (Mosser, 2003). The diverse biological functions of activated macrophages play central roles in inflammation and host defense response. A comprehensive discussion of macrophage plasticity and the role of this cell type are discussed in Chapter 6.

Macrophages are professional phagocytes capable of ingesting large amounts of small particles and debris ($<5\,\mu m$), while larger particle sizes ($>10\,\mu m$) cannot be internalized. The inability of macrophages to phagocytose supra-cellular sized foreign objects leads to "frustrated phagocytosis" around such large objects (Mosser, 2003), releasing mediators of degradation such as reactive oxygen intermediates (ROIs, oxygen free radicals) or degradative enzymes around the biomaterial surface (Henson, 1971). This inflammatory reaction, prolonged if the foreign body (i.e., biomaterial) resists degradation and phagocytic clearance, also correlates with the formation of multinucleated giant cells known as foreign body giant cells (FBGCs) (Xia and Triffitt, 2006). As discussed in detail in Chapter 2, cell–cell fusion of monocytes and macrophages to form multinucleate FBGCs requires a series of highly orchestrated biochemical and cellular events around the implant (Chen et al., 2007a). FBGCs display an antigenic phenotype similar to monocytes and macrophages formed from the fusion of monocyte-derived macrophages (Athanasou and Quinn, 1990). Formation of these cells is a histological hallmark of the FBR, although the precise role for FBGCs in the FBR is still unresolved. Their presence is generally localized to the implant surface and correlates with increased fibroblast presence around the implant and the encapsulation of the biomaterial (Shive and Anderson, 1997). Further understanding of dynamics and interactions of immune system components with inflammatory cells at implants is crucial for designing controls for these events to improve the host response, tissue integration, safety, biocompatibility, and function of these devices (Anderson et al., 2008).

THE HOST IMMUNE RESPONSE

The human body's response to implanted biomaterials is governed by its immune system, broadly classified into innate and adaptive immunity, sourced primarily by lymphoid organs (see Chapters 6, 7, and 8). Innate immunity is host intrinsic, natural immunity while adaptive immunity is acquired immune sensitivity and specificity over time due to exposure to foreign antigens, including pathogens and foreign materials. Implanted biomaterials are known to be antigenic, serving as adjuvants and primers of antigen-processing and -presenting cells (APCs) (Babensee, 2008; Yoshida and Babensee, 2004; Mikos et al., 1998). Implants also adsorb many proteins, including immunoglobulins, which prime immune cells (Ziats et al., 1990). Implants also ubiquitously activate complement as a potent immune cell stimulus. Hence, actual immunogenic and immune-stimulating aspects of implants contribute to the both innate and adaptive aspects of the host FBR.

Biological scaffold materials comprising processed mammalian ECM, typically allogeneic-or xenogenically derived tissues, elicit both innate and acquired immune host response (Badylak and Gilbert, 2008). Implantation of engineered cellular biomaterial hybrids elicits adaptive immune reactions toward the cellular component that influences the host response to the material component. Degradation products and surface alterations to the biomaterial also trigger both inflammatory and immune responses (Franz et al., 2011). Lymphocytes and plasma cells are involved principally in immune reactions and as key mediators of antibody production and delayed hypersensitive responses (Ratner, 2004). Lymphocytes play critical roles in the FBR; adherent lymphocytes predominantly associate with macrophages or FBGCs rather than the implant surface (Brodbeck et al., 2005). Danger signals (e.g., alarmins) released from damaged tissue are recognized by cells of the innate immune system (e.g., macrophages and dendritic cells, DCs) via pattern recognition receptors (PRR) such as scavenger receptors, Toll-like receptors, and C-type lectins, which stimulate both inflammation and immunity (Franz et al., 2011; Kono and Rock, 2008).

Several types of macrophages participate in implant immune responses: classically activated macrophages in early acute phases and regulatory and wound healing macrophages in the chronic resolution stage (Porcheray et al., 2005). Different macrophage populations are generated in response to either endogenous stimuli released by damaged cells or innate immune cells following injury or infection or to adaptive immune signals produced by antigen-specific immune cells. Activated macrophages are triggered by interferon-γ (IFN-γ) released by T helper 1 (Th1) cells during adaptive immunity, or by natural killer (NK) cells during innate immunity, and by TNF-α produced by APCs (Martinez et al., 2008). Wound healing macrophages are generated in response to IL-4 produced by basophils, mast cells, and granulocytes in early innate immune responses or by Th2 cells during adaptive immune responses. Both innate and acquired immune system cells can produce IL-4 and IL-13 which also prompt FBGC formation. IL-4 programs macrophages to down-regulate pro-inflammatory mediators and to promote wound healing processes by contributing to the production of ECM and by activation of fibroblasts. Although wound healing macrophages exert anti-inflammatory activities, they are not capable of down-regulating immune responses (Martinez et al., 2009). Regulatory macrophages also arise during innate and adaptive immune responses, triggered in response to a variety of signals including apoptotic cells, prostaglandins (PGs), IL-10, immune complexes, and glucocorticoids. Regulatory macrophages limit inflammation and dampen immune responses by releasing high levels of IL-10, a potent immunosuppressive cytokine (Mosser, 2003). Macrophages also present antigens to immune-competent cells (Mosser and Edwards, 2008). The various phenotypic profiles of macrophages are described in Chapter 6.

As shown in Chapter 7, DCs are also key players in host innate and adaptive immunity, producing adaptive immune responses through their antigen presentation and T-cell priming capabilities. Contacting biomaterials, activated DCs express an immunogenic phenotype known to be similar to that presented by LPS-activated DCs, characterized by increased expression of co-stimulatory molecules (CD80/CD86), and the DC maturation marker CD83 (Babensee, 2008). Based on the PRR profiles, DC maturation can be promoted or inhibited, leading to immunity or tolerance, respectively (Lutz and Schuler, 2002). Biomaterial-matured DCs are capable of promoting T-cell proliferation and secrete inflammatory cytokines (TNF-α and IL-6) known to further amplify DC maturation (Frick et al., 2010). Cross talk between NK cells and DCs mediates DC maturation, shaping the immune response (Moretta et al., 2008).

COMPLEMENT ACTIVATION

The unique ability of the complement system to discriminate "non-self" is an important mechanism in the body's defense against infection and foreign bodies, including medical devices. The complement system comprises more than 30 plasma and membrane-bound proteins (receptors and regulators) functioning either as enzymes or binding proteins (Nilsson et al., 2007). Complement activation destroys and removes foreign substances, either by direct lysis or by mediating leukocyte function in inflammation and innate immunity. The cascade is initiated via three different activation pathways:

1. Classical pathway triggered by the formation of antigen–antibody complexes
2. Mannose-binding lectin pathway trigged by specific carbohydrates on the surface of microorganisms
3. Alternative pathway triggered directly by foreign surfaces such as implants/biomaterials (Roos et al., 2001).

The main event in convergence of the multiple complement activation pathways is enzymatic cleavage of inactive C3 zymogen into active C3b and C3a by C3 convertase enzymes. Complement activation also occurs in various steps in the wound healing process (Janeway et al., 2001).

Implanted biomaterials activate complement commonly via the alternative pathway (Nilsson et al., 2007) to initiate an inflammatory response, observed to occur during cardiopulmonary bypass, hemodialysis, and with catheters and prosthetic vascular grafts. Complement activation and its subsequent reactions also produce adverse side effects during blood/material interactions with IMDs (Anderson et al., 2008). Complement activation releases C3a, C4a, and C5a peptide fragments, which are anaphylatoxins. These peptides are humoral messengers that bind to specific receptors on neutrophils, monocytes, macrophages, mast cells, and smooth muscle cells (Markiewski et al., 2007). They induce a variety of cellular responses such as chemotaxis, vasodilatation, cell activation, and cell adhesion. Cell surface expression of adhesion molecules is modulated by inflammatory agents including leukocyte adhesion molecules (C5a, LTB4) and endothelial adhesion molecules (IL-1). In the acute inflammation phase, increased leukocytic adhesion leads to specific interactions between complementary adhesion molecules present on the leukocyte and endothelial surfaces (Pober and Cotran, 1990).

Membrane-based integrin receptors expressed by monocytes/macrophages bind complement fragment C3bi and fibrinogen (McNally and Anderson, 2002). The complement components provide initial adhesion to multiple protein ligands participating in receptor–ligand binding and monocyte adhesion. In particular, complement activation on fibrinogen-adsorbed surfaces has been suggested as the primary adhesion event (McNally and Anderson, 1994). IL-4-induced FBGCs are characterized by integrin expression, indicating the potential interactions of complement C3b fragments, fibrin, fibrinogen, and fibronectin. Within minutes to hours following implantation of a medical device, a provisional matrix consisting of fibrin is produced by activation of both coagulation and thrombosis systems, and inflammatory products, released by the complement system, with activated platelets, inflammatory cells, and endothelial cells (Clark et al., 1982). Factor X and vitronectin are found at sites of FBR from biomaterial implantations (Anderson et al., 2008).

The most common complement pathway, the alternative pathway, does not require formation of antibody or immune complexes and is activated by any foreign surface, such as fungal, bacterial polysaccharides, lipopolysaccharides (endotoxin), particle and biomaterial surfaces (Gorbet and Sefton, 2004). Various complement products (C3b, C4b, and iC3b) bind to particles, surfaces, bacteria, and immune complexes in a process called opsonization, facilitating uptake by inflammatory cells (Ricklin et al., 2010). During phagocytosis and opsonization processes, both host IgG and complement-activated fragment C3b adsorb onto biomaterials and are then bound by neutrophils and macrophages with their corresponding cell membrane receptors (Ekdahl et al., 2011). Neutrophils adherent to complement-coated and immunoglobulin-coated nonphagocytosable surfaces release enzymes that trigger inflammation based on the size, surface properties, and biomaterial properties of the implant (Bridges and Garcia, 2008). Complement activation also results in bacterial cell lysis when the terminal attack complex is inserted into the cell membrane (Rus et al., 2005).

Biomaterials are usually classified as '"activating" or "nonactivating" surfaces (Kazatchkine and Carreno, 1988). On an nonactivating surface, negatively charged groups such as carboxyl, sulfate, sialic acid-containing glycoproteins, and bound proteoglycans (i.e., heparans, chondroitins) appear to promote high-affinity association between bound C3b and Factor H (Gorbet and Sefton, 2004). The activating surface is characterized by the presence of nucleophiles such as hydroxyl and amino groups that allow covalent binding of C3b and promote formation of C3 and C5 convertases. Some activating materials generate high levels of both C3b and C5b-9, while others generate high C3b but little C5b-9. However, even low amounts of C5b-9 are able to activate leukocytes and thus a low terminal complement activating material may still induce a significant inflammatory response (Colman, 2006). In addition to overlap with immune-stimulating cascades, complement also intersects the coagulation cascade to modulate each other's activity in the presence of a biomaterial (Markiewski et al., 2007).

THE COAGULATION CASCADE

The surgical placement of implants creates wounds and most wounds bleed, activating the native blood coagulation cascade and exposing IMDs to several thousand blood proteins. Blood coagulation involves a tightly regulated, cascading series of proteolytic reactions resulting in the formation of a cross-linked fibrin clot. The two pathways of coagulation (intrinsic and extrinsic) are independent of each other until they converge to a common terminal pathway resulting in fibrin clot formation by the enzymatic action of thrombin on fibrinogen. Factor XIII is activated by thrombin, which cross-links and stabilizes the newly formed fibrin clot into an insoluble fibrin gel (Ratner, 2004; Gorbet and Sefton, 2004). The key penultimate enzyme, thrombin, is formed following a cascade of blood-based reactions activated upon surface contact of an IMD or foreign body. Initiation of clotting occurs either by surface-mediated protease reactions or through tissue factor (TF) expression by cells at the site of vascular injury. Blood contact with a biomaterial represents a potential stimulus to induce TF expression by monocytes, resulting in blood coagulation through the extrinsic system. Plasma Factor VII (FVII) then binds to TF on cell membranes and requires activation by FVIIa to form a TF–VIIa complex. Coagulation initiated by a TF-dependent extrinsic pathway leads to production of FXa by the FIXa–FVIIIa complex, resulting in thrombin generation (Amara et al., 2008).

The intrinsic pathway is initiated by contact activation of high molecular weight kininogen (HMWK), prekallikrein, and Factor XII with surfaces that are negatively charged, a common result of adsorbed protein layer (Schmaier, 1997). The Vroman effect on blood-exposed biomaterial surfaces leads to fibrinogen replacement over time on surfaces by HMWK, linking the intrinsic pathway to biomaterial-based thrombosis mechanisms. However, adsorption of many other proteins to surfaces can also induce coagulation activation. Leukocytes are required for the TF-dependent pathway. Additionally, platelet activation is often presumed to occur via thrombin generation due to activation of the intrinsic coagulation cascade or by the release of adenosine diphosphate (ADP) from damaged red blood cells or platelets.

Development of thrombosis in aged individuals causes clinical events including deep vein thrombosis and pulmonary embolism (PE) due to the progressive increase in plasma concentrations of some coagulation factors (e.g., factors V, VII, VIII, and IX, fibrinogen) (Abbate et al., 1993; Previtali et al., 2011). Studies have shown a significant increase in fibrinogen concentration in the aged population (65–79 years) compared to younger populations (47–54 years) with the fibrinogen concentration increasing at a rate of 10 mg/dL per decade of age (Kannel et al., 1987). Fibrinogen-adsorbed implants show robust levels of macrophage adhesion and activation. High levels of plasma proteins cause the bridging of platelets via their glycoprotein IIb–IIa complex that serves as a direct substrate of the clot by increasing blood viscosity. Along with an increase in number, an increase in platelet reactivity with aging has also been demonstrated and activated platelets are known to accelerate thrombin generation (Previtali et al., 2011). Platelets of 60-year-old or older individuals aggregate more in response to ADP and collagen than platelets from younger individuals (Kasjanovova and Balaz, 1986). An increase in markers of platelet activation such as plasma β-thromboglobulin (a protein stored in the α-granules of platelets) and platelet membrane phospholipids increased in addition to binding of PDGF to arteries (Bastyr et al., 1990).

As shown in Figure 11.1, coagulation, thrombosis, infection, and inflammatory responses are coupled in host reactions to implanted biomaterial surfaces through wounding, the plasma protein adsorption profile, host inflammatory cell recruitment and competence, and infectious complications. The effect of aging on each of these contributing, interactive responses to IMDs is recognized anecdotally, but mechanisms remain poorly understood. Contributions of physiological redox homeostasis—the complex interactive balance of oxidative and reductive physiological processes elicited enzymatically and biochemically—normally control inflammatory and healing pathways (Droge, 2002). Imbalance in redox processes is associated with aging, disease, and foreign body reactions (FBR). Hence, as clarified in detail below, their collective implications as critical processes in aged responses to IMDs are apparent. Further sections below provide anecdotal insights into the variations caused by aging in each of these responses and their cellular mediators.

AGING-RELATED CHANGES IN INFLAMMATION, IMMUNE RESPONSE, COAGULATION, AND COMPLEMENT ACTIVATION

Age-related changes in both hemostasis and compromised, delayed wound healing in elderly patients are clinically acknowledged (Guo and Dipietro, 2010). Recruitment of inflammatory cells such as monocytes, macrophages, and lymphocytes is observed to be delayed at wound sites, with cell numbers peaking at day 84 in aged populations instead of day 7 for monocytes, and at day 21 for lymphocytes in younger populations. However, increased numbers of matured macrophages and a strong expression of activation marker E-selectin was observed in aged populations when compared to a lower number and decreased expression in younger patients (Ashcroft et al., 1998). Optimal wound healing requires both appropriate macrophage infiltration and phagocytic activity. Age-related changes have also been reported for T-cell infiltration into wounds, with alterations in wound chemokine content and concurrent decline in wound macrophage phagocytic function (Swift et al., 2001). Murine model studies report alterations in inflammatory cell content and elevation of MCP-1 levels in wounds of aged mice. Chemokines including MIP-2, MIP-1a, MIP-1b, and eotaxin tended to decline with age (Swift et al., 2001).

The normal aging process involves accumulation of genetic mutations, oxidative and cellular stresses, mitochondrial dysfunction, increased apoptosis, telomere length dysfunction, and differential gene expression that result in changes in cellular functions in wound healing processes (Kapetanaki et al., 2013). These cumulative genetic changes are also likely involved in common age-related "inflammatory diseases" such as metabolic syndromes, diabetes, sarcopenia, dementia, atherosclerosis, cancer, and osteoporosis (McGeer and McGeer, 1999). Metabolic syndromes, referring to a cluster of clinical factors, e.g., insulin resistance, hyperinsulinemia, high blood glucose, hypertension, and dyslipidemia with elevated triglycerides and low HDL levels are associated with both elderly populations and compromised wound healing (Hoffmann et al., 2007). Cause–effect relationships in these syndromes regarding healing are complex, and neither well understood nor well clinically controlled. Recent studies indicate that chronic up-regulation of pro-inflammatory mediators (e.g., TNF-α, IL-1β, IL-6, cyclooxygenase-2 (COX-2), inducible nitric oxide synthase (iNOS)) is induced during aging, resulting

Pathways of ROS production and clearance

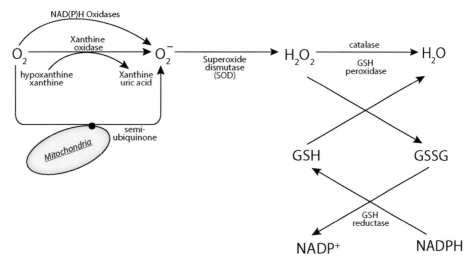

Figure 11.2 The molecular basis for biochemical oxygen free radical ROS generation through host-regulated production of nitric oxide and other oxygen free radicals, and host mitigation as a natural phenomenon in host redox balance. *(Adapted from Droge, 2002, with permission.)*

from age-related redox imbalance and sustained presence of reactive oxygen and nitrogen species (ROS and RNS, respectively). Figure 11.2 shows the molecular basis for ROS generation and mitigation as a natural phenomenon.

ROS include the important superoxide radical O_2^- and nonradical oxygen species singlet oxygen ($^1O_2$), hydrogen peroxide, and peroxynitrite anion ($ONOO^-$); hydrogen peroxide converts into the highly reactive hydroxyl radical (•OH). RNS include nitrosonium cation (NO^+), nitroxyl anion (NO^-), or peroxynitrite ($ONOO^-$), all resulting from oxidation of one of the guanido-nitrogen atoms of L-arginine by the endogenous enzyme, NOS. The most important radicals in biological regulation are ROS molecule superoxide and RNS species, NO. ROS and RNS are produced normally at low concentrations as part of the homeostatic redox balance as required by normal redox signaling used in many biochemical pathways. A redox balance is normally provided by intracellular antioxidant enzymes including superoxide dismutase (SOD), catalase, glutathione peroxidase, peroxiredoxin, and sulfiredoxin, and low molecular weight antioxidants such as glutathione, α-tocopherol (vitamin E), β-carotene, and ascorbate (vitamin C). Antioxidants as natural reducing equivalents act in tandem to produce a balance between the rates of ROS/RNS production and rates of their clearance by various antioxidant compounds and enzymes. Figure 11.3 shows how ROS signaling works and interacts with antioxidant species in balance.

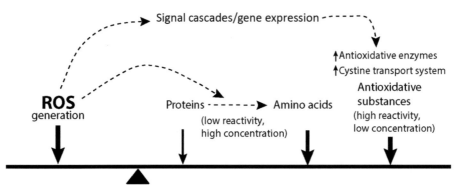

Figure 11.3 Balance between ROS production and various types of free radical scavengers that facilitate redox balance and homeostasis. Local tissue steady-state concentrations of ROS are determined by opposing rates of ROS production and respective clearance. Host free radical scavenging mechanisms use molecular reducing equivalents (antioxidant capacity) to neutralize oxidative burden. Prominent antioxidant enzymes (e.g., SOD, glutathione peroxidase, catalase, and thioredoxin) and nonenzymatic antioxidant small molecules (e.g., vitamins C and E, glutathione) are potent ROS scavengers but are present at relatively low concentrations in cells. Some amino acids and proteins are also ROS scavengers and are less potent that classical antioxidants but their cumulative intracellular concentration is much higher (i.e., >0.1 M). Local consumption of host reducing equivalents without elimination of oxidative stimuli leads to tissue oxidative stress. *(Adapted from Droge, 2002, with permission.)*

Depletion of endogenous antioxidants allows RNS and ROS to increase, altering the cell's normal redox condition and leading to oxidative stress. Eventually, with healing or elimination of disease, reducing equivalents are typically restored in tissues, oxidative stimulus is eliminated and the redox balance returns to homeostasis. Chronic unresolved inflammation, however, results in redox dysregulation, chronic depletion of antioxidants, maintenance of high ROS and RNS concentrations and production, and abnormal redox imbalance (Figure 11.4).

Sustained oxidative stress from continual unabated ROS and RNS production and production of pro-inflammatory mediators around IMDs are a natural part of the host FBR (Chung et al., 2009). Hence, ROS and RNS production is sustained around implants (Chung et al., 2009). ROS is often a transient product of normal inflammatory activities, serving to prompt many pro-inflammatory signaling pathways, including the nuclear factor-κB (NF-κB) signaling pathway involved in redox homeostasis through transcriptional regulation (Figure 11.5) (Chung et al., 2009).

Moderate, temporal changes in ROS and RNS are normal and critical to regulatory processes in physiological signaling, including protection of cells against oxidative stress. However, age-induced oxidative stress provoked by sustained redox imbalance and excess ROS and RNS activity is considered to be among the major factors contributing

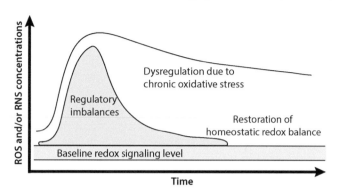

Figure 11.4 Local tissue redox balance depends on both magnitude and duration of ROS or RNS concentration changes at tissue and implant sites. ROS and RNS amounts in living tissues normally present at relatively low steady-state levels. Host-regulated increase in superoxide or nitric oxide free radical production as a natural response to insult leads to a temporary oxidative stress as a normal consequence, and redox imbalance as the basis of host tissue redox regulation. Sustained, persistent production of excessive amounts of ROS or RNS produces changes in local cellular signal transduction and gene expression to accommodate the increased local redox stress that eventually can produce a new elevated redox set point upon reestablishing redox homeostasis and or pathological conditions under chronic oxidative stress. *(Adapted from Droge, 2002, with permission.)*

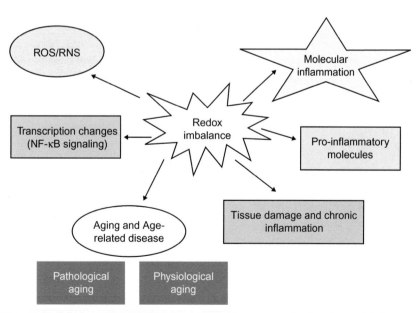

Figure 11.5 Oxidative stress consequences in a tissue site proposed to be responsible for age-related and homeostatic physiological functions.

to aging (Rahman, 2007). The "free radical theory of aging" refers to the toxic effects of sustained RNS and ROS presence during redox imbalance. This imbalance increases exponentially with age, paralleled by decline in the intrinsic cellular repair machinery (Beckman and Ames, 1998). ROS and RNS can normally be detoxified within the cell by several antioxidants, using both enzymatic and nonenzymatic mechanisms. In aging, systemic imbalance among the sophisticated antioxidant system and ROS and RNS presence results in generation of excess in free radicals that overwhelms host cellular antioxidant defenses (Cencioni et al., 2013). Often this balance in elderly patients is never normally reestablished; the high oxidative stress remains unresolved, serving to compromise other host repair and homeostatic mechanisms.

The consequences of increased ROS and RNS may include direct damage to DNA and apoptosis, among others (Barja, 2004). For example, macrophages in inflammatory sites can produce copious amounts of hydrogen peroxide ($\sim$2–6 $\times$ 10^{-14} mol/h/cell) in their oxidative burst reaction to foreign bodies, reaching local tissue sites concentrations of 10–100 μM (Droge, 2002). Accommodating reductive enzymatic processes normally serve to reestablish local redox balance to resolve this inflammatory assault. However, redox imbalance is prolonged in the presence of unresolved FBR (e.g., in response to nondegradable biomaterials). Additionally, aging compromises the oxidative and reductive enzymatic and biochemical pathways to hinder such rebalance. Sustained, unresolved activation of the cellular network of NF-κB dependent, pro-inflammatory molecules appears to be a molecular mechanism underlying numerous age-related diseases including dementia, cardiovascular disease, cancer, obesity, metabolic syndrome, and osteoporosis (Yu and Chung, 2006). Numerous studies support sustained, perhaps aberrant inflammatory pathway activation with altered redox imbalance as a primary factor underlying age-related diseases and aging processes (Chung et al., 2009). Chronic up-regulation of pro-inflammatory mediators (e.g., TNF-α, IL-1β, IL-6, COX-2, iNOS) is related to redox imbalance that activates many pro-inflammatory signaling pathways, including the NF-κB signaling pathway (Figure 11.5) (Brod, 2000). This age-related redox imbalance is caused by weakened antioxidative defense systems and continually increasing production of radical reactive species (e.g., ROS/RNS) (Kim et al., 2002). Overproduced and unregulated ROS/RNS during aging (Figure 11.4) are instrumental factors in immune system activation mediated in past by overreactive macrophages in the inflammatory process (Kim et al., 2002; Zou et al., 2004; Chung et al., 2006). That redox homeostasis is altered without normal physiological stabilization, or even reset to a higher level of oxidative stress in aging is a growing concept (Droge, 2002).

Clinical evidence supporting the age-related sustained unresolved inflammatory state hypothesis is based on two established findings, namely dysregulation of the immune system with age and altered redox status during aging (Chung et al., 2002). Excessive and unregulated ROS and RNS during aging are a major causative factor in immune system activation as exemplified by overreactive macrophages in the inflammatory process (Chung et al., 2006). Relationships between oxidative stress and inflammation are closely related to the well-recognized biosynthetic pathway of PGs that produces various reactive species (Koh et al., 2005). Redox imbalance significantly attenuates NF-κB, TNF-α and TNF-β, interleukins (IL-1β, IL-2, and IL-6), chemokines (IL-8 and Regulated on Activation, Normal T Cell Expressed and Secreted (RANTES)), and adhesion molecules (Zou et al., 2004). COX activity and the production of TXA2 and PGI2 are also increased during aging. Pro-inflammatory proteins, such as cellular adhesion molecules (CAMs) (e.g., VCAM-1, ICAM-1, and P- and E-selectins), are all up-regulated during aging (Zou et al., 2004). Aging is also associated with increased levels of inflammatory markers such as high-sensitivity C-reactive proteins used for risk assessment in the primary prevention of cardiovascular disease (Koh et al., 2005; Ridker, 2001). It is notable that many immune functional regulators in redox processing of wound healing are also key players in the FBR. Therefore, while a paucity of clinical data cofounds the direct correlation of inflammatory state redox dysregulation in the aged with implant-associated exacerbation of these pathways, redox dysregulation in the aged must interfere with or alter typical FBR cascades as well. How this results in marked changes of the FBR in the aged implanted patient is generally unreported.

Regarding hemostasis, aging correlates with increased plasma levels of fibrinogen, FVII, and FVIII, known to be risk factors for thrombotic disease (Franchini, 2006). Increased arterial thromboembolism in the elderly may be attributed to modifications of platelet membrane lipid composition, increased in the cholesterol/phospholipid ratio and a decrease in linoleic acid with possible related changes in cell membrane fluidity. Clinical evidence supports thromboembolic risks with age: the incidence of PE increases from 120 in 100,000 persons per year in the 65–69 years age group to more than 700 in 100,000 subjects per year in the 85 years and older group (Silverstein et al., 1998). Similarly, the frequency of myocardial infarction and stroke increases significantly with age (American Heart Association 2000, 2001; Wilkerson and Sane, 2002). Fibrinolytic activity is impaired in the elderly, likely due to reduced tissue plasminogen activator activity and increased plasminogen activator inhibitor 1 (Abbate et al., 1993).

Aging and cell senescence

Implants are prone to infection years after implantation even when surrounded by innumerable implant-resident macrophages as part of the host FBR. Additionally, pathogen inoculum necessary to produce an implant infection is orders of magnitude less than that required for infection in the absence of an implant; the reasons for which are poorly understood (Moriarty et al., 2014). Clearly, the FBR produces an infection-tolerant tissue niche that is distinct from normal tissue wounding and exhibits compromised immune competence. The local implant environment could adversely influence the implant-associated macrophage phenotype, proliferative capacity, activation states, sensitivity to infectious cues, and ability to neutralize pathogens. Additionally, macrophage senescence and quiescence is recently reported (Holt and Grainger, 2012), reducing these cells' ability to phagocytose around implants. Additionally, increased intracellular ROS production is known to induce cellular senescence (Colavitti and Finkel, 2005). Hence, sustained redox dysregulation (vida supra, Figures 11.4 and 11.5) around implants and in the aged both should therefore promote macrophage senescence and their reduced or otherwise altered activation. Little direct evidence for this hypothesis is available for the aged or implanted patient.

Cellular senescence occurs due to irreversible cell cycle arrest triggered by a variety of cellular damage or stress inducers, including disease, DNA damage, chromatin disruption, oncogene activation, oxidative stress, telomere dysfunction and attrition (Jun and Lau, 2010; Collado et al., 2007), and environmental and nutritional factors (Rodier and Campisi, 2011; Jeyapalan and Sedivy, 2008). Senescent cells are arrested to mitogenic stimulation but remain viable and metabolically active. In addition, senescent cells show widespread changes in chromatin organization and gene expression (Kuilman and Peeper, 2009). Accumulated DNA mutations or disrupted gene expression results in premature aging due to redox imbalance and ROS accumulation (Chen et al., 2007b).

Senescent cells express a senescence-associated secretory phenotype (SASP), leading to changes that include secretion of numerous pro-inflammatory cytokines (IL-1, IL-6, IL-8), chemokines, growth factors (MCP2, MCP4, MIP-1a, MIP-3a), ECM-degrading proteases (matrix metalloproteinases, MMPs), and down-regulated expression of ECM components (e.g., collagen) (Coppe et al., 2008; Young and Narita, 2009; Campisi, 2013; Coppe et al., 2011; Zhang, 2007; Lim, 2006). The link between the Hayflick limit (number of divisions that cells complete upon reaching the end of their replicative life span) and aging was largely made on the basis that replicatively senescent cells appeared to be degenerate, although they remained viable and metabolically active (Hayflick, 1965; Hayflick and Moorhead, 1961; Campisi, 2011). Therefore, senescent cells may have diverse and context-dependent effects on tissue pathologies (Irani et al., 1997). Although senescent cells have been found in various noncancerous pathologies and aging-related diseases, their roles in these contexts have not been thoroughly investigated (Jun and Lau, 2010). Effects of senescent cells and SASP include creating local and systemic inflammation, disrupting normal tissue structure and function leading to occurrence of cancer with aging (Schraml and Grillari, 2012; Provinciali et al., 2013). Senescent cells can also disrupt normal tissue structures and function (Campisi, 2013). These senescence-mediated effects are hypothesized to cause or contribute to age-related changes (Gredilla and Barja, 2005) affecting intimal thickening and medial hypertrophy of pulmonary arteries (Karanjawala and Lieber, 2004; Lu et al., 2004) leading to pulmonary hypertension, and aging of the skin leading to epidermal thinning and loss of collagen (Melov et al., 2001). Endothelial cell senescence is associated with endothelial dysfunction and vulnerability to atherosclerotic lesions.

Skin wound healing involving rapid synthesis and deposition of ECM to maintain tissue integrity is also known to have self-limiting wound healing due to myofibroblast senescence (Jun and Lau, 2010). Myofibroblasts are naturally driven into senescence at late stages of wound healing, thereby converting these ECM-producing cells into ECM-degrading cells and imposing a self-limiting control on fibrogenesis (Scheid et al., 2000). Myofibroblast senescence is triggered by dynamically expressed matricellular protein, CCN1 (also known as CYR61), through membrane integrin signaling (Kim et al., 2013). Using biomarkers, senescent cells have been detected *in vivo* in a variety of tissues in a number of different organisms including rodents, primates, and humans. *In vivo* studies have also found an age-associated increase in the occurrence of senescent cells in normal tissues (Herbig and Sedivy, 2006; Ressler et al., 2006). There is also evidence indicating that progressive telomere shortening, a biomarker of cellular aging, occurs in human blood vessels, which may be related to age-associated vascular diseases. Thus, vascular cell senescence *in vivo* may contribute to the pathogenesis in vascular aging (Minamino and Komuro, 2007).

Based on these effects, many possible cell senescence-induced relationships to the FBR in aged, implanted patients might be considered, including redox dysregulation and senescence in macrophage populations around the implant site, poor vascularization associated with endothelial cell dysfunction, and collagen matrix alterations (possibly both local reduction and also uncontrolled up-regulation depending on balances of different dysfunctional contributions *in situ*). Alterations to numerous spatial and temporal dynamic and interactive effects that influence cell–cell signaling in normal wound healing and also in the FBR are not known in the elderly.

Aging and nutritional effects on physiology

Normal wound healing requires adequate nutrition. Malnutrition impedes the proper progression of wound healing processes resulting in chronic nonhealed wounds (Stechmiller, 2010). FBRs around IMDs are also an example of a chronic nonhealed wound as well. Malnutrition can negatively affect wound healing by prolonging the inflammatory phase, decreasing fibroblast proliferation, and altering collagen synthesis (Arnold and Barbul, 2006; Campos et al., 2008). Malnutrition prolongs the inflammatory phase by reducing the proliferation of fibroblasts and formation of collagen as well as reducing wound tensile strength and angiogenesis. Malnutrition also places the patient at risk for infection by decreasing T-cell function, phagocytic activity, and complement and antibody levels (Campos et al., 2008). Host response to an IMD in the context of the FBR exhibits several distinctions to those of malnutrition, including over-expression of collagen from abundant recruited fibroblasts, and enhanced inflammatory markers.

Elderly populations often suffer from malnutrition due to several factors such as alterations in their diet, reduced food consumption, loss of appetite, decreased energy requirements, loss of teeth, and poor digestion/metabolism. Malnutrition is caused by reduced availability of macro- and micronutrients to the body. The ability of older adults to accurately regulate energy intake is impaired due to delayed rate of absorption of mac-ronutrients and numerous hormonal and metabolic mediators of energy regulation that change with aging (Roberts and Rosenberg, 2006). Micronutrients have been known to contribute directly to the functioning of homeostatic mechanisms such as antioxidant activity, immune, and inflammatory systems (Mocchegiani et al., 2008). Some micro-nutrients (e.g., zinc, copper, selenium) play an important role in maintaining homeo-static mechanisms as redox enzyme cofactors in redox balance and by influencing several genes that regulate immune and inflammatory responses (Mocchegiani et al., 2008; Mocchegiani et al., 2012). Zinc has been identified as indirectly responsible for the inhibi-tion of NF-κB via the TNF-receptor-associated factor pathway (Prasad, 2008). Lastly, body adipose composition changes substantially with age, reducing defense against infection (Rosenberg and Miller, 1992). Since IMDs intrinsically have enhanced infection propen-sity, implants in aged patients might be predicted to infect more often as they are suscepti-ble to higher incidence of diabetes and other medical comorbidities (Patel et al., 2007; Lai et al., 2007). Nonetheless, little clinical data are yet available to compare infections rates for different types of implants as a function of age or comorbidities. In hip and knee implant procedures, increased risk of infection is attributed to both the incidence of diabetes and greater number of medical comorbidities (at least three). (Patel et al., 2007; Lai et al., 2007) Since the incidence of both diabetes and comorbidities naturally increase with increasing age, infection incidence would be presumed to follow this trend with age as well.

AGING AND IMMUNE FUNCTIONAL CHANGES: IMMUNOSENESCENCE AND CHANGES IN CELL FUNCTIONS, SIGNALING, AND CELL–CELL INTERACTIONS

Immunosenescence is defined as the state of dysregulated immune function that con-tributes to the increased susceptibility of the elderly to infection and, possibly, to auto-immune disease and cancer (Castle, 2000). Aging alters both innate (monocytes, NK, DCs) and adaptive (B- and T-lymphotypes) immunity (Weiskopf et al., 2009). The clini-cal consequences of immunosenescence include increased susceptibility to infection, malignancy, and autoimmunity, decreased response to vaccination and impaired wound healing (Castelo-Branco and Soveral, 2014). Several factors such as lifestyle, infections, and physiological changes in the innate aging process and risk factors for age-associated diseases all influence the dysregulated immune response (Licastro et al., 2005).

The age-related changes in innate per cell unit activity of NK cells is related to diminished target binding due to inefficiency in cell signaling (Solana et al., 2012). Impaired activation of NK cells leads to impaired response to cytokines (IL-2, IL-12, IFN-α, IFN-β, or IFN-γ) and stimulation of NK cells to produce lymphokine-activated killer (LAK) cells that lyse cells resistant to NK cell lysis (Chakravarti and Abraham, 1999). PMN cells (neutrophils) that are an important component of the first line of defense and the first inflammatory cells recruited to tissue sites in response to inflammation or infection have shown reduced activity in older individuals (Castle, 2000). PMN cell functional cascades are suppressed in older individuals resulting in enhanced apoptosis and impaired killing by single PMN cells (Tortorella et al., 1998). PMN cell function is further compromised in elderly with hyperglycemia (with increased glycosylation of surface molecules or high lipid levels with altered membrane fluidity) (Castle, 2000). As all of these cells are prominent in normal wound healing as well as FBR processes, their functional impairment has profound implications for altering wound healing, immune competence, and the FBR. Specific details for FBR distinctions from younger patients remain unknown; however, growing evidence for age-associated defects in immune response is seen in aged individuals (Ponnappan and Ponnappan, 2011).

Gene variants that are apparently neutral at young age show a greatly different biological role at old and very old age in terms of apoptosis, cell proliferation, and cell senescence (De Benedictis and Franceschi, 2006). Though the number and phagocytic capacity of neutrophils is well preserved in the elderly, certain other functional characteristics of neutrophils from elderly individuals, such as ROS superoxide anion production, chemotaxis, and apoptosis in response to certain stimuli, are reduced (Fulop et al., 2004).

Macrophages play an important role in the initiation of inflammatory responses, elimination of pathogens, manipulation of the adaptive immune response and reparation of damaged tissue and function as "pathogen sensors" (Plowden et al., 2004). Although inflammatory cytokines such as IL-6 are elevated in the plasma of aged animals and humans, the production of inflammatory cytokines by peritoneal macrophages from mice and rats decreases with age (Plowden et al., 2004). Impaired IFN-γ production by macrophages and NK cells has shown to increase susceptibility to parasitic infection in aged mice due to impaired activation of tissue macrophages (De Martinis et al., 2006). Other investigators have demonstrated impaired tumor lysis or decreased nitric oxide synthetase (iNOS) levels from direct activation of macrophages in aged mice by IFN-γ and that endotoxin activation of PMN cell function is suppressed in older individuals resulting in enhanced apoptosis and impaired killing by single PMN cells (Burns and Goodwin, 1997). A nonspecific increase in production of pro-inflammatory proteins (i.e., increase in stimulated production of IL-6, IL-8, and TNF-α and decreased IL-1 production) is observed in the aged population (Ginaldi et al., 2001). Functionally impaired wound healing described in aged mice was reversed when macrophages from young mice were transferred to the aged mice (Burns and Goodwin, 1997).

A result of old age is a decrease in adaptive immunity and increased low-grade chronic inflammatory status from poor redox balance, referred to as "inflamm-aging." This impacts the internal physiology by changing its composition and functional capacity over time. This change is not in immune cells but also in their "microenvironment" or niche (Franceschi et al., 2000). It is well documented that both the T- and B-lymphocyte compartments of the adaptive immune system deteriorate progressively with advancing age (Stout and Suttles, 2005). Age-related changes in T-cell cytokines other than IL-2 and IL-10 have demonstrated a much more varied response, especially for IFN-γ and IL-4 (Bernstein et al., 1999). Age-related decline in T-cell functional changes are thought to result in a shift in the phenotype of circulating T-cells with reduction in the number of naive T-cells (CD45RA$^+$CD4$^+$cells) and relative accumulation of memory T-cells (CD45RO$^+$CD4$^+$ cells) of stimulation (Chakravarti and Abraham, 1999). Similarly, B-cells from older individuals show impaired activation and proliferation that may also be related to changes in co-stimulatory molecule expression (LeMaoult et al., 1997).

Immunosenescence and age-associated factors altering macrophage function are numerous; age-related dysfunction results from normal functional adaptation to these changes. Host macrophages maintain functional plasticity during this dysregulation. Age-related changes in macrophage function may be reversible rather than intrinsic based on the stimuli (e.g., oxidative stress) reduces macrophage capabilities to respond. However, antioxidants have shown some ability to improve responses to inflammatory stimuli (Stout and Suttles, 2005).

Growing evidence indicates age-associated defects in non-T-cells contributing to reduced immune competence in aged individuals. DCs are the major APCs responsible for initiating adaptive immune responses (Miller, 1991). APCs from chronically ill elderly show impaired antigen presentation associated with increased IL-10 and decreased IL-12 levels, suggesting a compromised immune response as a consequence of a double-hit impairment in both T-cells and APCs (Castle et al., 1999). Production of GM-CSF, a key DC growth factor, has been found to diminish in the elderly due to the impaired ability of DCs to differentiate after interaction with T-cells. DCs may have an impaired capacity to cross tissue barriers and to trigger IFN-γ or IL-10 from T-cells (Rhee et al., 2014; Steinman, 2001).

Immunosenescence is functionally recognized by multiple alterations in hematopoiesis, immune cell development and differentiation, and diverse cell functions in elderly, immunosuppressed, and chronically ill individuals (Thoman and Weigle, 1989). Immunosenescence is currently a prognostic factor for human longevity, and thus a more sophisticated understanding of resulting immune dysfunction will enhance clinical solutions for the elderly population (Sansoni et al., 2008). To date, lack of clinical correlations or reports clouds any rational understanding of how immunosenescence links to implant responses and eventual FBR, especially in the elderly patient.

Aging-related wound repair

Aging skin exhibits reduced dermal thickness, decline in collagen content, and a loss of elasticity (Farage et al., 2008). However, the clinical impact of these changes in acute wound healing is small compared to healing in chronic wounds in the elderly population and more related to comorbidities than age alone (Gist et al., 2009).

Epithelialization changes are slower in aged populations with epidermal growth factor and keratinocytes exhibiting reduced activity (Barrientos et al., 2008). Fibroblasts are responsible for the synthesis, deposition, and remodeling of the ECM. Fibroblast proliferation and collagen remodeling responsible for wound-site contraction is delayed in elderly patients and the contracted tissue, or scar tissue, is functionally inferior due to aging (Knowlton, 2004) Fibroblast-based synthesis and reorganization of the ECM are impaired due to reduced biosynthetic/functional response of these cells to stimulation by growth factors with aging. Studies on repair of dermal wounds and myocardial infracts in young and aged mice show that dermal collagen remodeling is slower in aged animals during early stage of tissue repair (Reed et al., 2006). As wound repair is a multistep process consisting of hemostasis, inflammatory cell infiltration, tissue regrowth, and remodeling, age-induced changes in any or all of the interactive pathways will change wound healing dynamics. In aged individuals, this progression of events is altered, resulting in wounds that heal more slowly than wounds in the young. The impact on chronic host responses to IMDs is therefore analogous: aggravated unresolved healing pathways around foreign bodies must be altered in the aged compared to more exuberant responses in the young. How these changes are manifest is not well understood. For example, dermal collagen deposition is slower in the aged (*vida supra*) and excessive type I collagen deposition is promoted in the FBR, but how these two opposing effects balance each other in the aged implanted patient is unknown.

Aging of connective tissue increases collagen type I content in the ECM, whereas collagen type III proteoglycans and elastin fiber content all decrease (Mays et al., 1988; Huang et al., 2007). Collagen production, as measured by hydroxyproline content, is decreased with aging (Viljanto, 1969), shown to be primarily a deficit of type I collagen (Reed et al., 2000). In laying down a new collagen framework, the existing ECM must be degraded, a process mediated by MMPs. Chronic nonhealing wounds show increased levels of MMP expression (Salo et al., 1994). Additionally, delayed healing in the aged has been shown to result from over-expression of MMPs, and under-expression of tissue inhibitors of metalloproteinases (TIMPs) (Wysocki et al., 1993). The delay in wound closure also results in an increased incidence of infection and medical complications and comorbidities common in the older population (e.g., diabetes, vascular disease) (Halasz, 1968). As a consequence of aging and impaired repair capacity, the ECM composition changes and the dynamic interaction between cells and their environment is damaged. The effect of intrinsic and extrinsic aging is a progressive loss of function, increased vulnerability to the environment, and decreased homeostatic capability (Kapetanaki et al., 2013).

In addition to cellular and molecular level influences on subcutaneous wound healing process in aging individuals (Guo and Dipietro, 2010), a number of structural and functional changes occur in aging tissue. Histological changes in skin with aging such as flattening of the dermal–epidermal junction, giving the appearance of atrophy

(Kurban and Bhawan, 1990). In addition, the time for keratinocytes to migrate from the basal layer to the skin surface, a key process in repair, increases by 50% in aged individuals (Gilchrest et al., 1982). With age, there is a flattening of the rete ridges resulting in decreased surface contact between the dermis and epidermis, which promotes separation of the dermal–epidermal junction with laterally applied tension (Montagna and Carlisle, 1979). The cellular content of the dermis, consisting of fibroblasts, mast cells, and macrophages, decreases with age (Swift et al., 2001) in addition to decreases in the number and function of APCs (e.g., Langerhans, DCs and mast cells) in aged skin (Bernstein et al., 1996). The protein content of the dermis, primarily collagen, is decreased with age as a result of both decreased production and increased degradation. The quality of the collagen that remains is altered, with fewer organized, rope-like bundles and a greater degree of disorganization (Lavker et al., 1987). The quantity of elastin, a determinant of skin elasticity, is fairly constant with age. However, like collagen, elastin in the aged dermis displays a disordered morphology, resulting in decreased elasticity of the skin (Gerstein et al., 1993). Along with these changes, blood flow, and dermal lymphatic drainage decreases with increasing age, diminishing the ability to clear the wound of pathogens and also inhibiting wound contraction (Lavker et al., 1987). Altered cell–fibronectin interactions may contribute to abnormal tissue remodeling by stimulating fibroblast proliferation, myofibroblast differentiation, and epithelial–mesenchymal transition, or facilitating local deposition of other matrix components, such as collagens. Increased MMP expression with age may increase susceptibility to tissue injury, prompting increased leukocyte migration and further tissue damage, indicating that aging leads to changes in the expression of TGF-β and ECM composition with important implications in the repair process (Sueblinvong et al., 2012).

Aging alters different phases of the healing process with increased pro-inflammatory cytokine productions (Shaw et al., 2013), decreased levels of growth factors, diminished cell proliferation and migration, and diminished ECM secretion during the wound healing process. Aged endothelial cells secrete less nitric oxide, a vasoactive mediator which is accompanied by decreased capillary permeability at the site of injury, decreased neutrophil numbers in contrast to an increase in leukocytes (Polverini et al., 1977). Endothelial CAM up-regulation may also be responsible for several vascular diseases that manifest with age. The proliferative phase of dermal wound repair in young and aged mice showed substantial differences due to delayed re-epithelialization, collagen synthesis, and angiogenesis in aged mice compared with young mice. Aged mice contain significantly reduced angiogenic mediators such as fibroblast growth factor-2 (FGF-2) and vascular endothelial growth factor (VEGF) compared to younger mice (Swift et al., 1999). Reduced levels of TGF-β1, and key matrix protein, type I collagen, in the ECM also contribute to impaired angiogenesis in aged mice (Reed et al., 1998). Studies in rat models with incisional wounds (with impaired wound healing due to aging or glucocorticoid administration) show that intravenously administered recombinant human transforming growth factor-β1 (rhTGF-β1) altered cellular responses that influence the wound healing cascade and resulted in improved wound healing ability (Beck et al., 1993). Adipose changes also cannot be ignored in wound healing in the elderly patient: altered subcutaneous fat distributions and decline in skin capillary surface area are also observed in aged populations. Data about the role of angiogenesis with aging are conflicting in the literature, with a majority of studies indicating a decrease (Holm-Pedersen and Viidik, 1972) in angiogenesis with age and others showing increases (Passaniti et al., 1992). Wound capillary ingrowth is delayed in aged animals due to reduced levels of angiogenic factors (e.g., FGF, VEGF, and TGF-β) (Rivard et al., 1999).

Epigenetic influences in aging

New studies demonstrate the appearance of age-associated diseases with both genetic and epigenetic changes in the host genome. Epigenetics involves the ability of somatically acquired and, in some cases, trans-generationally inherited chromatin modifications to alter gene expression but without altering DNA coding (Berger et al., 2009; Skinner, 2011). Epigenetic mechanisms can induce flexible, short-term gene silencing (i.e., through histone tail modifications), and more stable, longer-term gene expression (i.e., through DNA methylation). Overall, epigenomic control relies on a diverse number of histone-modifying complexes, DNA methylation enzymes, and noncoding RNAs that regulate chromatin structure and thereby its expression (Illi et al., 2009). An epigenetic trait is a stably heritable phenotype resulting from transient changes in a chromosome without changing the actual DNA sequence. Epigenetic changes during aging include both DNA methylation and histone acetylation reactions that lead to "dys-differentiation," declining multi-potency of adult stem cells with changes in their total numbers and irreversible alterations (Oberdoerffer et al., 2008). Various epigenetic changes have emerged as important new mechanisms by which cells change during development and cellular differentiation without permanent genetic alterations, and in response to environmental stimuli and stress (Berger et al., 2009). Tight control of this network is normally sustained for all biological processes; as shown in Figure 11.6, any dysregulation of the network as is found in tissue redox imbalance and unresolved oxidative stress is associated with disease and aging (Berdasco and Esteller, 2010).

Host epigenetic processing at specific targets and markers is proposed to orchestrate cellular and organismal homeostasis. Alteration of epigenetic mechanisms may lead to accumulation of functional errors and to ageing-associated diseases, such as cancer. Indeed, aged organisms present a peculiarly modified epigenome (Cencioni et al., 2013). Aging is characterized by accumulating effects of oxidative stress. It is also correlated with specific histone modifications (Cencioni et al., 2013). Global hypo-methylation witnessed in the aged genome is correlated with the normal accumulation of ROS and RNS damage and also decreased DNA methylation enzyme

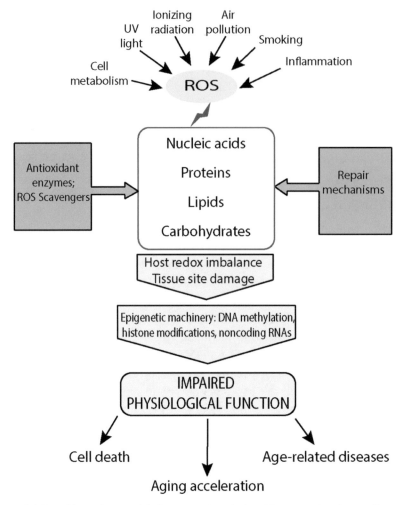

Figure 11.6 Origins of host tissue oxidative stress, its relationships to molecular mediators of redox balance, the epigenetic response, and aging phenomena associated with sustained oxidative insult and redox imbalance from sustained oxygen free radical (ROS and RNS) generation. *(Adapted from Cencioni et al., 2013, with permission.)*

activity. Hence, epigenetic machinery may represent an additional oxidative stress sensor involved in the progressive homeostasis and functional impairment characteristic of aging, contributing to the cellular senescence common to cell and tissue degeneration. Aging therefore presents specific epigenetic markers that together define what could be called the "aging epigenome." Epigenetic modifications could also reflect physiological or pathological processes experienced when initiating age-associated diseases (Cencioni et al., 2013).

No evidence to date suggests that host response to implants produces or induces epigenetic changes in local tissue sites as are now associated with aging and various pathologies. Additionally, specific epigenetic controls or dysregulation of the FBR are also unknown. Host genetics are integrally linked to epigenetic regulation so that general patterns important to wound healing and aging may be difficult to elucidate. However, since the implant site is a site of chronic inflammation, high ROS production, and redox imbalance, it is likely that epigenetic responses to this environment are naturally prompted and spontaneous. While epigenetics is increasingly linked to aging physiological control, that local epigenetic controls can also be used to modulate the FBR is logical and a promising, attractive new approach for IMD wound-site manipulation.

Aging and stem cell renewal

Stem cells are tissue regenerative tools fundamental to the body's ability to repair and self-renew with advancing age (Conboy and Rando, 2005). These cells exhibit the potential for self-renewal and importantly persist throughout the host life span in a diverse range of tissues (Behrens et al., 2014), maintaining homeostasis (Krishna et al., 2011). They are generally highly proliferative; adult stem cells in particular have a finite replicative life span that is determined to a large degree by telomere attrition (Wright and Shay, 2002). Nonetheless, their self-renewal capacity declines with age and is strongly influenced by genetics on their rate of aging (Roobrouck et al., 2008). Fundamentally, genomic integrity maintenance is heterogeneous and imperfect, meaning that criteria for self-renewal must not be overly restrictive or stringent (Reya et al., 2001). Adult stem cell capacity to resist, detect, and repair changes in the genome (e.g., telomere shortening and mutation accumulation) facilitates their ability to participate in tissue homeostasis and repair across an organism's life span (Reya et al., 2001). Stem cells experience the same aging stress factors that introduce genotypic and phenotypic changes associated with cellular "wear and tear" in other somatic cells. However, their intrinsic, robust ability to detect and resist damage, and continuously produce progeny with properties akin to parental cells sets them apart, importantly the distinction between replicative and chronological aging (Lepperdinger, 2009; Waterstrat and Van Zant, 2009).

Stem cell function is regulated at increasing levels of complexity, from cell-autonomous regulation to regulation by the local cellular environment (Sjoqvist et al., 2014), the surrounding tissue, the systemic milieu of the organism, and ultimately, the external environment (Wysocki et al., 1993). Cells resident in the bone marrow compartment is sensitive and responsive to changes in their niche, which in turn is responsive to changes in the global systemic milieu (Sharpless and DePinho, 2007). It appears intuitive therefore that ecological interactions in bone marrow niches are critical to resident stem cell function. Additionally, the aged tissue microenvironment to which exogenous stem cells are transplanted presents an inhibitory effect. Thus, diminished mesenchymal stem cell (MSC) function associated with natural aging may be due to deleterious changes at the niche level (Jones and Wagers, 2008). *Ex vivo* MSCs from aged rodents and humans show alterations in their expression of stemness and pluripotency-associated genes, indicating an age-associated collective loss of pluripotency-associated genes by MSCs and other bone-marrow-derived stem cells. This includes very small embryonic-like stem cells (VSELs), multi-potent adult progenitor cells, and marrow isolated multi-lineage inducible (MIAMI) cells, suggestive of broad molecular level sensitivity to aberrant changes across their niche (Yew et al., 2011; Asumda and Chase, 2011). Hence, specific age-associated alterations as a consequence of changes in the ecological niche environment will have consequences for MSC function and self-renewal (Asumda and Chase, 2011). Stem cells contribute primarily at an intermediate level of tissue homeostasis and repair, and might therefore participate negligibly to aging phenotypes for tissues with extremely low cellular turnover (Flurkey et al., 2001).

Suppression of adult stem cell proliferation by systemic milieu in aged animals limits tissue regenerative potential and possibly promotes senescence or apoptosis (Hornsby, 2002). Correlations with cellular aging such as telomere shortening have been shown to accompany decline in stem cell functions in both serial transplantation and natural aging (Liu and Rando, 2011). Multi-lineage differentiation, cytokine, paracrine, anti-apoptotic, and angiogenic capacity is fundamentally age compromised in MSCs (Song et al., 2010). However, the idea that stem cells display age-related function impairments remains controversial. Stem cells age differentially. Growth arrest and resultant cellular senescence displayed after a specific number of population doublings alone are not sufficient to completely compromise stem cell functionality *in vivo*. *Ex vivo* adult stem cells isolated from aged donors display characteristic features of both chronological and replicative aging typified by the accumulation of damaged proteins, enzymes, and cellular components required for efficient DNA replication and repair (Cameron, 1972). Other characteristic features are stress-related genome instability, loss of function, and changes in patterns of immunophenotype markers, gene, and protein expression (Yu et al., 2011). The "two-hit" model of leukemogenesis (Greaves, 2002) suggests that the aging of an individual can create cellular conditions conducive or permissive to acute myeloid leukemia development. Such conditions, either in conjunction with an initial mutation or alone and over a lifetime, include exposure to environmental insults, accumulated DNA damage, and/or decreased immune system surveillance (Bell and Van Zant, 2004). But these conditions are different for each individual. The DNA damage model of aging postulates that aging is a direct result of long-term accumulation of deleterious alterations in DNA structure (Garinis et al., 2008). As DNA damages, down-regulation of stemness genes and sustained telomerase activity reflect intrinsic aging; MSC function and self-renewal may also be affected by the changes in the ecological microenvironment (Asumda, 2013).

Declining tissue homeostasis or repair efficiency with age could arise from age-related changes in the numbers or properties of stem cells, in their local environment or niche, in the systemic milieu of the organism that influences all cells, or any combination of these (Harrison et al., 1977). Changes within the niche could include redox imbalance and oxidative stress, ROS and RNS profiles, alterations in ECM amount and composition, changes in cell membrane proteins and lipids in cells that directly contact stem cells, and changes in diverse soluble paracrine and endocrine factors that constitute the systemic milieu (*vida infra*). Stem cell functionality is influenced by systemic changes including oxidative stress, immunological and endocrine changes, and, in the case of tissue injury or disease, changes in factors released from damaged cells and the host inflammatory response that accompany such damage (Rando, 2006). Thus, even in the absence of significant aging effects within stem cells themselves, stem cell functionality could exhibit age-related decline due to decrements in the signals within the local and systemic environment that modulate the function of either stem cells or their progeny. Generally, the effects of age on isolated stems cells are compared using *in vitro* assays of growth, differentiation, apoptosis, transformation, and senescence. These assays naturally lack the complexity and comprehensive character that these cells experience *in vivo*. One study identified the implant-site presence of different primitive and stem cell populations (i.e., Lin^-Sca-1^+, Lin^-CD34^+, Lin^-c-kit^+, and Lin^-CD271^+) during FBR, possessing hematopoietic or mesenchymal colony-forming capacity. The authors concluded that the MSC colonies from tissue were able to differentiate into the adipo-, osteo-, and myofibroblastic lineages (Vranken et al., 2008). Histology and quantitative histomorphometry have shown reduced fracture healing with aging, involving decreased proliferation and differentiation of stem cells lining the bone surface. Aging periosteal progenitor cells have exhibited reduced regenerative responsiveness to bone injury in aged mice compared to young mice (Yukata et al., 2014). Transplantation of MSCs from young donors delays aging in female mice and results in significantly lower loss of bone density, demonstrating some control over tissue regenerative responses (Shen et al., 2011).

Bone-marrow-derived stem cells, hematopoietic stem cells (HSCs) and MSCs also show exhibit age-induced changes. MSCs derived from elderly humans have different morphology, increased production of ROS and oxidative damage, and DNA methylation changes affecting cell differentiation, slower proliferation rate in culture and shorter telomeres. A large fraction stain positive for senescence-associated β-galactosidase (Roobrouck et al., 2008). Aging mice have shown a senescence-related increase in fibrocyte mobilization, quiescent MSCs escape DNA damage checkpoints and several repair pathways that are cell cycle dependent, and that result in the accumulation of DNA damage during aging, ultimately resulting in rapid stem cell depletion or exhaustion (Lavasani et al., 2012). Human MSCs from aged donors did not perform as well as those from young donors: MSCs from old donors fail to differentiate in vitro into neuroectodermal cells, and early passage MSCs are more efficient in promoting the proliferation and maintenance of hematopoietic progenitor cells (Hermann et al., 2010). Aged HSCs seem to be less effective at homing and engrafting, suggesting that intrinsic aging of HSCs can be validated by this type of analysis (Sudo et al., 2000). The extent of intrinsic aging of HSCs also seems to be strain dependent, as determined by competitive-repopulation studies (Morrison et al., 1996). Thus, it appears that the diminished regenerative potential of aged musculoskeletal stem cells (i.e., satellite stem cells) is not primarily due to intrinsic aging of satellite cells, but rather to effects of the aged environment on satellite cell function (Charge and Rudnicki, 2004).

MSCs are immune privileged and immunosuppressive; surface immune antigens are present at minimal levels (Bernardo and Fibbe, 2012). This unique immunophenotype provides these cells a selective advantage fundamental to their clinical appeal. T-lymphocyte proliferation is suppressed, immunogenic major histocompatibility complex (MHC)-Ia expression is marginal, and immunosuppressive MHC-Ib is upregulated. However, MSCs appear to lose their immune privilege properties with advancing age. Whether natural aging exacerbates MSC immunogenicity remains a controversial open question (Uccelli et al., 2008). *In vivo* aging leads to impaired MSC morphology, migration potential, and mitochondrial and cytoskeletal function. The resultant old MSCs display a spread morphology, flattened, and enlarged with nuclei that appear larger than normal (Yu et al., 2011; Asumda, 2013). Proximity between MSCs and stem, and nonstem cells within the three-dimensional bone marrow micromilieu affect MSC function and self-renewal (Yew et al., 2011). Decline in MSC function is typified by the inability to repair injury, and proliferate or differentiate into multiple lineages (Conboy and Rando, 2005). Evidence of declining MSC activity and function both in humans and rodents has been attributed to aging (Asumda and Chase, 2011; Hermann et al., 2010).

Aging and host response to infection

All IMDs, from transient, easily inserted and retrieved contact lenses, urinary and peripheral vascular catheters and endotracheal tubes, to more permanently surgically implanted cardiac valves, embolic coils, vascular grafts, hip, knee and shoulder joints, pacemakers, coronary stents, hernia meshes, and plastic surgery augmentation devices suffer from recognized risks of "device-related" or "implant-associated" infections significantly higher than normal surgical site or wound infections (Wu and Grainger, 2006). IMDs create a local niche with enhanced propensity for tissue and bloodstream infections associated with inserted or IMDs (von Eiff et al., 2005). Importantly, foreign-body-related infections, particularly catheter-related infections, significantly contribute to the increasing clinical problem of nosocomial infections, with substantial treatment costs, morbidities, and mortality (Busscher et al., 2012; Grainger et al., 2013).

Most clinical infections in critically ill aged patients are associated with IMDs. Additionally, the clinical combination of an increasingly aging population and consistently growing numbers and diversities of inserted medical devices escalates the occurrence of infectious complications related to medical devices (Busscher et al., 2012; Grainger et al., 2013;

Kojic and Darouiche, 2004). Many reasons are attributed to increased susceptibility to infection in this patient cohort, including those also associated with reduced inflammatory and immune competences (*vida infra*). Epidemiological factors, immunosenescence, and malnutrition, as well as a large number of age-associated physiological and anatomical alterations associated with chronic oxidative stresses and repair, compromise facilitate infections (Shimada, 1985). Infection then leads to further enhanced inflammation, pathogen-dependent tissue destruction, accelerated cellular aging through increased turnover, and physiological stresses not easily ameliorated by aging defense and homeostatic processes (Phair et al., 1988). Infections in the elderly are frequent, severe, and complicated due to distinct features with respect to clinical presentation, laboratory results, microbial epidemiology, treatment, and infection control (High, 2002).

The majority of device infections in elderly patients are catheter-related, including central venous catheters (CVC), peripherally inserted central venous catheter (PICC), and urinary catheters, and contributions as well from ventilator-associated pneumonia (VAP) endotracheal tubes (Yokoe et al., 2008). Contamination of these inserted, transient medical devices most likely occurs by inoculation with only a few microorganisms, possibly commensal microbes from the patient's skin or mucous membranes during incision and implantation. Most bloodstream infections originate from indwelling vascular catheters, and most cases of pneumonia are associated with mechanical ventilation (Weinstein, 2001).

Latent or chronic infection contributes to or exacerbates the aging process by adding direct tissue destruction and oxidative stresses to already redox-imbalanced tissue milieu (Franceschi et al., 2000). Pathogens that cause chronic infections usually are capable of avoiding host immune response, and through their manipulation of cell and tissue function, sustain aging-promoting stress responses. Host immune-mediated phenomena that promote bacterial persistence are manifested by the reduced complement-mediated opsonic activity and decreased bactericidal activity of leukocyte infiltrates in tissues surrounding the implanted device (Zimmerli et al., 1982). The most studied immune mediator inhibiting persistence of already adherent bacteria on a device surface is IFN-γ. This immune mediator reduces the intracellular persistence of *Staphylococcus epidermidis* living within macrophage phagosomes around catheters subcutaneously implanted in mice and inhibits catheter colonization (Boelens et al., 2000). IFN-γ may exert this protective antibacterial effect by inducing MHC-II proteins on phagocytic cells, activating mononuclear phagocytes, and regulating humoral immune response (Weinstein, 2001). Nonetheless, IFN-γ production is reduced in aging humans, compromising this mechanism and enhancing IMD infection susceptibility (Desai et al., 2010; Michaud et al., 2013).

Sustained inflammatory responses in tissue beds surrounding IMDs (*vida infra* and details in several other chapters in this book) produce local oxidative stresses that remain unresolved for the implant's lifetime *in situ*. This interactive scenario, including

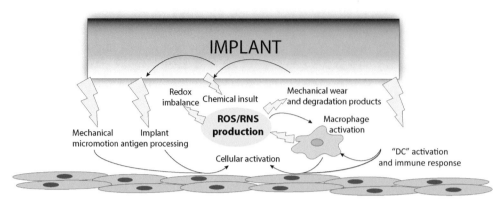

Figure 11.7 Schematic mechanism for oxidative stress generation by chemical or mechanical stimuli from an implanted biomaterial in a tissue bed. Direct and indirect effects of implant wounding, mechanical irritation, and chemical release (e.g., leachates and antigens) on local cell populations produce ROS/RNS generation. Tissue-resident and recruited cells (e.g., acute PMNs) produce ROS via enzymatic pathways that then attract macrophage infiltrates that produce more ROS. Elevated ROS over longer time periods consumes local reducing equivalents and produces redox imbalance that can degrade the implant as well as initiate chronic inflammatory processes. Sustained, persistent oxidative stress from implant-generated ROS/RNS without reestablishing local redox balance leads to chronic inflammation, FBR, and other possible implant-associated infection issues and pathologies. *(Adapted from Cochran and Dziubla, 2012.)*

contributions from both biochemical and mechanical implant stimuli that result in redox signaling and oxidative stress, are shown in Figure 11.7.

Neutrophil oxidative exhaustion, phagocytic frustration, and sustained ROS/RNS production near the implant result with concomitant redox dysregulation around the implant that alters typical healing outcomes. Typical levels of pro-inflammatory cytokines are also abnormal for physiological healing processes around IMDs. Mass transport, neovascularization, and metabolic processes around solid implants are reduced, impacting normal immune, inflammatory, and homeostatic processes associated with healing and reestablishing proper redox balance. Chronic altered cellular responses from infiltrating myofibroblasts produce excessive collagen as an increasing impermeable barrier that further isolates the implant from host physiology and defense sentinels. Reduced phagocytic capacity from resident host phagocytes (e.g., monocyte/macrophage populations) limits pathogen clearance. The "race for the surface" around the implant favors pathogen survival and proliferation in this implant niche (Busscher et al., 2012; Gristina, 1987; Gristina et al., 1987). Correlations between the FBR and implant infections have been intimated for some time (Brunstedt et al., 1995), but beyond clinical correlations, little actual evidence supports direct connections between foreign body infection niches and the FBR's lack of effective host tissue integration or tissue compatibility with an implanted biomaterial surface (Gristina et al., 1990).

Nonetheless, this entire chronological series of FBR physiological and tissue-site events *in situ* is altered in aged patients (*vida infra*). Cellular activities and normal healing and immunological cascades are slowed or compromised. Infection susceptibility is intrinsically enhanced. Increased incidence of cardiac device infection was observed in elderly patients compared to patients who were about 40 years old (Mueller et al., 1990). Increased implant complications and adverse events are also observed in the aged with prosthetic joint, vascular graft and indwelling transurethral catheter infections, endotracheal-tube-associated ventilator infections, and pneumonia in addition to higher rates of *methicillin-resistant Staphylococcus aureus*, and nosocomial infections causing serious clinical implications and mortality (Guggenbichler et al., 2011). Delayed wound healing is observed after total hip replacement surgeries in the elderly due to malnutrition that is difficult to correct than at a younger age (Hebuterne et al., 2001; Guo et al., 2010). Reasons for these increased infection rates and delayed wound healing in the aged populations can be attributed to age-related changes in many host tissue-resident factors already discussed (*vida infra*) and typical age-related comorbidities (e.g., diabetes, atherosclerosis). Whether the FBR is changed in the aged patient and how this further increases host vulnerability to infection should be better understood to mitigate the effects of the contributing factors. The logical conclusion from increasing implant placements into elderly and increasing infection incidence is that aging alters the FBR and that aging adversely impacts host infection resistance, so that aging results in more implant-centered infections. Clinical data to support this idea are scarce.

CONCLUSIONS

Many aspects of physiological homeostasis, including decreased metabolic processes, reduced cell activation, sustained oxidative insult, cumulative molecular and cellular damage, reduced vascular permeability, reduced collagen turnover and remodeling, increased and often imbalanced secretion of inflammatory mediators, delayed infiltration of macrophages and lymphocytes, impaired macrophage functions, and decreased secretion of growth factors lead to increased infections, loss of function, delayed wound healing, and decreased wound strength in aged individuals. Aging-associated altered FBR to IMDs cannot be attributed to any single cell, cytokine, or a regulatory mechanism, since it is a complex multifactorial phenomenon that is the result of several diverse factors including the surrounding tissue microenvironment, host health status, nutrition, and possibly host genetics all working in tandem and influencing wound healing, response to tissue insult, and implant integration. Perhaps the global inability of a host to effectively mitigate ongoing and cumulative oxidative stress damage as the hallmark of aging is also the most direct influence of how the aged are affected by such stress around an implant. Antioxidant-releasing implants are now under development as a local approach to combat uncontrolled oxidative implant-induced stress and the FBR complications in implant healing (Potter et al., 2014; Schweikl et al., 2007; Udipi et al., 2000; Gopinath et al., 2004; Gomathi et al., 2003; Merrell et al., 2009; Tian, 2013).

Many other studies have examined the role of therapeutic options for wound healing in aged populations. Systemically or topically applied growth factors as therapeutics such as TGF-β1, basic FGF (bFGF), PDGF, and others have been shown to offer some benefit in various animal models for wound healing lacking implants (Broadley et al., 1989; Mustoe et al., 1987; Lind, 1998). Ultimately, results from studies in humans have been largely inconsistent with preclinical promise or disappointing: clear clinical recommendations on the use of exogenous therapeutic growth factors lack consensus, either with or in the absence of implanted devices.

Some synthetic biomaterials have shown to promote DC maturation by developing a tolerogenic phenotype resulting in DC tolerance and induced T-cell tolerance (Yoshida and Babensee, 2004). Immunogenic DCs may prolong the immune response to biomaterials and delay wound healing. However, tolerogenic DCs are capable of down-regulating the immune cells and resolving inflammation. Thus, induction of tolerogenic DCs by rationally designing implant surface chemistry appears as a new promising strategy for modulating immune responses to biomaterials, possibly improving biocompatibility and integration (Rutella et al., 2006).

Animal models provide most of the current understanding for the physiological aspects of aging, wound healing, and implant responses. These models are also useful for establishing pharmacological responses and for measuring toxicities of wound-site reactions and products (Thomas, 2001). However, animal models generally have few reliable direct and predictive comparisons to human healing efficiency due to age, type of implant, anatomical, physiological, immunological, and biomechanical differences. Angiogenesis has been studied in either avian chorioallantoic membrane or rabbit corneas, whereas wound tensile strength has been evaluated in a rat linear incision model. Most implant studies are performed in rodent dermis and bone. Rodent bone and skin both differ structurally from human bone and skin and differ in the rate of healing. Collagen deposition begins in rodents on the fifth day of wounding and accumulates rapidly over 36 days. In contrast, collagen accumulation in human wounds is much slower. Hence, parallelization of wound healing models in aged mouse versus elderly human is not accurate and generalized (Harding et al., 2002). Many other aspects of animal models (e.g., animal reactions to anesthesia, distinct metabolic demands, unknown ROS and RNS production, intrinsic aging, different mechanical loading) complicate their direct extrapolation to human use.

Ultimately, the need to better understand complex interactions of host response and biomaterial implants in order to control their functions prompts the need for improved clarity of the possible roles of device engineering and host immune-modulation by new biomaterials (Hubbell et al., 2009). Implant-tissue integration has long been demanded by clinicians to resolve long-standing problems. That this cannot yet be reliably accomplished in younger, more healing-prone patient cohorts preempt the ability to produce success in aged, healing compromised patients, often with other confounding comorbidities. Precise bioactive control of the tissue microenvironment is likely required for effective regeneration and repair of the wound during implant. This tissue integration control would consider different pathways and altered physiological processes in aged patients compared to younger cohorts. Hence, directly addressing the implant response in aged patients would best rely on understanding the specific biochemical and cellular changes that accompany aging and their specific impacts on the FBR. Little of this is currently known.

Strategies for repairing injury and conditioning sites for implants in aged might also be improved by locally delivered therapeutics. Such therapeutics have traditionally included recombinant growth factors, anti-fibrotic, angiogenic, and antimicrobial drugs (Avula and Grainger, 2013; Wu and Grainger, 2006; Brooks et al., 2012), but more recently shift to delivery strategies using antioxidants, cellular delivery around the implant to aid implant integration, ease oxidative burden, and promote angiogenesis. However, single therapeutic agents typically address isolated aspects of the very complex FBR problem, and specifically for the aged, do not appreciate subtle and dramatic changes in homeostatic processes and cumulative stresses characteristic of aging.

Comprehensive approaches successful for addressing the specific requirements of implants in aged patients must first be informed by aging physiology, tissue site-specific functional and healing requirements distinct from younger populations, and the consequences of cumulative oxidative stresses that compromise cellular functions, tissue healing, infection resistance, regenerative capacities, and immune competence that characterize aged tissue beds. Decision points for future improved, age-specific implant designs and wound care regimens following medical implantation in the elderly could be a logical consequence.

ACKNOWLEDGMENT

The authors acknowledge support from National Institutes of Health award 1R01 EB000894 (DWG).

REFERENCES

Abbate, R., Prisco, D., Rostagno, C., Boddi, M., Gensini, G.F., 1993. Age-related changes in the hemostatic system. Int. J. Clin. Lab. Res. 23, 1–3.

Amara, U., Rittirsch, D., Flierl, M., Bruckner, U., Klos, A., Gebhard, F., et al., 2008. Interaction between the coagulation and complement system. Adv. Exp. Med. Biol. 632, 71–79.

American Heart Association 2000, 2001. Heart and Stroke Statistical Update. American Heart Association, Dallas, TX.

Anderson, J.M., Patel, J.D., 2013. Chapter 7. In: Moriarty, F., Zaat, S., Busscher, H. (Eds.), Biomaterial Dependent Characteristics of the Foreign Body Response and S. Epidermidis Biofilm Interactions, in Medical Device Associated Infection Springer, pp. 114–150.

Anderson, J.M., 1988. Inflammatory response to implants. ASAIO Trans. 34, 101–107.

Anderson, J.M., 2001. Biological responses to materials. Annu. Rev. Mater. Res. 31, 81–110.

Anderson, J.M., Rodriguez, A., Chang, D.T., 2008. Foreign body reaction to biomaterials. Semin. Immunol. 20, 86–100.

Arnold, M., Barbul, A., 2006. Nutrition and wound healing. Plast. Reconstr. Surg. 117, 42S–58S.

Ashcroft, G.S., Horan, M.A., Ferguson, M.W., 1998. Aging alters the inflammatory and endothelial cell adhesion molecule profiles during human cutaneous wound healing. Lab. Invest. 78, 47–58.

Asumda, F.Z., 2013. Age-associated changes in the ecological niche: implications for mesenchymal stem cell aging. Stem Cell Res. Ther. 4, 47.

Asumda, F.Z., Chase, P.B., 2011. Age-related changes in rat bone-marrow mesenchymal stem cell plasticity. BMC Cell Biol. 12, 44.

Athanasou, N.A., Quinn, J., 1990. Immunophenotypic differences between osteoclasts and macrophage polykaryons: immunohistological distinction and implications for osteoclast ontogeny and function. J. Clin. Pathol. 43, 997–1003.

Avula, M.A., Grainger, D.W., 2013. Addressing medical device challenges with drug/device combination. In: Siegal, R., Lyu, S.P. (Eds.), Drug-Device Combinations for Chronic Diseases John Wiley & Sons, New York, NY.

Babensee, J.E., 2008. Interaction of dendritic cells with biomaterials. Semin. Immunol. 20, 101–108.

Badylak, S.F., Gilbert, T.W., 2008. Immune response to biologic scaffold materials. Semin. Immunol. 20, 109–116.

Bamford, C.H., Cooper, S.L., Tsuruta, T. (Eds.), 1992. The Vroman Effect VSP, Germany.

Barja, G., 2004. Free radicals and aging. Trends Neurosci. 27, 595–600.

Barrientos, S., Stojadinovic, O., Golinko, M.S., Brem, H., Tomic-Canic, M., 2008. Growth factors and cytokines in wound healing. Wound Repair Regen. 16, 585–601.

Bastyr III, E.J., Kadrofske, M.M., Vinik, A.I., 1990. Platelet activity and phosphoinositide turnover increase with advancing age. Am. J. Med. 88, 601–606.

Beck, L.S., Deguzman, L., Lee, W.P., Xu, Y., Siegel, M.W., Amento, E.P., 1993. One systemic administration of transforming growth factor-beta 1 reverses age- or glucocorticoid-impaired wound healing. J. Clin. Invest. 92, 2841–2849.

Beckman, K.B., Ames, B.N., 1998. The free radical theory of aging matures. Physiol. Rev. 78, 547–581.

Behrens, A., van Deursen, J.M., Rudolph, K.L., Schumacher, B., 2014. Impact of genomic damage and ageing on stem cell function. Nat. Cell Biol. 16, 201–207.

Bell, D.R., Van Zant, G., 2004. Stem cells, aging, and cancer: inevitabilities and outcomes. Oncogene 23, 7290–7296.

Berdasco, M., Esteller, M., 2010. Aberrant epigenetic landscape in cancer: how cellular identity goes awry. Dev. Cell 19, 698–711.

Berger, S.L., Kouzarides, T., Shiekhattar, R., Shilatifard, A., 2009. An operational definition of epigenetics. Genes Dev. 23, 781–783.

Bernardo, M.E., Fibbe, W.E., 2012. Safety and efficacy of mesenchymal stromal cell therapy in autoimmune disorders. Ann. N.Y. Acad. Sci. 1266, 107–117.

Bernstein, E., Kaye, D., Abrutyn, E., Gross, P., Dorfman, M., Murasko, D.M., 1999. Immune response to influenza vaccination in a large healthy elderly population. Vaccine 17, 82–94.

Bernstein, E.F., Chen, Y.Q., Kopp, J.B., Fisher, L., Brown, D.B., Hahn, P.J., et al., 1996. Long-term sun exposure alters the collagen of the papillary dermis. Comparison of sun-protected and photoaged skin by northern analysis, immunohistochemical staining, and confocal laser scanning microscopy. J. Am. Acad. Dermatol. 34, 209–218.

Boccardi, V., Paolisso, G., 2014. Telomerase activation: a potential key modulator for human healthspan and longevity. Ageing Res. Rev. 15, 1–5.

Boelens, J.J., Dankert, J., Murk, J.L., Weening, J.J., van der Poll, T., Dingemans, K.P., et al., 2000. Biomaterial-associated persistence of *Staphylococcus epidermidis* in pericatheter macrophages. J. Infect. Dis. 181, 1337–1349.

Bridges, A.W., Garcia, A.J., 2008. Anti-inflammatory polymeric coatings for implantable biomaterials and devices. J. Diabetes Sci. Technol. 2, 984–994.

Broadley, K.N., Aquino, A.M., Woodward, S.C., Buckley-Sturrock, A., Sato, Y., Rifkin, D.B., et al., 1989. Monospecific antibodies implicate basic fibroblast growth factor in normal wound repair. Lab. Invest. 61, 571–575.

Brod, S.A., 2000. Unregulated inflammation shortens human functional longevity. Inflamm. Res. 49, 561–570.

Brodbeck, W.G., Macewan, M., Colton, E., Meyerson, H., Anderson, J.M., 2005. Lymphocytes and the foreign body response: lymphocyte enhancement of macrophage adhesion and fusion. J. Biomed. Mater. Res. A 74, 222–229.

Brooks, B., Brooks, A., Grainger, D.W., 2012. Antimicrobial technologies in preclinical and clinical medical devices. In: Moriarty, T.F., Zaat, S.A.J., Busscher, H.J. (Eds.), Biomaterials Associated Infection: Immunological Aspects and Antimicrobial Strategies Springer Verlag, New York, NY, pp. 307–354.

Broughton II, G., Janis, J.E., Attinger, C.E., 2006. The basic science of wound healing. Plast. Reconstr. Surg. 117, 12S–34S.

Brunstedt, M.R., Sapatnekar, S., Rubin, K.R., Kieswetter, K.M., Ziats, N.P., Merritt, K., et al., 1995. Bacteria/blood/material interactions. I. Injected and preseeded slime-forming *Staphylococcus epidermidis* in flowing blood with biomaterials. J. Biomed. Mater. Res. 29, 455–466.

Burns, E.A., Goodwin, J.S., 1997. Immunodeficiency of aging. Drugs Aging 11, 374–397.

Busscher, H.J., van der Mei, H.C., Subbiahdoss, G., Jutte, P.C., van den Dungen, J.J., Zaat, S.A., et al., 2012. Biomaterial-associated infection: locating the finish line in the race for the surface. Sci. Transl. Med. 4, 153rv10.

Cameron, I.L., 1972. Cell proliferation and renewal in aging mice. J. Gerontol. 27, 162–172.

Campisi, J., 2011. Cellular senescence: putting the paradoxes in perspective. Curr. Opin. Genet. Dev. 21, 107–112.

Campisi, J., 2013. Aging, cellular senescence, and cancer. Annu. Rev. Physiol. 75, 685–705.

Campos, A.C., Groth, A.K., Branco, A.B., 2008. Assessment and nutritional aspects of wound healing. Curr. Opin. Clin. Nutr. Metab. Care 11, 281–288.

Castelo-Branco, C., Soveral, I., 2014. The immune system and aging: a review. Gynecol. Endocrinol. 30, 16–22.

Castle, S.C., 2000. Clinical relevance of age-related immune dysfunction. Clin. Infect. Dis. 31, 578–585.

Castle, S.C., Uyemura, K., Crawford, W., Wong, W., Klaustermeyer, W.B., Makinodan, T., 1999. Age-related impaired proliferation of peripheral blood mononuclear cells is associated with an increase in both IL-10 and IL-12. Exp. Gerontol. 34, 243–252.

Cencioni, C., Spallotta, F., Martelli, F., Valente, S., Mai, A., Zeiher, A.M., et al., 2013. Oxidative stress and epigenetic regulation in ageing and age-related diseases. Int. J. Mol. Sci. 14, 17643–17663.

Chakravarti, B., Abraham, G.N., 1999. Aging and T-cell-mediated immunity. Mech. Ageing Dev. 108, 183–206.

Charge, S.B., Rudnicki, M.A., 2004. Cellular and molecular regulation of muscle regeneration. Physiol. Rev. 84, 209–238.

Chen, E.H., Grote, E., Mohler, W., Vignery, A., 2007a. Cell–cell fusion. FEBS Lett. 581, 2181–2193.

Chen, J.H., Hales, C.N., Ozanne, S.E., 2007b. DNA damage, cellular senescence and organismal ageing: causal or correlative? Nucleic Acids Res. 35, 7417–7428.

Chung, H.Y., Kim, H.J., Kim, K.W., Choi, J.S., Yu, B.P., 2002. Molecular inflammation hypothesis of aging based on the anti-aging mechanism of calorie restriction. Microsc. Res. Tech. 59, 264–272.

Chung, H.Y., Sung, B., Jung, K.J., Zou, Y., Yu, B.P., 2006. The molecular inflammatory process in aging. Antioxid. Redox Signal. 8, 572–581.

Chung, H.Y., Cesari, M., Anton, S., Marzetti, E., Giovannini, S., Seo, A.Y., et al., 2009. Molecular inflammation: underpinnings of aging and age-related diseases. Ageing Res. Rev. 8, 18–30.

Clark, R.A., Lanigan, J.M., Dellapelle, P., Manseau, E., Dvorak, H.F., Colvin, R.B., 1982. Fibronectin and fibrin provide a provisional matrix for epidermal cell migration during wound reepithelialization. J. Invest. Dermatol. 79, 264–269.

Cochran, D., Dziubla, T.D., 2012. Antioxidant polymers for tuning biomaterial biocompatibility: from drug delivery to tissue engineering. In: Cirilo, G., Lemma, F. (Eds.), Antioxidant Polymers: Synthesis, Properties, and Applications. John Wiley & Sons, New York, NY, pp. 459–484.

Colavitti, R., Finkel, T., 2005. Reactive oxygen species as mediators of cellular senescence. IUBMB Life 57, 277–281.

Collado, M., Blasco, M.A., Serrano, M., 2007. Cellular senescence in cancer and aging. Cell 130, 223–233.

Colman, R.W., 2006. Hemostasis and Thrombosis: Basic Principles and Clinical Practice. Lippincott Williams & Wilkins. <http://www.reportsnreports.com/reports/142514-the-outlook-for-medical-devices-worldwide.html>.

Conboy, I.M., Rando, T.A., 2005. Aging, stem cells and tissue regeneration: lessons from muscle. Cell Cycle 4, 407–410.

Coppe, J.P., Patil, C.K., Rodier, F., Sun, Y., Munoz, D.P., Goldstein, J., et al., 2008. Senescence-associated secretory phenotypes reveal cell-nonautonomous functions of oncogenic RAS and the p53 tumor suppressor. PLoS Biol. 6, 2853–2868.

Coppe, J.P., Rodier, F., Patil, C.K., Freund, A., Desprez, P.Y., Campisi, J., 2011. Tumor suppressor and aging biomarker p16(INK4a) induces cellular senescence without the associated inflammatory secretory phenotype. J. Biol. Chem. 286, 36396–36403.

De Benedictis, G., Franceschi, C., 2006. The unusual genetics of human longevity. Sci. Aging Knowledge Environ. 2006 (10), pe20.

De Martinis, M., Franceschi, C., Monti, D., Ginaldi, L., 2006. Inflammation markers predicting frailty and mortality in the elderly. Exp. Mol. Pathol. 80, 219–227.

Desai, A., Grolleau-Julius, A., Yung, R., 2010. Leukocyte function in the aging immune system. J. Leukoc. Biol. 87, 1001–1009.

Droge, W., 2002. Free radicals in the physiological control of cell function. Physiol. Rev. 82, 47–95.

Ekdahl, K.N., Lambris, J.D., Elwing, H., Ricklin, D., Nilsson, P.H., Teramura, Y., et al., 2011. Innate immunity activation on biomaterial surfaces: a mechanistic model and coping strategies. Adv. Drug Deliv. Rev. 63, 1042–1050.

Eming, S.A., Krieg, T., Davidson, J.M., 2007. Inflammation in wound repair: molecular and cellular mechanisms. J. Invest. Dermatol. 127, 514–525.

Farage, M.A., Miller, K.W., Elsner, P., Maibach, H.I., 2008. Intrinsic and extrinsic factors in skin ageing: a review. Int. J. Cosmet. Sci. 30, 87–95.

Flurkey, K., Papaconstantinou, J., Miller, R.A., Harrison, D.E., 2001. Lifespan extension and delayed immune and collagen aging in mutant mice with defects in growth hormone production. Proc. Natl. Acad. Sci. USA. 98, 6736–6741.

Franceschi, C., Bonafe, M., Valensin, S., Olivieri, F., De Luca, M., Ottaviani, E., et al., 2000. Inflamm-aging. An evolutionary perspective on immunosenescence. Ann. N.Y. Acad. Sci. 908, 244–254.

Franchini, M., 2006. Hemostasis and aging. Crit. Rev. Oncol. Hematol. 60, 144–151.

Franz, S., Rammelt, S., Scharnweber, D., Simon, J.C., 2011. Immune responses to implants—a review of the implications for the design of immunomodulatory biomaterials. Biomaterials 32, 6692–6709.

Frick, J.S., Grunebach, F., Autenrieth, I.B., 2010. Immunomodulation by semi-mature dendritic cells: a novel role of Toll-like receptors and interleukin-6. Int. J. Med. Microbiol. 300, 19–24.

Fujiwara, N., Kobayashi, K., 2005. Macrophages in inflammation. Curr. Drug Targets Inflamm. Allergy 4, 281–286.

Fulop, T., Larbi, A., Douziech, N., Fortin, C., Guerard, K.P., Lesur, O., et al., 2004. Signal transduction and functional changes in neutrophils with aging. Aging Cell 3, 217–226.

Garinis, G.A., van der Horst, G.T., Vijg, J., Hoeijmakers, J.H., 2008. DNA damage and ageing: new-age ideas for an age-old problem. Nat. Cell Biol. 10, 1241–1247.

Gerstein, A.D., Phillips, T.J., Rogers, G.S., Gilchrest, B.A., 1993. Wound healing and aging. Dermatol. Clin. 11, 749–757.

Gilchrest, B.A., Murphy, G.F., Soter, N.A., 1982. Effect of chronologic aging and ultraviolet irradiation on Langerhans cells in human epidermis. J. Invest. Dermatol. 79, 85–88.

Ginaldi, L., Loreto, M.F., Corsi, M.P., Modesti, M., De Martinis, M., 2001. Immunosenescence and infectious diseases. Microbes Infect. 3, 851–857.

Gist, S., Tio-Matos, I., Falzgraf, S., Cameron, S., Beebe, M., 2009. Wound care in the geriatric client. Clin. Interv. Aging 4, 269–287.

Global Population Ageing, 2011. Peril or Promise. World Economic Forum, Geneva.

Gomathi, K., Gopinath, D., Rafiuddin Ahmed, M., Jayakumar, R., 2003. Quercetin incorporated collagen matrices for dermal wound healing processes in rat. Biomaterials 24, 2767–2772.

Gopinath, D., Ahmed, M.R., Gomathi, K., Chitra, K., Sehgal, P.K., Jayakumar, R., 2004. Dermal wound healing processes with curcumin incorporated collagen films. Biomaterials 25, 1911–1917.

Aging and the Host Response to Implanted Biomaterials 307

Gorbet, M.B., Sefton, M.V., 2004. Biomaterial-associated thrombosis: roles of coagulation factors, complement, platelets and leukocytes. Biomaterials 25, 5681–5703.

Grainger, D.W., van der Mei, H.C., Jutte, P.C., van den Dungen, J.J., Schultz, M.J., van der Laan, B.F., et al., 2013. Critical factors in the translation of improved antimicrobial strategies for medical implants and devices. Biomaterials 34, 9237–9243.

Greaves, M., 2002. Childhood leukaemia. BMJ 324, 283–287.

Gredilla, R., Barja, G., 2005. Minireview: the role of oxidative stress in relation to caloric restriction and longevity. Endocrinology 146, 3713–3717.

Gristina, A.G., 1987. Biomaterial-centered infection: microbial adhesion versus tissue integration. Science 237, 1588–1595.

Gristina, A.G., Hobgood, C.D., Webb, L.X., Myrvik, Q.N., 1987. Adhesive colonization of biomaterials and antibiotic resistance. Biomaterials 8, 423–426.

Gristina, A.G., Naylor, P.T., Myrvik, Q.N., 1990. Biomaterial-centered infections: microbial adhesion versus tissue integration Pathogenesis of Wound and Biomaterial-Associated Infections. Springer-Verlag London Limited.

Guggenbichler, J.P., Assadian, O., Boeswald, M., Kramer, A., 2011. Incidence and clinical implication of nosocomial infections associated with implantable biomaterials—catheters, ventilator-associated pneumonia, urinary tract infections. GMS Krankenhhyg Interdiszip 6, Doc18.

Guo, J.J., Yang, H., Qian, H., Huang, L., Guo, Z., Tang, T., 2010. The effects of different nutritional measurements on delayed wound healing after hip fracture in the elderly. J. Surg. Res. 159, 503–508.

Guo, S., Dipietro, L.A., 2010. Factors affecting wound healing. J. Dent. Res. 89, 219–229.

Halasz, N.A., 1968. Dehiscence of laparotomy wounds. Am. J. Surg. 116, 210–214.

Harding, K.G., Morris, H.L., Patel, G.K., 2002. Science, medicine and the future: healing chronic wounds. BMJ 324, 160–163.

Harrison, D.E., Astle, C.M., Doubleday, J.W., 1977. Cell lines from old immunodeficient donors give normal responses in young recipients. J. Immunol. 118, 1223–1227.

Hayflick, L., 1965. The limited *in vitro* lifetime of human diploid cell strains. Exp. Cell Res. 37, 614–636.

Hayflick, L., Moorhead, P.S., 1961. The serial cultivation of human diploid cell strains. Exp. Cell Res. 25, 585–621.

Hebuterne, X., Bermon, S., Schneider, S.M., 2001. Ageing and muscle: the effects of malnutrition, re-nutrition, and physical exercise. Curr. Opin. Clin. Nutr. Metab. Care 4, 295–300.

Henson, P.M., 1971. The immunologic release of constituents from neutrophil leukocytes. II. Mechanisms of release during phagocytosis, and adherence to nonphagocytosable surfaces. J. Immunol. 107, 1547–1557.

Herbig, U., Sedivy, J.M., 2006. Regulation of growth arrest in senescence: telomere damage is not the end of the story. Mech. Ageing Dev. 127, 16–24.

Hermann, A., List, C., Habisch, H.J., Vukicevic, V., Ehrhart-Bornstein, M., Brenner, R., et al., 2010. Age-dependent neuroectodermal differentiation capacity of human mesenchymal stromal cells: limitations for autologous cell replacement strategies. Cytotherapy 12, 17–30.

High, K.P., 2002. Infection in an ageing world. Lancet Infect. Dis. 2, 655.

Hoffmann, R., Stellbrink, E., Schroder, J., Grawe, A., Vogel, G., Blindt, R., et al., 2007. Impact of the metabolic syndrome on angiographic and clinical events after coronary intervention using bare-metal or sirolimus-eluting stents. Am. J. Cardiol. 100, 1347–1352.

Holm-Pedersen, P., Viidik, A., 1972. Tensile properties and morphology of healing wounds in young and old rats. Scand. J. Plast. Reconstr. Surg. 6, 24–35.

Holt, D.J., Grainger, D.W., 2012. Senescence and quiescence induced compromised function in cultured macrophages. Biomaterials 33, 7497–7507.

Hornsby, P.J., 2002. Cellular senescence and tissue aging *in vivo*. J. Gerontol. A Biol. Sci. Med. Sci. 57, B251–B256.

Hu, W.J., Eaton, J.W., Ugarova, T.P., Tang, L., 2001. Molecular basis of biomaterial-mediated foreign body reactions. Blood 98, 1231–1238.

Huang, K., Mitzner, W., Rabold, R., Schofield, B., Lee, H., Biswal, S., et al., 2007. Variation in senescent-dependent lung changes in inbred mouse strains. J. Appl. Physiol. (1985) 102, 1632–1639.

Hubbell, J.A., Thomas, S.N., Swartz, M.A., 2009. Materials engineering for immunomodulation. Nature 462, 449–460.

Illi, B., Colussi, C., Grasselli, A., Farsetti, A., Capogrossi, M.C., Gaetano, C., 2009. NO sparks off chromatin: tales of a multifaceted epigenetic regulator. Pharmacol. Ther. 123, 344–352.

Irani, K., Xia, Y., Zweier, J.L., Sollott, S.J., Der, C.J., Fearon, E.R., et al., 1997. Mitogenic signaling mediated by oxidants in Ras-transformed fibroblasts. Science 275, 1649–1652.

Janeway, C., Travers, P., Walport, M., Capra, J.D., 2001. Immunobiology: The Immune System in Health and Disease. Churchill Livingstone, Garland Publishing, New York.

Jenney, C.R., Anderson, J.M., 2000. Adsorbed serum proteins responsible for surface dependent human macrophage behavior. J. Biomed. Mater. Res. 49, 435–447.

Jeyapalan, J.C., Sedivy, J.M., 2008. Cellular senescence and organismal aging. Mech. Ageing Dev. 129, 467–474.

Jones, D.L., Wagers, A.J., 2008. No place like home: anatomy and function of the stem cell niche. Nat. Rev. Mol. Cell Biol. 9, 11–21.

Jun, J.I., Lau, L.F., 2010. Cellular senescence controls fibrosis in wound healing. Aging (Albany NY) 2, 627–631.

Kannel, W.B., Wolf, P.A., Castelli, W.P., D'agostino, R.B., 1987. Fibrinogen and risk of cardiovascular disease. The Framingham Study. JAMA 258, 1183–1186.

Kapetanaki, M.G., Mora, A.L., Rojas, M., 2013. Influence of age on wound healing and fibrosis. J. Pathol. 229, 310–322.

Karanjawala, Z.E., Lieber, M.R., 2004. DNA damage and aging. Mech. Ageing Dev. 125, 405–416.

Kasjanovova, D., Balaz, V., 1986. Age-related changes in human platelet function in vitro. Mech. Ageing Dev. 37, 175–182.

Kazatchkine, M.D., Carreno, M.P., 1988. Activation of the complement system at the interface between blood and artificial surfaces. Biomaterials 9, 30–35.

Kim, H.J., Jung, K.J., Yu, B.P., Cho, C.G., Choi, J.S., Chung, H.Y., 2002. Modulation of redox-sensitive transcription factors by calorie restriction during aging. Mech. Ageing Dev. 123, 1589–1595.

Kim, K.H., Chen, C.C., Monzon, R.I., Lau, L.F., 2013. Matricellular protein CCN1 promotes regression of liver fibrosis through induction of cellular senescence in hepatic myofibroblasts. Mol. Cell Biol. 33, 2078–2090.

Knowlton E.W., 2004. Method for treatment of tissue. US Patent 20,040,206,365.

Koh, J.M., Khang, Y.H., Jung, C.H., Bae, S., Kim, D.J., Chung, Y.E., et al., 2005. Higher circulating hsCRP levels are associated with lower bone mineral density in healthy pre- and postmenopausal women: evidence for a link between systemic inflammation and osteoporosis. Osteoporos. Int. 16, 1263–1271.

Kojic, E.M., Darouiche, R.O., 2004. Candida infections of medical devices. Clin. Microbiol. Rev. 17, 255–267.

Kono, H., Rock, K.L., 2008. How dying cells alert the immune system to danger. Nat. Rev. Immunol. 8, 279–289.

Kramer, D.B., Xu, S., Kesselheim, A.S., 2012. How does medical device regulation perform in the United States and the European Union? A systematic review. PLoS Med. 9, e1001276.

Krishna, K.A., Krishna, K.S., Berrocal, R., Tummala, A., Rao, K.S., Rao, K.R., 2011. A review on the therapeutic potential of embryonic and induced pluripotent stem cells in hepatic repair. J. Nat. Sci. Biol. Med. 2, 141–144.

Kuilman, T., Peeper, D.S., 2009. Senescence-messaging secretome: SMS-ing cellular stress. Nat. Rev. Cancer 9, 81–94.

Kurban, R.S., Bhawan, J., 1990. Histologic changes in skin associated with aging. J. Dermatol. Surg. Oncol. 16, 908–914.

Lai, K., Bohm, E.R., Burnell, C., Hedden, D.R., 2007. Presence of medical comorbidities in patients with infected primary hip or knee arthroplasties. J. Arthroplasty 22, 651–656.

Lavasani, M., Robinson, A.R., Lu, A., Song, M., Feduska, J.M., Ahani, B., et al., 2012. Muscle-derived stem/progenitor cell dysfunction limits healthspan and lifespan in a murine progeria model. Nat. Commun. 3, 608.

Lavker, R.M., Zheng, P.S., Dong, G., 1987. Aged skin: a study by light, transmission electron, and scanning electron microscopy. J. Invest. Dermatol. 88, 44s–51s.

Lemaoult, J., Szabo, P., Weksler, M.E., 1997. Effect of age on humoral immunity, selection of the B-cell repertoire and B-cell development. Immunol. Rev. 160, 115–126.

Lepperdinger, G., 2009. Open-ended question: is immortality exclusively inherent to the germline?—A mini-review. Gerontology 55, 114–117.

Licastro, F., Candore, G., Lio, D., Porcellini, E., Colonna-Romano, G., Franceschi, C., et al., 2005. Innate immunity and inflammation in ageing: a key for understanding age-related diseases. Immun. Ageing 2, 8.

Lim, C.S., 2006. Cellular senescence, cancer, and organismal aging: a paradigm shift. Biochem. Biophys. Res. Commun. 344, 1–2.

http://www.reportsnreports.com/reports/142514-the-outlook-for-medical-devices-worldwide.html.

Lind, M., 1998. Growth factor stimulation of bone healing. Effects on osteoblasts, osteomies, and implants fixation. Acta Orthop. Scand. Suppl. 283, 2–37.

Liu, L., Rando, T.A., 2011. Manifestations and mechanisms of stem cell aging. J. Cell Biol. 193, 257–266.

Lu, T., Pan, Y., Kao, S.Y., Li, C., Kohane, I., Chan, J., et al., 2004. Gene regulation and DNA damage in the ageing human brain. Nature 429, 883–891.

Lutz, M.B., Schuler, G., 2002. Immature, semi-mature and fully mature dendritic cells: which signals induce tolerance or immunity? Trends Immunol. 23, 445–449.

Markiewski, M.M., Nilsson, B., Ekdahl, K.N., Mollnes, T.E., Lambris, J.D., 2007. Complement and coagulation: strangers or partners in crime? Trends Immunol. 28, 184–192.

Martin, P., Leibovich, S.J., 2005. Inflammatory cells during wound repair: the good, the bad and the ugly. Trends Cell Biol. 15, 599–607.

Martinez, F.O., Sica, A., Mantovani, A., Locati, M., 2008. Macrophage activation and polarization. Front. Biosci. 13, 453–461.

Martinez, F.O., Helming, L., Gordon, S., 2009. Alternative activation of macrophages: an immunologic functional perspective. Annu. Rev. Immunol. 27, 451–483.

Mays, P.K., Bishop, J.E., Laurent, G.J., 1988. Age-related changes in the proportion of types I and III collagen. Mech. Ageing Dev. 45, 203–212.

Mcgeer, P.L., Mcgeer, E.G., 1999. Inflammation of the brain in Alzheimer's disease: implications for therapy. J. Leukoc. Biol. 65, 409–415.

Mcnally, A.K., Anderson, J.M., 1994. Complement C3 participation in monocyte adhesion to different surfaces. Proc. Natl. Acad. Sci. USA. 91, 10119–10123.

Mcnally, A.K., Anderson, J.M., 2002. Beta1 and beta2 integrins mediate adhesion during macrophage fusion and multinucleated foreign body giant cell formation. Am. J. Pathol. 160, 621–630.

Melov, S., Doctrow, S.R., Schneider, J.A., Haberson, J., Patel, M., Coskun, P.E., et al., 2001. Lifespan extension and rescue of spongiform encephalopathy in superoxide dismutase 2 nullizygous mice treated with superoxide dismutase-catalase mimetics. J. Neurosci. 21, 8348–8353.

Merrell, J.G., Mclaughlin, S.W., Tie, L., Laurencin, C.T., Chen, A.F., Nair, L.S., 2009. Curcumin-loaded poly(epsilon-caprolactone) nanofibres: diabetic wound dressing with anti-oxidant and anti-inflammatory properties. Clin. Exp. Pharmacol. Physiol. 36, 1149–1156.

Michaud, M., Balardy, L., Moulis, G., Gaudin, C., Peyrot, C., Vellas, B., et al., 2013. Proinflammatory cytokines, aging, and age-related diseases. J. Am. Med. Dir. Assoc. 14, 877–882.

Mikos, A.G., Mcintire, L.V., Anderson, J.M., Babensee, J.E., 1998. Host response to tissue engineered devices. Adv. Drug Deliv. Rev. 33, 111–139.

Miller, R.A., 1991. Aging and immune function. Int. Rev. Cytol. 124, 187–215.

Minamino, T., Komuro, I., 2007. Vascular cell senescence: contribution to atherosclerosis. Circ. Res. 100, 15–26.

Mocchegiani, E., Malavolta, M., Muti, E., Costarelli, L., Cipriano, C., Piacenza, F., et al., 2008. Zinc, metallothioneins and longevity: interrelationships with niacin and selenium. Curr. Pharm. Des. 14, 2719–2732.

Mocchegiani, E., Costarelli, L., Giacconi, R., Piacenza, F., Basso, A., Malavolta, M., 2012. Micronutrient (Zn, Cu, Fe)–gene interactions in ageing and inflammatory age-related diseases: implications for treatments. Ageing Res. Rev. 11, 297–319.

Montagna, W., Carlisle, K., 1979. Structural changes in aging human skin. J. Invest. Dermatol. 73, 47–53.

Moretta, A., Marcenaro, E., Parolini, S., Ferlazzo, G., Moretta, L., 2008. NK cells at the interface between innate and adaptive immunity. Cell Death Differ. 15, 226–233.

Moriarty, T.F., Richards, R.G., Grainger, D.W., 2014. Challenges in linking preclinical anti-microbial research strategies with clinical outcomes for device-associated infections. Eur. Cells Mater. 28, 112–128.

Morrison, S.J., Wandycz, A.M., Akashi, K., Globerson, A., Weissman, I.L., 1996. The aging of hematopoietic stem cells. Nat. Med. 2, 1011–1016.

Mosser, D.M., 2003. The many faces of macrophage activation. J. Leukoc. Biol. 73, 209–212.

Mosser, D.M., Edwards, J.P., 2008. Exploring the full spectrum of macrophage activation. Nat. Rev. Immunol. 8, 958–969.

Mueller, X., Sadeghi, H., Kappenberger, L., 1990. Complications after single versus dual chamber pacemaker implantation. Pacing Clin. Electrophysiol. 13, 711–714.

Mustoe, T.A., Pierce, G.F., Thomason, A., Gramates, P., Sporn, M.B., Deuel, T.F., 1987. Accelerated healing of incisional wounds in rats induced by transforming growth factor-beta. Science 237, 1333–1336.

Nilsson, B., Ekdahl, K.N., Mollnes, T.E., Lambris, J.D., 2007. The role of complement in biomaterial-induced inflammation. Mol. Immunol. 44, 82–94.

Oberdoerffer, P., Michan, S., Mcvay, M., Mostoslavsky, R., Vann, J., Park, S.K., et al., 2008. SIRT1 redistribution on chromatin promotes genomic stability but alters gene expression during aging. Cell 135, 907–918.

Passaniti, A., Taylor, R.M., Pili, R., Guo, Y., Long, P.V., Haney, J.A., et al., 1992. A simple, quantitative method for assessing angiogenesis and antiangiogenic agents using reconstituted basement membrane, heparin, and fibroblast growth factor. Lab. Invest. 67, 519–528.

Patel, V.P., Walsh, M., Sehgal, B., Preston, C., Dewal, H., Di Cesare, P.E., 2007. Factors associated with prolonged wound drainage after primary total hip and knee arthroplasty. J. Bone Joint Surg. Am. 89 (1), 33–38.

Phair, J.P., Hsu, C.S., Hsu, Y.L., 1988. Ageing and infection. Ciba Found. Symp. 134, 143–154.

Plowden, J., Renshaw-Hoelscher, M., Engleman, C., Katz, J., Sambhara, S., 2004. Innate immunity in aging: impact on macrophage function. Aging Cell 3, 161–167.

Pober, J.S., Cotran, R.S., 1990. Cytokines and endothelial cell biology. Physiol. Rev. 70, 427–451.

Polverini, P.J., Cotran, P.S., Gimbrone JR., M.A., Unanue, E.R., 1977. Activated macrophages induce vascular proliferation. Nature 269, 804–806.

Ponnappan, S., Ponnappan, U., 2011. Aging and immune function: molecular mechanisms to interventions. Antioxid. Redox Signal. 14, 1551–1585.

Porcheray, F., Viaud, S., Rimaniol, A.C., Leone, C., Samah, B., Dereuddre-Bosquet, N., et al., 2005. Macrophage activation switching: an asset for the resolution of inflammation. Clin. Exp. Immunol. 142, 481–489.

Potter, K.A., Jorfi, M., Householder, K.T., Foster, E.J., Weder, C., Capadona, J.R., 2014. Curcumin-releasing mechanically adaptive intracortical implants improve the proximal neuronal density and blood–brain barrier stability. Acta Biomater. 10, 2209–2222.

Prasad, A.S., 2008. Zinc in human health: effect of zinc on immune cells. Mol. Med. 14, 353–357.

Previtali, E., Bucciarelli, P., Passamonti, S.M., Martinelli, I., 2011. Risk factors for venous and arterial thrombosis. Blood Transfus. 9, 120–138.

Provinciali, M., Cardelli, M., Marchegiani, F., Pierpaoli, E., 2013. Impact of cellular senescence in aging and cancer. Curr. Pharm. Des. 19, 1699–1709.

Rahman, K., 2007. Studies on free radicals, antioxidants, and co-factors. Clin. Interv. Aging 2, 219–236.

Rando, T.A., 2006. Stem cells, ageing and the quest for immortality. Nature 441, 1080–1086.

Ratner, B.D., 2004. Biomaterials Science: An Introduction to Materials in Medicine. Elsevier Academic Press, Amsterdam; Boston, MA.

Raymond Brood, L.C., Daniels, N., Davison, G.C., et.al., 2012 Global Population Ageing: Peril or Promise? In: Bloom, D, (Ed.), World Economic Forum.

Reed, M.J., Corsa, A., Pendergrass, W., Penn, P., Sage, E.H., Abrass, I.B., 1998. Neovascularization in aged mice: delayed angiogenesis is coincident with decreased levels of transforming growth factor beta1 and type I collagen. Am. J. Pathol. 152, 113–123.

Reed, M.J., Corsa, A.C., Kudravi, S.A., Mccormick, R.S., Arthur, W.T., 2000. A deficit in collagenase activity contributes to impaired migration of aged microvascular endothelial cells. J. Cell. Biochem. 77, 116–126.

Reed, M.J., Karres, N., Eyman, D., Vernon, R.B., Edelberg, J.M., 2006. Age-related differences in repair of dermal wounds and myocardial infarcts attenuate during the later stages of healing. In Vivo 20, 801–806.

Report to Congress, 2012. Aging Services Technology Study. Available online: <http://aspe.hhs.gov/daltcp/reports/2012/astsrptcong.cfm>. Office of the Assistant Secretary for Planning and Evaluation Report, Department of Human and Health Services.

Ressler, S., Bartkova, J., Niederegger, H., Bartek, J., Scharffetter-Kochanek, K., Jansen-Durr, P., et al., 2006. p16INK4A is a robust in vivo biomarker of cellular aging in human skin. Aging Cell 5, 379–389.

Reya, T., Morrison, S.J., Clarke, M.F., Weissman, I.L., 2001. Stem cells, cancer, and cancer stem cells. Nature 414, 105–111.

Rhee, I., Zhong, M.C., Reizis, B., Cheong, C., Veillette, A., 2014. Control of dendritic cell migration, T cell-dependent immunity, and autoimmunity by protein tyrosine phosphatase PTPN12 expressed in dendritic cells. Mol. Cell Biol. 34, 888–899.

Ricklin, D., Hajishengallis, G., Yang, K., Lambris, J.D., 2010. Complement: a key system for immune surveillance and homeostasis. Nat. Immunol. 11, 785–797.

Ridker, P.M., 2001. High-sensitivity C-reactive protein: potential adjunct for global risk assessment in the primary prevention of cardiovascular disease. Circulation 103, 1813–1818.

Rivard, A., Fabre, J.E., Silver, M., Chen, D., Murohara, T., Kearney, M., et al., 1999. Age-dependent impairment of angiogenesis. Circulation 99, 111–120.

Roberts, S.B., Rosenberg, I., 2006. Nutrition and aging: changes in the regulation of energy metabolism with aging. Physiol. Rev. 86, 651–667.

Rodier, F., Campisi, J., 2011. Four faces of cellular senescence. J. Cell Biol. 192, 547–556.

Roobrouck, V.D., Ulloa-Montoya, F., Verfaillie, C.M., 2008. Self-renewal and differentiation capacity of young and aged stem cells. Exp. Cell Res. 314, 1937–1944.

Roos, A., Bouwman, L.H., van Gijlswijk-Janssen, D.J., Faber-Krol, M.C., Stahl, G.L., Daha, M.R., 2001. Human IgA activates the complement system via the mannan-binding lectin pathway. J. Immunol. 167, 2861–2868.

Rosenberg, I.H., Miller, J.W., 1992. Nutritional factors in physical and cognitive functions of elderly people. Am. J. Clin. Nutr. 55, 1237S–1243S.

Rossi, D.J., Jamieson, C.H., Weissman, I.L., 2008. Stems cells and the pathways to aging and cancer. Cell 132, 681–696.

Rot, A.A., von Andrian, U.H., 2004. Chemokines in innate and adaptive host defense: basic chemokinese grammar for immune cells. Annu. Rev. Immunol. 22, 891–928.

Rus, H., Cudrici, C., Niculescu, F., 2005. The role of the complement system in innate immunity. Immunol. Res. 33, 103–112.

Rutella, S., Danese, S., Leone, G., 2006. Tolerogenic dendritic cells: cytokine modulation comes of age. Blood 108, 1435–1440.

Salo, T., Makela, M., Kylmaniemi, M., Autio-Harmainen, H., Larjava, H., 1994. Expression of matrix metalloproteinase-2 and -9 during early human wound healing. Lab. Invest. 70, 176–182.

Sansoni, P., Vescovini, R., Fagnoni, F., Biasini, C., Zanni, F., Zanlari, L., et al., 2008. The immune system in extreme longevity. Exp. Gerontol. 43, 61–65.

Scheid, A., Wenger, R.H., Christina, H., Camenisch, I., Ferenc, A., Stauffer, U.G., et al., 2000. Hypoxia-regulated gene expression in fetal wound regeneration and adult wound repair. Pediatr. Surg. Int. 16, 232–236.

Schmaier, A.H., 1997. Contact activation: a revision. Thromb. Haemost. 78, 101–107.

Schraml, E., Grillari, J., 2012. From cellular senescence to age-associated diseases: the miRNA connection. Longev. Healthspan 1, 10.

Schweikl, H., Hartmann, A., Hiller, K.A., Spagnuolo, G., Bolay, C., Brockhoff, G., et al., 2007. Inhibition of TEGDMA and HEMA-induced genotoxicity and cell cycle arrest by N-acetylcysteine. Dent. Mater. 23, 688–695.

Sharpless, N.E., Depinho, R.A., 2007. How stem cells age and why this makes us grow old. Nat. Rev. Mol. Cell Biol. 8, 703–713.

Shaw, A.C., Goldstein, D.R., Montgomery, R.R., 2013. Age-dependent dysregulation of innate immunity. Nat. Rev. Immunol. 13, 875–887.

Shen, J., Tsai, Y.T., Dimarco, N.M., Long, M.A., Sun, X., Tang, L., 2011. Transplantation of mesenchymal stem cells from young donors delays aging in mice. Sci. Rep. 1, 67.

Shimada, K., 1985. Ageing and host responses: infection. Nihon Naika Gakkai Zasshi 74, 1353–1356.

Shive, M.S., Anderson, J.M., 1997. Biodegradation and biocompatibility of PLA and PLGA microspheres. Adv. Drug Deliv. Rev. 28, 5–24.

Silverstein, M.D., Heit, J.A., Mohr, D.N., Petterson, T.M., O'fallon, W.M., Melton III, L.J., 1998. Trends in the incidence of deep vein thrombosis and pulmonary embolism: a 25-year population-based study. Arch. Intern. Med. 158, 585–593.

Simchi, A., Tamjid, E., Pishbin, F., Boccaccini, A.R., 2011. Recent progress in inorganic and composite coatings with bactericidal capability for orthopaedic applications. Nanomedicine 7, 22–39.

Singer, A.J., Clark, R.A., 1999. Cutaneous wound healing. N. Engl. J. Med. 341, 738–746.

Sjoqvist, S., Jungebluth, P., Lim, M.L., Haag, J.C., Gustafsson, Y., Lemon, G., et al., 2014. Experimental orthotopic transplantation of a tissue-engineered oesophagus in rats. Nat. Commun. 5, 3562.

Skinner, M.K., 2011. Environmental epigenetic transgenerational inheritance and somatic epigenetic mitotic stability. Epigenetics 6, 838–842.

Solana, R., Tarazona, R., Gayoso, I., Lesur, O., Dupuis, G., Fulop, T., 2012. Innate immunosenescence: effect of aging on cells and receptors of the innate immune system in humans. Semin. Immunol. 24, 331–341.

Song, H., Song, B.W., Cha, M.J., Choi, I.G., Hwang, K.C., 2010. Modification of mesenchymal stem cells for cardiac regeneration. Expert Opin. Biol. Ther. 10, 309–319.

Stechmiller, J.K., 2010. Understanding the role of nutrition and wound healing. Nutr. Clin. Pract. 25, 61–68.

Steinman, R.M., 2001. Dendritic cells and the control of immunity: enhancing the efficiency of antigen presentation. Mt. Sinai. J. Med. 68, 160–166.

Stout, R.D., Suttles, J., 2005. Immunosenescence and macrophage functional plasticity: dysregulation of macrophage function by age-associated microenvironmental changes. Immunol. Rev. 205, 60–71.

Sudo, K., Ema, H., Morita, Y., Nakauchi, H., 2000. Age-associated characteristics of murine hematopoietic stem cells. J. Exp. Med. 192, 1273–1280.

Sueblinvong, V., Neujahr, D.C., Mills, S.T., Roser-Page, S., Ritzenthaler, J.D., Guidot, D., et al., 2012. Predisposition for disrepair in the aged lung. Am. J. Med. Sci. 344, 41–51.

Swift, M.E., Kleinman, H.K., Dipietro, L.A., 1999. Impaired wound repair and delayed angiogenesis in aged mice. Lab. Invest. 79, 1479–1487.

Swift, M.E., Burns, A.L., Gray, K.L., Dipietro, L.A., 2001. Age-related alterations in the inflammatory response to dermal injury. J. Invest. Dermatol. 117, 1027–1035.

Tang, L., Jennings, T.A., Eaton, J.W., 1998. Mast cells mediate acute inflammatory responses to implanted biomaterials. Proc. Natl. Acad. Sci. USA. 95, 8841–8846.

Thoman, M.L., Weigle, W.O., 1989. The cellular and subcellular bases of immunosenescence. Adv. Immunol. 46, 221–261.

Thomas, D.R., 2001. Age-related changes in wound healing. Drugs Aging 18, 607–620.

Tian, L., 2013. Vitamin Blended Implants to Boost Shoulder Joint Lifespan? <http://healthcare.globaldata.com/media-center/press-releases/medical-devices/vitamin-blended-implants-to-boost-shoulder-joint-lifespan>Globaldata.

Tortorella, C., Piazzolla, G., Spaccavento, F., Pece, S., Jirillo, E., Antonaci, S., 1998. Spontaneous and Fas-induced apoptotic cell death in aged neutrophils. J. Clin. Immunol. 18, 321–329.

Uccelli, A., Moretta, L., Pistoia, V., 2008. Mesenchymal stem cells in health and disease. Nat. Rev. Immunol. 8, 726–736.

Udipi, K., Ornberg, R.L., Thurmond II, K.B., Settle, S.L., Forster, D., Riley, D., 2000. Modification of inflammatory response to implanted biomedical materials in vivo by surface bound superoxide dismutase mimics. J. Biomed. Mater. Res. 51, 549–560.

Viljanto, J., 1969. A sponge implantation method for testing connective tissue regeneration in surgical patients. Acta Chir. Scand. 135, 297–300.

von Eiff, C., Jansen, B., Kohnen, W., Becker, K., 2005. Infections associated with medical devices: pathogenesis, management and prophylaxis. Drugs 65, 179–214.

Vranken, I., De Visscher, G., Lebacq, A., Verbeken, E., Flameng, W., 2008. The recruitment of primitive Lin− Sca-1+, CD34+, c-kit+ and CD271+ cells during the early intraperitoneal foreign body reaction. Biomaterials 29, 797–808.

Waterstrat, A., Van Zant, G., 2009. Effects of aging on hematopoietic stem and progenitor cells. Curr. Opin. Immunol. 21, 408–413.

Weinstein, R.A., 2001. Device-related infections. Clin. Infect. Dis. 33, 1386.

Weiskopf, D., Weinberger, B., Grubeck-Loebenstein, B., 2009. The aging of the immune system. Transpl. Int. 22, 1041–1050.

WHO. Ageing and Life Course. 2012. <http://www.who.int/ageing/about/facts/en/>, 2014 (accessed 02.25.14).

Wilkerson, W.R., Sane, D.C., 2002. Aging and thrombosis. Semin. Thromb. Hemost. 28, 555–568.

Wright, W.E., Shay, J.W., 2002. Historical claims and current interpretations of replicative aging. Nat. Biotechnol. 20, 682–688.

Wu, P., Grainger, D.W., 2006. Drug/device combinations for local drug therapies and infection prophylaxis. Biomaterials 27, 2450–2467.

Wysocki, A.B., Staiano-Coico, L., Grinnell, F., 1993. Wound fluid from chronic leg ulcers contains elevated levels of metalloproteinases MMP-2 and MMP-9. J. Invest. Dermatol. 101, 64–68.

Xia, Z., Triffitt, J.T., 2006. A review on macrophage responses to biomaterials. Biomed. Mater. 1, R1–R9.

Yew, T.L., Chiu, F.Y., Tsai, C.C., Chen, H.L., Lee, W.P., Chen, Y.J., et al., 2011. Knockdown of p21(Cip1/Waf1) enhances proliferation, the expression of stemness markers, and osteogenic potential in human mesenchymal stem cells. Aging Cell 10, 349–361.

Yokoe, D.S., Mermel, L.A., Anderson, D.J., Arias, K.M., Burstin, H., Calfee, D.P., et al., 2008. A compendium of strategies to prevent healthcare-associated infections in acute care hospitals. Infect. Control Hosp. Epidemiol. 29 (Suppl. 1), S12–S21.

Yoshida, M., Babensee, J.E., 2004. Poly(lactic-co-glycolic acid) enhances maturation of human monocyte-derived dendritic cells. J. Biomed. Mater. Res. A 71, 45–54.

Young, A.R., Narita, M., 2009. SASP reflects senescence. EMBO Rep. 10, 228–230.

Yu, B.P., Chung, H.Y., 2006. Adaptive mechanisms to oxidative stress during aging. Mech. Ageing Dev. 127, 436–443.

Yu, J.M., Wu, X., Gimble, J.M., Guan, X., Freitas, M.A., Bunnell, B.A., 2011. Age-related changes in mesenchymal stem cells derived from rhesus macaque bone marrow. Aging Cell 10, 66–79.

Yukata, K., Xie, C., Li, T.-F., Takahata, M., Hoak, D., Kondabolu, S., et al., 2014. Aging periosteal progenitor cells have reduced regenerative responsiveness to bone injury and to the anabolic actions of PTH 1-34 treatment. Bone 62, 79–89.

Zdolsek, J., Eaton, J.W., Tang, L., 2007. Histamine release and fibrinogen adsorption mediate acute inflammatory responses to biomaterial implants in humans. J. Transl. Med. 5, 31.

Zhang, H., 2007. Molecular signaling and genetic pathways of senescence: its role in tumorigenesis and aging. J. Cell. Physiol. 210, 567–574.

Ziats, N.P., Pankowsky, D.A., Tierney, B.P., Ratnoff, O.D., Anderson, J.M., 1990. Adsorption of Hageman factor (factor XII) and other human plasma proteins to biomedical polymers. J. Lab. Clin. Med. 116, 687–696.

Zimmerli, W., Waldvogel, F.A., Vaudaux, P., Nydegger, U.E., 1982. Pathogenesis of foreign body infection: description and characteristics of an animal model. J. Infect. Dis. 146, 487–497.

Zou, Y., Jung, K.J., Kim, J.W., Yu, B.P., Chung, H.Y., 2004. Alteration of soluble adhesion molecules during aging and their modulation by calorie restriction. FASEB J. 18, 320–322.

CHAPTER 12

Host Response to Orthopedic Implants (Metals and Plastics)

Zhenyu Yao[1], Tzu-Hua Lin[1], Jukka Pajarinen[1], Taishi Sato[1] and Stuart Goodman[1,2]
[1]Department of Orthopaedic Surgery, Stanford University, Stanford, CA, USA
[2]Department of Bioengineering, Stanford University, Stanford, CA, USA

Contents

Host Response to Biomaterials.
DOI: http://dx.doi.org/10.1016/B978-0-12-800196-7.00012-8

INTRODUCTION—EPIDEMIOLOGY AND BASIC CONCEPTS/ DEFINITIONS

Structural biomaterials including metals, plastics, and ceramics are frequently used in orthopedic surgery, for fixation of fractures, for reconstructive purposes in joint replacement, spinal diseases and deformities, and in numerous other orthopedic subspecialties. According to the United States Bone and Joint Decade publication "The Burden of Musculoskeletal Diseases," in 2007, there were over 1 million joint replacements in the United States. The majority of which were hip and knee procedures, at a total cost of approximately $50 billion (United States Bone and Joint Initiative, 2011). The CDC (2010) recorded 332,000 total hip replacements and 719,000 total knee replacements in 2010. By 2030, Kurtz et al. (2007) estimates that more than 570,000 primary total hip replacements and 3.5 million primary total knee replacements will be performed in the United States. In 2010, there were 671,000 admissions to hospital for fractures; 438,000 of these required open reduction and internal fixation (Control, 2010). Between 1998 and 2008, the number of discharges with a diagnosis of spinal fusion in the United States increased 2.4-fold from 174,223 to 413,171 (Rajaee et al., 2012). These procedures are virtually always accompanied by internal fixation. Other orthopedic subspecialties such as sports medicine, foot and ankle, orthopedic oncology, and pediatrics use implants such as screws, wires, rods, external fixation devices, partial/total joint replacements (TJRs), and others. Indeed, the use of implants in orthopedic surgery has revolutionized the care of patients, relieving pain and facilitating more normal function and activity.

Orthopedic implants must be deemed safe and effective prior to their introduction to the marketplace and therefore first undergo extensive preclinical and clinical investigation. In the United States, the Food and Drug Administration (FDA) regulates the approval, manufacturing, and labeling of orthopedic devices. In Europe, the European Commission awards the CE mark to approved medical devices. Other nations have their own regulatory bodies for implants or recognize the FDA and/or CE approval status. In addition, for implants to yield a constructive benefit to society, they must be cost-effective. An implant that is both safe and effective will not garner widespread use if its production and marketing costs are exorbitant and the patient or insurance company does not approve its purchase.

When discussing safety and efficacy of implants, it should be noted that all implants surgically placed within the body generate an acute inflammatory response. Thus, there are at least two components that determine the biological reaction to an implanted bio-material in the short and long term. The first component is the acute inflammatory reaction that accompanies the surgical intervention itself. The concept of surgically induced tissue injury as an unavoidable component of the host response to biomaterial implantation has been mentioned several times in this textbook (see Chapters 2, 3, 5, and 9). The severity of the acute inflammatory response is determined, in part, by the location and type of surgical procedure, the surgical technique used, and the biological "makeup" (genetically determined) of the host. The second component has to do with the implant used and its relationship to the host. Important factors include the size and shape of the implant, the composition, surface roughness, surface chemistry, surface energy, as well as its degradability including the production of fragments, particles, ions, and other by-products. The function of an implant may change with time. For example, a load sharing femoral intramedullary nail will see much less load once the fracture has united; loading of spinal instrumentation is dramatically relieved once fusion has occurred.

The term "biocompatibility" is important when considering the host response to orthopedic implants (Goodman et al., 2009). The definition of biocompatibility is rather controversial and has changed significantly during the past 50 years. Prof. David Williams' early definition was as follows: "The state of mutual coexistence between a biomaterial and the physiological environment such that neither has an undesirable effect on the other" (Williams, 1980). Later, Dr. Williams modified this definition: "Biocompatibility refers to the ability of a biomaterial to perform its desired function with respect to a medical therapy, without eliciting any undesirable local or systemic effects in the recipient or beneficiary of that therapy, but generating the most appropriate beneficial cellular or tissue response in that specific situation, and optimizing the clinically relevant performance of that therapy" (Williams, 2008). According to the International Union of Pure and Applied Chemistry, the definition of biocompatibility is the "ability to be in contact with a living system without producing an adverse effect" (Vert et al., 2012). In more pragmatic terms, the term "biocompatibility" is used more in reference to the outcome (favorable or adverse) of a series of biological tests performed under standardized testing protocols. See also "biocompatibility" versus "biotolerability" in Chapter 3.

Many biomaterials for orthopedic use are implanted within bone. These implants need definitive anchorage to avoid displacement under physiologic day-to-day loading. Originally, implants were grouted into place with cement, such as polymethylmethacrylate (PMMA) (see below). However, an alternative approach was introduced in which the bone was mechanically prepared to precise measurements so that it could accept a specific sized implant without the use of a grout. The term "osseointegration" originated with the experimental work of Brånemark's group in Gothenburg Sweden. The idea was "to endeavor to achieve a direct contact between living bone and implant, hoping in this way to improve the long-term function of the prosthetic device" (Albrektsson et al., 1981). Brånemark's group emphasized the use of threaded, unalloyed titanium, with a defined finish and geometry, placed within bone using meticulous surgical technique and a subsequent period of 3–4 months without loading to allow for adequate bone healing (Albrektsson et al., 1981). They showed direct implant–bone contact could be achieved at the light and transmission electron microscope levels. This group had extensive experience with titanium implants screwed into the mandible and maxilla as a platform to repair edentulous oral conditions (Adell et al., 1981). Over a period of approximately four decades, osseointegrated implants have found their way into many oral–facial and musculoskeletal applications, including joint replacement (Branemark et al., 2001). In this respect, the definition of osseointegration has been modified to mean that "there is no progressive relative movement between the implant and the bone with which it has direct contact"… and that "this anchorage can persist under all normal conditions of loading" (Branemark et al., 2001). Osseointegration is thought to be due to precise surgical technique and the use of a titanium implant that has an oxide layer, thus forming a hydrated titanium peroxy matrix (Branemark et al., 2001).

Osseointegration still remains a chief concept for the stabilization of joint replacements today. However, cementless implants for joint replacement currently are not screwed into place; instead, the bone is prepared to accept a slightly oversized implant that is "press fit" (usually by 1–2 mm) into the surrounding bone bed (Mai et al., 2010). Other methods have been added to obtain mechanical and biological stability, including porous coating, roughened surfaces, and splines to obtain bone ingrowth. Porous coating attempts to provide a mechanical interlock between the prosthesis and bone by creating pores on a portion of the implant surface using metal beads, wires, or a more structured cancellous bone-like surface (Mai et al., 2010; Bobyn et al., 1980; Patil et al., 2009; Galante, 1985). Usually this surface coating is sintered or plasma sprayed onto the implant circumferentially to avoid longitudinal channels for ingress of wear debris and inflammatory factors, capable of initiating bone loss (periprosthetic osteolysis) (Bobyn et al., 1995). The tissue growing into the pores is cancellous-like woven bone that matures, as well as stress-oriented fibrous tissue (Cook et al., 1988; Engh et al., 1993). Coatings such as hydroxyapatite (HA) have been added on the surface of some implants with/without porous coating. These HA coatings act as osteoconductive materials (Epinette and Manley, 2008). The use of HA coatings is somewhat controversial, and at least two meta-analyses have shown no additive benefit to HA over porous coating alone for primary total hip arthroplasty (Gandhi et al., 2009; Goosen et al., 2009).

Loose implants are not adequately fixed to bone, such that they migrate under physiological loads. This migration causes pain and limits function. By definition, loose cementless implants are not osseointegrated. Although the term "implant failure" may include many different causes including infection, breakage or dissociation of the parts, wear of the bearing surface with/without periprosthetic osteolysis, or adverse tissue reactions, failure is commonly used to denote a painful, migrating, loose prosthesis that is not functioning appropriately.

JOINT REPLACEMENT

Cemented joint replacements

The first highly successful joint replacement was the Low Friction Arthroplasty of the hip introduced by Sir John Charnley (1979). These hip replacements consisted of a stainless steel, one piece femoral component with a 22.25 mm femoral head that articulated with a socket made of high-density polyethylene. These implants were fixed in place with a grouting material, acrylic cement, or PMMA. This method was introduced to Charnley by Prof. Dennis Smith, then a Lecturer at the Turner Dental School in Manchester (The John Charnley Research Institute, 2009). Together, Charnley and Smith optimized the chemical and mechanical properties of bone cement for orthopedic applications (Charnley, 1970a, 1979; The John Charnley Research Institute, 2009).

Charnley originally used a cemented femoral component with a large femoral head (>40 mm in diameter) that articulated with a thin polytetrafluorethylene (Fluon) socket. The large ball size and suboptimal wear characteristics of the polymer lead to high frictional torque, the generation of wear particles, and an aggressive chronic inflammatory and foreign body response (FBR) leading to synovitis, osteolysis, and loosening. The final Low Friction Arthroplasty was a scientific optimization of engineering, material, and biological principles, and still remains a cornerstone for implant surgery today.

One of Charnley's achievements was monitoring the biocompatibility of the new hip replacement throughout the lifetime of the prosthesis. Through careful periodic clinical and radiological assessments, as well as histological analysis of femora with implants at postmortem, the biological reaction to a cemented prosthesis was described in detail. During the initial implantation of a cemented prosthesis, there is death of bone from the surgical procedure and a subsequent acute inflammatory reaction that extends to a radius of approximately 500 μm. This inflammatory reaction resolves over the next few weeks, with formation of fibrous tissue, fibrocartilage, and woven bone which undergoes remodeling adjacent to the cement mantle (Charnley, 1970b, 1979). In some areas, new bone is found directly abutting the cement, with integration of the cement within the interstices of the bony trabecula. As the bone remodels with age, the endosteal bone is resorbed and new lamella of bone are laid down by the periosteum. The remnant endosteum develops a neocortex around the cement mantle, connected to the more peripheral cortex by spicules of bone (Charnley, 1979; Maloney et al., 1989).

Particulate debris from cemented implants with conventional polyethylene generally consisted of fragments of bone cement, shards and submicron particles of polyethylene, and more rarely, metal particulates. Although the cement mantle can retain its fixation properties for many years, periprosthetic osteolysis can be seen in areas where the biological reaction to fractured cement has initiated a chronic inflammatory reaction, also known as "cement disease" (Jones and Hungerford, 1987; Willert et al., 1990a). More commonly though, periprosthetic osteolysis with cemented or hybrid hip and knee replacements was due to wear of conventional polyethylene (Willert et al., 1990b; Schmalzried et al., 1992; Campbell et al., 1995; Maloney et al., 1990a; Fornasier et al., 1991; Ingham and Fisher, 2000). This wear process undermines the bony support of the implant and can lead to prosthetic loosening due to failure of fixation. Histologically this failure of fixation is associated with a classic "pseudosynovial membrane" that can produce high levels of pro-inflammatory factors (Ingham and Fisher, 2000; Goldring et al., 1983; Goodman et al., 1989; Mandelin et al., 2005; Kadoya et al., 1996). The interface of loose cemented implants is laden with macrophages, scattered lymphocytes, and other cells in a fibrous tissue stroma (Revell, 2008). There is a great deal of heterogeneity in the tissue all histologically, histochemically, and biochemically depending on the anatomic site from which the sample is biopsied (Goodman et al., 1996). This chronic inflammatory reaction to wear debris can lead to bone destruction (periprosthetic osteolysis), jeopardizing the long-term stability of the implant (Maloney et al., 1990a; Fornasier et al., 1991; Kadoya et al., 1996; Santavirta et al., 1990a; Tallroth et al., 1989). However, many cemented implants last for decades without substantial degradation of the interfaces.

Cementless joint replacements

Cementless joint replacements rely on an initial "press fit" to obtain primary mechanical stability; this fit is often supplemented with screws, splines, surface coatings, or other mechanisms to obtain more sustaining long-term integration with host bone (Figure 12.1). Autopsy retrieval studies have demonstrated successful osseointegration

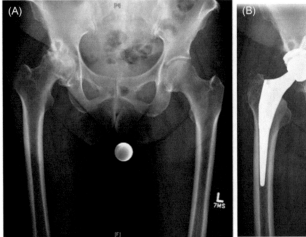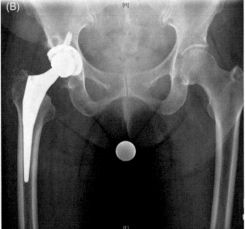

Figure 12.1 *Cementless total hip replacement.* (A) A severely arthritic left hip with no cartilage remaining, peripheral osteophytes and cyst formation in the femoral head and acetabulum. (B) Post cementless total hip replacement using a porous-coated acetabular component and screws, a cementless porous-coated stem, and a cobalt–chrome femoral head and highly cross-liked polyethylene liner.

of retrieved cementless hip implants in bone; however, much of the porous coating may be filled with oriented fibrous tissue instead of bone (Cook et al., 1988; Engh et al., 1993; Jacobs et al., 1999; Maloney et al., 1996). The characteristics of the patient, the implant, surgical technique, and the biomechanical environment determine the extent to which the surrounding bone undergoes remodeling. In cases of distally fixed stiff implants, adverse bone remodeling occurs with marked adverse remodeling such as disappearance of the proximal femur after hip replacement, the so-called stress shielding (Maloney et al., 1996). Although this adverse remodeling may be marked, it does not generally lead to loosening of the implant or pain (McAuley et al., 1998). In fact, when a cementless prosthesis has undergone extensive osseointegration, it is common to see proximal stress shielding (rounding off of the proximal-medial calcar femorale), osteopenia, and more distal oblique struts of bone connecting the cortex to the distal porous coating, the so-called spot welds.

Polyethylene debris can migrate along cementless interfaces, especially those without porous coating leading to progressive bone loss and periprosthetic osteolysis. Such osteolysis can occur even with well-fixed implants (Maloney et al., 1990b) and can lead to subsequent loosening of implants. With cyclic loading of the joint, waves of joint fluid, wear particles, and inflammatory mediators can be distributed widely around the prosthesis (Aspenberg and Van der Vis, 1998a,b) (Figures 12.2 and 12.3). Retrieval studies of tissues from cementless implants with osteolysis have shown a chronic inflammatory and FBR to polyethylene wear particles (Goodman et al., 1998; Kim et al., 1993).

Loose implants, whether cemented or cementless, often migrate, creating reactive remodeling in the surrounding bone, irrespective of wear particles. The resultant pressure on the endosteum at the point of contact leads to bone resorption on the inner cortex and new bone formation externally (Greenfield and Bechtold, 2008).

Metallic particles

Particles of polymers, ceramics, and other nonmetallic debris less than approximately 10 μm are phagocytosed by macrophages and other cells, activating these cells to produce pro-inflammatory factors (Willert and Semlitsch, 1977). Larger particles that can't be phagocytosed are surrounded by mono- and multinucleate giant cells ("frustrated phagocytosis"). See Chapter 2 for a more detailed description. The above reactions constitute a nonspecific, nonantigenic chronic inflammatory and foreign body reaction that may lead to periprosthetic osteolysis. Cobalt–chrome metal particles are different. These particles are in the nanometer range and are in far greater number from metal-on-metal (MoM) bearings than metal-on-polyethylene hip replacements. Metal particles can stimulate both the innate and adaptive immune system. In other words, metal particles can be phagocytosed and activate macrophages in a nonspecific manner (innate immune system), and can combine with serum proteins to form a hapten

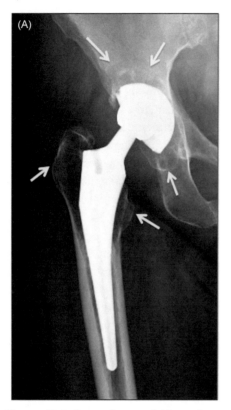
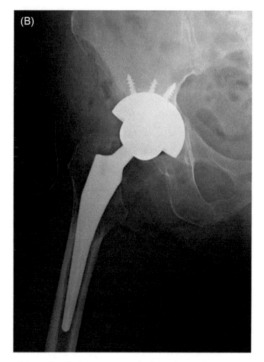

Figure 12.2 *Cementless total hip replacement with polyethylene wear and periprosthetic oste-olysis.* (A) Note the eccentric position of the femoral head in the cup, indicating polyethylene wear. Surrounding the cup and in the proximal femur, the biological reaction to wear particles has led to bone destruction called osteolysis (arrows). (B) Revision surgery has consisted of changing the entire cup and femoral head, and bone grafting of the deficient acetabular bed. Note a larger modular femoral head has been used to increase stability of the hip.

to activate the T lymphocyte dominated adaptive immune system. This latter biological mechanism is thought to constitute a type IV cell-mediated immune reaction and can result in nonloose implants with progressive, often severe soft tissue and bone destruction (Willert et al., 2005; Hallab et al., 2008). Cobalt–chrome metal particles, in sufficient numbers, have been shown to result in cytotoxicity, metal hypersensitivity, and pseudotumor formation (Gill et al., 2012). Pseudotumors are solid or cystic periarticular masses that have large areas of inflammation and tissue necrosis. Although perivascular lymphocytic cuffing is often seen in retrieved tissues from these implants, this histopathological finding is not specific for MoM implants and can be seen with metal-on-polyethylene prostheses as well (Fujishiro et al., 2011). Metal particles can be generated from other sources around hip and knee replacements, such as at the head–neck

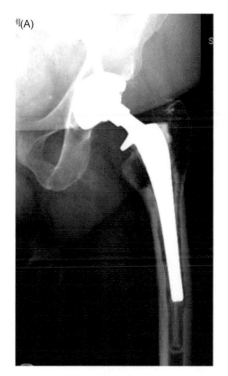
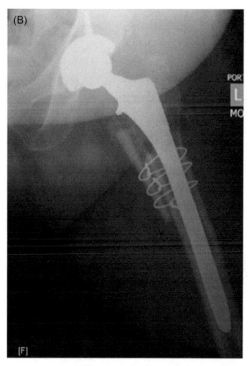

Figure 12.3 *Hybrid hip replacement with "cement disease."* (A) This total hip replacement has a well-fixed cementless acetabular component and a loose cemented stem. Note the bone destruction around the loose stem, which has changed position. (B) Immediate postoperative radiograph shows that a longer, porous-coated stem has been placed in the cleaned femoral canal. A femoral strut graft and wires buttresses the most severely deficient area on the femur. The modular acetabular plastic liner and femoral head have also been changed.

or neck–stem articulation in modular hip replacements, or when the plastic has been completely worn through, and a metal surface subsequently articulates with the underlying opposing metal backing. Titanium particles appear to be less stimulatory of these reactions compared to cobalt–chrome particles. See Chapter 8.

Clinical aspects of infection

Infection is one of the leading causes of failure of joint replacements. Infection severely compromises the function and durability of prosthetic joints (Vegari and Parvizi, 2011). A recent international consensus meeting has reviewed and reported the principle controversies surrounding infection of joint replacements (Parvizi et al., 2013). Infection of an implant bed can't be eradicated without extracting the prosthesis and thoroughly debriding the implant bed and all infected bone and soft tissue. The necessity for implant extraction is due to the fact that bacteria in the tissue fluid adjacent to artificial implants reside both in planktonic form and in the biofilm on the implant as sessile, dormant bacteria that may become activated at any time. Thus, total elimination of the infection necessitates removal of the implant.

Acute bacterial infection of a prosthesis is accompanied by an acute inflammatory reaction. Histologically, the tissues are edematous and contain polymorphonuclear leukocytes and bacteria. Chronic infection is usually more indolent, and the periprosthetic tissues are often filled with infected granulation tissue. There may be new periosteal bone formation around the prosthesis or areas of inflammation-associated osteolysis. Many infections have an acute on chronic component (i.e., "chronic active").

The pro-inflammatory factor profile of tissues from infected implants is similar to that of tissues from implants with particle-associated periprosthetic osteolysis (Pajarinen et al., 2010a). Prosthetic infection is associated with activation of Toll-like receptors (TLRs) which are part of the innate immune system. This mechanism involves the recognition of pathogen-associated molecular patterns (PAMPs) of bacteria, fungi, and viruses by pattern recognition receptors (PRRs) on cell membranes. This interaction activates a complex pro-inflammatory cascade that destroys the pathogen and reestablishes homeostasis to ensure survival of the organism. Previous research has demonstrated that retrieved implants frequently harbor PAMPs on their surfaces (Greenfield et al., 2005). These aspects are discussed in more detail below and in Chapters 7 and 8.

OTHER CLINICAL SCENARIOS

Implants are used in virtually every orthopedic subspecialty. Fractures of the upper and lower extremities are reduced and stabilized by plates and screws, intramedullary devices, wires, etc. Similarly, devices have been designed for spine fracture reduction and fixation, as well as the correction of spinal deformities. Arthroplasties of the upper and lower extremities are used with increasing frequency. Disk replacements in the cervical and lumbar spine are also being performed (Cason and Herkowitz, 2013; Jacobs et al., 2013). In general, these implants are composed of metal alloys, including stainless steel, cobalt–chrome, titanium, and tantalum, nonbiodegradable polymers, such as polyethylene, PMMA, polyaryletherketones (PAEKs), among others, and biodegradable polymers such as poly-L-lactic acid (PLLA), co-poly lactic acid/glycolic acid (PLGA), and numerous other biopolymers as scaffolds for orthopedic tissue engineering.

The basic biological, biomechanical, and material principles of bone and soft tissue healing are applicable to all subspecialties that employ implants (Bong et al., 2007; Marsell and Einhorn, 2011). In addition, preclinical biological and biomechanical testing must be comprehensive for the specific anatomical application prior to introduction of the device to the marketplace (Gardner et al., 2012). This approach will hopefully limit complications such as suboptimal surgical technique and placement of devices, mechanical failure of the device, adverse tissue reactions, and others. Although bioabsorbable fixation devices were enticing, an increased incidence of adverse tissue reactions was often noted with some materials, such as polyglycolic acid (Bostman and Pihlajamaki, 2000).

Spinal disk replacement with a nonbiodegradable implant is a new application, although the procedure is still controversial (Cason and Herkowitz, 2013; Jacobs et al., 2013). Wear particle debris from intervertebral disk replacements may have more serious consequences than debris in more peripheral joints because of the close proximity of neural structures (Jacobs et al., 2006; Baxter et al., 2013; Punt et al., 2012, 2009).

IMMUNE RESPONSES TO BIOMATERIALS FOR ORTHOPEDIC APPLICATIONS—PRECLINICAL STUDIES

Acute inflammation

Implantation of biomaterials is always accompanied by injury due to the surgical procedure (Wilson et al., 2005). Injury to the tissue or organ initiates an acute inflammatory reaction in addition to the specific reaction to the biomaterial itself. These events primarily activate the nonspecific innate immune system. The characteristics of the reaction are identified by, and dependent upon, several factors including the extent of injury, protein absorption, coagulation, complement activation, and migration of leukocytes to the area. See Chapter 5.

Protein adsorption

After first contact with tissue, proteins from the blood and interstitial fluid immediately adsorb to the material surface prior to interacting with host cells. This layer of proteins determines the tissue reaction to the implant and guides the inflammatory cascade to the formation of a transient provisional matrix, complement activation, and migration of leukocytes to the surgical site (Wilson et al., 2005; Andersson et al., 2002; Gorbet and Sefton, 2004). Conversely, the physicochemical properties of the biomaterial implant including the composition, size, shape, surface roughness, surface chemistry, hydrophobicity, and surface charge influence the types, concentrations, and conformations of the adsorbed proteins on the surface. These proteins subsequently determine the adhesion and survival of cells, especially polymorphonuclear neutrophils, monocytes, macrophages, and foreign body giant cells (FBGCs) (Hunt et al., 1996; DeFife et al., 1999). The presence of adsorbed protein such as albumin, fibrinogen, complement, fibronectin (Fn), vitronectin, and γ-globulin determine and modulate cell adhesion and intercellular interactions on the implant surface, thereby influencing the subsequent wound healing response. This protein adsorption phenomenon is the equivalent of the Vroman effect for biomaterials in contact with blood. See Chapters 3, 5, and 8 for further details.

Coagulation

The intrinsic and extrinsic coagulation cascades are initiated by Factor XII (FXII) and tissue factor (TF). The intrinsic coagulation is induced by contact activation of FXII on negatively charged substrates followed by a downstream cascade of protein reactions resulting in the activation of prothrombin to thrombin (Gorbet and Sefton, 2004; Schmaier, 1997). Activation of FXII has been shown to be catalyzed by surface contact with biomaterials (Zhuo et al., 2006). Although activated FXII on the material surface initiates the generation of thrombin, the amount produced is not sufficient to induce clot formation (Sperling et al., 2009). Blood coagulation on biomaterials has been recently shown to require the combination of both contact activation and platelet adhesion and activation (Sperling et al., 2009; Fischer et al., 2010a).

Thrombin is one of the most important activators of platelets. The minute amount of thrombin resulting from FXII activates platelets to release mediators of the coagulation system and exposes negatively charged phospholipids, thus providing the necessary catalytic surface for the coagulation cascade (Sperling et al., 2009; Heemskerk et al., 2002). Subsequent thrombin production activates platelets and the coagulation cascade on biomaterial surfaces (Johne et al., 2006). Fibrinogen also absorbs to biomaterials (Tang, 1998). Integrin bonding domains on phagocytes are activated by fibrinogen/fibrin adhered to biomaterials, further initiating the inflammatory response and blood clot formation (Hu et al., 2001). Besides thrombin and fibrinogen, TF expressed on damaged cells or activated leukocytes can activate attached platelets (Fischer et al., 2010b).

Complement activation

Upon contact with biomaterials, three distinct pathways, the alternative, the classical, and the lectin pathway, can activate complement. All of the pathways converge at the level of C3 convertase activation that mediates the formation and release of the anaphylatoxins C3 and C5a (Sarma and Ward, 2011). Complement activation is always associated with the biomaterial adsorbed protein layer. Attached IgG has been demonstrated to bind C1q resulting in the assembly of C1, the first enzyme of the classical pathway that promotes the initiation of classical C3 convertase (Tengvall et al., 2001). C3 adsorbed to the biomaterial surface promotes the assembly of the initiating C3 convertase of the alternative pathway (Andersson et al., 2005). C3 convertase generates C3b that binds to the biomaterial protein layer to form more C3 convertase (Andersson et al., 2002; Nilsson et al., 2007). Once the complement cascade has been initiated, high amounts of C3a and C5a are generated at the implantation site (Andersson et al., 2005). Both anaphylatoxins can contribute to the onset of inflammatory responses at the implantation site through their multitude of effector functions including triggering mast cell degranulation, increasing vascular permeability, attracting and activating granulocytes and monocytes, and inducing the release of granulocyte-reactive oxygen species (Sarma and Ward, 2011). The coagulation cascade and complement system closely interact on the biomaterial surface and modulate each other activities (Fischer et al., 2010b).

Inflammatory cells

Leukocytes migrate from the blood vessels to the perivascular tissues at the implantation site (Henson and Johnston, 1987; Lehrer et al., 1988; Malech and Gallin, 1987). These leukocytes accumulate through a series of processes including margination, adhesion, emigration, phagocytosis, and extracellular release of leukocyte contents. Cell adhesion and activation on biomaterial surfaces primarily interact with the adsorbed proteins. Protein ligands of integrins which represent the major adhesion receptors of leukocytes include fibrinogen, factor X, iC3b, Fn, and vitronectin (Hynes, 2002; Lowell and Berton, 1999). Initial adhesion and spreading of phagocytes are achieved through b2 integrins (Hu et al., 2001; McNally and Anderson, 1994) which in turn leads to a change in the receptor profile including the up-regulation and enabling of further integrins (Hynes, 2002). Mast cell degranulation and associated histamine release have been shown to play a role in directing polymorphonuclear leukocytes and monocytes to implanted biomaterials in mice and human (Tang et al., 1998; Zdolsek et al., 2007). Interleukin-4 (IL-4) and IL-13 are also released from mast cells during the degranulation process and play significant roles in determining the extent of the subsequent foreign body reaction. Polymorphonuclear leukocytes represent a source of immunoregulatory signals which are synthesized upon activation (Scapini et al., 2000). IL-8 is among the most prominent of these chemokines. The primary target of IL-8 is polymorphonuclaer leukocytes. With some materials such as chitosan, granulocyte migration may be prolonged due to persistent autocrine polymorphonuclear leukocytes attraction by IL-8 (Hidaka et al., 1999; VandeVord et al., 2002; Park et al., 2009).

Activated polymorphonuclear leukocytes also secrete monocyte chemotactic protein-1 (MCP-1, also called CCL2) and macrophage inflammatory protein-1 (MIP-1) (Kobayashi et al., 2005). Both chemokines are known as potent chemoattractants and activation factors for monocytes, macrophages, immature dendritic cells, and lymphocytes (Yamashiro et al., 2001). Increased release of these chemokines by polymorphonuclear leukocytes suppresses further polymorphonuclear leukocyte infiltration in favor of mononuclear cell influx (Gilroy et al., 2004). Due to a lack of further activation signals, polymorphonuclear leukocytes undergo apoptosis after having fulfilled their roles as phagocytes and are subsequently engulfed by macrophages (Gilroy et al., 2004). Macrophage phagocytosis of apoptotic PMNs has been shown to promote a phenotypic shift in macrophage phenotype toward an anti-inflammatory and immunoregulatory form. See Chapter 6. This macrophage phenotype shift may be critical in limiting the severity and duration of the inflammatory process. Thus, within the first 2 days after biomaterial implantation, polymorphonuclear leukocytes typically disappear from surgical sites (Anderson et al., 2008).

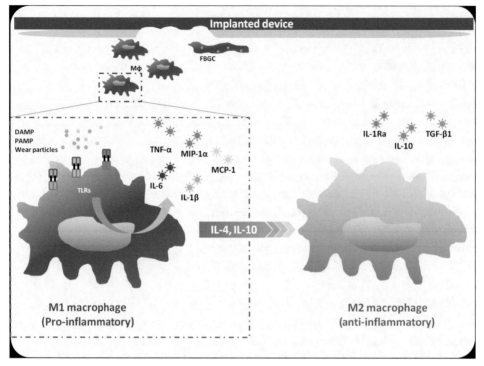

Figure 12.4 *Macrophage polarization in relation to orthopedic biomaterials and their by-products.*

Chronic inflammation induced by implanted biomaterials

Excessive generation of wear particles can lead to chronic inflammation, which involves the secretion of multiple cytokines from macrophages and FBGC. The biological response of immune effector cells to the particles is dependent on the particle composition (Ingham and Fisher, 2000), dose (Green et al., 2000; Chiu et al., 2009), and size (Green et al., 2000, 1998; Wang, A. et al., 1996; Hallab et al., 2011). Smaller particles (<1 μm) are phagocytosed by macrophages, whereas larger sized particles (>10 μm) are generally surrounded by many macrophages and FBGCs (frustrated phagocytosis) (Ingham and Fisher, 2005). The activated macrophages secrete cytokines, chemokines, and other factors that recruit more macrophages to the local area, induce osteoclast maturation, and eventually cause periprosthetic osteolysis (Ingham and Fisher, 2005) (Figure 12.4).

Recognition of wear particles by TLRs

The innate immune response can be activated by PRRs on or within cells, in the presence of chemical sequences called bacterial-derived PAMPs (described earlier) and host-derived damage-associated molecular patterns (DAMPs). These molecular patterns are "danger signals" resulting from invasion of the host by pathogens or result from cellular trauma due to adverse stimuli. These DAMPs and PAMPs can adhere to the surface of implanted devices or be associated with the generated wear particles, and are recognized by PRRs such as TLRs (Greenfield et al., 2005; Bennewitz and Babensee, 2005; Kido et al., 2004; Rogers and Babensee, 2010; Nalepka et al., 2006; Xing et al., 2006; Tatro et al., 2007). TLR2 and TLR4 are most relevant to wear particle-induced inflammation and osteolysis (Gu et al., 2012). Increased TLR2, TLR4, TLR5, and TLR9 expressions were found in monocyte/macrophages from aseptically loose periprosthetic tissues and septic synovial membranes around total hip implants (Tamaki et al., 2009). TLR2 and TLR5 expression was found to be significantly higher than TLR4 and TLR9. In *in vitro* studies, titanium particles coated by lipopolysaccharide (LPS) stimulated increased TLR2 expression in rat bone-marrow-derived macrophages (Hirayama et al., 2011). However, the expression of TLR4, TLR5, and RLT9 was decreased, suggesting a homeostatic protective mechanism to contain the adverse stimulus. In experimental mouse models, TLR2 expression was increased in the synovial membranes of knee joints injected with ultrahigh molecular weight polyethylene (UHMWPE) particles (Paulus et al., 2013). TLR2 and TLR4 expressions were both increased in a cavarial model injected with UHMWPE particles (Valladares et al., 2013). In contrast, the number of TLR positive cells was reduced in the mouse femur exposed to titanium particles (Pajarinen et al., 2010b). In transgenic animal studies, titanium particle-induced tumor necrosis factor-α (TNF-α) expression by macrophages was significantly reduced in both TLR2 and TLR4 deficient mice (Greenfield et al., 2010). However, osteolysis using the mouse cavarial model was only partially reduced, suggesting that the TLR2 and TLR4 independent pathways may contribute to titanium particle-induced osteolysis.

The requirement of PAMP in wear particle-induced TLR activation may depend on the particle characteristics and the experimental model used. Greenfield et al. (2010) showed that titanium particle-induced inflammatory responses and osteolysis required the presence of bacterial-derived PAMP. Pearl et al. (2011) demonstrated that TNF-α secretion was reduced in mouse macrophages from MyD88 deficient mice or by the presence of MyD88 inhibitors when the cells were stimulated by PMMA. Reduction of osteolysis was also observed in the MyD88 deficient mice using a particle-exposed cavarial model. These results suggest that PMMA particles without PAMP can activate macrophages and induce osteolysis in a TLR pathway-dependent manner.

Macrophages and secreted cytokines

Periprosthetic osteolysis is associated with a granulomatous reaction that is rich in macrophages and wear debris (Ingham and Fisher, 2005). The presence of macrophages correlates with the amount of wear debris in tissues from implants with aseptic loosening (Maloney et al., 1990b; Santavirta et al., 1990b). Submicron-sized wear particles are phagocytosed leading to increased production of cytokines by macrophages.

Increased TNF-α, IL-1, and IL-6 levels were found in the interfacial tissue from hip replacements with osteolysis (Chiba et al., 1994). Chemokines including MCP-1 and MIP-1α were also detected by immunohistochemistry in periprosthetic granulomatous tissue (Nakashima et al., 1999a). Increased prostaglandin E2 (PGE2) was found in tissues from loose implants compared to those which were well fixed (Nakashima et al., 1999a). Increased growth factor and matrix metalloproteinase expression was also noted in tissues from cases exhibiting osteolysis. However, there is no consistent relationship that directly correlates the degree of osteolysis with the amount of any specific inflammatory factor (Ingham and Fisher, 2005).

In vitro studies of macrophages and wear particles have proven to be very useful, as many factors such as the particle characteristics and cell type can be standardized. In one study, mouse macrophages exposed to endotoxin-free titanium particles showed no induction of TNF-α (Greenfield et al., 2010). In contrast, the expression of TNF-α and MCP-1 was increased in mouse macrophages exposed to endotoxin-free PMMA particles (Pearl et al., 2011; Yao et al., 2013). A recent study using cytokine arrays showed that when mouse bone marrow macrophages and human THP-1 macrophage cells were exposed to endotoxin-free UHMWPE particles, chemokines including MCP-1, MIP-1α, IL-8, CXCL1, and the pro-inflammatory cytokine TNF-α were increased (Lin et al., 2014).

Recent murine studies suggested that TNF-α could be a valuable target to mitigate particle-induced osteolysis. Using the mouse cavarial model, osteolysis induced by PMMA (Merkel et al., 1999) or titanium (Schwarz et al., 2000c; Merkel et al., 1999) particles were both reduced in the TNF-α receptor type I knockout mice or mice treated with TNF-α receptor antagonist, despite persistently high levels of TNF-α. However, a pilot study in 20 patients with TJRs and osteolysis showed no significant benefit by treatment using a TNF-α receptor antagonist (Schwarz et al., 2003); these findings may due to the limited number of patients in the study or potential compensated roles of other inflammatory cytokines. Alternatively, suppression of macrophage functions may be achieved via interruption of macrophage infiltration, blockage of inflammatory signaling, or modulation of macrophage polarization. The details of macrophage targeting therapy are described in the section "Local Biologic Modulation to Wear Particles."

Adaptive immune response to metals
Introduction
There is little question that the innate immune system is involved in the host response to implanted orthopedic materials, with macrophages playing a key role in the initiation, propagation, and resolution of this biomaterial-induced inflammation. In contrast, the role of adaptive immunity to implanted orthopedic materials is less clear. While the innate immune system interacts directly with the biomaterial and/or the proteins

bound to its surface via complement activation and direct recognition by various PRRs, T-cells can recognize their corresponding antigen only if presented to them by a professional antigen-presenting cell.

Antigen presentation and T-cell activation is a complex, multistep process that is initiated by dendritic cell activation due to recognition of a danger signal molecule, antigen internalization and processing via the endolysosomal route, migration of the dendritic cell to local lymphatic tissue, up-regulation of co-stimulatory molecules, and finally presentation of the processed antigen as a part of the major histocompatibility complex (MHC) II. See Chapter 7 for more details regarding the role of dendritic cells in the host response. If the antigen is presented with a sufficient set of co-stimulatory molecules (that are regulated by the extent of dendritic cell stimulation by danger signal molecules), the naïve T helper cell becomes activated and clonally expands. The cytokines secreted by the activated dendritic cell during antigen presentation further regulate T-cell polarization into phenotypes such as Th1, Th2, Th17, or T-reg. These immunocompetent CD4$^+$ T helper cells migrate to the area of inflammation where they regulate the inflammatory reaction and chemotaxis as well as the actions of innate immune cells such as macrophages, by secreting chemokines and cytokines including CCL2, CCL3, CCL4, TNF-α, IL-17, IFN-γ, IL-4, and IL-10 while cytotoxic CD8$^+$ T-cells induce the apoptosis of transformed or virus-infected cells. In contrast to T-cells, naïve B-cells can directly recognize their corresponding antigen without presentation but to differentiate into mature antibody producing plasma cell, B-cells still need a signal from CD4$^+$ T helper cell already activated by the antigen-presenting dendritic cell. See Chapters 7 and 8 for additional details regarding antigen-presenting cells.

Thus, the involvement of the adaptive immune response, either T- or B-cell-mediated, in the host response to inorganic orthopedic materials seems unlikely. Although sensitization against PMMA has been described, there is little evidence that adaptive immunity is involved in the host response to typical orthopedic polymers (Goodman, 2007). For example, in animal models, the foreign body reaction to implanted polyethylene or PMMA particles is not dependent on the existence of T lymphocytes (Goodman et al., 1994; Jiranek et al., 1995; Taki et al., 2005). Furthermore, although osteolytic lesions developing due to PMMA or polyethylene wear around joint replacements containing scattered T lymphocytes, it is not clear whether these cells are active participants to the inflammatory process or just innocent bystanders (Li et al., 2001; Baldwin et al., 2002; Arora et al., 2003). B-cells and plasma cells are notably absent from these lesions, and it has even been suggested, although not thoroughly validated, that the presence of B-cells and plasma cells in the periimplant tissues might indicate subclinical implant infection (Pajarinen et al., 2010a); while the aseptic foreign body reaction to polymer wear products probably does not provide a sufficient stimulus to activate the adaptive immune response, implant-associated biofilm that occasionally releases danger signal molecules and presentable foreign antigens might do so.

Type IV delayed-type hypersensitivity

In contrast to orthopedic polymers, metal ions can function as effective allergens and activate adaptive, cell-mediated, immune responses by forming haptens with proteins in biological fluids. Solubilized metal ions bind to host proteins, altering their conformation so that they become immunogenic and are recognized as foreign when presented to the T lymphocyte population. Furthermore, metal ions can induce conformational changes to the MHC molecule itself causing it to be recognized as foreign similar to organ transplant rejection. Metal ions can also activate T-cell receptors directly in the manner of super antigens. However, hapten formation is the archetypal way in which metals are able to activate adaptive immune responses.

The best characterized example of this phenomenon, known as type IV or delayed-type hypersensitivity reaction, is nickel-induced contact dermatitis (Schmidt and Goebeler, 2011). Nickel ions are released from metal alloys in contact with the skin and sweat. Ions activate dermal dendritic cells, which present ion–protein complexes to T lymphocytes in the local lymph node. T lymphocytes are activated, assume Th1 polarization, and migrate to the area of inflammation where they regulate the function of macrophages presenting similar haptens in their MHC II molecules. In addition to forming haptens, nickel ions also activate TLR4 signaling in dendritic cells (Schmidt et al., 2010). Thus nickel ions are able to produce both immune-reactive neo-antigens and provide the required danger signal to initiate dendritic cell maturation and antigen presentation, possibly explaining why nickel is such an effective and prevalent allergen. In addition to nickel, cobalt, chrome, and several other metal ions are known to induce contact dermatitis via similar mechanisms. However, although reports of titanium hypersensitivity do exist, it is a rare phenomenon.

Delayed-type hypersensitivity and orthopedic implants

It has long been speculated that a type IV hypersensitivity reaction could develop against metal ions released from the metal alloys commonly used in orthopedics, such as stainless steel and cobalt–chrome (releasing mainly cobalt, chromium, and nickel ions) or titanium alloy. Although there are incidental reports describing the development of an allergic reaction against implants used in fracture fixation (Cramers and Lucht, 1977; Thomas et al., 2000, 2006), the interest in the possibility of metal allergy has been renewed by the unexpected early failures of MoM joint replacements and the peculiar tissue responses that characterize these failures. These adverse reactions to MoM implants have been attributed to the unique wear characteristics of metal bearing surfaces with generation of large amounts of nano-sized metal particles, corrosion of these particles, and subsequent release of metal ions. Indeed, high levels of cobalt and chrome have been described not only in periprosthetic tissues but also in the blood and urine of MoM joint replacement recipients (De Smet et al., 2008; Hart et al., 2011; Skipor et al., 2002); furthermore cases of alleged systemic cobalt toxicity with severe cardiac and neurological manifestations have been described (Tower, 2010; Allen et al., 2014). Widespread dissemination of metal wear particles, e.g., to local lymph nodes, has been reported (Urban et al., 2000).

The osteolytic lesions developing around joint replacements due to polyethylene or PMMA wear particles have traditionally been composed of sheet-like macrophages, some scattered T lymphocytes, and large areas of fibrosis (Santavirta et al., 1990a; Willert and Semlitsch, 1977; Mirra et al., 1982). In contrast, the adverse tissue response developing around MoM implants is characterized by the development of large cystic or solid pseudotumors sometimes with considerable bone loss. Large areas of necrosis and macrophage as well as T, B lymphocyte and plasma cell infiltrates are typically seen histologically. Perivascular T lymphocyte infiltrates have been described as characteristic of the adverse reaction to MoM implants and been considered as histopathological evidence of a metal hypersensitivity reaction (Willert et al., 2005; Davies et al., 2005; Korovessis et al., 2006; Campbell et al., 2010). In agreement with this assumption, an association between periprosthetic tissue metal content and the type of inflammatory cell infiltration was recently described; high cobalt and chrome concentration was associated with nodular lymphocyte infiltrates whereas macrophage infiltrates predominated in tissues with low metal content (Lohmann et al., 2013). However, other reports have found no clear link between tissue metal content and the type of inflammatory reaction while still others have described that perivascular lymphocyte infiltrates are, in fact, found also from considerable number of adverse tissue reactions that are caused by conventional, non-MoM TJR implants (Fujishiro et al., 2011; Ng et al., 2011).

Alterations in the peripheral blood lymphocyte populations have been described in MoM implant recipients. Typically a decrease either in the total number of circulating T lymphocytes or in the $CD8^+$ cytotoxic subpopulation has been reported (Granchi et al., 2003; Hart et al., 2009). It has been suggested that this relative lymphopenia might be due to increased lymphocyte recruitment to inflamed periprosthetic tissue, although decreased lymphocyte proliferation and viability (see below) might also explain the phenomenon. Increased reactivity of peripheral blood lymphocytes against cobalt and chrome ions in patients with either non-MoM or MoM implants has also been described and the magnitude of this metal ion-induced lymphocyte activation has in some studies correlated to blood cobalt and chromium levels (Granchi et al., 1999; Hallab et al., 2004, 2005, 2008). Typically metal-reactive lymphocytes have exhibited a Th1 type of response, fitting the theory of metal hypersensitivity (Granchi et al., 1999; Hallab et al., 2008). In an interesting case report, cobalt-reactive Th1 lymphocytes were isolated from periprosthetic tissue surrounding a wrist joint replacement implant (Thomssen et al., 2001). Although these reports would seem to indicate the development of metal-reactive lymphocyte populations due to metal ions released from conventional or MoM joint replacement implants, contradictory reports that could not find increased reactivity to metal ions also exist (Kwon et al., 2010). Overall the wider meaning of these findings remains to be determined.

In vitro and *in vivo* *effects of orthopedic metals in adaptive immunity*

In addition to these clinical observations, there are *in vitro* and *in vivo* studies investigating the effects that cobalt, chromium, and titanium ions or nano-sized particles have on cells of the adaptive immune system. Titanium ions increased the proliferation and enhanced the activation and receptor activator nuclear factor kappa B (RANKL) production of phytohemagglutinin-activated human peripheral blood mononuclear cells (Cadosch et al., 2010). Another study found that titanium and chromium ions formed complexes with serum proteins and were able to activate peripheral blood mononuclear cells; chromium ions and the fraction of larger serum proteins were more stimulatory than titanium ions or the fraction of smaller serum proteins (Hallab et al., 2001). However, several contradictory observations describing metal-ion-induced enhancement of lymphocyte activation have been made. For example, retrieved micron-sized titanium particles had no effect on the proliferation or the production of IL-2 from activated peripheral blood lymphocytes; of interest, similar particles had an activating effect on peripheral blood-derived macrophages (Kohilas et al., 1999). In addition cobalt–chrome nanoparticles did not activate dendritic cells or B lymphocytes *in vitro* and reduced the proliferation of activated T lymphocytes (Ogunwale et al., 2009). In another study, it was found that titanium, chromium, and cobalt ions all inhibited human peripheral blood T and B lymphocyte activation and the production of inflammatory cytokines, while cytotoxicity was not observed (Wang, J.Y. et al., 1996). Similar effects were reported for activated and nonactivated human peripheral blood T lymphocytes in which cobalt and chromium ions at clinically relevant concentrations inhibited the proliferation and cytokine production of lymphocytes, and induced lymphocyte apoptosis at higher ion concentrations (Akbar et al., 2011). Another study reported that cobalt, chromium, and various other metal ions had a cytotoxic effect on the human T lymphocyte Jurkat cell line, with metal ions inducing both apoptosis and cell necrosis; interestingly these effects were not associated with DNA damage (Caicedo et al., 2008). Wang et al. (1997a) performed a series of *in vitro* and *in vivo* studies with titanium and cobalt–chrome particles and ions. These metals/ions inhibited cytokine release from cultured and activated murine T lymphocytes as well as IgG production from activated B lymphocytes with cobalt–chrome having more clear-cut effect than titanium. Interestingly very similar immunosuppressive effects on T lymphocyte cytokine production and B lymphocyte IgG production were observed *in vivo* when titanium or cobalt–chrome particles were injected into the mouse peritoneal cavity and the proliferation, cytokine release, and IgG production of activated splenic T and B lymphocytes were analyzed in subsequent weeks.

Taken together, the majority of these studies suggest that cobalt, chromium and, to lesser extent, titanium ions have suppressive rather than stimulatory effects on T and B lymphocyte activation and proliferation, with higher ion concentrations having cytotoxic effects. However, these studies have not really investigated the immunogenicity of these metal ions but investigated how metal ions modulate lymphocyte action. Relatively little is known about the actions of nano-sized metal particles. In this regard, a recent study by Brown et al. (2013) may have shed further light on these issues. Nano- or micron-sized cobalt–chrome particles at clinically relevant dosages were repeatedly injected into mouse knee joints at 0, 6, 12, and 18 weeks. Both types of particles were rapidly transported to local lymph nodes with minimal inflammatory infiltrates at the joint tissue itself. Interestingly mice injected with micron-sized, but not nano-sized, particles developed cobalt-, chrome-, and nickel-reactive Th1 lymphocytes. In contrast, there was increased abnormal DNA breakage observed in bone marrow cells and even brain cells in the nanoparticle group. It was suggested that micron-sized particles are phagocytosed with endogenous proteins by antigen-presenting cells, corroded in the acidic environment of phagolysosomes to release metal ions which then form haptens with endogenous peptides, and are finally presented to T lymphocytes by MHC II molecules. In contrast, nano-sized particles enter the cell outside the phagolysosomal route and cause DNA damage via mechanisms that are poorly understood.

Clinical metal allergy and TJR survivorship

The relationship of metal allergy and conventional and MoM implant survivorship has been investigated in several clinical studies. In a recent meta-analysis, although the occurrence of metal allergy was more common in patients with MoM implants, the detection of the allergy did not reliably predict implant failure (Granchi et al., 2012). Thus the extent to which adaptive immune responses participate in the development of pseudotumors and to other adverse reactions to MoM implants still remains a subject for further studies. The question of why metal allergy is relatively common but only occasionally contributes to implant failures might reflect tissue-specific immune response, i.e., the type and extent of the adaptive immune response is tuned to meet the needs of the specific tissue microenvironment (Matzinger, 2007; Matzinger and Kamala, 2011). In this case, it is probable that the detection of *dermal* metal allergy does not comprehensively reflect the immunological microenvironment of the periimplant tissue. For example, multinucleated epidermal giant cells are found exclusively in the skin and may be only involved in a local allergic phenomenon.

Other effects of metal wear

In addition to the potential of activating an adaptive type IV hypersensitivity, several other means by which metal particles and a large metal ion load can cause adverse host responses have been reported. For example, metal ions display dose-dependent cytotoxic effects on macrophages, osteoblasts, and fibroblasts (Gill et al., 2012; Billi and Campbell, 2010). Dose- and time-dependent increases in macrophage mortality have been reported, with smaller ion concentrations being associated with macrophage apoptosis and larger ones with necrosis (Catelas et al., 2005). The cytotoxic effects of various metal ions might explain the extensive necrotic areas developing around MoM joint replacements; the intracellular danger signal molecules released during cell necrosis provide the danger signal necessary to initiate dendritic cell maturation and antigen presentation ultimately leading to activation of adaptive immunity. Metal ions and larger (micron-sized) metal particles can also activate macrophages and the innate immune system in a manner very similar to polymeric wear, presumably via such mechanisms as recognition via PRRs, induction of endosomal damage, and activation of intracellular danger sensing mechanisms (Taki et al., 2005; Shanbhag et al., 1995; Nakashima et al., 1999b; Caicedo et al., 2009, 2013). Importantly, up-regulation of co-stimulatory molecules in macrophages by metal ions and particles have been described (Caicedo et al., 2010). Other effects that have been attributed to metal ions include suppression of osteoblast function, with alteration of the osteoprotegerin (OPG)/RANKL ratio to favor osteoclastogenesis (Wang et al., 1997b; Fleury et al., 2006; Andrews et al., 2011; Zijlstra et al., 2012).

Finally, Ninomiya et al. (2013) recently reported that cobalt ions activated vascular endothelial cells to produce chemokines and adhesion molecules with increased lymphocyte adherence and endothelial transmigration. It is possible that the perivascular lymphocyte infiltrates described around MoM implants might be, in fact, caused by cobalt-induced endothelial activation and increased recruitment of lymphocytes. Recently it was reported that, in analogy to nickel ions, TLR4 signaling is also directly activated by cobalt ions (Tyson-Capper et al., 2013; Konttinen and Pajarinen, 2013); this observation might explain how cobalt ions are recognized by macrophages and other cells and how the ions elicit cell activation and inflammatory responses, providing a direct mechanistic link between the activation of the innate and adaptive immune systems (Figure 12.5).

MODULATING THE HOST RESPONSE TO ORTHOPEDIC IMPLANTS

Implantation of an orthopedic device initiates a host reaction associated with the implant and leads to the generation of wear particles and other by-products. The reaction is typically divided into sequential stages that follow in continuous manner and can be recognized by typical periimplant histology (Anderson, 1993; Luttikhuizen et al., 2006). Although most materials evoke an innate nonspecific, nonantigenic host immune response, macrophages and dendritic cells may process and present potential antigenic stimuli to cells of the adaptive immune system. Whether innate or adaptive (antigenic) immune responses are activated, macrophages are key regulators because of the great number of biologically active products they produce (Johnston, 1988).

Although the chronic inflammatory reaction to implant degradation products is primarily a local phenomenon, several research groups demonstrated migration of systemically delivered reporter macrophages and mesenchymal cells to the site of

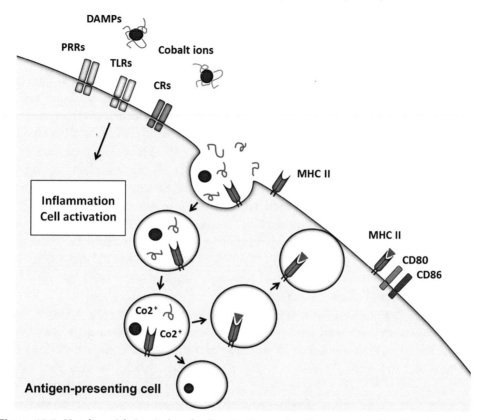

Figure 12.5 *Metal particle/ion-induced cell activation and antigen presentation.* Metal particles in biological fluids are coated with host proteins, such as complement fragments and possibly by danger signal molecules (DAMP) released from necrotic cells and fragmented extra cellular matrix, while metal ions form haptens with host proteins. Protein-coated metallic wear particles are recognized by cell surface receptors, such as complement receptors (CRs) and various PRRs. In addition, nickel and cobalt ions can directly induce TLR4 signaling. Signaling via these receptors induces an inflammatory reaction and cell activation followed by migration to local lymphatic tissue and the up-regulation of MHC II and co-stimulatory molecules such as CD80 and CD86. Signaling via various PRRs also induces phagocytosis of metal particles or metal ions in complexes with host proteins. These are processed along the endolysosomal route, leading to corrosion of the metal particles with further release of metal ions and formation of haptens. Haptens are then bound to MHC II and transported back to the cell surface. Finally these neo-antigens are presented to T lymphocytes in the local lymphatic tissue and, if the expression of co-stimulatory molecules is sufficient, the adaptive immune system is activated.

inflammation induced by biomaterial by-products (Fritton et al., 2012; Gibon et al., 2012b; Ren et al., 2011, 2008; Schepers et al., 2006). Thus, systemic or local interference of inflammatory pathways and inhibition of inflammatory macrophage migration might mitigate the inflammatory reaction to orthopedic biomaterials.

Systemic modulation of wear particle-induced osteolysis

Typically, as wear particles and other by-products are released from prostheses and other orthopedic implants, local tissue macrophages initiate an inflammatory reaction both regionally and systemically that responds to the adverse stimuli. Cell signaling processes will be triggered which will induce osteoclasts to effect periprosthetic bone resorption (Ingham and Fisher, 2005). The host response can be modulated pharmacologically through the systemic use of anti-inflammatory and related agents such as bisphosphonates, vitamins, anti-TNF-α/IL-1 agents, and others (Shanbhag, 2006; Schwarz et al., 2000a). Anti-inflammatory agents have proved effective for the treatment of osteolysis in animal models. Pentoxifylline, etanercept, and other anti-TNF-α therapies have been reported to diminish particle-induced osteolysis in mouse models (Schwarz et al., 2000a,b; Childs et al., 2001). Pentoxifylline, a potent oral TNF-α inhibitor, has been used in the treatment of peripheral vascular disease. *In vitro* studies showed that this drug reduced the inflammatory response of isolated monocytes from healthy subjects to wear particle exposure. However, the effects of pentoxyfylline in patients with osteolysis have not been elucidated (Pollice et al., 2001).

Currently, there are no drugs/agents specifically approved for the systemic treatment of wear particle-induced osteolysis and aseptic loosening. Potential systemic therapies to modulate the host response to wear particles can be arbitrarily categorized into three potential strategies. The first is bisphosphonate-like agents, which induce osteoclast apoptosis by blocking the mevalonate pathway of isoprenoid biosynthesis and have been widely used as bone resorption inhibition agents to treat osteoporosis (Bone et al., 2004). In addition to inhibiting osteoclastic bone resorption, bisphosphonates can stimulate proliferation of human osteoblast-like cells (Im et al., 2004). Bisphosphonates also stimulate the formation of osteoblast precursors and mineralized nodules in mouse and human bone marrow cultures thereby promoting early osteoblastogenesis (Giuliani et al., 1998). Because of the capability of blocking excessive osteoclast activity in osteoporosis and their anabolic effect on osteoblasts (Im et al., 2004; Giuliani et al., 1998; Tsuchimoto et al., 1994; von Knoch, F. et al., 2005), bisphosphonates have been considered as potential therapeutic agents in the treatment of wear particle-induced osteolysis. The results from animal studies have been encouraging. Alendronate inhibited wear particle-induced osteolysis in rat, canine, and murine models (Schwarz et al., 2000a; Millett et al., 2002; Shanbhag et al., 1997). Direct administration of zoledronic acid after surgery also suppressed particle-induced osteolysis using the mouse calvarial model (von Knoch, M. et al., 2005). Despite promising results in animal models, the clinical effectiveness of bisphosphonates in the treatment of patients with osteolysis is limited and contradictive (Maccagno et al., 1994; Ralston et al., 1989; Eggelmeijer et al., 1996). Although it is possible that the doses used were inadequate to block osteolysis, or other administration routes or long-term therapy might be necessary, studies in humans suggest that bisphosphonates may be less effective for the treatment against particle-induced osteolysis than against generalized osteoporosis. In addition to potentially inhibiting osteoclast-mediated bone resorption associated with particle disease, bisphosphonates have been shown to induce pathologic femoral fractures, mandibular lesions, impairment of fracture healing, and other adverse effects (Orozco and Maalouf, 2012). The potential long-term effects of bisphosphonates on other normal bones (if given for localized osteolysis around a joint replacement) have not been adequately investigated either.

The second potential strategy to mitigate osteolysis is to target known pro-inflammatory cytokines including TNF-α and IL-1 using medications such as etanercept, infliximab, and others (Maini et al., 1995; Moreland et al., 1997), or interfere with the RANK/RANKL/nuclear factor kappa B (NF-κB) signaling pathway more downstream (Childs et al., 2002; Dai et al., 2004; Ulrich-Vinther et al., 2002). Interference with a single cytokine has been successful in animals but not in humans, possibly due to the redundancy of the inflammatory cascade. The costs of these agents are also prohibitive. Persistent systemic inhibition of specific inflammatory cytokines or NF-κB results in generalized immune deficiency that can lead to opportunistic infections and cancer, such as lymphoma. Another novel approach is the delivery of these therapies using gene therapy (Wang, H. et al., 2013). However, these treatments should be approached with great caution.

Inhibition of mature osteoclast function is another a third therapeutic strategy for osteolysis and includes inhibitors for cathepsin K (Bossard et al., 1999; Lark et al., 2002; Shakespeare et al., 2003), the osteoclast ATPase proton pump (Visentin et al., 2000), the vitronectin receptor (Lark et al., 2001), and src tyrosine kinase and other factors. Bone normally undergoes continuous remodeling. The balance between bone resorption and formation is responsible for adult skeletal homeostasis (Rodan, 1998). The major concern of sustained systemic usage of these inhibitors is that perturbation of normal bone remodeling through continuous osteoclast inhibition may adversely affect the mechanical quality of bone (making bone both stiffer and more brittle) and impair fracture healing.

In summary, although the systemic approaches to modulating wear particle-induced periprosthetic osteolysis have been encouraging in animal studies, the safety, efficacy, and cost-effectiveness in humans have not been substantiated. Furthermore, it is questionable as to whether systemic treatment of primarily a localized issue is the optimal strategy.

Local coatings to enhance osseointegration and mitigate infection

The innate immune system protects the organism from adverse stimuli that can potentially lead to injury. However, acute inflammation also initiates a series of events leading to repair and reestablishment of homeostasis. Clearly, a balance between inflammation and repair must be reached to ensure survival of the organism. Ideally, systems should be developed to abort/modulate acute inflammation, avoid chronic inflammation and fibrosis, and initiate the reparative phase concurrently.

Previously, the primary aim of orthopedic implants was to provide simple mechanical stabilization to maintain optimal alignment and function of bone and decrease unwanted shear stress after an injury such as a fracture (Carter et al., 1998). The biological aspects of the implant were a by–product of stable internal/external fixation of the device to the surrounding bone and soft tissue. The concept purports that bone will "heal by itself" if appropriately stabilized. However, in the United States, there are approximately 600,000 fractures with delayed union and 100,000 cases of nonunion each year (Bishop et al., 2012). Cementless joint replacements do not always osseointegrate with the surrounding bone, which may cause implant migration and loosening (Aro et al., 2012). Furthermore, spinal fusion is not always a certainty (Raizman et al., 2009). Recently, biologic coatings have been incorporated into orthopedic implants in order to modulate the surrounding biological milieu. The mechanical and biological aspects of bone healing are closely interrelated and ultimately determine the final clinical outcome. The dilemma is how to modulate the biological environment of the implant bed to help ensure a more robust bone healing response. Although systemic pharmacological or biological treatments to accomplish this goal have been considered, local strategies have many advantages including local targeted anatomic delivery of specific biologics to the injury site, low overall dosage requirements, and mitigation of potentially serious systemic adverse effects. Local modulation of orthopedic implants involves two tasks: to improve implant osseointegration for joint replacement and to mitigate local infection.

Calcium phosphate-like materials coating

Bone is a composite structure composed of cells, protein (mainly collagen and other signaling proteins), and inorganic mineral. The mineral portion of bone constitutes about 50% of its weight and is mainly composed of carbonated HA. HA is chemically similar to the apatite of the host's bone and is a source of calcium and phosphate to the healing interface (Geesink et al., 1988). Coating the surface with HA can improve osseointegration of a cementless metallic prosthesis (de Groot et al., 1987; Geesink et al., 1987). Sintered HA can form tight bonds with living bone with little degradation of the HA layer (Ducheyne et al., 1990, 1980). However, suboptimal fatigue properties of sintered HA have led to the development of thinner coatings ($\sim$30–100 μm) for application to a titanium implant substrate via plasma spraying. Other techniques of HA coating include sputtering, pulse layer deposition, and electrostatic multilayer assemblies fabricated using the layer-by-layer technique (He et al., 2012). The shear strength of HA plasma-sprayed titanium alloy implants in animal models is similar to the shear strength of cortical bone (Geesink et al., 1988). Osteoblasts form osteoid directly on the HA surface coating, suggesting that the bone–implant interface is bonded both chemically and biologically to the HA. Traditionally, HA coatings have been thought of as osteoconductive. However, calcium phosphate biomaterials with certain three-dimensional geometries have been shown to bind endogenous bone morphogenetic proteins (BMPs), and therefore some have designated these materials as osteoinductive (LeGeros, 2002).

HA coatings have been shown to enhance new bone formation on an implant surface with a line-to-line fit, and in situations where there are gaps of 1–2 mm. In canine studies, new bone formation was found even at distances of 400 µm from the HA surface, suggesting a gradient effect on the osteoconductive properties of HA (Soballe, 1993). Furthermore, the presence of an HA coating prevents the formation of fibrous tissue that would normally result due to micromovements of an uncoated titanium implant (Soballe et al., 1993).

The two main methods of bio-resorption of HA coatings include one that is solution mediated (dissolution) and another that is cell mediated via phagocytosis (Jarcho, 1981; Sun et al., 2002). The HA coatings undergo variable resorption which is dictated by numerous chemical, biological, and mechanical factors including the composition and physicochemical properties of the coating, the anatomical location, and whether micromotion is present at the interface with bone (Soballe et al., 1999). Increased crystallinity appears to slow resorption of HA and decrease bone ingrowth (Overgaard et al., 1999). Mechanical instability hastens HA dissolution (Soballe, 1993).

HA coatings not only enhance osseointegration but function to seal the interface from wear particles and macrophage-associated periprosthetic osteolysis (Rahbek et al., 2001; Geesink, 2002). Studies of total hip replacements have shown improved fixation with a decrease in radiolucencies around HA-coated titanium alloy femoral components (Reikeras and Gunderson, 2003; Chambers et al., 2007), although others have shown no differences between coated and uncoated implants (Lee and Lee, 2007; Lombardi et al., 2006). A recent systematic review of randomized controlled trials of porous-coated femoral components with or without HA coating in primary cementless total hip replacement demonstrated no benefit of the HA coating (Goosen et al., 2009). However, reports of adverse events associated with HA coatings, which may fragment, migrate, and even cause increased polyethylene wear secondary to third body abrasive wear, have been reported (Bauer, 1995; Bloebaum et al., 1994; Morscher et al., 1998; Stilling et al., 2009). Many of these adverse events were found with first generation thicker HA coatings and may be less relevant to current implants with thinner more uniform HA coatings.

Recently, HA coatings have been used as a method for delivery of growth factors, bioactive molecules, and DNA (He et al., 2012; Choi and Murphy, 2010; Saran et al., 2011). For example, HA coatings augmented with BMP-7 placed on segmental femoral diaphyseal replacement prostheses improved bone ingrowth in a canine extra-cortical bone-bridging model. Titanium alloy plasma-sprayed porous HA coatings infiltrated with collagen, recombinant human bone morphogenetic protein (rhBMP-2), and RGD peptide improved mesenchymal stem cell (MSC) adhesion, proliferation and differentiation *in vitro*, and increased bone formation in ectopic muscle and intra-osseous locations *in vivo* (He et al., 2012). Another group used HA nanoparticles complexed with chitosan into nanoscale nondegradable electrostatic multilayers which were capped with a degradable poly(β-amino ester)-based film incorporating physiological amounts of rhBMP-2 (Shah et al., 2012). Plasmid DNA bound to calcium phosphate coatings deposited on poly-lactide-co-glycolide was released according to the properties of the mineral and solution environment (Choi and Murphy, 2010). These methods of delivery of bioactive molecules extend the function of HA as a novel coating to enhance new bone formation on orthopedic implants. However, the biologics added to HA must be introduced at the appropriate time (some are heat sensitive) and dose, and their release kinetics from the HA has to be carefully optimized.

In summary, HA coatings provide an osteoconductive and (arguably) osteoinductive approach for enhancement of bone formation on orthopedic implants. These biological properties may be augmented by adding growth factors and other molecules to produce a truly osteoinductive platform. Questions related to the necessity and efficacy of HA coatings in different anatomic sites, the robustness of HA coatings to withstand physiological loads without fragmentation, and problems related to third body wear by HA particles limit their more widespread use.

Bisphosphonate coatings

Bisphosphonate coatings have been used to enhance implant fixation and bone ingrowth at the implant site. *In vitro* and *in vivo* studies have been carried out to determine the elution characteristics and the effects on the surrounding bone (Bobyn et al., 2005; Tanzer et al., 2005). Zoledronic acid coating improved bone ingrowth in a canine porous-coated implant model; zoledronate grafted onto HA coatings on titanium implants in rat condyles demonstrated dose–response effects on periimplant bone density (Bobyn et al., 2005; Tanzer et al., 2005; Peter et al., 2005). Using stainless-steel-coated and -uncoated screws in rat tibias, an *N*-bisphosphonate, pamidronate, was immobilized onto fibrinogen, and *N*-bisphosphonate, ibandronate, was adsorbed on top of this layer. Pullout force (28%) and pullout energy (90%) were increased after 2 weeks, compared to uncoated screws (Tengvall et al., 2004). A companion study using coated screws in rats found that HA improved bone–implant attachment, whereas the two bisphosphonate coatings together improved fixation by increasing the amount of surrounding bone (Agholme et al., 2012). A recent study incorporating a rabbit intramedullary tibial rod model examined the periimplant bone using histomorphometric methods, push-out mechanical tests, and serum bone turnover markers (Niu et al., 2012). Alendronate and HA improved bone–implant contact, bone mass, and bone mineral density around the rod. A composite coating of risedronate and HA had similar effects; however, this combination had a greater effect on bones remote from the implant. Long-term observation and careful dosing requirements are necessary to determine whether these effects are temporary or more sustained to avoid any adverse systemic effects.

Biomolecule coatings

In addition to HA coating, a number of biomolecules have been used to coat the surface of an implant to promote osteoinduction. Large proteins or glycosaminoglycans such as collagen and chondroitin sulfate provide a biomimetic coating on the surface of an implant that can improve integration (Mathews et al., 2011; Rammelt et al., 2006). Growth factors are potential biomolecules for implant coatings due to their ability to decrease inflammation, enhance stem cell differentiation, induce blood vessel formation, and act as chemoattractants for circulating osteoprogenitors (Crouzier et al., 2009; Liu et al., 2005; Macdonald et al., 2011). In addition to using whole protein molecules, small peptides may enhance adhesion or bone formation by local osteoblasts (Auernheimer et al., 2005; Elmengaard et al., 2005; Wojtowicz et al., 2010). Compared to the use of whole proteins, the smaller size peptides potentially allow higher concentration of specific biological cues to be incorporated into the coating. As an alternative to using proteins or peptides, DNA molecules have been incorporated into implant coatings; these molecules can translocate into the cell nucleus to express sequence-specific mRNAs which can produce proteins over the course of 1–2 weeks (Dupont et al., 2012; Ito et al., 2005). The major advantage of oligonucleotide delivery is the ability to specifically regulate intracellular events leading to increased or decreased homologous protein production. However, one disadvantage is the instability of such biomolecules *in vivo*.

In summary, the future of bioactive molecule coating technology will depend on the specific structure and function of the molecule to be delivered, the rate of release and presentation to cells, the rate of degradation, and of course the host response.

Coatings to mitigate the FBR and infection

Insertion of an implant of any type within the body including bone evokes an inflammatory and (usually) limited foreign body reaction (Anderson et al., 2008). During use of an orthopedic implant, wear particles, and other by-products are generated from the bearing surfaces of joint replacements, and nonarticulating implant surfaces that impinge or fret (e.g., screws in a plate for fracture fixation or spinal stabilization). Depending on the anatomic location, the number and characteristics of the wear by-products and the host's ability to distribute, isolate, or detoxify the particles, these wear by-products may be benign or harmful. A localized foreign body and chronic inflammatory reaction may occur, resulting in bone destruction (osteolysis) (Hallab and Jacobs, 2009). If this process continues without resolution, it will jeopardize the long-term stability of the implant.

Infection is one of the leading causes of failure of joint replacements. Bacterial colonization and biofilm formation on the implanted device may lead to acute and chronic infection of the underlying bone and the adjacent soft tissues (Gristina, 1987). Biofilm on the implant surface protects the microorganisms from the host immune system and antibiotic therapy (Hetrick and Schoenfisch, 2006; Harris and Richards, 2006; Dunne, 2002; van de Belt et al., 2001; Danon et al., 1989), which may lead to persistence of infection despite continued aggressive antibiotic treatment. These events can lead to delayed bone healing, nonunion of fractures, and implant loosening. Treatment often necessitates surgical removal of the device in addition to prolonged courses of antibiotic therapy, both systemic and local. Thus orthopedic implant infection is a substantial healthcare burden and leads to prolonged patient suffering, and substantial morbidity and even mortality.

Orthopedic implants must provide mechanical stability and be biologically acceptable to the adjacent bone and soft tissue. With regard to integration of orthopedic implants, Gristina coined the phrase "race for the surface," implying that host cells and bacteria compete to adhere, replicate, and colonize the implant surface. Ideally, the race is won by host cells, which provide a stable interface with implant integration while "defending" the implant surface from invading bacteria by vigorous immune competence (Gristina, 1987).

Orthopedic devices are expected to stimulate host tissue integration and prevent microbial adhesion and colonization. However, the balance between these two requirements is often challenging. Biomaterial surfaces that facilitate host cell adhesion, spreading, and growth are also favorable to microorganisms that share many of the same adhesive mechanisms as host cells (Johansson et al., 1997; Fowler et al., 2000). On the other hand, surfaces and coatings designed to prevent bacterial colonization and biofilm formation may not effectively integrate with host tissues. Thus, the challenge is to develop new infection-resistant coatings without impairing local host immune competence or the potential for tissue integration.

Coatings to mitigate infection and the foreign body reaction can be categorized as passive or active depending on whether there are antibacterial agents delivered locally. Passive coatings, which do not release antibacterial agents to the surrounding tissues, may impede bacterial adhesion and kill bacteria upon contact. In contrast, active coatings release preincorporated bactericidal agents such as antibiotics, antiseptics, silver ions, and growth factors/chemokines/peptides to down-regulate infection actively.

Passive coatings

Implant surface physiochemical characteristics such as surface roughness and chemistry, hydrophilicity, and surface energy, potential, and conductivity play crucial roles in the initial bacterial adhesion and subsequent biofilm formation. Modification of these surface properties is a relatively simple and economic way to limit bacterial colonization.

Ultraviolet light irradiation can lead to a "spontaneous" increase in wettability on titanium dioxide, which can inhibit bacterial adhesion without compromising the desired response of bone-forming cells on a titanium alloy implant (Gallardo-Moreno et al., 2009; Yu et al., 2003). Anti-adhesive surfaces can also be achieved by modifying the crystalline structure of the surface oxide layer. The modified crystalline anatase-type titanium oxide layer reduces bacterial attachment without affecting cell metabolic activity (Del Curto et al., 2005).

In addition, polymer coatings such as the hydrophilic poly(methacrylic acid), poly(ethylene oxide), and protein-resistant poly(ethylene glycol) can inhibit adhesion of bacteria to a titanium implant (Zhang, F. et al., 2008; Harris et al., 2004; Kaper et al., 2003; Kingshott et al., 2003). Although these coatings may impair osteoblast function on the surface of implant, use of bioactive molecules such as sericin and RGD (Arg-Gly-Asp) motif with the immobilization technique can restore or improve the impaired cell function.

In summary, passive coatings are preferred as long as their antibacterial ability is strong enough to prevent biofilm formation. Unfortunately, the effectiveness of passive coatings for repelling bacterial adhesion is limited and varies greatly depending on the bacterial species (Hetrick and Schoenfisch, 2006). Development of alternatives to the traditional surface-modifying preventive approaches is required. Biosurfactants and microbial amphiphilic compounds inhibit bacterial adhesion and retard biofilm formation, and are thus potentially useful as a new generation of anti-adhesive and antimicrobial coatings for medical implants (Rivardo et al., 2009; Rodrigues et al., 2006). However, their use has been limited by their relatively high production costs and technical difficulties of binding them to implant surfaces.

Active coatings

Coatings with antibiotics Systemic prophylactic antibiotics have been administered routinely to patients who receive implants to prevent infection. However, systemic antibiotics have relatively low drug concentration at the target site and potential toxicity. Thus, local administration of antibiotics around the implant has attracted attention. Buchholz and Engelbrecht (1970) first incorporated antibiotics into bone cement to give local antibiotic prophylaxis in cemented total joint arthroplasty. Antibiotic-loaded bone cement can decrease the revision, aseptic loosening, and deep infection rates of cemented total hip arthroplasties when combined with systemic administration (Engesaeter et al., 2003). With the increasing use of cementless implants worldwide, the use of antibiotic-loaded bone cement has diminished dramatically, providing a unique opportunity for the development of new antibacterial technologies.

Gentamicin, an aminoglycoside antibiotic, has a relatively broad antibacterial spectrum and is thermostable. Gentamicin is one of the most widely used antibiotics in antibiotic-loaded cement and antibiotics-loaded coatings on titanium implants (van de Belt et al., 2001; Alt et al., 2006). In addition, cephalothin, carbenicillin, amoxicillin, cefamandol, tobramycin, and vancomycin have been used in coatings on orthopedic implants (Stigter et al., 2004, 2002; Radin et al., 1997).

Calcium phosphate coatings are potential carriers of antibiotics and bioactive molecules (Gautier et al., 2001, 2000). Antibiotics have been loaded into porous HA coatings on titanium implants. The antibiotic HA coatings exhibit significant improvement in infection prophylaxis compared with standard HA coatings *in vivo* (Alt et al., 2006), but there are still many unresolved issues with respect to antibiotic incorporation into the HA coating and the release kinetics. The antibiotics cannot be incorporated into the calcium phosphate coating during its formation because of the extremely high processing temperature such as that encountered in plasma spraying. Moreover, physical absorption of these drugs onto the surface of calcium phosphates limits the loaded amount and release characteristics. Antibiotic loading by a dipping method leads to a burst release of the antibiotics that constitutes 80–90% of the antibiotic released from the coating within the first 60 min (Radin et al., 1997; Yamamura et al., 1992).

Biodegradable polymers and sol–gel coatings are also utilized for controlled release antibiotic-laden coatings on titanium implants. The release of the antibiotics from these biodegradable coatings is slower than from HA coatings. The optimized layer-by-layer self-assembly coating technique can also significantly slow the release of antibiotics. However, the elution kinetics of antibiotics from the coating is still too fast to be clinically acceptable (Radin and Ducheyne, 2007). The ideal antibiotic delivery coating method should release antibiotics prophylactically at optimal effective levels (to kill bacteria yet spare adjacent normal tissues) for a sufficiently long period of time (perhaps days to 1–2 weeks) to prevent potential infection and then cease to minimize antibiotic resistance. The effects of antibiotics should not interfere with integration of the implant with the surrounding tissues (Antoci et al., 2007).

Coatings impregnated with nonantibiotic agents (silver, organic agents, bioactive molecules, cytokines/chemokines) Due to the risk of antibiotic resistance associated with antibiotic-loaded coatings, nonantibiotic agents in the coating become attractive alternatives. Among the various dopants, silver is the most well-known agent due to its broad antibacterial spectrum (both gram-negative and -positive bacteria), inhibition of bacterial adhesion, long-lasting antibacterial effect, being less prone to development of resistance, easy and stable administration by a variety of well-established techniques such as plasma immersion ion implantation and physical vapor deposition (Ewald et al., 2006; Zhang, W. et al., 2008). Other inorganic antimicrobial agents including copper, fluorine, calcium, nitrogen, and zinc have also been studied on titanium implant surfaces. Silver-containing HA coating can effectively inhibit bacterial adhesion and growth without compromising the activity of osteoblasts and epithelial cells (Ewald et al., 2006; Chen et al., 2006). Silver ions generated by anodization can inhibit bacterial growth effectively. Silver-coated titanium screws can prevent implant-associated bone infection when anodically polarized (Secinti et al., 2008; Spadaro et al., 1974). Studies have shown that silver coatings have excellent biocompatibility and are less prone to the development of resistance in the host (Percival et al., 2005; Bosetti et al., 2002). *In vivo* studies have shown that silver coatings do not have local or systemic adverse effects (Hardes et al., 2007; Gosheger et al., 2004). The underlying mechanisms are still unclear. Although silver is very attractive as an antimicrobial reagent, further information is needed regarding long-term tissue toxicity and exact bactericidal mechanisms.

Several organic bioactive agents such as hyaluronic acid and chitosan possess the ability to prevent bacterial adhesion and/or bacterial proliferation and activity (Singla and Chawla, 2001) (Chua et al., 2008). However, one report showed that osteoblast adhesion is impaired by the presence of the hyaluronic acid chains (Chua et al., 2008). There is still insufficient *in vivo* evidence indicating that these molecules support osseointegration better than, for example, calcium phosphate (Bumgardner et al., 2007).

As stated earlier, macrophages constitute the primary line of innate immune defense against most bacterial pathogens in the early stage of infection and play an essential role in the late cell mediated immune response. Local injection of activated macrophages significantly reduces the mortality of patients with infection (Danon et al., 1989; Goldmann et al., 2004). To attract macrophages to the site of infection, one possible strategy is to design a nano-coating system which delivers essential chemoattractant proteins such as MCP-1, IL-12, and others to the local site. Li et al. (2010) demonstrated that the local application of MCP-1 and IL-12 through nano-coating on intramedullary stainless steel Kirschner wires significantly prevented infection. However, recruited and activated macrophages can also synthesize and release pro-inflammatory cytokines that may lead to further tissue destruction. Additional *in vivo* studies investigating the optimal release kinetics and time course are required to evaluate these local nano-coating systems in the treatment of infection.

Multifunctional coatings Recently, the concept of multiple functionalities for surface coating of implants has been explored (Chen et al., 2006; Brohede et al., 2009; Bruellhoff et al., 2010; Muszanska et al., 2011; Smith et al., 2012). As stated above, osseointegration is very important in the success of orthopedic devices implanted within bone. However, biomaterial surfaces that facilitate host cell adhesion, spreading, and growth also favor similar processes by bacteria. Infecting microorganisms share many of the same adhesive mechanisms as host tissue cells, such as extracellular matrix (ECM) protein Fn (Johansson et al., 1997). This molecule, which is frequently used to coat implants to improve the immobilization rate of antibiotics/antimicrobial peptides, can also be recognized by staphylococci by its Fn-binding proteins (Fowler et al., 2000). On the other hand, surfaces and coatings designed to inhibit bacterial colonization frequently do not effectively integrate with host tissues. These multi-functional coatings should be easily applied, efficacious, have optimal temporal and dosing release profiles, demonstrate no local and systemic toxicity, not interfere with (or possibly even facilitate) adjacent tissue integration and be cost-effective. While no one strategy has dominated the marketplace, active ongoing research will undoubtedly produce a coating technology that will mitigate the occurrence of commonly found implant infections.

Local biologic modulation to wear particles

Interfering with ongoing migration of monocyte/macrophages to the implant site by modulating the chemokine–receptor axis

Macrophages phagocytose by-products from implants which stimulate complex systemic, paracrine, and autocrine cell interactions that lead to an inflammatory reaction. These events are mediated by pro-inflammatory factors released locally into the adjacent tissues (Jacobs et al., 2008; Tuan et al., 2008) and can lead to bone resorption (osteolysis) (Bauer, 2002; Sabokbar et al., 1998). Wear debris also interfere with mesenchymal cell proliferation, differentiation, and function (Wang et al., 2002; Chiu et al., 2006, 2007). With regard to implants, these events disturb the homeostatic balance between bone formation and degradation. By-products of implant wear inhibit osseointegration leading to implant micromotion and prosthesis loosening.

MCP-1 (human gene 17q11.2) belongs to the g-chemokine subfamily (C-C chemokines) and is an immediate early stress-responsive factor (Goodman et al., 2005). Once released in the bloodstream, MCP-1 binds its receptors (G-protein-coupled receptors) CCR2A and CCR2B (human gene ID 1231), with preference for CCR2B expressed by monocytes and activated natural killer (NK) lymphocyte cells (Deshmane et al., 2009; Proudfoot et al., 2000). Huang et al. (2010) *in vitro* challenged murine macrophages (RAW 264.7) with clinically relevant polymer particles (PMMA and UHMWPE) and demonstrated that MCP-1 was released at fourfold higher than the level of constitutional secretion. In addition, the conditioned media-induced chemotaxis of human macrophages (THP-1) and MSCs; this chemotactic effect could be blocked with MCP-1 neutralizing antibody. Other studies showed similar results using human macrophages or fibroblasts exposed to titanium and PMMA particles (Nakashima et al., 1999a; Yaszay et al., 2001). High levels of MCP-1 and MIP-1α (also called CCL3) were found after exposure to particles and the chemotactic activity of cells could be blocked by neutralizing antibodies to MCP-1 or MIP-1α antibody. The chemotactic activity and subsequent activation of macrophages can be interrupted by using mutant MCP-1 protein called 7ND which lacks the N-terminal amino acids 2 through 8 in the sequence (Yao et al., 2013; Keeney et al., 2013). The effect of chemokines released from cells appears to be dependent on the particle type (Nakashima et al., 1999a; Huang et al., 2010; Yaszay et al., 2001).

Ren et al. (2011, 2008, 2010) injected macrophages labeled by bioluminescent optical reporter genes into the tail vein of mice and showed systemic trafficking of these cells to the femoral shaft where PMMA or UHMWPE particles were injected. Using similar techniques, Gibon et al. (2012a,b) demonstrated systemic interference with the MCP-1-CCR-2 ligand–receptor axis by injection of an MCP-1 receptor antagonist (acting on the CCR2B receptor), which decreased trafficking of exogenously injected macrophages and osteolysis associated with local polyethylene particle infusion. This indicated that the MCP-1-CCR2 ligand–receptor axis is strongly involved in particle-induced periprosthetic osteolysis. Furthermore, systemic trafficking of MSCs in the presence of UHMWPE particles was inhibited by the interruption of the MIP-1α-CCR1 ligand–receptor axis (Gibon et al., 2012a). These data suggest that strategies that interfere with cell migration/recruitment may provide a potential method for modulating the inflammatory reaction to orthopedic implants and their by-products. Indeed, the concept of local anti-MCP-1 therapy has already been successfully employed in drug-eluting coronary stents (Schepers et al., 2006; Ohtani et al., 2004; Kitamoto et al., 2003; Egashira et al., 2007; Kitamoto and Egashira, 2002; Nakano et al., 2007).

Altering the functional activities of local macrophages by targeting macrophage polarization

Concept of macrophage activation and polarization

Macrophages are highly heterogeneous and display remarkable plasticity and can rapidly change their function in response to local microenvironmental signals. This plasticity makes macrophages key regulators of inflammation, immunity, and tissue regeneration; modulation of macrophage activation state is an attractive target for a wide variety of therapeutic intervention (Galli et al., 2011; Ma et al., 2003; Murray and Wynn, 2011). Unlike T-cells, which undergo extensive epigenetic modification during differentiation, macrophages seem to retain their plasticity and respond to environmental signals (Stout et al., 2005).

Currently, macrophage activation is best understood in the framework known as macrophage polarization (Murray and Wynn, 2011; Martinez et al., 2008; Mosser and Edwards, 2008). Mirroring the well-known polarization of the T helper (Th) lymphocytes (Mosmann et al., 1986), the macrophage polarization paradigm dictates that in response to Th1 or Th2 cell-derived cytokines, macrophages assume two distinct phenotypes known as M1 and M2, or "classically" and "alternatively" activated macrophages. Although macrophage plasticity probably represents more of a continuum of macrophage polarization states rather than the strict dichotomy suggested by the original macrophage polarization model, this paradigm is still a useful framework for simplifying complex, poorly understood macrophage characteristics (Martinez et al., 2008; Mosser and Edwards, 2008; Geissmann et al., 2010). See Chapter 6 for more details regarding macrophage phenotypes and factors that affect macrophage phenotypes.

Residual mature macrophages are contained throughout the body and are responsible for the removal of apoptotic cells, participate to the regulation of tissue homeostasis, and perform various tissue-specific functions (Murray and Wynn, 2011). M1 pro-inflammatory macrophages are induced upon exposure to Th1 cytokines such as IFN-γ secreted by NK or Th1 cells, and other activators, including TNF or TLR ligands, such as LPS (Ma et al., 2003; Mosser and Edwards, 2008). In addition, macrophage polarization induced by Th2 cytokines such as IL-4 and IL-13 become anti-inflammatory pro-healing/repair M2 macrophages (Martinez et al., 2009; Gordon and Taylor, 2005).

In classical M1 macrophage activation, IFN-γ binds to an IFN-γ receptor, which then signals via intermediary molecules to induce the transcription of M1-related genes (Schroder et al., 2004; Lawrence and Natoli, 2011; Liu and Yang, 2013). In addition, danger signal molecules (DAMPs), released from invading pathogens or damaged cells or ECM, can be recognized by certain TLRs, leading to NF-κB activation and to production of type I interferon and other pro-inflammatory factors (Akira and Takeda, 2004; Kawai and Akira, 2010). This activation pathway can act in an auto- and paracrine manner, and can partially substitute for IFN-γ in inducing the M1 phenotype (Mosser and Edwards, 2008). In this M1 macrophage activation process, IFN-γ usually acts synergistically with TNF. Other cytokines, such as IL-1β and granulocyte macrophage colony-stimulating factor (GM-CSF), also play a role as modulators of macrophage activation. After activated by Th1 cells/cytokines, M1 macrophages become effector cells in cell-mediated immunity and in the Th1 cell responses, e.g., with greatly enhanced capability to kill intracellular microbes/pathogens (Galli et al., 2011; Ma et al., 2003; Murray and Wynn, 2011; Martinez et al., 2008; Mosser and Edwards, 2008). M1 activation is further characterized by production of high levels of IL-12 that supports a developing Th1 response; production of other pro-inflammatory cytokines (TNF-α, IL-1β, IL-6, and IL-23); inhibition of anti-inflammatory cytokine production; and production of inflammatory chemokines (CCL2, CCL3, CCL4, IL-8, CXCL9, CXCL10, and CXCL11) that recruit neutrophils, monocytes, and activated Th1 lymphocytes (Martinez et al., 2008). Thus, M1 macrophages are important components of host defense, but their activation can't go unregulated as this can lead to host–tissue damage and autoimmune diseases (Zhang and Mosser, 2008; Szekanecz and Koch, 2007).

In the presence of Th2 cell cytokines, e.g., IL-4 or IL-13, M0 or M1 macrophages can be activated in an alternative way, and switch to the M2 phenotype (Lawrence and Natoli, 2011; Liu and Yang, 2013; Ricote et al., 1998; Pascual et al., 2005). The IL-4 receptor also uses other less well-characterized signaling pathways that lead to activation of the peroxisome proliferator-activated receptor-γ (PPAR-γ) and phosphoinositide 3-kinase, that have a direct effect on the transcription of M2-related genes. PPAR-γ also exerts a direct suppressive effect on the production of inflammatory cytokines mediated by STAT1, activator protein-1 (AP-1) and NF-κB. These alternatively activated macrophages are a functionally heterogeneous group of cells including M2a, M2b (combination with TLR stimulus), and M2c (stimulated with IL-10, TGF-β, or glucocorticoids) that participate in a wide range of physiological and pathological processes such as Th2-polarized responses, allergy, parasite immunity, tissue healing, homoeostasis, and fibrosis (Martinez et al., 2009; Gordon and Taylor, 2005). The latter two alternative M2 macrophage phenotypes are distinguished by a lack of ECM production and high levels of IL-10 production; they are primarily considered to perform immunosuppressive or modulatory functions (Martinez et al., 2008).

Modulation of macrophage polarization to mitigate wear particle-induced osteolysis

Orthopedic implant-derived wear particles have been shown to cause macrophage activation and inflammation *in vitro* and *in vivo* (Ren et al., 2011, 2008, 2010; Ingham and Fisher, 2005; Nich et al., 2013). This macrophage dominated infiltrate is composed primarily of the M1 pro-inflammatory phenotype (Tuan et al., 2008; Martinez et al., 2008). M1 macrophages can be transformed into the M2 phenotype by exposure to IL-4 (Martinez et al., 2008; Mosser and Edwards, 2008; Mantovani et al., 2004; Mantovani, 2008; Ho and Sly, 2009). As described earlier, M2 macrophages down-regulate pro-inflammatory mediators and provide signals for tissue repair and neovascularization (Martinez et al., 2008; Lolmede et al., 2009). Thus, sequential modulation of macrophage polarization favoring the M2 rather than the M1 phenotype is a feasible strategy to reduce chronic inflammation near the implant, improve bone apposition, and decrease wear particle-induced bone loss.

Trindade et al. (1999b) showed the anti-inflammatory effects of IL-4 treatment on PMMA particle-induced cytokine release by macrophages (TNF-α, IL-1β, and GM-CSF); this inhibitory effect was dose-dependent. Other studies showed similar suppressive effect of IL-4 using human peripheral blood monocytes stimulated with titanium alloy (Ti) wear particles (Im and Han, 2001). Pajarinen et al. (2013) showed that, in comparison to M0 macrophages, the overall chemotactic and inflammatory responses to Ti particles were greatly enhanced upon challenge of M1 macrophages but effectively suppressed when M2 macrophages were challenged. The mode in which macrophages responded to particle stimuli was dependent on the polarization status of the macrophages; induction of M2 polarization might limit particle-induced macrophage activation (Pajarinen et al., 2013). Rao et al. (2012) found that IL-4 administration after PMMA particle challenge was sufficient to reduce particle-induced TNF-α production in mouse bone-marrow-derived macrophages. Antonios et al. (2013) reported that these effects were more prominent if IL-4 was applied to the cells before, rather than concurrently with the PMMA stimulus; the production of the anti-inflammatory cytokine IL-1 receptor antagonist (IL-1Ra) was highest if macrophages had first passed from the M0 to the M1 state before being further polarized into an M2 phenotype.

Using a mouse calvarial model of particle-induced osteolysis, Rao et al. (2013) observed that daily IL-4 injections to the subcutaneous bursa overlying the calvaria significantly reduced polyethylene particle-induced osteolysis. In addition, prior IL-4 treatment reduced particle-induced TNF-α and RANKL production from calvarial samples cultured *ex vivo*. Increased M1 to M2 ratio was observed in polyethylene particle-treated group while in IL-4 treatment returned this ratio to that of negative controls. Thus, IL-4 treatment reduced particle-induced osteolysis by modulating macrophage activation from M1 toward M2-like macrophage phenotype. Using the murine air pouch model of polyethylene particle-induced osteolysis, Wang, Y. et al. (2013) observed that daily IL-4 or IL-13 injections reduced particle-induced bone collagen loss and the bone surface area covered by tartrate-resistant acid phosphatase (TRAP)-positive osteoclasts. A corresponding reduction in the production of RANKL and TRAP and increase in OPG production was observed in IL-4-treated groups. Interestingly, these effects were more pronounced if both IL-4 and IL-13 were administered rather than IL-4 or IL-13 alone.

Several studies reported that the inflammatory responses to wear particles were exacerbated if macrophages had first been polarized into M1 macrophages (Pajarinen et al., 2013; Trindade et al., 1999a). Pretreatment of IFN-α enhanced the production of TNF-α and IL-6 from human monocytes stimulated with PMMA particles (Trindade et al., 1999a). These observations raise some interesting points. It is tempting to speculate that chronic, low-grade inflammation in other anatomic locations caused by atherosclerosis, metabolic syndrome, periodontitis, or other conditions might predetermine the systemic M1–M2 balance of macrophages and thus the mode that local macrophages react to wear particles. These other conditions may impact the susceptibility of an individual to develop aseptic osteolysis. Future studies should explore the correlation among individual patient characteristics, macrophage polarization, and the reaction to orthopedic implants and their by-products.

Taken together, current *in vitro* and *in vivo* studies suggest that macrophage polarization is an essential factor that determines how macrophages respond to biomaterials; local modulation of the macrophage phenotype appears to be a potential means to limit biomaterial wear particle-induced inflammation and subsequent osteolysis. However, there are still many questions with respect to this paradigm, e.g., there are differences in macrophage polarization between mice and humans which may limit direct interspecies translation (Mantovani et al., 2004).

Modulating the production and release of pro-inflammatory factors

Currently, there are no clinically successful nonsurgical treatments for wear particle-induced periprosthetic osteolysis. Blocking individual pro-inflammatory factors systemically or locally has been unsuccessful clinically. These treatments have been downstream in the inflammatory cascade and have been directed toward a specific late biological event, such as excessive production of prostaglandins or TNF, or osteoclast function (Ren et al., 2008). The above treatments have been ineffective because there is much redundancy in the inflammatory cascade, and both bone formation and resorption are adversely affected by wear by-products.

The inflammatory reaction to orthopedic wear debris is mediated primarily by the transcription factor NF-κB, a critical signaling molecule in the activation of pro-inflammatory genes (Ren et al., 2003). NF-κB is highly conserved among species (Xu et al., 2009) and is activated by stress, injury, inflammatory cytokines, reactive oxygen intermediates, microbial by-products, chemical agents, and other noxious stimuli (Yamanaka et al., 2011; Kumar et al., 2004). Activation of NF-κB is via two pathways: the classical (canonical) pathway that involves inhibitor of κB proteins and the alternative (noncanonical) pathway that involves proteolytic processing of NF-κB2/p100 REL protein. In both pathways, proteins translocate from the cytoplasm into the nucleus to regulate the transcription of numerous target genes for pro-inflammatory cytokines, chemokines, cell-adhesion molecules, acute phase response proteins, immunoregulatory molecules, and transcription factors.

Systemic modulation of NF-κB, or blockade of specific subunits of the NF-κB pathway, has been proposed to abrogate particle-induced inflammation and osteolysis (Yamanaka et al., 2011; Ren et al., 2006, 2004; Cheng and Zhang, 2008; Akisue et al., 2002; Peng et al., 2008); however, these interventions are impractical and/or require systemic delivery and possible adverse consequences on other organs. Furthermore, their effects on osteoprogenitor cells have not been thoroughly investigated. Thus the translational potential for these interventions is limited. Local modulation of NF-κB activity such as delivery of an NF-κB inhibitor appears to be a potential strategy. The intervention is far upstream biologically and therefore will down-regulate numerous pro-inflammatory and osteoclastogenic pathways implicated in particle-induced osteolysis.

The NF-κB transactivation process includes nuclear translocation, specific DNA binding to the target sequence, and enhancement of target gene transcription. Among these, suppression of the DNA-binding ability via decoy oligodeoxynucleotide (ODN) is one of the most potent and specific ways to suppress NF-κB transactivation. ODNs can be used as "decoy" cis-elements to block the binding of nuclear factors to promoter regions of targeted genes, resulting in the inhibition of gene activation (Nakagami et al., 2006). Decoy ODNs are short synthesized duplex DNAs that mimic the transcription response element and can specifically suppress transcription factor activity via competitive binding with endogenous protein (Osako et al., 2012). Synthetic NF-κB decoy ODNs are readily incorporated into monocyte/macrophage lineage cells and appear to leave stromal and osteoblast cell function intact (Shimizu et al., 2009). *In vitro* and *in vivo* studies have shown that local application of ODNs can prevent bone loss and promote tissue healing in diseases such as periodontitis and rheumatoid arthritis (Shimizu et al., 2009; Tomita, T. et al., 2000). Thus, local application of NF-κB decoy ODNs provides a clear opportunity to mitigate particle-induced inflammation and osteolysis. This intervention could potentially decrease pro-inflammatory factor production by monocyte/macrophage lineage cells, and decrease osteoclast-mediated osteolysis.

Application of decoy ODNs has been shown to prevent NF-κB transactivation of pro-inflammatory cytokine genes in primary cultured macrophage (Dinh et al., 2011). In addition, NF-κB decoy ODNs have been investigated for the treatment of periodontitis, inflammatory arthritis, chronic obstructive pulmonary disease and cardiovascular disease, etc. (Greenfield et al., 2005; Shimizu et al., 2009; Tomita, N. et al., 2000; Desmet et al., 2004; Egashira et al., 2008).

Anatomically, wear particle-induced osteolysis is generally a confined disease so that local treatment such as local treatment of NF-κB decoy ODN could be an ideal way to minimize potential adverse effects on the normal host immune system (de Poorter et al., 2005). However, in order to optimize the strategy, the delivery route, timing and dosage, as well as potential toxicity must be considered carefully. In addition, since the NF-κB decoy ODN intervention is far upstream, blocking the activity in a confined microenvironment may also suppress other NF-κB-dependent pathways, especially the protective effects on osteolysis. The type I collagen in osteoprogenitor cells and IL-10 secreted by MSCs are both targeted by NF-κB (Ollivere et al., 2012; Shi et al., 2010; Cao et al., 2006). In addition, suppression of NF-κB activity may unexpectedly enhance cytokine expression owing to enhanced AP-1 transactivation (Stein et al., 1993) or block the negative feedback regulator, TNF-α-induced protein 3 (Lee et al., 2000). Further preclinical studies are necessary to establish the efficacy and safety of local delivery of NF-κB decoy ODN for the treatment of periprosthetic osteolysis.

SUMMARY AND FUTURE DIRECTIONS

Biomaterials implanted in the body for orthopedic applications assume a specific functional role that is determined by the surgical procedure, the characteristics of the host and the physical–chemical properties of the biomaterial, and any by-products. Despite exhaustive preclinical studies, the intended use and outcome of the implanted biomaterial may not be realized. The acute inflammatory reaction that always accompanies the surgical procedure may potentially alter the features of the implant, its function, or performance *in vivo*. More recently, the so-called minimally invasive surgical procedures have been explored to mitigate the accompanying tissue destruction and inflammatory reaction that may occur with more extensive surgical exposures and tissue dissections. Indeed, chronic inflammation and fibrosis may encapsulate the biomaterial, isolating it and inadvertently altering its ultimate purpose or performance.

With regard to orthopedic implants, acute infection is virtually impossible to eradicate without removal of the device and aggressive debridement and systemic/local antibiotics. Low-grade chronic infection is often unsuspected and harder to diagnose. The acidic conditions that accompany infection alter the local microenvironment and are generally less conducive to normal cellular function.

How can one help ensure that an orthopedic device implanted in the body produces its intended purpose without adverse consequences? First, careful meticulous preoperative planning will suggest the use of a specific device and surgical technique to obtain a particular realizable goal for the appropriate patient. Immunocompromised patient scenarios such as inflammatory arthritis, diabetes, cancer, and other diagnoses may suggest alternative medical strategies or surgical techniques, such as the use of specific prophylactic antibiotics. Gentle handling of the tissues will limit tissue necrosis and subsequent inflammation. Avoidance of specific medications (such as nonsteroidal anti-inflammatory medications which interfere with bone healing) may be indicated. More recently, systemic and/or local modulation of the inflammatory response or intended biological reaction has been suggested and explored. The choice of specific materials, geometries, topologies, etc. can determine the biological and clinical fate of the device. For example, the recent use of porous metals with roughened surfaces has enhanced initial implant stability in revision joint replacements with compromised bone stock, thus providing a more favorable biological environment for enhanced bone ingrowth. Implant coatings and drug delivery devices to prevent infection or alter the local biological milieu are currently being investigated. These combination products have great potential to modulate the biological processes leading to incorporation of the device. For example, local elution of antibiotics can potentially be combined with an osteoconductive implant coating such as HA to both prevent infection and facilitate implant osseointegration. These and other strategies need rigorous preclinical testing prior to limited clinical trials in order to determine safety and efficacy. If successful, these enhancements may further improve the outcome and longevity of orthopedic implants.

REFERENCES

Adell, R., Lekholm, U., Rockler, B., Branemark, P.I., 1981. A 15-year study of osseointegrated implants in the treatment of the edentulous jaw. Int. J. Oral Surg. 10 (6), 387–416.

Agholme, F., Andersson, T., Tengvall, P., Aspenberg, P., 2012. Local bisphosphonate release versus hydroxyapatite coating for stainless steel screw fixation in rat tibiae. J. Mater. Sci. Mater. Med. 23 (3), 743–752.

Akbar, M., Brewer, J.M., Grant, M.H., 2011. Effect of chromium and cobalt ions on primary human lymphocytes in vitro. J. Immunotoxicol. 8 (2), 140–149.

Akira, S., Takeda, K., 2004. Toll-like receptor signalling. Nat. Rev. Immunol. 4 (7), 499–511.

Akisue, T., Bauer, T.W., Farver, C.F., Mochida, Y., 2002. The effect of particle wear debris on NFkappaB activation and pro-inflammatory cytokine release in differentiated THP-1 cells. J. Biomed. Mater. Res. 59 (3), 507–515.

Albrektsson, T., Branemark, P.I., Hansson, H.A., Lindstrom, J., 1981. Osseointegrated titanium implants. Requirements for ensuring a long-lasting, direct bone-to-implant anchorage in man. Acta Orthop. Scand. 52 (2), 155–170.

Allen, L.A., Ambardekar, A.V., Devaraj, K.M., Maleszewski, J.J., Wolfel, E.E., 2014. Clinical problem-solving. Missing elements of the history. N. Engl. J. Med. 370 (6), 559–566.

Alt, V., Bitschnau, A., Osterling, J., Sewing, A., Meyer, C., Kraus, R., et al., 2006. The effects of combined gentamicin–hydroxyapatite coating for cementless joint prostheses on the reduction of infection rates in a rabbit infection prophylaxis model. Biomaterials 27 (26), 4627–4634.

Anderson, J.M., 1993. Chapter 4 Mechanisms of inflammation and infection with implanted devices. Cardiovasc. Pathol. 2 (3, Suppl.), 33–41.

Anderson, J.M., Rodriguez, A., Chang, D.T., 2008. Foreign body reaction to biomaterials. Semin. Immunol. 20 (2), 86–100.

Andersson, J., Ekdahl, K.N., Larsson, R., Nilsson, U.R., Nilsson, B., 2002. C3 adsorbed to a polymer surface can form an initiating alternative pathway convertase. J. Immunol. 168 (11), 5786–5791.

Andersson, J., Ekdahl, K.N., Lambris, J.D., Nilsson, B., 2005. Binding of C3 fragments on top of adsorbed plasma proteins during complement activation on a model biomaterial surface. Biomaterials 26 (13), 1477–1485.

Andrews, R.E., Shah, K.M., Wilkinson, J.M., Gartland, A., 2011. Effects of cobalt and chromium ions at clinically equivalent concentrations after metal-on-metal hip replacement on human osteoblasts and osteoclasts: implications for skeletal health. Bone 49 (4), 717–723.

Antoci Jr., V., Adams, C.S., Hickok, N.J., Shapiro, I.M., Parvizi, J., 2007. Antibiotics for local delivery systems cause skeletal cell toxicity in vitro. Clin. Orthop. Relat. Res. 462, 200–206.

Antonios, J.K., Yao, Z., Li, C., Rao, A.J., Goodman, S.B., 2013. Macrophage polarization in response to wear particles in vitro. Cell. Mol. Immunol. 10 (6), 471–482.

Aro, H.T., Alm, J.J., Moritz, N., Makinen, T.J., Lankinen, P., 2012. Low BMD affects initial stability and delays stem osseointegration in cementless total hip arthroplasty in women: a 2-year RSA study of 39 patients. Acta Orthop. 83 (2), 107–114.

Arora, A., Song, Y., Chun, L., Huie, P., Trindade, M., Smith, R.L., et al., 2003. The role of the TH1 and TH2 immune responses in loosening and osteolysis of cemented total hip replacements. J. Biomed. Mater. Res. A 64 (4), 693–697.

Aspenberg, P., van der Vis, H., 1998a. Fluid pressure may cause periprosthetic osteolysis. Particles are not the only thing. Acta Orthop. Scand. 69 (1), 1–4.

Aspenberg, P., Van der Vis, H., 1998b. Migration, particles, and fluid pressure. A discussion of causes of prosthetic loosening. Clin. Orthop. Relat. Res. (352), 75–80.

Auernheimer, J., Zukowski, D., Dahmen, C., Kantlehner, M., Enderle, A., Goodman, S.L., et al., 2005. Titanium implant materials with improved biocompatibility through coating with phosphonate-anchored cyclic RGD peptides. Chembiochem 6 (11), 2034–2040.

Baldwin, L., Flanagan, B.F., McLaughlin, P.J., Parkinson, R.W., Hunt, J.A., Williams, D.F., 2002. A study of tissue interface membranes from revision accord knee arthroplasty: the role of T lymphocytes. Biomaterials 23 (14), 3007–3014.

Bauer, T.W., 1995. Hydroxyapatite: coating controversies. Orthopedics 18 (9), 885–888.

Bauer, T.W., 2002. Particles and periimplant bone resorption. Clin. Orthop. Relat. Res. (405), 138–143.

Baxter, R.M., Macdonald, D.W., Kurtz, S.M., Steinbeck, M.J., 2013. Severe impingement of lumbar disc replacements increases the functional biological activity of polyethylene wear debris. J. Bone Joint Surg. Am. 95 (11), e751–e759.

Bennewitz, N.L., Babensee, J.E., 2005. The effect of the physical form of poly(lactic-co-glycolic acid) carriers on the humoral immune response to co-delivered antigen. Biomaterials 26 (16), 2991–2999.

Billi, F., Campbell, P., 2010. Nanotoxicology of metal wear particles in total joint arthroplasty: a review of current concepts. J. Appl. Biomater. Biomech. 8 (1), 1–6.

Bishop, J.A., Palanca, A.A., Bellino, M.J., Lowenberg, D.W., 2012. Assessment of compromised fracture healing. J. Am. Acad. Orthop. Surg. 20 (5), 273–282.

Bloebaum, R.D., Beeks, D., Dorr, L.D., Savory, C.G., DuPont, J.A., Hofmann, A.A., 1994. Complications with hydroxyapatite particulate separation in total hip arthroplasty. Clin. Orthop. Relat. Res. (298), 19–26.

Bobyn, J.D., Jacobs, J.J., Tanzer, M., Urban, R.M., Aribindi, R., Sumner, D.R., et al., 1995. The susceptibility of smooth implant surfaces to periimplant fibrosis and migration of polyethylene wear debris. Clin. Orthop. Relat. Res. (311), 21–39.

Bobyn, J.D., Pilliar, R.M., Cameron, H.U., Weatherly, G.C., 1980. The optimum pore size for the fixation of porous-surfaced metal implants by the ingrowth of bone. Clin. Orthop. Relat. Res. (150), 263–270.

Bobyn, J.D., Hacking, S.A., Krygier, J.J., Harvey, E.J., Little, D.G., Tanzer, M., 2005. Zoledronic acid causes enhancement of bone growth into porous implants. J. Bone Joint Surg. Br. 87 (3), 416–420.

Bone, H.G., Hosking, D., Devogelaer, J.P., Tucci, J.R., Emkey, R.D., Tonino, R.P., et al., 2004. Ten years' experience with alendronate for osteoporosis in postmenopausal women. N. Engl. J. Med. 350 (12), 1189–1199.

Bong, M.R., Kummer, F.J., Koval, K.J., Egol, K.A., 2007. Intramedullary nailing of the lower extremity: biomechanics and biology. J. Am. Acad. Orthop. Surg. 15 (2), 97–106.

Bosetti, M., Masse, A., Tobin, E., Cannas, M., 2002. Silver coated materials for external fixation devices: in vitro biocompatibility and genotoxicity. Biomaterials 23 (3), 887–892.

Bossard, M.J., Tomaszek, T.A., Levy, M.A., Ijames, C.F., Huddleston, M.J., Briand, J., et al., 1999. Mechanism of inhibition of cathepsin K by potent, selective 1, 5-diacylcarbohydrazides: a new class of mechanism-based inhibitors of thiol proteases. Biochemistry 38 (48), 15893–15902.

Bostman, O.M., Pihlajamaki, H.K., 2000. Adverse tissue reactions to bioabsorbable fixation devices. Clin. Orthop. Relat. Res. (371), 216–227.

Branemark, R., Branemark, P.I., Rydevik, B., Myers, R.R., 2001. Osseointegration in skeletal reconstruction and rehabilitation: a review. J. Rehabil. Res. Dev. 38 (2), 175–181.

Brohede, U., Forsgren, J., Roos, S., Mihranyan, A., Engqvist, H., Stromme, M., 2009. Multifunctional implant coatings providing possibilities for fast antibiotics loading with subsequent slow release. J. Mater. Sci. Mater. Med. 20 (9), 1859–1867.

Brown, C., Lacharme-Lora, L., Mukonoweshuro, B., Sood, A., Newson, R.B., Fisher, J., et al., 2013. Consequences of exposure to peri-articular injections of micro- and nano-particulate cobalt–chromium alloy. Biomaterials 34 (34), 8564–8580.

Bruellhoff, K., Fiedler, J., Moller, M., Groll, J., Brenner, R.E., 2010. Surface coating strategies to prevent biofilm formation on implant surfaces. Int. J. Artif. Organs 33 (9), 646–653.

Buchholz, H.W., Engelbrecht, H., 1970. Depot effects of various antibiotics mixed with Palacos resins. Chirurg 41 (11), 511–515.

Bumgardner, J.D., Chesnutt, B.M., Yuan, Y., Yang, Y., Appleford, M., Oh, S., et al., 2007. The integration of chitosan-coated titanium in bone: an in vivo study in rabbits. Implant Dent. 16 (1), 66–79.

Cadosch, D., Sutanto, M., Chan, E., Mhawi, A., Gautschi, O.P., von Katterfeld, B., et al., 2010. Titanium uptake, induction of RANK-L expression, and enhanced proliferation of human T-lymphocytes. J. Orthop. Res. 28 (3), 341–347.

Caicedo, M., Jacobs, J.J., Reddy, A., Hallab, N.J., 2008. Analysis of metal ion-induced DNA damage, apoptosis, and necrosis in human (Jurkat) T-cells demonstrates Ni2+ and V3+ are more toxic than other metals: Al3+, Be2+, Co2+, Cr3+, Cu2+, Fe3+, Mo5+, Nb5+, Zr2+. J. Biomed. Mater. Res. A 86 (4), 905–913.

Caicedo, M.S., Desai, R., McAllister, K., Reddy, A., Jacobs, J.J., Hallab, N.J., 2009. Soluble and particulate Co–Cr–Mo alloy implant metals activate the inflammasome danger signaling pathway in human macrophages: a novel mechanism for implant debris reactivity. J. Orthop. Res. 27 (7), 847–854.

Caicedo, M.S., Pennekamp, P.H., McAllister, K., Jacobs, J.J., Hallab, N.J., 2010. Soluble ions more than particulate cobalt–alloy implant debris induce monocyte costimulatory molecule expression and release of proinflammatory cytokines critical to metal-induced lymphocyte reactivity. J. Biomed. Mater. Res. A 93 (4), 1312–1321.

Caicedo, M.S., Samelko, L., McAllister, K., Jacobs, J.J., Hallab, N.J., 2013. Increasing both CoCrMo-alloy particle size and surface irregularity induces increased macrophage inflammasome activation in vitro potentially through lysosomal destabilization mechanisms. J. Orthop. Res. 31 (10), 1633–1642.

Campbell, P., Ma, S., Yeom, B., McKellop, H., Schmalzried, T.P., Amstutz, H.C., 1995. Isolation of predominantly submicron-sized UHMWPE wear particles from periprosthetic tissues. J. Biomed. Mater. Res. 29 (1), 127–131.

Campbell, P., Ebramzadeh, E., Nelson, S., Takamura, K., De Smet, K., Amstutz, H.C., 2010. Histological features of pseudotumor-like tissues from metal-on-metal hips. Clin. Orthop. Relat. Res. 468 (9), 2321–2327.

Cao, S., Zhang, X., Edwards, J.P., Mosser, D.M., 2006. NF-kappaB1 (p50) homodimers differentially regulate pro- and anti-inflammatory cytokines in macrophages. J. Biol. Chem. 281 (36), 26041–26050.

Carter, D.R., Beaupre, G.S., Giori, N.J., Helms, J.A., 1998. Mechanobiology of skeletal regeneration. Clin. Orthop. Relat. Res. 355 (Suppl.), S41–S55.

Cason, G.W., Herkowitz, H.N., 2013. Cervical intervertebral disc replacement. J. Bone Joint Surg. Am. 95 (3), 279–285.

Catelas, I., Petit, A., Vali, H., Fragiskatos, C., Meilleur, R., Zukor, D.J., et al., 2005. Quantitative analysis of macrophage apoptosis vs. necrosis induced by cobalt and chromium ions *in vitro*. Biomaterials 26 (15), 2441–2453.

Chambers, B., St Clair, S.F., Froimson, M.I., 2007. Hydroxyapatite-coated tapered cementless femoral components in total hip arthroplasty. J. Arthroplasty 22 (4, Suppl. 1), 71–74.

Charnley, J., 1970a. Acrylic Cement in Orthopaedic Surgery. S. Livingston Ltd, Edinburgh.

Charnley, J., 1970b. The reaction of bone to self-curing acrylic cement. A long-term histological study in man. J. Bone Joint Surg. Br. 52 (2), 340–353.

Charnley, J., 1979. Low Friction Arthroplasty of the Hip. Springer-Verlag, New York, NY.

Chen, W., Liu, Y., Courtney, H.S., Bettenga, M., Agrawal, C.M., Bumgardner, J.D., et al., 2006. *In vitro* antibacterial and biological properties of magnetron co-sputtered silver-containing hydroxyapatite coating. Biomaterials 27 (32), 5512–5517.

Cheng, T., Zhang, X., 2008. NFκB gene silencing inhibits wear particles-induced inflammatory osteolysis. Med. Hypotheses 71 (5), 727–729.

Chiba, J., Rubash, H.E., Kim, K.J., Iwaki, Y., 1994. The characterization of cytokines in the interface tissue obtained from failed cementless total hip arthroplasty with and without femoral osteolysis. Clin. Orthop. Relat. Res. (300), 304–312.

Childs, L.M., Goater, J.J., O'Keefe, R.J., Schwarz, E.M., 2001. Efficacy of etanercept for wear debris-induced osteolysis. J. Bone Miner. Res. 16 (2), 338–347.

Childs, L.M., Paschalis, E.P., Xing, L., Dougall, W.C., Anderson, D., Boskey, A.L., et al., 2002. *In vivo* RANK signaling blockade using the receptor activator of NF-κB:Fc effectively prevents and ameliorates wear debris-induced osteolysis via osteoclast depletion without inhibiting osteogenesis. J. Bone Miner. Res. 17 (2), 192–199.

Chiu, R., Smith, R.L., Goodman, S.B., 2006. Polymethylmethacrylate particles inhibit osteoblastic differentiation of bone marrow osteoprogenitor cells. J. Biomed. Mater. Res. A 77 (4), 850–856.

Chiu, R., Ma, T., Smith, R.L., Goodman, S.B., 2007. Kinetics of polymethylmethacrylate particle-induced inhibition of osteoprogenitor differentiation and proliferation. J. Orthop. Res. 25 (4), 450–457.

Chiu, R., Ma, T., Smith, R.L., Goodman, S.B., 2009. Ultrahigh molecular weight polyethylene wear debris inhibits osteoprogenitor proliferation and differentiation *in vitro*. J. Biomed. Mater. Res. A 89 (1), 242–247.

Choi, S., Murphy, W.L., 2010. Sustained plasmid DNA release from dissolving mineral coatings. Acta Biomater. 6 (9), 3426–3435.

Chua, P.H., Neoh, K.G., Kang, E.T., Wang, W., 2008. Surface functionalization of titanium with hyaluronic acid/chitosan polyelectrolyte multilayers and RGD for promoting osteoblast functions and inhibiting bacterial adhesion. Biomaterials 29 (10), 1412–1421.

Center for Disease Control, 2010. Number of All-Listed Procedures for Discharges from Short-Stay Hospitals, by Procedure Category and Age. United States.

Cook, S.D., Thomas, K.A., Haddad Jr., R.J., 1988. Histologic analysis of retrieved human porous-coated total joint components. Clin. Orthop. Relat. Res. (234), 90–101.

Cramers, M., Lucht, U., 1977. Metal sensitivity in patients treated for tibial fractures with plates of stainless steel. Acta Orthop. Scand. 48 (3), 245–249.

Crouzier, T., Ren, K., Nicolas, C., Roy, C., Picart, C., 2009. Layer-by-layer films as a biomimetic reservoir for rhBMP-2 delivery: controlled differentiation of myoblasts to osteoblasts. Small 5 (5), 598–608.

Dai, S., Hirayama, T., Abbas, S., Abu-Amer, Y., 2004. The IkappaB kinase (IKK) inhibitor, NEMO-binding domain peptide, blocks osteoclastogenesis and bone erosion in inflammatory arthritis. J. Biol. Chem. 279 (36), 37219–37222.

Danon, D., Kowatch, M.A., Roth, G.S., 1989. Promotion of wound repair in old mice by local injection of macrophages. Proc. Natl. Acad. Sci. USA. 86 (6), 2018–2020.

Davies, A.P., Willert, H.G., Campbell, P.A., Learmonth, I.D., Case, C.P., 2005. An unusual lymphocytic perivascular infiltration in tissues around contemporary metal-on-metal joint replacements. J. Bone Joint Surg. Am. 87 (1), 18–27.

DeFife, K.M., Colton, E., Nakayama, Y., Matsuda, T., Anderson, J.M., 1999. Spatial regulation and surface chemistry control of monocyte/macrophage adhesion and foreign body giant cell formation by photochemically micropatterned surfaces. J. Biomed. Mater. Res. 45 (2), 148–154.

de Groot, K., Geesink, R., Klein, C.P., Serekian, P., 1987. Plasma sprayed coatings of hydroxylapatite. J. Biomed. Mater. Res. 21 (12), 1375–1381.

de Poorter, J.J., Tolboom, T.C., Rabelink, M.J., Pieterman, E., Hoeben, R.C., Nelissen, R.G., et al., 2005. Towards gene therapy in prosthesis loosening: efficient killing of interface cells by gene-directed enzyme prodrug therapy with nitroreductase and the prodrug CB1954. J. Gene Med. 7 (11), 1421–1428.

De Smet, K., De Haan, R., Calistri, A., Campbell, P.A., Ebramzadeh, E., Pattyn, C., et al., 2008. Metal ion measurement as a diagnostic tool to identify problems with metal-on-metal hip resurfacing. J. Bone Joint Surg. Am. 90 (Suppl. 4), 202–208.

Del Curto, B., Brunella, M.F., Giordano, C., Pedeferri, M.P., Valtulina, V., Visai, L., et al., 2005. Decreased bacterial adhesion to surface-treated titanium. Int. J. Artif. Organs 28 (7), 718–730.

Deshmane, S.L., Kremlev, S., Amini, S., Sawaya, B.E., 2009. Monocyte chemoattractant protein-1 (MCP-1): an overview. J. Interferon. Cytokine Res. 29 (6), 313–326.

Desmet, C., Gosset, P., Pajak, B., Cataldo, D., Bentires-Alj, M., Lekeux, P., et al., 2004. Selective blockade of NF-kappa B activity in airway immune cells inhibits the effector phase of experimental asthma. J. Immunol. 173 (9), 5766–5775.

Dinh, T.D., Higuchi, Y., Kawakami, S., Yamashita, F., Hashida, M., 2011. Evaluation of osteoclastogenesis via NFkappaB decoy/mannosylated cationic liposome-mediated inhibition of pro-inflammatory cytokine production from primary cultured macrophages. Pharm. Res. 28 (4), 742–751.

Ducheyne, P., Hench, L.L., Kagan, A. 2nd, Martens, M., Bursens, A., Mulier, J.C., 1980. Effect of hydroxyapatite impregnation on skeletal bonding of porous coated implants. J. Biomed. Mater. Res. 14 (3), 225–237.

Ducheyne, P., Beight, J., Cuckler, J., Evans, B., Radin, S., 1990. Effect of calcium phosphate coating characteristics on early post-operative bone tissue ingrowth. Biomaterials 11 (8), 531–540.

Dunne Jr., W.M., 2002. Bacterial adhesion: seen any good biofilms lately? Clin. Microbiol. Rev. 15 (2), 155–166.

Dupont, K.M., Boerckel, J.D., Stevens, H.Y., Diab, T., Kolambkar, Y.M., Takahata, M., et al., 2012. Synthetic scaffold coating with adeno-associated virus encoding BMP2 to promote endogenous bone repair. Cell Tissue Res. 347 (3), 575–588.

Egashira, K., Nakano, K., Ohtani, K., Funakoshi, K., Zhao, G., Ihara, Y., et al., 2007. Local delivery of anti-monocyte chemoattractant protein-1 by gene-eluting stents attenuates in-stent stenosis in rabbits and monkeys. Arterioscler. Thromb. Vasc. Biol. 27 (12), 2563–2568.

Egashira, K., Suzuki, J., Ito, H., Aoki, M., Isobe, M., Morishita, R., 2008. Long-term follow up of initial clinical cases with NF-kappaB decoy oligodeoxynucleotide transfection at the site of coronary stenting. J. Gene Med. 10 (7), 805–809.

Eggelmeijer, F., Papapoulos, S.E., van Paassen, H.C., Dijkmans, B.A., Valkema, R., Westedt, M.L., et al., 1996. Increased bone mass with pamidronate treatment in rheumatoid arthritis. Results of a three-year randomized, double-blind trial. Arthritis Rheum. 39 (3), 396–402.

Elmengaard, B., Bechtold, J.E., Soballe, K., 2005. *In vivo* study of the effect of RGD treatment on bone ongrowth on press-fit titanium alloy implants. Biomaterials 26 (17), 3521–3526.

Engesaeter, L.B., Lie, S.A., Espehaug, B., Furnes, O., Vollset, S.E., Havelin, L.I., 2003. Antibiotic prophylaxis in total hip arthroplasty: effects of antibiotic prophylaxis systemically and in bone cement on the revision rate of 22,170 primary hip replacements followed 0–14 years in the Norwegian Arthroplasty Register. Acta Orthop. Scand. 74 (6), 644–651.

Engh, C.A., Zettl-Schaffer, K.F., Kukita, Y., Sweet, D., Jasty, M., Bragdon, C., 1993. Histological and radiographic assessment of well functioning porous-coated acetabular components. A human postmortem retrieval study. J. Bone Joint Surg. Am. 75 (6), 814–824.

Epinette, J.A., Manley, M.T., 2008. Uncemented stems in hip replacement—hydroxyapatite or plain porous: does it matter? Based on a prospective study of HA Omnifit stems at 15-years minimum follow-up. Hip Int. 18 (2), 69–74.

Ewald, A., Gluckermann, S.K., Thull, R., Gbureck, U., 2006. Antimicrobial titanium/silver PVD coatings on titanium. Biomed. Eng. Online 5, 22.

Fischer, M., Sperling, C., Werner, C., 2010a. Synergistic effect of hydrophobic and anionic surface groups triggers blood coagulation *in vitro*. J. Mater. Sci. Mater. Med. 21 (3), 931–937.

Fischer, M., Sperling, C., Tengvall, P., Werner, C., 2010b. The ability of surface characteristics of materials to trigger leukocyte tissue factor expression. Biomaterials 31 (9), 2498–2507.

Fleury, C., Petit, A., Mwale, F., Antoniou, J., Zukor, D.J., Tabrizian, M., et al., 2006. Effect of cobalt and chromium ions on human MG-63 osteoblasts *in vitro*: morphology, cytotoxicity, and oxidative stress. Biomaterials 27 (18), 3351–3360.

Fornasier, V., Wright, J., Seligman, J., 1991. The histomorphologic and morphometric study of asymptomatic hip arthroplasty. A postmortem study. Clin. Orthop. Relat. Res. (271), 272–282.

Fowler, T., Wann, E.R., Joh, D., Johansson, S., Foster, T.J., Hook, M., 2000. Cellular invasion by *Staphylococcus aureus* involves a fibronectin bridge between the bacterial fibronectin-binding MSCRAMMs and host cell beta1 integrins. Eur. J. Cell Biol. 79 (10), 672–679.

Fritton, K., Ren, P.G., Gibon, E., Rao, A.J., Ma, T., Biswal, S., et al., 2012. Exogenous MC3T3 preosteoblasts migrate systemically and mitigate the adverse effects of wear particles. Tissue Eng. Part A 18 (23–24), 2559–2567.

Fujishiro, T., Moojen, D.J., Kobayashi, N., Dhert, W.J., Bauer, T.W., 2011. Perivascular and diffuse lymphocytic inflammation are not specific for failed metal-on-metal hip implants. Clin. Orthop. Relat. Res. 469 (4), 1127–1133.

Galante, J., 1985. Bone ingrowth in porous materials. American Academy of Orthopaedic Surgeons. Park Ridge.

Gallardo-Moreno, A.M., Pacha-Olivenza, M.A., Saldana, L., Perez-Giraldo, C., Bruque, J.M., Vilaboa, N., et al., 2009. *In vitro* biocompatibility and bacterial adhesion of physico-chemically modified Ti6Al4V surface by means of UV irradiation. Acta Biomater. 5 (1), 181–192.

Galli, S.J., Borregaard, N., Wynn, T.A., 2011. Phenotypic and functional plasticity of cells of innate immunity: macrophages, mast cells and neutrophils. Nat. Immunol. 12 (11), 1035–1044.

Gandhi, R., Davey, J.R., Mahomed, N.N., 2009. Hydroxyapatite coated femoral stems in primary total hip arthroplasty: a meta-analysis. J. Arthroplasty 24 (1), 38–42.

Gardner, M.J., Silva, M.J., Krieg, J.C., 2012. Biomechanical testing of fracture fixation constructs: variability, validity, and clinical applicability. J. Am. Acad. Orthop. Surg. 20 (2), 86–93.

Gautier, H., Daculsi, G., Merle, C., 2001. Association of vancomycin and calcium phosphate by dynamic compaction: *in vitro* characterization and microbiological activity. Biomaterials 22 (18), 2481–2487.

Gautier, H., Merle, C., Auget, J.L., Daculsi, G., 2000. Isostatic compression, a new process for incorporating vancomycin into biphasic calcium phosphate: comparison with a classical method. Biomaterials 21 (3), 243–249.

Geesink, R.G., 2002. Osteoconductive coatings for total joint arthroplasty. Clin. Orthop. Relat. Res. (395), 53–65.

Geesink, R.G., de Groot, K., Klein, C.P., 1987. Chemical implant fixation using hydroxyl-apatite coatings. The development of a human total hip prosthesis for chemical fixation to bone using hydroxyl-apatite coatings on titanium substrates. Clin. Orthop. Relat. Res. (225), 147–170.

Geesink, R.G., de Groot, K., Klein, C.P., 1988. Bonding of bone to apatite-coated implants. J. Bone Joint Surg. Br. 70 (1), 17–22.

Geissmann, F., Gordon, S., Hume, D.A., Mowat, A.M., Randolph, G.J., 2010. Unravelling mononuclear phagocyte heterogeneity. Nat. Rev. Immunol. 10 (6), 453–460.

Gibon, E., Ma, T., Ren, P.G., Fritton, K., Biswal, S., Yao, Z., et al., 2012a. Selective inhibition of the MCP-1-CCR2 ligand–receptor axis decreases systemic trafficking of macrophages in the presence of UHMWPE particles. J. Orthop. Res. 30 (4), 547–553.

Gibon, E., Yao, Z., Rao, A.J., Zwingenberger, S., Batke, B., Valladares, R., et al., 2012b. Effect of a CCR1 receptor antagonist on systemic trafficking of MSCs and polyethylene particle-associated bone loss. Biomaterials 33 (14), 3632–3638.

Gill, H.S., Grammatopoulos, G., Adshead, S., Tsialogiannis, E., Tsiridis, E., 2012. Molecular and immune toxicity of CoCr nanoparticles in MoM hip arthroplasty. Trends Mol. Med. 18 (3), 145–155.

Gilroy, D.W., Lawrence, T., Perretti, M., Rossi, A.G., 2004. Inflammatory resolution: new opportunities for drug discovery. Nat. Rev. Drug Discov. 3 (5), 401–416.

Giuliani, N., Pedrazzoni, M., Negri, G., Passeri, G., Impicciatore, M., Girasole, G., 1998. Bisphosphonates stimulate formation of osteoblast precursors and mineralized nodules in murine and human bone marrow cultures *in vitro* and promote early osteoblastogenesis in young and aged mice *in vivo*. Bone 22 (5), 455–461.

Goldmann, O., Rohde, M., Chhatwal, G.S., Medina, E., 2004. Role of macrophages in host resistance to group A streptococci. Infect. Immun. 72 (5), 2956–2963.

Goldring, S.R., Schiller, A.L., Roelke, M., Rourke, C.M., O'Neil, D.A., Harris, W.H., 1983. The synovial-like membrane at the bone–cement interface in loose total hip replacements and its proposed role in bone lysis. J. Bone Joint Surg. Am. 65 (5), 575–584.

Goodman, S., Wang, J.S., Regula, D., Aspenberg, P., 1994. T-lymphocytes are not necessary for particulate polyethylene-induced macrophage recruitment. Histologic studies of the rat tibia. Acta Orthop. Scand. 65 (2), 157–160.

Goodman, S.B., 2007. Wear particles, periprosthetic osteolysis and the immune system. Biomaterials 28 (34), 5044–5048.

Goodman, S.B., Knoblich, G., O'Connor, M., Song, Y., Huie, P., Sibley, R., 1996. Heterogeneity in cellular and cytokine profiles from multiple samples of tissue surrounding revised hip prostheses. J. Biomed. Mater. Res. 31 (3), 421–428.

Goodman, S.B., Chin, R.C., Chiou, S.S., Schurman, D.J., Woolson, S.T., Masada, M.P., 1989. A clini-cal–pathologic–biochemical study of the membrane surrounding loosened and nonloosened total hip arthroplasties. Clin. Orthop. Relat. Res. (244), 182–187.

Goodman, S.B., Huie, P., Song, Y., Schurman, D., Maloney, W., Woolson, S., et al., 1998. Cellular profile and cytokine production at prosthetic interfaces. Study of tissues retrieved from revised hip and knee replacements. J. Bone Joint Surg. Br. 80 (3), 531–539.

Goodman, S.B., Trindade, M., Ma, T., Genovese, M., Smith, R.L., 2005. Pharmacologic modulation of periprosthetic osteolysis. Clin. Orthop. Relat. Res. (430), 39–45.

Goodman, S.B., Gomez Barrena, E., Takagi, M., Konttinen, Y.T., 2009. Biocompatibility of total joint replacements: a review. J. Biomed. Mater. Res. A 90 (2), 603–618.

Goosen, J.H., Kums, A.J., Kollen, B.J., Verheyen, C.C., 2009. Porous-coated femoral components with or without hydroxyapatite in primary uncemented total hip arthroplasty: a systematic review of random-ized controlled trials. Arch. Orthop. Trauma. Surg. 129 (9), 1165–1169.

Gorbet, M.B., Sefton, M.V., 2004. Biomaterial-associated thrombosis: roles of coagulation factors, comple-ment, platelets and leukocytes. Biomaterials 25 (26), 5681–5703.

Gordon, S., Taylor, P.R., 2005. Monocyte and macrophage heterogeneity. Nat. Rev. Immunol. 5 (12), 953–964.

Gosheger, G., Hardes, J., Ahrens, H., Streitburger, A., Buerger, H., Erren, M., et al., 2004. Silver-coated megaendoprostheses in a rabbit model—an analysis of the infection rate and toxicological side effects. Biomaterials 25 (24), 5547–5556.

Granchi, D., Ciapetti, G., Stea, S., Savarino, L., Filippini, F., Sudanese, A., et al., 1999. Cytokine release in mononuclear cells of patients with Co–Cr hip prosthesis. Biomaterials 20 (12), 1079–1086.

Granchi, D., Savarino, L., Ciapetti, G., Cenni, E., Rotini, R., Mieti, M., et al., 2003. Immunological changes in patients with primary osteoarthritis of the hip after total joint replacement. J. Bone Joint Surg. Br. 85 (5), 758–764.

Granchi, D., Cenni, E., Giunti, A., Baldini, N., 2012. Metal hypersensitivity testing in patients undergoing joint replacement: a systematic review. J. Bone Joint Surg. Br. 94 (8), 1126–1134.

Green, T., Fisher, J., Stone, M., Wroblewski, B., Ingham, E., 1998. Polyethylene particles of a "critical size" are necessary for the induction of cytokines by macrophages *in vitro*. Biomaterials 19 (24), 2297–2302.

Green, T., Fisher, J., Matthews, J., Stone, M., Ingham, E., 2000. Effect of size and dose on bone resorption activity of macrophages by *in vitro* clinically relevant ultra high molecular weight polyethylene particles. J. Biomed. Mater. Res. 53 (5), 490–497.

Greenfield, E.M., Bechtold, J., 2008. What other biologic and mechanical factors might contribute to oste-olysis? J. Am. Acad. Orthop. Surg. 16 (Suppl. 1), S56–S62.

Greenfield, E.M., Bi, Y., Ragab, A.A., Goldberg, V.M., Nalepka, J.L., Seabold, J.M., 2005. Does endotoxin contribute to aseptic loosening of orthopedic implants? J. Biomed. Mater. Res. B Appl. Biomater. 72 (1), 179–185.

Greenfield, E.M., Beidelschies, M.A., Tatro, J.M., Goldberg, V.M., Hise, A.G., 2010. Bacterial pathogen-associated molecular patterns stimulate biological activity of orthopaedic wear particles by activating cognate Toll-like receptors. J. Biol. Chem. 285 (42), 32378–32384.

Gristina, A.G., 1987. Biomaterial-centered infection: microbial adhesion versus tissue integration. Science 237 (4822), 1588–1595.

Gu, Q., Shi, Q., Yang, H., 2012. The role of TLR and chemokine in wear particle-induced aseptic loosening. J. Biomed. Biotechnol. 2012, 596870.

Hallab, N.J., Jacobs, J.J., 2009. Biologic effects of implant debris. Bull. NYU Hosp. Jt. Dis. 67 (2), 182–188.

Hallab, N.J., Mikecz, K., Vermes, C., Skipor, A., Jacobs, J.J., 2001. Differential lymphocyte reactivity to serum-derived metal–protein complexes produced from cobalt-based and titanium-based implant alloy degradation. J. Biomed. Mater. Res. 56 (3), 427–436.

Hallab, N.J., Anderson, S., Caicedo, M., Skipor, A., Campbell, P., Jacobs, J.J., 2004. Immune responses correlate with serum-metal in metal-on-metal hip arthroplasty. J. Arthroplasty 19 (8, Suppl. 3), 88–93.

Hallab, N.J., Anderson, S., Stafford, T., Glant, T., Jacobs, J.J., 2005. Lymphocyte responses in patients with total hip arthroplasty. J. Orthop. Res. 23 (2), 384–391.

Hallab, N.J., Caicedo, M., Finnegan, A., Jacobs, J.J., 2008. Th1 type lymphocyte reactivity to metals in patients with total hip arthroplasty. J. Orthop. Surg. 3, 6.

Hallab, N.J., McAllister, K., Brady, M., Jarman-Smith, M., 2011. Macrophage reactivity to different polymers demonstrates particle size- and material-specific reactivity: PEEK-OPTIMA((R)) particles versus UHMWPE particles in the submicron, micron, and 10 micron size ranges. J. Biomed. Mater. Res. B Appl. Biomater.

Hardes, J., Ahrens, H., Gebert, C., Streitbuerger, A., Buerger, H., Erren, M., et al., 2007. Lack of toxicological side-effects in silver-coated megaprostheses in humans. Biomaterials 28 (18), 2869–2875.

Harris, L.G., Richards, R.G., 2006. Staphylococci and implant surfaces: a review. Injury 37 (Suppl. 2), S3–14.

Harris, L.G., Tosatti, S., Wieland, M., Textor, M., Richards, R.G., 2004. *Staphylococcus aureus* adhesion to titanium oxide surfaces coated with non-functionalized and peptide-functionalized poly(L-lysine)-grafted-poly(ethylene glycol) copolymers. Biomaterials 25 (18), 4135–4148.

Hart, A.J., Skinner, J.A., Winship, P., Faria, N., Kulinskaya, E., Webster, D., et al., 2009. Circulating levels of cobalt and chromium from metal-on-metal hip replacement are associated with CD8+ T-cell lymphopenia. J. Bone Joint Surg. Br. 91 (6), 835–842.

Hart, A.J., Sabah, S.A., Bandi, A.S., Maggiore, P., Tarassoli, P., Sampson, B., et al., 2011. Sensitivity and specificity of blood cobalt and chromium metal ions for predicting failure of metal-on-metal hip replacement. J. Bone Joint Surg. Br. 93 (10), 1308–1313.

He, J., Huang, T., Gan, L., Zhou, Z., Jiang, B., Wu, Y., et al., 2012. Collagen-infiltrated porous hydroxyapatite coating and its osteogenic properties: *in vitro* and *in vivo* study. J. Biomed. Mater. Res. A 100 (7), 1706–1715.

Heemskerk, J.W., Bevers, E.M., Lindhout, T., 2002. Platelet activation and blood coagulation. Thromb. Haemost. 88 (2), 186–193.

Henson, P.M., Johnston Jr., R.B., 1987. Tissue injury in inflammation. Oxidants, proteinases, and cationic proteins. J. Clin. Invest. 79 (3), 669–674.

Hetrick, E.M., Schoenfisch, M.H., 2006. Reducing implant-related infections: active release strategies. Chem. Soc. Rev. 35 (9), 780–789.

Hidaka, Y., Ito, M., Mori, K., Yagasaki, H., Kafrawy, A.H., 1999. Histopathological and immunohistochemical studies of membranes of deacetylated chitin derivatives implanted over rat calvaria. J. Biomed. Mater. Res. 46 (3), 418–423.

Hirayama, T., Tamaki, Y., Takakubo, Y., Iwazaki, K., Sasaki, K., Ogino, T., et al., 2011. Toll-like receptors and their adaptors are regulated in macrophages after phagocytosis of lipopolysaccharide-coated titanium particles. J. Orthop. Res. 29 (7), 984–992.

Ho, V.W., Sly, L.M., 2009. Derivation and characterization of murine alternatively activated (M2) macrophages. Methods Mol. Biol. 531, 173–185.

Hu, W.J., Eaton, J.W., Ugarova, T.P., Tang, L., 2001. Molecular basis of biomaterial-mediated foreign body reactions. Blood 98 (4), 1231–1238.

Huang, Z., Ma, T., Ren, P.G., Smith, R.L., Goodman, S.B., 2010. Effects of orthopedic polymer particles on chemotaxis of macrophages and mesenchymal stem cells. J. Biomed. Mater. Res. A 94 (4), 1264–1269.

Hunt, J.A., Flanagan, B.F., McLaughlin, P.J., Strickland, I., Willia, D.F., 1996. Effect of biomaterial surface charge on the inflammatory response: evaluation of cellular infiltration and TNF alpha production. J. Biomed. Mater. Res. 31 (1), 139–144.

Hynes, R.O., 2002. Integrins: bidirectional, allosteric signaling machines. Cell 110 (6), 673–687.

Im, G.I., Han, J.D., 2001. Suppressive effects of interleukin-4 and interleukin-10 on the production of proinflammatory cytokines induced by titanium–alloy particles. J. Biomed. Mater. Res. 58 (5), 531–536.

Im, G.I., Qureshi, S.A., Kenney, J., Rubash, H.E., Shanbhag, A.S., 2004. Osteoblast proliferation and maturation by bisphosphonates. Biomaterials 25 (18), 4105–4115.

Ingham, E., Fisher, J., 2000. Biological reactions to wear debris in total joint replacement. Proc. Inst. Mech. Eng. Part H, J. Eng. Med. 214 (1), 21–37.

Ingham, E., Fisher, J., 2005. The role of macrophages in osteolysis of total joint replacement. Biomaterials 26 (11), 1271–1286.

The John Charnley Research Institute. 2009 <http://charnleyresearch.co.uk>.

Ito, H., Koefoed, M., Tiyapatanaputi, P., Gromov, K., Goater, J.J., Carmouche, J., et al., 2005. Remodeling of cortical bone allografts mediated by adherent rAAV-RANKL and VEGF gene therapy. Nat. Med. 11 (3), 291–297.

Jacobs, J.J., Campbell, P.A., Konttinen, T.Y., 2008. How has the biologic reaction to wear particles changed with newer bearing surfaces? J. Am. Acad. Orthop. Surg. 16 (Suppl. 1), S49–S55.

Jacobs, J.J., Patterson, L.M., Skipor, A.K., Hall, D.J., Urban, R.M., Black, J., et al., 1999. Postmortem retrieval of total joint replacement components. J. Biomed. Mater. Res. 48 (3), 385–391.

Jacobs, J.J., Hallab, N.J., Urban, R.M., Wimmer, M.A., 2006. Wear particles. J. Bone Joint Surg. Am. 88 (Suppl. 2), 99–102.

Jacobs, W.C., van der Gaag, N.A., Kruyt, M.C., Tuschel, A., de Kleuver, M., Peul, W.C., et al., 2013. Total disc replacement for chronic discogenic low back pain: a Cochrane review. Spine (Phila Pa 1976) 38 (1), 24–36.

Jarcho, M., 1981. Calcium phosphate ceramics as hard tissue prosthetics. Clin. Orthop. Relat. Res. 157, 259–278.

Jiranek, W., Jasty, M., Wang, J.T., Bragdon, C., Wolfe, H., Goldberg, M., et al., 1995. Tissue response to particulate polymethylmethacrylate in mice with various immune deficiencies. J. Bone Joint Surg. Am. 77 (11), 1650–1661.

Johansson, S., Svineng, G., Wennerberg, K., Armulik, A., Lohikangas, L., 1997. Fibronectin–integrin interactions. Front. Biosci. 2, d126–d146.

Johne, J., Blume, C., Benz, P.M., Pozgajova, M., Ullrich, M., Schuh, K., et al., 2006. Platelets promote coagulation factor XII-mediated proteolytic cascade systems in plasma. Biol. Chem. 387 (2), 173–178.

Johnston, R.B., 1988. Monocytes and macrophages. N. Engl. J. Med. 318 (12), 747–752.

Jones, L.C., Hungerford, D.S., 1987. Cement disease. Clin. Orthop. Relat. Res. (225), 192–206.

Kadoya, Y., Revell, P.A., al-Saffar, N., Kobayashi, A., Scott, G., Freeman, M.A., 1996. Bone formation and bone resorption in failed total joint arthroplasties: histomorphometric analysis with histochemical and immunohistochemical technique. J. Orthop. Res. 14 (3), 473–482.

Kaper, H.J., Busscher, H.J., Norde, W., 2003. Characterization of poly(ethylene oxide) brushes on glass surfaces and adhesion of *Staphylococcus epidermidis*. J. Biomater. Sci. Polym. Ed. 14 (4), 313–324.

Kawai, T., Akira, S., 2010. The role of pattern-recognition receptors in innate immunity: update on Toll-like receptors. Nat. Immunol. 11 (5), 373–384.

Keeney, M., Waters, H., Barcay, K., Jiang, X., Yao, Z., Pajarinen, J., et al., 2013. Mutant MCP-1 protein delivery from layer-by-layer coatings on orthopedic implants to modulate inflammatory response. Biomaterials 34 (38), 10287–10295.

Kido, A., Pap, G., Nagler, D.K., Ziomek, E., Menard, R., Neumann, H.W., et al., 2004. Protease expression in interface tissues around loose arthroplasties. Clin. Orthop. Relat. Res. (425), 230–236.

Kim, K.J., Rubash, H.E., Wilson, S.C., D'Antonio, J.A., McClain, E.J., 1993. A histologic and biochemical comparison of the interface tissues in cementless and cemented hip prostheses. Clin. Orthop. Relat. Res. (287), 142–152.

Kingshott, P., Wei, J., Bagge-Ravn, D., Gadegaard, N., Gram, L., 2003. Covalent attachment of poly(ethylene glycol) to surfaces, critical for reducing bacterial adhesion. Langmuir 19 (17), 6912–6921.

Kitamoto, S., Egashira, K., 2002. Gene therapy targeting monocyte chemoattractant protein-1 for vascular disease. J. Atheroscler. Thromb. 9 (6), 261–265.

Kitamoto, S., Egashira, K., Takeshita, A., 2003. Stress and vascular responses: anti-inflammatory therapeutic strategy against atherosclerosis and restenosis after coronary intervention. J. Pharmacol. Sci. 91 (3), 192–196.

Kobayashi, S.D., Voyich, J.M., Burlak, C., DeLeo, F.R., 2005. Neutrophils in the innate immune response. Arch. Immunol. Ther. Exp. (Warsz) 53 (6), 505–517.

Kohilas, K., Lyons, M., Lofthouse, R., Frondoza, C.G., Jinnah, R., Hungerford, D.S., 1999. Effect of prosthetic titanium wear debris on mitogen-induced monocyte and lymphoid activation. J. Biomed. Mater. Res. 47 (1), 95–103.

Konttinen, Y.T., Pajarinen, J., 2013. Adverse reactions to metal-on-metal implants. Nat. Rev. Rheumatol. 9 (1), 5–6.

Korovessis, P., Lyons, M., Lofthouse, R., Frondoza, C.G., Jinnah, R., Hungerford, D.S., 2006. Metallosis after contemporary metal-on-metal total hip arthroplasty. Five to nine-year follow-up. J. Bone Joint Surg. Am. 88 (6), 1183–1191.

Kumar, A., Takada, Y., Boriek, A.M., Aggarwal, B.B., 2004. Nuclear factor-kappaB: its role in health and disease. J. Mol. Med. 82 (7), 434–448.

Kurtz, S., Ong, K., Lau, E., Mowat, F., Halpern, M., 2007. Projections of primary and revision hip and knee arthroplasty in the United States from 2005 to 2030. J. Bone Joint Surg. Am. 89 (4), 780–785.

Kwon, Y.M., Thomas, P., Summer, B., Pandit, H., Taylor, A., Beard, D., et al., 2010. Lymphocyte proliferation responses in patients with pseudotumors following metal-on-metal hip resurfacing arthroplasty. J. Orthop. Res. 28 (4), 444–450.

Lark, M.W., Stroup, G.B., Dodds, R.A., Kapadia, R., Hoffman, S.J., Hwang, S.M., et al., 2001. Antagonism of the osteoclast vitronectin receptor with an orally active nonpeptide inhibitor prevents cancellous bone loss in the ovariectomized rat. J. Bone Miner. Res. 16 (2), 319–327.

Lark, M.W., Stroup, G.B., James, I.E., Dodds, R.A., Hwang, S.M., Blake, S.M., et al., 2002. A potent small molecule, nonpeptide inhibitor of cathepsin K (SB 331750) prevents bone matrix resorption in the ovariectomized rat. Bone 30 (5), 746–753.

Lawrence, T., Natoli, G., 2011. Transcriptional regulation of macrophage polarization: enabling diversity with identity. Nat. Rev. Immunol. 11 (11), 750–761.

Lee, J.M., Lee, C.W., 2007. Comparison of hydroxyapatite-coated and non-hydroxyapatite-coated noncemented total hip arthroplasty in same patients. J. Arthroplasty 22 (7), 1019–1023.

Lee, E.G., Boone, D.L., Chai, S., Libby, S.L., Chien, M., Lodolce, J.P., et al., 2000. Failure to regulate TNF-induced NF-kappaB and cell death responses in A20-deficient mice. Science 289 (5488), 2350–2354.

LeGeros, R.Z., 2002. Properties of osteoconductive biomaterials: calcium phosphates. Clin. Orthop. Relat. Res. (395), 81–98.

Lehrer, R.I., Ganz, T., Selsted, M.E., Babior, B.M., Curnutte, J.T., 1988. Neutrophils and host defense. Ann. Intern. Med. 109 (2), 127–142.

Li, T.F., Santavirta, S., Waris, V., Lassus, J., Lindroos, L., Xu, J.W., et al., 2001. No lymphokines in T-cells around loosened hip prostheses. Acta Orthop. Scand. 72 (3), 241–247.

Li, B., Jiang, B., Dietz, M.J., Smith, E.S., Clovis, N.B., Rao, K.M., 2010. Evaluation of local MCP-1 and IL-12 nanocoatings for infection prevention in open fractures. J. Orthop. Res. 28 (1), 48–54.

Lin, T.H., Yao, Z, Sato, T, Woo, D.K., Pajarinen, J., Goodman, S.B., 2014. Suppression of UHMWPE Wear Particle- induced Pro-Inflammatory Cytokine and Chemokine Production by Macrophages Using an NF-κB Decoy Oligodeoxynucleotide. Annual meeting, Society for Biomaterials.

Liu, G., Yang, H., 2013. Modulation of macrophage activation and programming in immunity. J. Cell. Physiol. 228 (3), 502–512.

Liu, Y., de Groot, K., Hunziker, E.B., 2005. BMP-2 liberated from biomimetic implant coatings induces and sustains direct ossification in an ectopic rat model. Bone 36 (5), 745–757.

Lohmann, C.H., Meyer, H., Nuechtern, J.V., Singh, G., Junk-Jantsch, S., Schmotzer, H., et al., 2013. Periprosthetic tissue metal content but not serum metal content predicts the type of tissue response in failed small-diameter metal-on-metal total hip arthroplasties. J. Bone Joint Surg. Am. 95 (17), 1561–1568.

Lolmede, K., Campana, L., Vezzoli, M., Bosurgi, L., Tonlorenzi, R., Clementi, E., et al., 2009. Inflammatory and alternatively activated human macrophages attract vessel-associated stem cells, relying on separate HMGB1- and MMP-9-dependent pathways. J. Leukoc. Biol. 85 (5), 779–787.

Lombardi Jr., A.V., Berend, K.R., Mallory, T.H., 2006. Hydroxyapatite-coated titanium porous plasma spray tapered stem: experience at 15 to 18 years. Clin. Orthop. Relat. Res. 453, 81–85.

Lowell, C.A., Berton, G., 1999. Integrin signal transduction in myeloid leukocytes. J. Leukoc. Biol. 65 (3), 313–320.

Luttikhuizen, D.T., Harmsen, M.C., Van Luyn, M.J., 2006. Cellular and molecular dynamics in the foreign body reaction. Tissue Eng. 12 (7), 1955–1970.

Ma, J., Chen, T., Mandelin, J., Ceponis, A., Miller, N.E., Hukkanen, M., et al., 2003. Regulation of macrophage activation. Cell. Mol. Life Sci. 60 (11), 2334–2346.

Maccagno, A., Di Giorgio, E., Roldan, E.J., Caballero, L.E., Perez Lloret, A., 1994. Double blind radiological assessment of continuous oral pamidronic acid in patients with rheumatoid arthritis. Scand. J. Rheumatol. 23 (4), 211–214.

Macdonald, M.L., Samuel, R.E., Shah, N.J., Padera, R.F., Beben, Y.M., Hammond, P.T., 2011. Tissue integration of growth factor-eluting layer-by-layer polyelectrolyte multilayer coated implants. Biomaterials 32 (5), 1446–1453.

Mai, K.T., Verioti, C.A., Casey, K., Slesarenko, Y., Romeo, L., Colwell Jr., C.W., 2010. Cementless femoral fixation in total hip arthroplasty. Am. J. Orthop. (Belle Mead NJ) 39 (3), 126–130.

Maini, R.N., Elliott, M.J., Brennan, F.M., Williams, R.O., Chu, C.Q., Paleolog, E., et al., 1995. Monoclonal anti-TNF alpha antibody as a probe of pathogenesis and therapy of rheumatoid disease. Immunol. Rev. 144, 195–223.

Malech, H.L., Gallin, J.I., 1987. Current concepts: immunology. Neutrophils in human diseases. N. Engl. J. Med. 317 (11), 687–694.

Maloney, W.J., Jasty, M., Burke, D.W., O'Connor, D.O., Zalenski, E.B., Bragdon, C., et al., 1989. Biomechanical and histologic investigation of cemented total hip arthroplasties. A study of autopsy-retrieved femurs after in vivo cycling. Clin. Orthop. Relat. Res. (249), 129–140.

Maloney, W.J., et al., 1990a. Bone lysis in well-fixed cemented femoral components. J. Bone Joint Surg. Br. 72 (6), 966–970.

Maloney, W.J., Jasty, M., Harris, W.H., Galante, J.O., Callaghan, J.J., 1990a. Endosteal erosion in association with stable uncemented femoral components. J. Bone Joint Surg. Am. 72 (7), 1025–1034.

Maloney, W.J., Jasty, M., Rosenberg, A., Harris, W.H., 1990b. Bone lysis in well-fixed cemented femoral components. J. Bone Joint Surg. Br. 72 (6), 966–970.

Mandelin, J., Liljestrom, M., Li, T.F., Ainola, M., Hukkanen, M., Salo, J., et al., 2005. Pseudosynovial fluid from loosened total hip prosthesis induces osteoclast formation. J. Biomed. Mater. Res. B Appl. Biomater. 74 (1), 582–588.

Mantovani, A., 2008. From phagocyte diversity and activation to probiotics: back to Metchnikoff. Eur. J. Immunol. 38 (12), 3269–3273.

Mantovani, A., Sica, A., Sozzani, S., Allavena, P., Vecchi, A., Locati, M., 2004. The chemokine system in diverse forms of macrophage activation and polarization. Trends Immunol. 25 (12), 677–686.

Marsell, R., Einhorn, T.A., 2011. The biology of fracture healing. Injury 42 (6), 551–555.

Martinez, F.O., Helming, L., Gordon, S., 2009. Alternative activation of macrophages: an immunologic functional perspective. Annu. Rev. Immunol. 27, 451–483.

Martinez, F.O., Sica, A., Mantovani, A., Locati, M., 2008. Macrophage activation and polarization. Front. Biosci. 13, 453–461.

Mathews, S., Bhonde, R., Gupta, P.K., Totey, S., 2011. A novel tripolymer coating demonstrating the synergistic effect of chitosan, collagen type 1 and hyaluronic acid on osteogenic differentiation of human bone marrow derived mesenchymal stem cells. Biochem. Biophys. Res. Commun. 414 (1), 270–276.

Matzinger, P., 2007. Friendly and dangerous signals: is the tissue in control? Nat. Immunol. 8 (1), 11–13.

Matzinger, P., Kamala, T., 2011. Tissue-based class control: the other side of tolerance. Nat. Rev. Immunol. 11 (3), 221–230.

McAuley, J.P., Culpepper, W.J., Engh, C.A., 1998. Total hip arthroplasty. Concerns with extensively porous coated femoral components. Clin. Orthop. Relat. Res. (355), 182–188.

McNally, A.K., Anderson, J.M., 1994. Complement C3 participation in monocyte adhesion to different surfaces. Proc. Natl. Acad. Sci. U.S.A. 91 (21), 10119–10123.

Merkel, K.D., Erdmann, J., McHugh, K., Abu-Amer, Y., Ross, F., Teitelbaum, S., 1999. Tumor necrosis factor-alpha mediates orthopedic implant osteolysis. Am. J. Pathol. 154 (1), 203–210.

Millett, P.J., Allen, M.J., Bostrom, M.P., 2002. Effects of alendronate on particle-induced osteolysis in a rat model. J. Bone Joint Surg. Am. 84-A (2), 236–249.

Mirra, J.M., Marder, R.A., Amstutz, H.C., 1982. The pathology of failed total joint arthroplasty. Clin. Orthop. Relat. Res. (170), 175–183.

Moreland, L.W., Baumgartner, S.W., Schiff, M.H., Tindall, E.A., Fleischmann, R.M., Weaver, A.L., et al., 1997. Treatment of rheumatoid arthritis with a recombinant human tumor necrosis factor receptor (p75)-Fc fusion protein. N. Engl. J. Med. 337 (3), 141–147.

Morscher, E.W., Hefti, A., Aebi, U., 1998. Severe osteolysis after third-body wear due to hydroxyapatite particles from acetabular cup coating. J. Bone Joint Surg. Br. 80 (2), 267–272.

Mosmann, T.R., Cherwinski, H., Bond, M.W., Giedlin, M.A., Coffman, R.L., 1986. Two types of murine helper T cell clone. I. Definition according to profiles of lymphokine activities and secreted proteins. J. Immunol. 136 (7), 2348–2357.

Mosser, D.M., Edwards, J.P., 2008. Exploring the full spectrum of macrophage activation. Nat. Rev. Immunol. 8 (12), 958–969.

Murray, P.J., Wynn, T.A., 2011. Protective and pathogenic functions of macrophage subsets. Nat. Rev. Immunol. 11 (11), 723–737.

Muszanska, A.K., Busscher, H.J., Herrmann, A., van der Mei, H.C., Norde, W., 2011. Pluronic–lysozyme conjugates as anti-adhesive and antibacterial bifunctional polymers for surface coating. Biomaterials 32 (26), 6333–6341.

Nakagami, H., Tomita, N., Kaneda, Y., Ogihara, T., Morishita, R., 2006. Anti-oxidant gene therapy by NF kappa B decoy oligodeoxynucleotide. Curr. Pharm. Biotechnol. 7 (2), 95–100.

Nakano, K., Egashira, K., Ohtani, K., Zhao, G., Funakoshi, K., Ihara, Y., et al., 2007. Catheter-based adeno-virus-mediated anti-monocyte chemoattractant gene therapy attenuates in-stent neointima formation in cynomolgus monkeys. Atherosclerosis 194 (2), 309–316.

Nakashima, Y., Sun, D.H., Trindade, M.C., Chun, L.E., Song, Y., Goodman, S.B., et al., 1999a. Induction of macrophage C-C chemokine expression by titanium alloy and bone cement particles. J. Bone Joint Surg. Br. 81 (1), 155–162.

Nakashima, Y., Sun, D.H., Trindade, M.C., Maloney, W.J., Goodman, S.B., Schurman, D.J., et al., 1999b. Signaling pathways for tumor necrosis factor-alpha and interleukin-6 expression in human macro-phages exposed to titanium-alloy particulate debris *in vitro*. J. Bone Joint Surg. Am. 81 (5), 603–615.

Nalepka, J.L., Lee, M.J., Kraay, M.J., Marcus, R.E., Goldberg, V.M., Chen, X., et al., 2006. Lipopolysaccharide found in aseptic loosening of patients with inflammatory arthritis. Clin. Orthop. Relat. Res. 451, 229–235.

Ng, V.Y., Lombardi Jr., A.V., Berend, K.R., Skeels, M.D., Adams, J.B., 2011. Perivascular lymphocytic infiltra-tion is not limited to metal-on-metal bearings. Clin. Orthop. Relat. Res. 469 (2), 523–529.

Nich, C., Takakubo, Y., Pajarinen, J., Ainola, M., Salem, A., Sillat, T., et al., 2013. Macrophages—key cells in the response to wear debris from joint replacements. J. Biomed. Mater. Res. A 101 (10), 3033–3045.

Nilsson, B., Ekdahl, K.N., Mollnes, T.E., Lambris, J.D., 2007. The role of complement in biomaterial-induced inflammation. Mol. Immunol. 44 (1–3), 82–94.

Ninomiya, J.T., Kuzma, S.A., Schnettler, T.J., Krolikowski, J.G., Struve, J.A., Weihrauch, D., 2013. Metal ions activate vascular endothelial cells and increase lymphocyte chemotaxis and binding. J. Orthop. Res. 31 (9), 1484–1491.

Niu, S., Cao, X., Zhang, Y., Zhu, Q., Zhu, J., Zhen, P., 2012. Peri-implant and systemic effects of high-/ low-affinity bisphosphonate-hydroxyapatite composite coatings in a rabbit model with peri-implant high bone turnover. BMC Musculoskelet. Disord. 13, 97.

Ogunwale, B., Schmidt-Ott, A., Meek, R.M., Brewer, J.M., 2009. Investigating the immunologic effects of CoCr nanoparticles. Clin. Orthop. Relat. Res. 467 (11), 3010–3016.

Ohtani, K., Usui, M., Nakano, K., Kohjimoto, Y., Kitajima, S., Hirouchi, Y., ct al., 2004. Antimonocyte chemoattractant protein-1 gene therapy reduces experimental in-stent restenosis in hypercholesterolemic rabbits and monkeys. Gene Ther. 11 (16), 1273–1282.

Ollivere, B., Wimhurst, J.A., Clark, I.M., Donell, S.T., 2012. Current concepts in osteolysis. J. Bone Joint Surg. Br. 94 (1), 10–15.

Orozco, C., Maalouf, N.M., 2012. Safety of bisphosphonates. Rheum. Dis. Clin. North Am. 38 (4), 681–705.

Osako, M.K., Nakagami, H., Morishita, R., 2012. Modification of decoy oligodeoxynucleotides to achieve the stability and therapeutic efficacy. Curr. Top. Med. Chem. 12 (15), 1603–1607.

Overgaard, S., Bromose, U., Lind, M., Bunger, C., Soballe, K., 1999. The influence of crystallinity of the hydroxyapatite coating on the fixation of implants. Mechanical and histomorphometric results. J. Bone Joint Surg. Br. 81 (4), 725–731.

Pajarinen, J., Cenni, E., Savarino, L., Gomez-Barrena, E., Tamaki, Y., Takagi, M., et al., 2010a. Profile of toll-like receptor-positive cells in septic and aseptic loosening of total hip arthroplasty implants. J. Biomed. Mater. Res. A 94 (1), 84–92.

Pajarinen, J., Mackiewicz, Z., Pollanen, R., Takagi, M., Epstein, N.J., Ma, T., et al., 2010b. Titanium particles modulate expression of Toll-like receptor proteins. J. Biomed. Mater. Res. A 92 (4), 1528–1537.

Pajarinen, J., Kouri, V.P., Jamsen, E., Li, T.F., Mandelin, J., Konttinen, Y.T., 2013. The response of macrophages to titanium particles is determined by macrophage polarization. Acta Biomater. 9 (11), 9229–9240.

Park, C.J., Gabrielson, N.P., Pack, D.W., Jamison, R.D., Wagoner Johnson, A.J., 2009. The effect of chitosan on the migration of neutrophil-like HL60 cells, mediated by IL-8. Biomaterials 30 (4), 436–444.

Parvizi, J., Gehrke, T., Chen, A.F., 2013. Proceedings of the international consensus on periprosthetic joint infection. Bone Joint J. 95-B (11), 1450–1452.

Pascual, G., Fong, A.L., Ogawa, S., Gamliel, A., Li, A.C., Perissi, V., et al., 2005. A SUMOylation-dependent pathway mediates transrepression of inflammatory response genes by PPAR-gamma. Nature 437 (7059), 759–763.

Patil, N., Lee, K., Goodman, S.B., 2009. Porous tantalum in hip and knee reconstructive surgery. J. Biomed. Mater. Res. B Appl. Biomater. 89 (1), 242–251.

Paulus, A.C., Frenzel, J., Ficklscherer, A., Rossbach, B.P., Melcher, C., Jansson, V., et al., 2013. Polyethylene wear particles induce TLR 2 upregulation in the synovial layer of mice. J. Mater. Sci. Mater. Med. 25 (2)., 507–513.

Pearl, J.I., Ma, T., Irani, A.R., Huang, Z., Robinson, W.H., Smith, R.L., et al., 2011. Role of the Toll-like receptor pathway in the recognition of orthopedic implant wear-debris particles. Biomaterials 32 (24), 5535–5542.

Peng, X., Tao, K., Cheng, T., Zhu, J., Zhang, X., 2008. Efficient inhibition of wear debris-induced inflammation by locally delivered siRNA. Biochem. Biophys. Res. Commun. 377 (2), 532–537.

Percival, S.L., Bowler, P.G., Russell, D., 2005. Bacterial resistance to silver in wound care. J. Hosp. Infect. 60 (1), 1–7.

Peter, B., Pioletti, D.P., Laib, S., Bujoli, B., Pilet, P., Janvier, P., et al., 2005. Calcium phosphate drug delivery system: influence of local zoledronate release on bone implant osteointegration. Bone 36 (1), 52–60.

Pollice, P.F., Rosier, R.N., Looney, R.J., Puzas, J.E., Schwarz, E.M., O'Keefe, R.J., 2001. Oral pentoxifylline inhibits release of tumor necrosis factor-alpha from human peripheral blood monocytes: a potential treatment for aseptic loosening of total joint components. J. Bone Joint Surg. Am. 83-A (7), 1057–1061.

Proudfoot, A.E., Power, C.A., Wells, T.N., 2000. The strategy of blocking the chemokine system to combat disease. Immunol. Rev. 177, 246–256.

Punt, I.M., Cleutjens, J.P., de Bruin, T., Willems, P.C., Kurtz, S.M., van Rhijn, L.W., et al., 2009. Periprosthetic tissue reactions observed at revision of total intervertebral disc arthroplasty. Biomaterials 30 (11), 2079–2084.

Punt, I.M., Austen, S., Cleutjens, J.P., Kurtz, S.M., ten Broeke, R.H., van Rhijn, L.W., et al., 2012. Are periprosthetic tissue reactions observed after revision of total disc replacement comparable to the reactions observed after total hip or knee revision surgery? Spine (Phila Pa 1976) 37 (2), 150–159.

Radin, S., Ducheyne, P., 2007. Controlled release of vancomycin from thin sol–gel films on titanium alloy fracture plate material. Biomaterials 28 (9), 1721–1729.

Radin, S., Campbell, J.T., Ducheyne, P., Cuckler, J.M., 1997. Calcium phosphate ceramic coatings as carriers of vancomycin. Biomaterials 18 (11), 777–782.

Rahbek, O., Overgaard, S., Lind, M., Bendix, K., Bunger, C., Soballe, K., 2001. Sealing effect of hydroxy-apatite coating on peri-implant migration of particles. An experimental study in dogs. J. Bone Joint Surg. Br. 83 (3), 441–447.

Raizman, N.M., O'Brien, J.R., Poehling-Monaghan, K.L., Yu, W.D., 2009. Pseudarthrosis of the spine. J. Am. Acad. Orthop. Surg. 17 (8), 494–503.

Rajaee, S.S., Bae, H.W., Kanim, L.E., Delamarter, R.B., 2012. Spinal fusion in the United States: analysis of trends from 1998 to 2008. Spine (Phila Pa 1976) 37 (1), 67–76.

Ralston, S.H., Hacking, L., Willocks, L., Bruce, F., Pitkeathly, D.A., 1989. Clinical, biochemical, and radio-graphic effects of aminohydroxypropylidene bisphosphonate treatment in rheumatoid arthritis. Ann. Rheum. Dis. 48 (5), 396–399.

Rammelt, S., Illert, T., Bierbaum, S., Scharnweber, D., Zwipp, H., Schneiders, W., 2006. Coating of titanium implants with collagen, RGD peptide and chondroitin sulfate. Biomaterials 27 (32), 5561–5571.

Rao, A.J., Gibon, E., Ma, T., Yao, Z., Smith, R.L., Goodman, S.B., 2012. Revision joint replacement, wear particles, and macrophage polarization. Acta Biomater. 8 (7), 2815–2823.

Rao, A.J., Nich, C., Dhulipala, L.S., Gibon, E., Valladares, R., Zwingenberger, S., et al., 2013. Local effect of IL-4 delivery on polyethylene particle induced osteolysis in the murine calvarium. J. Biomed. Mater. Res. A 101 (7), 1926–1934.

Reikeras, O., Gunderson, R.B., 2003. Excellent results of HA coating on a grit-blasted stem: 245 patients followed for 8–12 years. Acta Orthop. Scand. 74 (2), 140–145.

Ren, W., Yang, S.Y., Fang, H.W., Hsu, S., Wooley, P.H., 2003. Distinct gene expression of receptor activator of nuclear factor-kappaB and rank ligand in the inflammatory response to variant morphologies of UHMWPE particles. Biomaterials 24 (26), 4819–4826.

Ren, W., Li, X.H., Chen, B.D., Wooley, P.H., 2004. Erythromycin inhibits wear debris-induced osteoclas-togenesis by modulation of murine macrophage NF-kappaB activity. J. Orthop. Res. 22 (1), 21–29.

Ren, W., Wu, B., Peng, X., Mayton, L., Yu, D., Ren, J., et al., 2006. Erythromycin inhibits wear debris-induced inflammatory osteolysis in a murine model. J. Orthop. Res. 24 (2), 280–290.

Ren, P.G., Lee, S.W., Biswal, S., Goodman, S.B., 2008. Systemic trafficking of macrophages induced by bone cement particles in nude mice. Biomaterials 29 (36), 4760–4765.

Ren, P.G., Huang, Z., Ma, T., Biswal, S., Smith, R.L., Goodman, S.B., 2010. Surveillance of systemic traffick-ing of macrophages induced by UHMWPE particles in nude mice by noninvasive imaging. J. Biomed. Mater. Res. A 94 (3), 706–711.

Ren, P.G., Irani, A., Huang, Z., Ma, T., Biswal, S., Goodman, S.B., 2011. Continuous infusion of UHMWPE particles induces increased bone macrophages and osteolysis. Clin. Orthop. Relat. Res. 469 (1), 113–122.

Revell, P.A., 2008. The combined role of wear particles, macrophages and lymphocytes in the loosening of total joint prostheses. J. R. Soc. Interface 5 (28), 1263–1278.

Ricote, M., Li, A.C., Willson, T.M., Kelly, C.J., Glass, C.K., 1998. The peroxisome proliferator-activated receptor-gamma is a negative regulator of macrophage activation. Nature 391 (6662), 79–82.

Rivardo, F., Turner, R.J., Allegrone, G., Ceri, H., Martinotti, M.G., 2009. Anti-adhesion activity of two biosurfactants produced by *Bacillus* spp. prevents biofilm formation of human bacterial pathogens. Appl. Microbiol. Biotechnol. 83 (3), 541–553.

Rodan, G.A., 1998. Bone homeostasis. Proc. Natl. Acad. Sci. USA. 95 (23), 13361–13362.

Rodrigues, L., Banat, I.M., Teixeira, J., Oliveira, R, 2006. Biosurfactants: potential applications in medicine. J. Antimicrob. Chemother. 57 (4), 609–618.

Rogers, T.H., Babensee, J.E., 2010. Altered adherent leukocyte profile on biomaterials in Toll-like receptor 4 deficient mice. Biomaterials 31 (4), 594–601.

Sabokbar, A., Pandey, R., Quinn, J.M., Athanasou, N.A., 1998. Osteoclastic differentiation by mononuclear phagocytes containing biomaterial particles. Arch. Orthop. Trauma. Surg. 117 (3), 136–140.

Santavirta, S., Konttinen, Y.T., Bergroth, V., Eskola, A., Tallroth, K., Lindholm, T.S., 1990b. Aggressive granulomatous lesions associated with hip arthroplasty. Immunopathological studies. J. Bone Joint Surg. Am. 72 (2), 252–258.

Santavirta, S., Hoikka, V., Eskola, A., Konttinen, Y.T., Paavilainen, T., Tallroth, K., 1990a. Aggressive granulomatous lesions in cementless total hip arthroplasty. J. Bone Joint Surg. Br. 72 (6), 980–984.

Saran, N., Zhang, R., Turcotte, R.E., 2011. Osteogenic protein-1 delivered by hydroxyapatite-coated implants improves bone ingrowth in extracortical bone bridging. Clin. Orthop. Relat. Res. 469 (5), 1470–1478.

Sarma, J.V., Ward, P.A., 2011. The complement system. Cell Tissue Res. 343 (1), 227–235.

Scapini, P., Lapinet-Vera, J.A., Gasperini, S., Calzetti, F., Bazzoni, F., Cassatella, M.A., 2000. The neutrophil as a cellular source of chemokines. Immunol. Rev. 177, 195–203.

Schepers, A., Eefting, D., Bonta, P.I., Grimbergen, J.M., de Vries, M.R., van Weel, V., et al., 2006. Anti-MCP-1 gene therapy inhibits vascular smooth muscle cells proliferation and attenuates vein graft thickening both *in vitro* and *in vivo*. Arterioscler. Thromb. Vasc. Biol. 26 (9), 2063–2069.

Schmaier, A.H., 1997. Contact activation: a revision. Thromb. Haemost. 78 (1), 101–107.

Schmalzried, T.P., Kwong, L.M., Jasty, M., Sedlacek, R.C., Haire, T.C., O'Connor, D.O., et al., 1992. The mechanism of loosening of cemented acetabular components in total hip arthroplasty. Analysis of specimens retrieved at autopsy. Clin. Orthop. Relat. Res. (274), 60–78.

Schmidt, M., Goebeler, M., 2011. Nickel allergies: paying the Toll for innate immunity. J. Mol. Med. (Berl) 89 (10), 961–970.

Schmidt, M., Raghavan, B., Muller, V., Vogl, T., Fejer, G., Tchaptchet, S., et al., 2010. Crucial role for human Toll-like receptor 4 in the development of contact allergy to nickel. Nat. Immunol. 11 (9), 814–819.

Schroder, K., Hertzog, P.J., Ravasi, T., Hume, D.A., 2004. Interferon-gamma: an overview of signals, mechanisms and functions. J. Leukoc. Biol. 75 (2), 163–189.

Schwarz, E.M., Looney, R.J., O'Keefe, R.J., 2000a. Anti-TNF-alpha therapy as a clinical intervention for periprosthetic osteolysis. Arthritis Res. 2 (3), 165–168.

Schwarz, E.M., Benz, E.B., Lu, A.P., Goater, J.J., Mollano, A.V., Rosier, R.N., et al., 2000b. Quantitative small-animal surrogate to evaluate drug efficacy in preventing wear debris-induced osteolysis. J. Orthop. Res. 18 (6), 849–855.

Schwarz, E.M., Lu, A.P., Goater, J.J., Benz, E.B., Kollias, G., Rosier, R.N., et al., 2000c. Tumor necrosis factor-alpha/nuclear transcription factor-kappaB signaling in periprosthetic osteolysis. J. Orthop. Res. 18 (3), 472–480.

Schwarz, E.M., Campbell, D., Totterman, S., Boyd, A., O'Keefe, R.J., Looney, R.J., 2003. Use of volumetric computerized tomography as a primary outcome measure to evaluate drug efficacy in the prevention of peri-prosthetic osteolysis: a 1-year clinical pilot of etanercept vs. placebo. J. Orthop. Res. 21 (6), 1049–1055.

Secinti, K.D., Ayten, M., Kahilogullari, G., Kaygusuz, G., Ugur, H.C., Attar, A., 2008. Antibacterial effects of electrically activated vertebral implants. J. Clin. Neurosci. 15 (4), 434–439.

Shah, N.J., Hong, J., Hyder, M.N., Hammond, P.T., 2012. Osteophilic multilayer coatings for accelerated bone tissue growth. Adv. Mater. 24 (11), 1445–1450.

Shakespeare, W.C., Metcalf 3rd, C.A., Wang, Y., Sundaramoorthi, R., Keenan, T., Weigele, M., et al., 2003. Novel bone-targeted Src tyrosine kinase inhibitor drug discovery. Curr. Opin. Drug Discov. Devel. 6 (5), 729–741.

Shanbhag, A.S., 2006. Use of bisphosphonates to improve the durability of total joint replacements. J. Am. Acad. Orthop. Surg. 14 (4), 215–225.

Shanbhag, A.S., Hasselman, C.T., Rubash, H.E., 1997. The John Charnley Award. Inhibition of wear debris mediated osteolysis in a canine total hip arthroplasty model. Clin. Orthop. Relat. Res. (344), 33–43.

Shanbhag, A.S., Jacobs, J.J., Black, J., Galante, J.O., Glant, T.T., 1995. Human monocyte response to particulate biomaterials generated *in vivo* and *in vitro*. J. Orthop. Res. 13 (5), 792–801.

Shi, Y., Hu, G., Su, J., Li, W., Chen, Q., Shou, P., et al., 2010. Mesenchymal stem cells: a new strategy for immunosuppression and tissue repair. Cell Res. 20 (5), 510–518.

Shimizu, H., Nakagami, H., Morita, S., Tsukamoto, I., Osako, M.K., Nakagami, F., et al., 2009. New treatment of periodontal diseases by using NF-kappaB decoy oligodeoxynucleotides via prevention of bone resorption and promotion of wound healing. Antioxid. Redox Signal. 11 (9), 2065–2075.

Singla, A.K., Chawla, M., 2001. Chitosan: some pharmaceutical and biological aspects—an update. J. Pharm. Pharmacol. 53 (8), 1047–1067.

Skipor, A.K., Campbell, P.A., Patterson, L.M., Anstutz, H.C., Schmalzried, T.P., Jacobs, J.J., 2002. Serum and urine metal levels in patients with metal-on-metal surface arthroplasty. J. Mater. Sci. Mater. Med. 13 (12), 1227–1234.

Smith, R.S., Zhang, Z., Bouchard, M., Li, J., Lapp, H.S., Brotske, G.R., et al., 2012. Vascular catheters with a nonleaching poly-sulfobetaine surface modification reduce thrombus formation and microbial attachment. Sci. Transl. Med. 4 (153), 153ra132.

Soballe, K., 1993. Hydroxyapatite ceramic coating for bone implant fixation. Mechanical and histological studies in dogs. Acta Orthop. Scand. Suppl. 255, 1–58.

Soballe, K., Hansen, E.S., Brockstedt-Rasmussen, H., Bunger, C., 1993. Hydroxyapatite coating converts fibrous tissue to bone around loaded implants. J. Bone Joint Surg. Br. 75 (2), 270–278.

Soballe, K., Overgaard, S., Hansen, E.S., Brokstedt-Rasmussen, H., Lind, M., Bunger, C., 1999. A review of ceramic coatings for implant fixation. J. Long Term Eff. Med. Implants 9 (1–2), 131–151.

Spadaro, J.A., Berger, T.J., Barranco, S.D., Chapin, S.E., Becker, R.O., 1974. Antibacterial effects of silver electrodes with weak direct current. Antimicrob. Agents Chemother. 6 (5), 637–642.

Sperling, C., Fischer, M., Maitz, M.F., Werner, C., 2009. Blood coagulation on biomaterials requires the combination of distinct activation processes. Biomaterials 30 (27), 4447–4456.

Stein, B., Baldwin Jr., A.S., Ballard, D.W., Greene, W.C., Angel, P., Herrlich, P., 1993. Cross-coupling of the NF-kappa B p65 and Fos/Jun transcription factors produces potentiated biological function. EMBO J. 12 (10), 3879–3891.

Stigter, M., de Groot, K., Layrolle, P., 2002. Incorporation of tobramycin into biomimetic hydroxyapatite coating on titanium. Biomaterials 23 (20), 4143–4153.

Stigter, M., Bezemer, J., de Groot, K., Layrolle, P., 2004. Incorporation of different antibiotics into carbonated hydroxyapatite coatings on titanium implants, release and antibiotic efficacy. J. Control. Release 99 (1), 127–137.

Stilling, M., Rahbek, O., Soballe, K., 2009. Inferior survival of hydroxyapatite versus titanium-coated cups at 15 years. Clin. Orthop. Relat. Res. 467 (11), 2872–2879.

Stout, R.D., Jiang, C., Matta, B., Tietzel, I., Watkins, S.K., Suttles, J., 2005. Macrophages sequentially change their functional phenotype in response to changes in microenvironmental influences. J. Immunol. 175 (1), 342–349.

Sun, L., Berndt, C.C., Khor, K.A., Cheang, H.N., Gross, K.A., 2002. Surface characteristics and dissolution behavior of plasma-sprayed hydroxyapatite coating. J. Biomed. Mater. Res. 62 (2), 228–236.

Szekanecz, Z., Koch, A.E., 2007. Macrophages and their products in rheumatoid arthritis. Curr. Opin. Rheumatol. 19 (3), 289–295.

Taki, N., Tatro, J.M., Nalepka, J.L., Togawa, D., Goldberg, V.M., Rimnac, C.M., et al., 2005. Polyethylene and titanium particles induce osteolysis by similar, lymphocyte-independent, mechanisms. J. Orthop. Res. 23 (2), 376–383.

Tallroth, K., Eskola, A., Santavirta, S., Konttinen, Y.T., Lindholm, T.S., 1989. Aggressive granulomatous lesions after hip arthroplasty. J. Bone Joint Surg. Br. 71 (4), 571–575.

Tamaki, Y., Takakubo, Y., Goto, K., Hirayama, T., Sasaki, K., Konttinen, Y.T., et al., 2009. Increased expression of toll-like receptors in aseptic loose periprosthetic tissues and septic synovial membranes around total hip implants. J. Rheumatol. 36 (3), 598–608.

Tang, L., 1998. Mechanisms of fibrinogen domains: biomaterial interactions. J. Biomater. Sci. Polym. Ed. 9 (12), 1257–1266.

Tang, L., Jennings, T.A., Eaton, J.W., 1998. Mast cells mediate acute inflammatory responses to implanted biomaterials. Proc. Natl. Acad. Sci. U.S.A. 95 (15), 8841–8846.

Tanzer, M., Karabasz, D., Krygier, J.J., Cohen, R., Bobyn, J.D., 2005. The Otto Aufranc Award: bone augmentation around and within porous implants by local bisphosphonate elution. Clin. Orthop. Relat. Res. 441, 30–39.

Tatro, J.M., Taki, N., Islam, A.S., Goldberg, V.M., Rimnac, C.M., Doerschuk, C.M., et al., 2007. The balance between endotoxin accumulation and clearance during particle-induced osteolysis in murine calvaria. J. Orthop. Res. 25 (3), 361–369.

Tengvall, P., Askendal, A., Lundstrom, I.I., 2001. Ellipsometric in vitro studies on the activation of complement by human immunoglobulins M and G after adsorption to methylated silicon. Colloids Surf. B Biointerfaces 20 (1), 51–62.

Tengvall, P., Skoglund, B., Askendal, A., Aspenberg, P., 2004. Surface immobilized bisphosphonate improves stainless-steel screw fixation in rats. Biomaterials 25 (11), 2133–2138.

Thomas, P., Summer, B., Sander, C.A., Przybilla, B., Thomas, M., Naumann, T., 2000. Intolerance of osteo-synthesis material: evidence of dichromate contact allergy with concomitant oligoclonal T-cell infiltrate and TH1-type cytokine expression in the peri-implantar tissue. Allergy 55 (10), 969–972.

Thomas, P., Bandl, W.D., Maier, S., Summer, B., Przybilla, B., 2006. Hypersensitivity to titanium osteosyn-thesis with impaired fracture healing, eczema, and T-cell hyperresponsiveness in vitro: case report and review of the literature. Contact Dermatitis 55 (4), 199–202.

Thomssen, H., Hoffmann, B., Schank, M., Hohler, T., Thabe, H., Meyer zum Buschenfelde, K.H., et al., 2001. Cobalt-specific T lymphocytes in synovial tissue after an allergic reaction to a cobalt alloy joint prosthesis. J. Rheumatol. 28 (5), 1121–1128.

Tomita, N., Morishita, R., Tomita, S., Gibbons, G.H., Zhang, L., Horiuchi, M., et al., 2000. Transcription factor decoy for NFkappaB inhibits TNF-alpha-induced cytokine and adhesion molecule expression in vivo. Gene Ther. 7 (15), 1326–1332.

Tomita, T., Takano, H., Tomita, N., Morishita, R., Kaneko, M., Shi, K., et al., 2000. Transcription factor decoy for NFkappaB inhibits cytokine and adhesion molecule expressions in synovial cells derived from rheumatoid arthritis. Rheumatology (Oxford) 39 (7), 749–757.

Tower, S.S., 2010. Arthroprosthetic cobaltism: neurological and cardiac manifestations in two patients with metal-on-metal arthroplasty: a case report. J. Bone Joint Surg. Am. 92 (17), 2847–2851.

Trindade, M.C., Lind, M., Goodman, S.B., Maloney, W.J., Schurman, D.J., Smith, R.L., 1999a. Interferon-gamma exacerbates polymethylmethacrylate particle-induced interleukin-6 release by human mono-cyte/macrophages in vitro. J. Biomed. Mater. Res. 47 (1), 1–7.

Trindade, M.C., Nakashima, Y., Lind, M., Sun, D.H., Goodman, S.B., Maloney, W.J., et al., 1999b. Interleukin-4 inhibits granulocyte-macrophage colony-stimulating factor, interleukin-6, and tumor necrosis factor-alpha expression by human monocytes in response to polymethylmethacrylate particle challenge in vitro. J. Orthop. Res. 17 (6), 797–802.

Tsuchimoto, M., Azuma, Y., Higuchi, O., Sugimoto, I., Hirata, N., Kiyoki, M., et al., 1994. Alendronate modulates osteogenesis of human osteoblastic cells in vitro. Jpn. J. Pharmacol. 66 (1), 25–33.

Tuan, R.S., Lee, F.Y., Konttinen, Y., Wilkinson, J.M., Smith, R.L., 2008. What are the local and systemic bio-logic reactions and mediators to wear debris, and what host factors determine or modulate the biologic response to wear particles? J. Am. Acad. Orthop. Surg. 16 (Suppl. 1), S33–S38.

Tyson-Capper, A.J., Lawrence, H., Holland, J.P., Deehan, D.J., Kirby, J.A., 2013. Metal-on-metal hips: cobalt can induce an endotoxin-like response. Ann. Rheum. Dis. 72 (3), 460–461.

Ulrich-Vinther, M., Carmody, E.E., Goater, J.J., S balle, K., O'Keefe, R.J., Schwarz, E.M., 2002. Recombinant adeno-associated virus-mediated osteoprotegerin gene therapy inhibits wear debris-induced osteolysis. J. Bone Joint Surg. Am. 84-A (8), 1405–1412.

United States Bone and Joint Initiative, 2011. The Burden of Musculoskeletal Diseases in the United States, second ed. Available from: <http://www.boneandjointburden.org>.

Urban, R.M., Jacobs, J.J., Tomlinson, M.J., Gavrilovic, J., Black, J., Peoc'h, M., 2000. Dissemination of wear particles to the liver, spleen, and abdominal lymph nodes of patients with hip or knee replacement. J. Bone Joint Surg. Am. 82 (4), 457–476.

Valladares, R.D., Nich, C., Zwingenberger, S., Li, C., Swank, K.R., Gibon, E., et al., 2013. Toll-like receptors-2 and 4 are overexpressed in an experimental model of particle-induced osteolysis. J. Biomed. Mater. Res. A. 102 (9), 3004–3011.

van de Belt, H., Neut, D., Schenk, W., van Horn, J.R., van der Mei, H.C., Busscher, H.J., 2001. Infection of orthopedic implants and the use of antibiotic-loaded bone cements. A review. Acta Orthop. Scand. 72 (6), 557–571.

VandeVord, P.J., Matthew, H.W., DeSilva, S.P., Mayton, L., Wu, B., Wooley, P.H., 2002. Evaluation of the biocompatibility of a chitosan scaffold in mice. J. Biomed. Mater. Res. 59 (3), 585–590.

Vegari, D.N., Parvizi, J., 2011. Joint arthroplasty and infection: where do we stand? J. Long Term Eff. Med. Implants 21 (3), 225–232.

Vert, M., Doi, Y., Hellwich, K.-H., Hess, M., Hodge, P., Kubisa, P., et al., 2012. Terminology for biorelated polymers and applications (IUPAC Recommendations 2012). Pure Appl. Chem. 84 (2), 377–410.

Visentin, L., Dodds, R.A., Valente, M., Misiano, P., Bradbeer, J.N., Oneta, S., et al., 2000. A selective inhibitor of the osteoclastic V-H(+)-ATPase prevents bone loss in both thyroparathyroidectomized and ovariec-tomized rats. J. Clin. Invest. 106 (2), 309–318.

von Knoch, F., Jaquiery, C., Kowalsky, M., Schaeren, S., Alabre, C., Martin, I., et al., 2005. Effects of bisphosphonates on proliferation and osteoblast differentiation of human bone marrow stromal cells. Biomaterials 26 (34), 6941–6949.

von Knoch, M., Wedemeyer, C., Pingsmann, A., von Knoch, F., Hilken, G., Sprecher, C., et al., 2005. The decrease of particle-induced osteolysis after a single dose of bisphosphonate. Biomaterials 26 (14), 1803–1808.

Wang, A., Essner, A., Stark, C., Dumbleton, J.H., 1996. Comparison of the size and morphology of UHMWPE wear debris produced by a hip joint simulator under serum and water lubricated conditions. Biomaterials 17 (9), 865–871.

Wang, J.Y., Tsukayama, D.T., Wicklund, B.H., Gustilo, R.B., 1996. Inhibition of T and B cell proliferation by titanium, cobalt, and chromium: role of IL-2 and IL-6. J. Biomed. Mater. Res. 32 (4), 655–661.

Wang, J.Y., Wicklund, B.H., Gustilo, R.B., Tsukayama, D.T., 1997a. Prosthetic metals impair murine immune response and cytokine release *in vivo* and *in vitro*. J. Orthop. Res. 15 (5), 688–699.

Wang, J.Y., Wicklund, B.H., Gustilo, R.B., Tsukayama, D.T., 1997b. Prosthetic metals interfere with the functions of human osteoblast cells *in vitro*. Clin. Orthop. Relat. Res. (339), 216–226.

Wang, M.L., Nesti, L.J., Tuli, R., Lazatin, J., Danielson, K.G., Sharkey, P.F., et al., 2002. Titanium particles suppress expression of osteoblastic phenotype in human mesenchymal stem cells. J. Orthop. Res. 20 (6), 1175–1184.

Wang, H., Jia, T.H., Zacharias, N., Gong, W., Du, H.X., Wooley, P.H., et al., 2013. Combination gene therapy targeting on interleukin-1beta and RANKL for wear debris-induced aseptic loosening. Gene Ther. 20 (2), 128–135.

Wang, Y., Wu, N.N., Mou, Y.Q., Chen, L., Deng, Z.L., 2013. Inhibitory effects of recombinant IL-4 and recombinant IL-13 on UHMWPE-induced bone destruction in the murine air pouch model. J. Surg. Res. 180 (2), e73–e81.

Willert, H.G., Semlitsch, M., 1977. Reactions of the articular capsule to wear products of artificial joint prostheses. J. Biomed. Mater. Res. 11 (2), 157–164.

Willert, H.G., Bertram, H., Buchhorn, G.H., 1990a. Osteolysis in alloarthroplasty of the hip. The role of bone cement fragmentation. Clin. Orthop. Relat. Res. (258), 108–121.

Willert, H.G., Bertram, H., Buchhorn, G.H., 1990b. Osteolysis in alloarthroplasty of the hip. The role of ultra-high molecular weight polyethylene wear particles. Clin. Orthop. Relat. Res. (258), 95–107.

Willert, H.G., Buchhorn, G.H., Fayyazi, A., Flury, R., Windler, M., Koster, G., et al., 2005. Metal-on-metal bearings and hypersensitivity in patients with artificial hip joints. A clinical and histomorphological study. J. Bone Joint Surg. Am. 87 (1), 28–36.

Williams, D.F., 1980. Fundamental Aspects of Biocompatibility. CRC Press, Boca Raton, FL.

Williams, D.F., 2008. On the mechanisms of biocompatibility. Biomaterials 29 (20), 2941–2953.

Wilson, C.J., Clegg, R.E., Leavesley, D.I., Pearcy, M.J., 2005. Mediation of biomaterial–cell interactions by adsorbed proteins: a review. Tissue Eng. 11 (1–2), 1–18.

Wojtowicz, A.M., Shekaran, A., Oest, M.E., Dupont, K.M., Templeman, K.L., Hutmacher, D.W., et al., 2010. Coating of biomaterial scaffolds with the collagen-mimetic peptide GFOGER for bone defect repair. Biomaterials 31 (9), 2574–2582.

Xing, Z., Pabst, M.J., Hasty, K.A., Smith, R.A., 2006. Accumulation of LPS by polyethylene particles decreases bone attachment to implants. J. Orthop. Res. 24 (5), 959–966.

Xu, J., Wu, H.F., Ang, E.S., Yip, K., Woloszyn, M., Zheng, M.H., et al., 2009. NF-kappaB modulators in osteolytic bone diseases. Cytokine Growth Factor Rev. 20 (1), 7–17.

Yamamura, K., Iwata, H., Yotsuyanagi, T., 1992. Synthesis of antibiotic-loaded hydroxyapatite beads and *in vitro* drug release testing. J. Biomed. Mater. Res. 26 (8), 1053–1064.

Yamanaka, Y., Karuppaiah, K., Aber-Amer, Y., 2011. Polyubiquitination events mediate PMMA particles activation of NF-κB pathway. J. Biol. Chem. 286 (27)., 23735–23741.

Yamashiro, S., Kamohara, H., Wang, J.M., Yang, D., Gong, W.H., Yoshimura, T., 2001. Phenotypic and functional change of cytokine-activated neutrophils: inflammatory neutrophils are heterogeneous and enhance adaptive immune responses. J. Leukoc. Biol. 69 (5), 698–704.

Yao, Z., Keeney, M., Lin, T.H., Pajarinen, J., Barcay, K., Waters, H., et al., 2014. Mutant monocyte chemoattractant protein 1 protein attenuates migration of and inflammatory cytokine release by macrophages exposed to orthopedic implant wear particles. J. Biomed. Mater. Res. A 102 (9), 3291–3297.

Yaszay, B., Trindade, M.C., Lind, M., Goodman, S.B., Smith, R.L., 2001. Fibroblast expression of C-C chemokines in response to orthopaedic biomaterial particle challenge *in vitro*. J. Orthop. Res. 19 (5), 970–976.

Yu, J.C., Ho, W., Lin, J., Yip, H., Wong, P.K., 2003. Photocatalytic activity, antibacterial effect, and photoinduced hydrophilicity of TiO_2 films coated on a stainless steel substrate. Environ. Sci. Technol. 37 (10), 2296–2301.

Zdolsek, J., Eaton, J.W., Tang, L., 2007. Histamine release and fibrinogen adsorption mediate acute inflammatory responses to biomaterial implants in humans. J. Transl. Med. 5, 31.

Zhang, F., Zhang, Z., Zhu, X., Kang, E.T., Neoh, K.G., 2008. Silk-functionalized titanium surfaces for enhancing osteoblast functions and reducing bacterial adhesion. Biomaterials 29 (36), 4751–4759.

Zhang, W., Luo, Y., Wang, H., Jiang, J., Pu, S., Chu, P.K., 2008. Ag and Ag/N_2 plasma modification of polyethylene for the enhancement of antibacterial properties and cell growth/proliferation. Acta Biomater. 4 (6), 2028–2036.

Zhang, X., Mosser, D.M., 2008. Macrophage activation by endogenous danger signals. J. Pathol. 214 (2), 161–178.

Zhuo, R., Siedlecki, C.A., Vogler, E.A., 2006. Autoactivation of blood factor XII at hydrophilic and hydrophobic surfaces. Biomaterials 27 (24), 4325–4332.

Zijlstra, W.P., Bulstra, S.K., van Raay, J.J., van Leeuwen, B.M., Kuijer, R., 2012. Cobalt and chromium ions reduce human osteoblast-like cell activity *in vitro*, reduce the OPG to RANKL ratio, and induce oxidative stress. J. Orthop. Res. 30 (5), 740–747.

CHAPTER 13

Host Response to Biomaterials for Pelvic Floor Reconstruction

William R. Barone[1], Steven D. Abramowitch[1,2] and Pamela A. Moalli[2]
[1]Department of Bioengineering, University of Pittsburgh, Pittsburgh, PA, USA
[2]Magee-Womens Research Institute, University of Pittsburgh, Pittsburgh, PA, USA

Contents

Host Response to Biomaterials.
DOI: http://dx.doi.org/10.1016/B978-0-12-800196-7.00013-X

INTRODUCTION

The overall aim of this chapter is to provide the reader with a perspective on the uses of biomaterials in the treatment of pelvic floor disorders. Specifically, this chapter will focus on the structure and function of the female pelvic floor, discuss several common pelvic floor disorders for which biomaterials are currently utilized, and the host response to biomaterials used in this anatomic site. While the concept of using biomaterials in pelvic floor reconstruction is far from novel, their use in this anatomic location has become an area of intense interest in recent decades. Despite the tremendous increase in use of materials to address pelvic floor dysfunction, many products have been met with controversy due to poor efficacy or relatively high complication rates. As such, there is a clear need to reevaluate and understand both the materials that are being used along with the host response to these materials. In addition, the effect of these variables and the overall function that these devices are expected to perform must be further understood.

In order to provide a complete understanding of biomaterial use in the pelvic floor, we first discuss the anatomy of the pelvic floor. By examining the gross and functional anatomy, we hope to provide insight into both the shortcomings and successes of current biomaterials, while examining effective uses for biomaterials under the constraints of this anatomy. Please note that this text will not provide an all-inclusive look at the pelvic floor, but rather focuses on providing the reader with sufficient anatomic background to understand our current knowledge of native pelvic floor support. Following this, we will discuss various pathologies that have become the focus for repair using biomaterials, again addressing anatomical features, the intended function of grafts under these conditions, and the effect of the host response upon outcome. Finally, we will examine the factors of biomaterials that influence the host response and discuss various challenges that must be considered for biomaterial use in the pelvic floor.

PELVIC FLOOR ANATOMY

The pelvic floor is a highly complex, interdependent network of soft tissue and bony structures that provide support to the vagina. In turn, the vagina provides support to a number of other pelvic organs. While this text will primarily focus on the nulliparous anatomy and changes relative to this reference, it should be noted that the anatomy of the pelvic floor is subject to change throughout a woman's lifetime. For instance, the positioning and composition of the vagina are likely altered during and after childbirth, though in many women these changes do not result in dysfunction. As such, the concepts and requirements of surgical reconstruction may be relative to the reference configuration that is considered.

Bony pelvis

In general, the viscera of the pelvic floor are contained within the bony pelvis, which serves as the base of attachment for much of the musculature and connective tissues that support the pelvic viscera. Points of articulation and their three-dimensional (3D) positioning appear to play a critical role for pelvic floor support and function, as skeletal abnormalities are highly associated with pelvic floor disorders. For instance, nearly 100% of women with a wide transverse outlet, short anterior–posterior diameter, and absent pubic symphysis develop pelvic organ prolapse (POP) (Muir et al., 2004). While dysfunction may be expected in such a dramatically altered pelvis, even subtle changes in pelvic diameter carry an increased risk for developing prolapse (Bent et al., 2008).

Outlining the pelvic cavity, the bony pelvis is comprised of the coxal bones (also known as the hip bones), sacrum, and coccyx. Each coxal bone is the fusion of three bones, with the ilium superiorly, the ischium inferiorly and posteriorly, and the pubis inferiorly and anteriorly. The two inferior bones form the acetabulum, which articulates with the head of the femur. In addition, the two coxal bones articulate anteriorly at the pubic symphysis, a cartilaginous joint at the pelvic midline. Finally, the sacrum consists of five fused vertebral bones that articulate bilaterally with the posterior ilium at the sacroiliac joint and inferiorly to the coccyx. When standing, the superior inlet plane of the normal female pelvis is approximately 60–65° from the horizontal plane (Bent et al., 2008). Points of attachment on these structures will be highlighted as necessary and can be found in Figure 13.1.

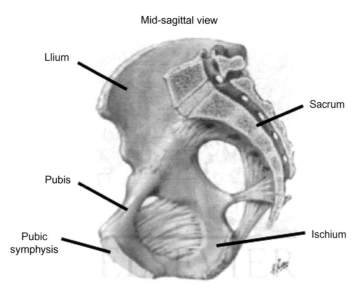

Mid-sagittal view

Llium

Sacrum

Pubis

Pubic symphysis

Ischium

Figure 13.1 A midsagittal cross section of the bony pelvis. The bony pelvis is comprised of coxal bones, sacrum, and coccyx with various ligaments connecting these bones, providing a stable outline for the pelvic organs. The coxal bone is formed by the fusion of the ilium, ischium, and pubis bones. The paired coxal bones articulate anteriorly and the pubic symphysis and posteriorly to the sacrum.

Musculature

While the superior outlet of the bony pelvis is open to the abdominal cavity, inferiorly it is largely closed by the pelvic floor musculature. Anteriorly is a group of skeletal muscles, including the obturator internus, that originate from the pubic ramus and function to stabilize and rotate the femur (Figure 13.2). Posteriorly, the performis muscles originate on the anterior sacrum, through the greater sciatic notch and act to externally rotate the thigh. Inferiorly is a group of muscles referred to as the pelvic diaphragm. The pelvic diaphragm consists of the levator ani muscles, coccygeus muscles, and fascia (Figure 13.2). Often the pelvic diaphragm is described as a "hammock-like" or "U-shaped" structure stretched between the pubis and coccyx with attachments along the lateral walls of the bony pelvis (Bent et al., 2008; Walters and Karram, 1993). The area contained within this U-shaped region is referred to as the urogenital hiatus and contains the urethra, vagina, and rectum (Figure 13.2). The levator ani fan out with broad attachments and create the posterior and lateral pelvic floor. Given the broad, fanning organization of the levator ani, this muscle is further divided into three parts according to their points of attachment. From medial to lateral, the components of the levator ani are the puborectalis, pubococcygeus, and iliococcygeus.

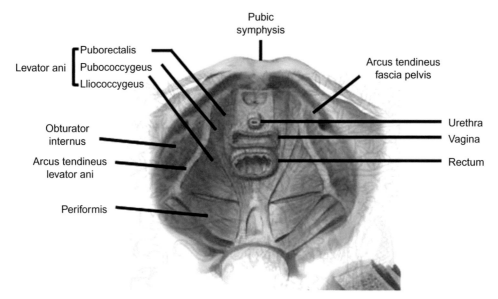

Figure 13.2 Superior view of the pelvic floor musculature. The muscles of the pelvic floor close the inferior aspect of the pelvis while providing support to various organs and stabilizing several bones including the femur and bony pelvis. These muscles also create a U-shaped cavity known as the urogenital hiatus, which contains the urethra, vagina, and rectum.

In many texts, the pelvic diaphragm is portrayed as a simple hammock structure lying in the horizontal plane that closes the inferior pelvic floor and provides a resting surface for the pelvic viscera. Specifically, Bent et al. (2008) state that the contraction of the pelvic diaphragm provides a horizontal plate on which the pelvic organs lie. However, given the horizontal offset of the bony pelvis and the basal tone of these muscles, their function appears more complex. Indeed, Bent et al. and others acknowledge that the resting tone of the pelvic floor muscles pull the distal vagina toward the pubic symphysis. A more representative orientation of the pelvic diaphragm can be observed upon magnetic resonance imaging (MRI) segmentation of the pelvic floor muscles. In our research center, we have observed that that these muscles have a noticeable horizontal offset, approaching the vertical plane, placing the musculature in a position to actively pull the pelvic viscera anteriorly toward the pubic symphysis. As such, the pelvic floor musculature appears to be a vital component in positioning the organs in this space. Increased vertical positioning of the pelvic diaphragm is also consistent with the observation of the change in vaginal orientation along its length. It is well known that the vagina does not form a straight line from the introitus to the sacrum, but rather the distal vagina is pulled anteriorly, while the proximal vagina is directed toward the sacrum more in line with the horizontal axis. The change in angle between proximal and distal vaginal axes is common in normal pelvic floor anatomy. As such, weakening of these muscles or defects in these structures may result in more posterior placement of the vagina, and alter the angle between the proximal and distal vagina. This change would then affect the positioning of other pelvic viscera, potentially placing them in a less optimal position, directly over the vaginal introitus. While this hypothetical scenario may or may not be related to pelvic floor disorders, this example readily demonstrates the integral behavior of pelvic floor structures and the impact of this musculature on viscera positioning.

Connective tissue

One of the primary components of pelvic floor support is connective tissues, typically arising from the fascia which covers the musculature and viscera. The connective tissue of the pelvic floor is a continuous, intricate web that covers and mechanically supports the vagina and the pelvic organs. These connective tissues suspend the organs of the pelvic floor through attachments to the pelvic sidewall. This support system is quite complex, as the composition, thickness, and strength of the connective tissues vary significantly based on their location.

In order to improve our understanding of the connective tissue support of the pelvic floor, DeLancey (1994) introduced a level-based system that conceptually divides connective tissue support based on location of attachment. This popular approach considers three levels of support for the pelvis with levels I, II, and III representing support

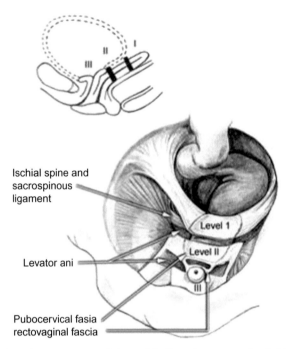

Ischial spine and
sacrospinous
ligament

Level 1

Level II

Levator ani

III

Pubocervical fasia
rectovaginal fascia

Figure 13.3 Connective tissue support of the pelvic floor is commonly divided into three distinct levels described by DeLancey. The proximal, middle, and distal aspects of the vagina are supported by levels I (*uterosacral ligaments*), II (*paravaginal attachments*), and III (*perineal body*), respectively. *Reprinted with permission from DeLancey (1994).*

for the proximal, middle, and distal portions of the vagina respectively (Figure 13.3). Level I structures consist of the cardinal and uterosacral ligaments and provide support to the uterus and upper vagina. It should be noted that these structures are quite dissimilar from other ligamentous structures throughout the body. As opposed to the dense, fibrous bundles that connect bones and consist primarily of collagen I, the ligaments of the pelvic floor are complex connective tissue structures that envelope neurovascular structures and attach the vagina to the bony pelvis. The composition of the uterosacral ligament varies along its length, ranging from fat and loose connective tissue at its attachment to the sacrum, to dense connective tissue in the midregion, to predominately muscle at the cervical attachment. The primary structural protein of the uterosacral ligament is collagen III, providing a combination of flexibility and strength (Gabriel et al., 2005). The paired uterosacral ligaments direct the vagina superiorly and posteriorly, providing support to the cervix and upper vagina (DeLancey, 1994). In its course to the sacrum, the uterosacral ligament fans out and attaches at sacral segments ranging from S1 to S4. Lateral stability of the vagina is maintained by the cardinal ligaments, which also insert along the paracervical ring, combining with the urterosac-ral ligaments. The cardinal ligaments also have a fan-like appearance, extending along to proximal third of the vagina and running laterally with broad attachments to the pelvic sidewall. Level II support provides additional lateral stabilization of the vagina. Level II consists of anterior and posterior portions of the endopelvic fascia, a loose connective tissue extending from the midvagina to the pelvic sidewall inserting into the acrus tendineous fascia pelvis. Finally, level III support arises from the fusion of the endopelvic fascia at the pubic symphysis (anterior) and perineal body (posterior) (Figure 13.3).

Additional connective tissue structures in the pelvic floor include the arcus tendin-eus levator ani and arcus tendineus fascia pelvis (ATFP), which are lateral condensa-tions of fascia with increased collagen content and organization relative to neighboring endopelvic fascia (Bent et al., 2008) (Figure 13.2). The arcus tendineus levator ani inserts at the pubic rami anteriorly and runs posteriorly to the ischial spine, provid-ing an anchor for the pubococcygeus and iliococcygeus muscles of the levator ani. Running parallel to the arcus tendineus lavator ani, the ATFP inserts at the pubic rami, just anterior to the arcus tendineus lavator ani and inserts posteriorly at the ischial spine. The ATFP is formed from the condensation of the parietal fascias, overlying the obturator internus and levator ani, and serves as the lateral attachment for the vagina anchoring the anterior vagina to the pelvic sidewall (Moalli et al., 2004). Bilateral sup-port from the ATFP helps fix the vagina in place. The ATFP is comprised of roughly 84% collagen, 13% elastin, and 3% smooth muscle. Collagen content is dominated by type III at 84%, while type I and type V are approximately 13% and 5%, respectively (Moalli et al., 2004). Given this composition, the ATFP is fairly flexible structure, dis-tending in response to increases in intra-abdominal pressure. Further, the ATFP is a sig-nificant contributor to pelvic floor support, allowing the vagina to resist the downward pressure applied via the bladder and urethra.

Pelvic floor viscera

The pelvic floor contains viscera which are part of the lower urinary and alimentary tracts. Urinary tract structures found within the pelvis include the ureters, bladder, and urethra. The ureters are approximately 12–15 cm within the pelvis (in addition to the 12–15 cm in the abdomen) and attach to the peritoneum of lateral pelvic wall prior to inserting into the superior aspect of the bladder. The bladder is a muscular organ that serves as a reservoir for urinary system. The bladder is quite distensible, ranging from a flat shape when empty to globular when full. Along the base of the bladder is the bladder neck, which acts to prevent the flow of urine and is thought to be opened via musculature (pubovesical muscle) during voiding. Extending from the bladder neck is the urethra, a muscular tube that is central to urinary continence. In the female

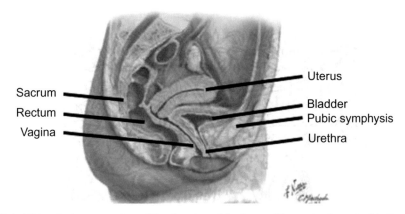

Sacrum

Rectum

Vagina

Uterus

Bladder

Pubic symphysis

Urethra

Figure 13.4 Midsagittal cross section of the female pelvic viscera. The vagina is central to these organs with the bladder and urethra anteriorly, the rectum posteriorly, and the uterus superiorly. The vagina is supported by several connective tissue structures and musculature (*levator ani*), in turn supporting many of the other viscera of the pelvic floor. *Reprinted with permission from Cosson et al. (2003).*

anatomy, the urethra is embedded in the adventitia of the anterior vaginal wall and has an external orifice just distal to the vaginal opening (Figure 13.4).

Urinary continence is highly dependent on both musculature and supportive structures. The musculature contribution arises from a sphincter mechanism, consisting of two components. The upper portion, known as the internal urethral sphincter mechanism, is comprised of urethral smooth muscle and detrusor muscle at the bladder base, which acts to shorten and widen the urethra, while contraction of circular smooth muscle provides resistance to flow (Walters and Karram, 1993). Distally, the external sphincter mechanism is formed by the sphincter urethrae, compressor urethrae, and urethrovaginal sphincter muscles. Together these three muscles function to maintain closure of the urethra and allow voluntary interruption of urine flow. In addition to these muscular contributions to continence, the urethra receives mechanical support from the pubourethral ligaments and the anterior vaginal wall (Figure 13.5). The vagina provides a sling-like base on which the urethra sits and is thought to provide a stable base upon which the bladder neck and urethra can be compressed. As such, disruption of vaginal support may lead to urinary incontinence (Figure 13.5). Multiple etiologies of urinary incontinence include the loss of volume and function of the urethral sphincter and loss of support to the urethra by the pubourethral ligaments and the vagina (Petros and Woodman, 2008).

The vagina, a hollow fibromuscular organ that extends from the perineum to the uterine cervix, is central to pelvic organ support (Figure 13.4). The vagina is composed of four distinct layers, consisting of a nonkeratinized stratified squamous epithelium, subepithelium (lamina propia), muscularis, and adventitia (Alperin and Moalli, 2006).

(A)   (B)

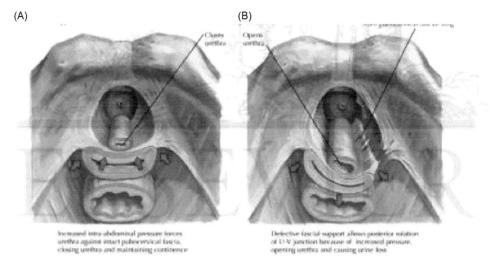

Figure 13.5 The vagina is central to pelvic floor support, with the urethra anteriorly and rectum posteriorly. The vagina is thought to provide a stable base on which the urethra is compressed to maintain continence (A). However defects in vaginal support, such as detachment from the arcus tendineus as illustrated here, may alter continence mechanisms as the urethra may not properly close (B).

The subepithelium and muscularis provide much of the mechanical integrity of the vaginal wall, as the subepithelium contains dense connective tissue, while the muscularis contains predominately smooth muscle. Conversely, the adventitia is primarily loose connective tissue. Collagen in the vagina has been found to have a whorled appearance and consists predominately of collagen III, though the expression of proteins varies from layer to layer (Moalli et al., 2005). In general, the anterior and posterior walls of the vagina are in contact with each other except near the uterine cervix. The lumen of the vagina also has a distinctive cross section along the long axis, ranging from diamond shaped near the introitus to an "h" or butterfly shaped at the midsection, to an oval shape near the cervix. The anterior vaginal wall is contiguous with the bladder base, and as previously mentioned, provides support for the urethra. Posteriorly, the vagina neighbors the rectum and perineal body. As such, the vagina is a crucial structure in terms of pelvic floor support, providing a stable base on which the pelvic organs largely passively rest. In turn, the vagina is supported bilaterally and apically by the aforementioned connective tissues and musculature. In a nonpathological state, the lower one-third of the vagina is approximately 45° from the horizontal (Sze et al., 2001). However, just above this, the vaginal angle makes a noticeable change and the proximal two-thirds of the vagina lie nearly horizontal, with the vaginal apex directed toward S2. The angle between these two vaginal axes has been found to be approximately 145° for the nonpathological anatomy (Sze et al., 2001).

PELVIC FLOOR DISORDERS

Pelvic floor dysfunction includes a number of pathologies, which vary in terms of symptoms and severity. These disorders include POP, urinary incontinence fecal incontinence, voiding dysfunction, defecatory dysfunction, and sexual dysfunction. In addition, these disorders are often exhibited concomitantly. While the exact etiology of many disorders is unknown, pelvic floor disorders are prevalent among women, affecting one-third of all premenopausal women and one-half of all postmenopausal women (Abramowitch et al., 2009). In many cases, dysfunction is thought to be the result of a loss of structural support to the pelvic organs, altering the mechanisms that are necessary for proper anatomical positioning, voiding, and sexual function. Surgical treatment of pelvic floor disorders aims to restore the support to the pelvic floor, reconstructing normal anatomy in order to restore proper function. While biomaterials may be used to treat several disorders, we will discuss their use in two of their most common applications: the treatment of urinary incontinence and POP (Jones et al., 2009).

Urinary incontinence

Urinary incontinence is a prevalent disorder among women, affecting 23–35% of adult women (Bent et al., 2008). There are various forms of incontinence including stress urinary incontinence (SUI) and urge incontinence. SUI is characterized by the loss of urine when pressure is exerted on the bladder by means of coughing, sneezing, laughing, exercising, or lifting a heavy object. Urge incontinence is used to describe a sudden urge to urinate followed by a loss of urine. While it is occasionally difficult to distinguish between the two, it is generally believed that SUI comprises 50% of all urinary incontinence cases, while 25% are urge, and the remaining 25% are mixed (Bent et al., 2008). However, the distribution between these three subtypes varies widely according to how they are defined (Bent et al., 2008).

The risk for developing urinary incontinence noticeably varies by sex, affecting roughly three times as many women relative to men (Bent et al., 2008; Walters and Karram, 1993). In addition, the likelihood of urinary incontinence increases with age, affecting 8–9% of those from ages 20–24 and plateauing at approximately 35% for those over the age of 54. The impact of age and sex is likely driven by many additional risk factors that stem from events that typically occur during a woman's life span. The most significant risk factor for development of urinary incontinence is pregnancy or childbirth. While continence issues during pregnancy are fairly common (30–60%), there is currently no manner to adequately distinguish those patients whose symptoms will resolve postpartum and those who will develop chronic urinary incontinence (Bent et al., 2008). Nonetheless it is has been found that urinary incontinence rates are higher among parous women relative to nulliparous women, regardless of age. In addition, there is uncertainty about the role of delivery mode in the development of incontinence. Many cite that vaginal delivery, rather than parity, increases the risk of developing pelvic floor disorders due to the injury induced by stretching of the muscles, nerves, and connective tissues. Several studies have argued that cesarean delivery provides a protective effect (Lukacz et al., 2006). However, this claim is refuted by similar studies showing that the mode of delivery (vaginal and cesarean) does not impact a woman's risk of developing pelvic floor disorders, suggesting that pregnancy alone is the primary risk factor (MacLennan et al., 2000). Despite these conflicting reports, it appears as though mechanical deformation of the pelvic floor tissues, either by long-term increases in pressure and distention via gestation or significant stretching to accommodate delivery, plays a role in development of pelvic floor disorders.

Menopausal status is another factor believed to play a significant role in the development of urinary incontinence, due to the dramatic drop in estrogen. Given the onset time at which menopause occurs within the life cycle, this factor may explain the significant increase in risk for incontinence with increasing age. It has been suggested that following the onset of menopause, vascularity and muscle function are decreased in the distal urethra, leading to incontinence, though this data remains unclear. Others have found that the collagen of the fascial tissues which support the urethra become mechanically inferior in the absence of hormones (Moalli et al., 2004), thereby altering the support of the urethra and spurring the development of urinary incontinence. Despite the potential effects of hormones, estrogen has not been found to be an effective treatment for urinary incontinence. It should be noted that initiation of estrogen therapy relative to the onset of menopause may be important to consider as hormone treatment started 10–15 years after menopause onset has been ineffective relative to initiation within 5–8 years for other pelvic floor disorders (Jones and Moalli, 2010).

Additionally, smoking and obesity have been associated with an elevated risk for developing urinary incontinence. Smoking is thought to decrease the quality of connective tissues and increase a woman's risk two- to threefold, though evidence linking tobacco use to the development of pelvic floor disorders is also conflicting. The effect of obesity has been documented in many studies, showing that women of moderate obesity (BMI 26–30) were 50% more likely to develop urinary incontinence relative to those with a BMI less than 26. Further, women with a BMI greater than 30 have a 66% increase in risk (Bent et al., 2008). These studies suggest that the increased abdominal pressure exhibited in overweight women significantly impacts the function of the pelvic floor.

While these risk factors are present for all types of urinary incontinence, much of the following text will focus on SUI. As such, these factors must be considered in terms of their impact on the mechanics of continence. In general, the bladder, urethra, and corresponding sphincter mechanisms must balance external pressures applied via increases in abdominal pressure. If these structures or mechanisms are compromised, application of pressure to the bladder may result in loss of urine. As discussed previously, continence is a complex function, relying on active resistance to flow provided by musculature and support provided by connective tissues. Thus, changes in connective tissue may impact support of the vagina, thereby altering the ability to close the urethra to resist urine flow.

Treatment using biomaterials: suburethral slings

One of the most common surgical repair procedures for SUI is the use of a suburethral sling. During this procedure, a graft is placed suburethrally, typically at the level of the midurethra or bladder neck (Figure 13.6). In this procedure, a strap of material is passed behind the symphysis pubis and fixed to the rectus fascia or pubic bone. While the precise mechanism explaining the efficacy of this procedure is unknown, it is thought that sling placement serves to reestablish the ureterovesicular junction and provide a stable base on which the urethra can be compressed. Although a variety of approaches and materials are currently used to treat SUI, it is widely accepted that the graft should be placed under "minimal tension" to prevent the development of additional voiding dysfunction such as obstruction with incomplete bladder emptying (Walters and Karram, 1993).

Biological materials

Treatment for SUI using biomaterials dates back to 1907, when the gracilis muscle flap was used as a suburethral sling (Bent et al., 2008; Walters and Karram, 1993). Throughout the early and mid–1900s, many sling procedures utilized autologous tissues, with nearly exclusive use of fascial tissues until the 1950s when nylon was used to construct the first synthetic sling (Walters and Karram, 1993). Procedures using autologous tissues have been found to have low complication rates, with cure rates varying

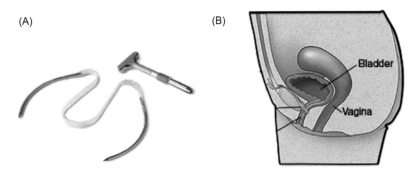

(A)   (B)

Bladder

Vagina

Figure 13.6 Contemporary suburethral slings are often comprised of synthetic materials, such as the polypropylene (A). Slings are placed on the posterior surface of the urethra, just anterior to the vagina (B). Note that the space between the urethra and vagina is exaggerated above to highlight sling placement as the distal urethra inserts into the anterior vagina. Slings may be placed abdominally or transvaginally.

between 70% and 100% (Iglesia et al., 1997). In addition, concerns of increased surgical time to harvest tissue, donor site morbidity, prolonged recovery, and pain at the harvesting site have decreased the appeal of autologous grafts.

In order to alleviate donor site morbidity and long surgical times, allograft use became popularized in the late 1990s for pubovaginal sling procedures (Moalli, 2006). Allografts for SUI slings are typically harvested from cadaveric fascia lata and are expected to provide the low complication benefits of autografts, while eliminating donor site morbidity. In order to reduce the risk for disease transmission and ensure adequate graft supply, harvested allografts are "processed" and often freeze-dried (Moalli, 2006). The goal of tissue processing is to eliminate infectious materials such as cells, bacteria, myobacteria, viruses, fungi, and spores. Generally, tissue processing is not standardized and varies from company to company, often with each company utilizing a unique procedure. However, tissue processing protocols, freeze-drying, and rehydration are believed to impact the mechanical properties of allografts (Hinton et al., 1992). Despite the promise of allografts in the pelvic floor, clinical use has suffered from high early failure rates, especially for freeze-dried grafts (Bent et al., 2008). In fact, allografts have been reported to be less effective than autologous fascia for sling procedures, with SUI returning within 6 months for 67% of allograft procedures and 21% of autologous grafts procedures (Soergel et al., 2001). More recently, xenografts have been examined for suburethral slings, though data regarding such materials is limited to animal models and small case series. In many cases, these slings are comprised of porcine non-cross-linked intestinal submucosa (SurgiSIS) or cross-linked porcine dermis (Pelvichol). Unfortunately, the host response to these materials is highly variable and long-term success rates have been poor with symptomatic recurrence often present within 12 months postoperatively (Mangera et al., 2013). Still, the application of xenografts for treatment of SUI and other pelvic floor disorders is relatively new and the potential of such devices is not yet fully understood. Indeed, the development of xenografts for urogynecological use remains an area of active research. An understanding of the effect of source tissue and the effects of different processing methods upon the host response to these biological materials in the pelvic floor region is lacking. Until such an understanding is acquired, the design and development of effective biological materials for pelvic floor disorders will likely make little progress.

Synthetic

Due to the relatively high recurrence rates associated with biological sling materials, synthetic grafts were developed based on mesh products already in use for abdominal hernia repair. Since their introduction, synthetic slings have been composed of a variety of materials including polypropylene (Marlex, Trelex), polyester (Mersilene), polytetrafluoroethylene (Teflon), expanded polytetrafluoroethylene (Gore-Tex), and silicone and have been met with a wide range of results (Iglesia et al., 1997). The main deterrent to synthetic mesh use in incontinence surgery is the risk of complications associated with the implantation of a permanent (i.e., nondegradable) foreign material. While the cure rate of synthetic mesh is often reported to be greater than 80%, historically complication rates have been found to range between 0% and 35%, though more contemporary procedures such as tension-free vaginal tape (TVT) have lowered this to 0–15% (Iglesia et al., 1997).

Following the introduction of the TVT procedure in late 1990s, synthetic sling use increased dramatically (US FDA, 2008). The increased use of these materials may be attributed to their consistent properties, elimination of disease transmission and donor site morbidity, and their relative low cost compared to biological devices. The prototype device is the TVT introduced by Ulmsten in 1996 (Ulmsten et al., 1996). Building upon DeLancey's concept of pelvic floor support, Petros and Ulmsten (1997) considered the relationship between the urethra and vagina. Thus, the goal of the TVT procedure was to reconstruct the pubourethral vesical ligament in order to restore urethral support. However, MRI studies examining the efficacy of this procedure have found that TVT does not restore this support. Rather, success was attributed to the restoration of a base (vagina) upon which the urethra could be compressed (Bent et al., 2008).

The TVT procedure utilizes a sling device, comprised of a knitted wide pore polypropylene mesh to reconstruct urethra support. The device is placed vaginally, through a midline incision to access the urethra and then introduced lateral to the urethra through the endopelvic fascia, coursing immediately behind the pubic bone and into the retropubic space exiting on the skin (retropubic approach). Alternatively, the sling can be delivered lateral to the urethra through the obturator foramen exiting the space between the vulva and the thigh, thus avoiding the retropubic space (transobturator approach). In 2008, the Trial of Mid-Urethral Slings (TOMUS) was initiated to determine the effect of anatomic location and compare efficacy and morbidity between these sites (Albo et al., 2008). This trial found that both approaches demonstrate good 12-month objective outcomes, with 80.8% and 77.7% objective success rates for retropubic and transobturator procedures respectively (Brubaker et al., 2011). The TOMUS trial also found that 42% of participants experienced at least one adverse effect within 2 years of surgical treatment, while 12% had serious adverse effects. Of these complications, 77% were found to occur within 6 months of surgery or during surgery. Overall, serious complications were more common in the retropubic group, nearly double that of the transobturator approach (15.1% vs. 8.4%). Further, several adverse effects were more characteristic of a given approach. For instance, bladder perforation and voiding dysfunction occurred only in retropubic cases, while neurological symptoms including numbness or weakness in the legs or pelvic area were more prominent in transobturator cases. Mesh erosion and exposure were not found to differ between the approaches with these complications occurring in 4.7% and 3% of retropubic and transobturator participants, respectively (Brubaker et al., 2011). While many of these complications may be related to surgical technique and route of delivery, new data suggests that an adverse host response to the material may play a role (Nolfi et al., 2014).

While each of these approaches has unique considerations, it is clear that the TVT procedure has dramatically impacted the clinical management of SUI, providing high cure rates and reducing complication rates. Aside from strong efficacy reports, perhaps the greatest accomplishment of the TVT procedure is that it has greatly reduced the morbidity of surgical treatment of SUI, as it is minimally invasive and does not require harvesting of graft tissues. Thus this simplified surgical procedure has greatly expedited patient recovery, as women undergoing the procedure can be discharged the same day after voiding (Brophy et al., 2001). Moreover, previous SUI slings were associated with significant complication rates, while the TVT is consistently reported to have low complication rates, including erosion rates ranging from 1% to 3% (Bent et al., 2008; Brophy et al., 2001; Abouassaly et al., 2004) and pain and injury to adjacent structures is less than 1% (Rodrigues Macield da Fonseca et al., 2013). Given the improvement in outcomes, TVT meshes appear to be responsible for the widespread acceptance of type I polypropylene mesh as the material of choice for pelvic floor reconstructions.

Based on the successes of the TVT, numerous companies developed similar products comprised of type I polypropylene mesh, though the knit pattern, mesh weight, pore size, and porosity of these products vary widely from vendor to vendor. Despite the same base material, the altered knit patterns used in manufacturing the products have been shown to significantly impact the mechanical behavior of these devices. Specifically, pore geometry (the shape of the repeating pore structures) and edge features (tanged vs. heat sealed) impact sling stiffness and permanent elongation following repeated mechanical loading (Moalli et al., 2008). In addition, these features greatly influence the characteristic uniaxial load-elongation curves for sling products. While most SUI slings exhibit a nonlinear load-elongation curve, several displayed a linear behavior until failure. It appears most probable that the shape of the load-elongation curve is a function of pore geometry and its orientation to the axis of loading. Pores whose fibers are less aligned with the axis of loading and have sufficient ability to rotate are likely to generate nonlinear loading curves as fibers are recruited to withstand mechanical forces. This logic follows from similar mathematical descriptions of collagen fiber recruitment developed by Lanir (1979). Conversely, pores whose fibers are aligned with the axis of loading, such as a square loaded along its orthogonal axes, or with rigid pores (i.e., little to no fiber rotation) would exhibit a purely linear response.

Lastly, there have been a limited number of slings that have combined biological and synthetic materials, though several of these products have been associated with suboptimal outcomes. One such device, Protogen, a woven, polyester sling coated with bovine collagen, saw incredibly high exposure rates, with 50% of meshes leading to exposure of the mesh through the vagina and more than 20% of meshes resulting in urethral erosion (Kobashi and Dmochowski, 1999). The primary problem is that many of these hybrid devices, such as Protogen, were comprised of Mersilene (polyester family), which is woven and as the fibers slide against each other, the pore size is reduced allowing the mesh to harbor bacteria resulting in bacterial proliferation and chronic infection. Thus, any potential benefit of a collagen coating may have been overshadowed by the underlying problems with Mersilene. Further, the clinical failure of Protogen may stem from other potential problems, such as using cross-linked collagen to coat the synthetic mesh. In addition, it is possible that coating may have significantly compromised the porosity of the synthetic mesh, though studies examining the impact of porosity on this composite mesh have not been completed. While it is clear that many factors such as material type, mesh construction techniques, biological variants, and the method of adhering biological components to synthetic products, the combined biological–synthetic products carry a stigma due to catastrophic clinical results such as those experienced with Protogen.

Pelvic organ prolapse

POP is characterized by the abnormal descent of the pelvic viscera into the vagina. This disorder arises from a lack of support to the vagina, allowing the walls cervix or other viscera to form a bulge into the vagina or even through the vagina resulting in eversion of the vagina. Symptoms of POP include urinary incontinence, voiding difficulty (urinary and defecatory), sensation of bulge in the vagina, pelvic pressure or pain, and sexual dysfunction (Walters and Karram, 1993). Given that the vagina is a central structure to the pelvic floor environment in terms of location and support, it is not surprising that vaginal support defects lead to prolapse, with prolapse often presenting as additional forms of pelvic dysfunction. While this general description is indicative of prolapse, the specific location at which prolapse occurs varies from patient to patient and may include the anterior vaginal wall, the posterior vaginal wall, and the vaginal apex. Prolapse of the anterior and posterior vaginal wall are characterized by bulging of the respective wall into the vaginal canal, while descent of the vaginal apex is characterized by movement of the cervix, or top of the vagina after a hysterectomy, distally toward and potentially beyond the hymen (Figure 13.7). In addition to variable appearance, there are various degrees of POP, with a range of four stages, characterized by the severity of prolapse. Classification of prolapse is determined using the POP quantification (POPQ) system. The POPQ system scores the severity of prolapse by measuring nine points on vagina and perineum using an ordinal staging system. Positions of these anatomical points are measured relative to the hymen. Stage 0 indicates ideal support, while stage IV signifies severe prolapse with complete eversion of the vagina. Of those suffering from prolapse, the majority have stages I and II, while only 3–9% have stage III or IV (Bent et al., 2008). Evaluation of prolapse using the POPQ staging system is crucial before reconstructive surgery, as it allows

(A)   (B)

(C)   (D)

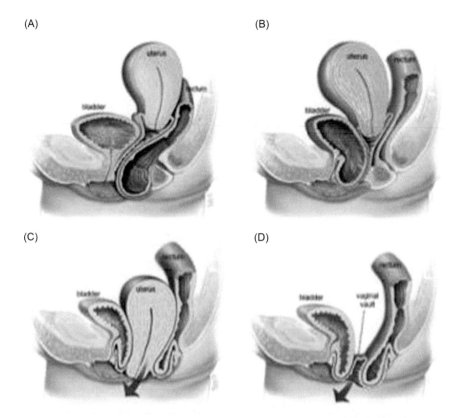

Figure 13.7 POP is characterized by the decent of the pelvic organs into the vaginal canal, though prolapse has several clinical presentations depending on the location of a patient's vaginal support defect: (A) posterior compartment prolapse (rectocele), (B) anterior compartment prolapse (cystocele), (C) uterine prolapse, and (D) vaginal vault prolapse.

clinicians to select procedures that address each patient's specific deficiencies in support (Lowder et al., 2008).

As with SUI, the primary risk factors for the development of POP are childbirth and aging. In addition, much of the same rationale is used to hypothesize how these processes degenerate or alter supportive structures. During pregnancy, stretching of the connective tissues and damage to the pelvic floor muscles are believed to impair vaginal support, allowing the viscera to descend. Others speculate that tearing of pelvic fascia and the perineum during vaginal delivery may destabilize vaginal support and initiate these weaknesses (Walters and Karram, 1993). Yet as with SUI, it is unclear whether pregnancy alone is permissive or vaginal delivery is requisite for the development of POP (Lukacz et al., 2006; MacLennan et al., 2000; Sze et al., 2002). Unfortunately these mechanisms are poorly understood as prolapse often develops years or decades after injury or insult due to childbirth. Regardless, studies report a 10% increase in POP occurrence for each birth, while others suggest a fourfold increase in risk with just one pregnancy and an eightfold increase with a second pregnancy (Mant et al., 1997). Aging has also been shown to greatly influence the development of POP, with an increased incidence of 30–50% each 10 years of age, eventually plateauing at age 70 (Bent et al., 2008). As mentioned with SUI, the impact of aging is virtually impossible to distinguish from the independent impact of menopause. Until recently the impact of menopause on the tissues of the pelvic floor was largely unknown. Additional perspectives on the effects of age on the host response can be found in Chapter 11.

In light of recent data, the impact of menopause on the connective tissues is believed to be significant. Specifically, Moalli et al. examined the impact of menopause on collagen of the ATFP, as separation of the vagina from the ATFP (a paravaginal defect) is the most common cause of anterior wall prolapse (DeLancey, 2002). Arcus biopsies from premenopausal and postmenopausal women were examined in addition to postmenopausal women who were receiving hormone therapy. Postmenopausal women were found to have decreases in both collagen I levels and the ratio of collagen $I/(III + V)$ compared to both premenopausal women and postmenopausal women receiving hormone therapy. These findings suggest that the ATFP is a weaker structure following menopause, with increased flexibility, as even small changes collagen subtypes can alter the tensile strength of tissues (Birk et al., 1990). Such remodeling of collagen subtypes may also result from mechanical stretch associated with childbirth or increases in intra-abdominal pressure associated with a woman's lifestyle. Further, the absence of hormones following menopause may alter the tissues response to such loading. Evidence for this paradigm follows from studies demonstrating the impact of hormones on the response of vaginal tissue upon mechanical loading. Zong et al. (2010a) found that hormone treatment returned collagenase activity to control levels, significantly lower than mechanically stimulated tissues without hormones. From this data it appears as though hormones provide a preventative mechanism for vaginal tissue, reducing the likelihood for maladaptive remodeling upon application of biomechanical forces.

Additional risk factors of note include hysterectomy and lifestyle, though data regarding the impact of hysterectomy on the development of POP is been unclear. Hysterectomy is generally believed to impact apical support of the vagina by disrupting the uterosacral and cardinal ligaments, though the incidence of prolapse is similar between those women who have undergone hysterectomy and the general population (Jones and Moalli, 2010; Olsen et al., 1997; Hendrix et al., 2002). Of lifestyle considerations, it appears that high-impact activities greatly increase the risk for developing prolapse. Specifically, this includes occupations during which women repeatedly lift or carry heavy objects. For example, a study of nursing assistants, whose duties included regular lifting of equipment, found that these women were 60% more likely to have prolapse compared to the general population (Hendrix et al., 2002). In addition, prolapse rates among nulliparous paratroopers are significantly higher than the general population (Larsen and Yavork, 2007). Intuitively these occupations lead to sustained and repetitive increases in intra-abdominal pressure and the data is consistent with observed trends in POP among obese patients (Jones and Moalli, 2010). The increased loading of the pelvic floor under these conditions may alter the connective tissues via damage or remodeling.

Despite the identification of several main risk factors, the cause of prolapse remains unclear. In order to more thoroughly understand this pathology, several studies have examined the morphology and composition of the vagina and its supportive structures in women with and without prolapse. Utilizing full thickness biopsies from the vaginal apex, women with prolapse were found to have significant increases in total collagen content, with amounts 49% greater than control levels (Moalli et al., 2005). Interestingly, postmenopausal controls receiving hormone supplements were similar to premenopausal controls. This increase was driven by a 37% rise in collagen III, the predominant collagen subtype of the vagina. In addition, women with prolapse were found to have increased levels of active matrix metalloprotease-9 (MMP-9), with a 28% increase in this collagenase. Elevated levels of active MMP-9 suggest that the vagina is actively remodeling in response to biomechanical stresses associated with prolapse rather than a cause of prolapse *per se* (Langberg et al., 1999; Kjaer et al., 2005). Previously, increased MMP-9 has been associated with remodeling in soft tissues such as the coronary artery and dermis (Gillard et al., 2004; Orringer et al., 2004). It should be noted that the above data was obtained using full thickness biopsies, whereas many studies do not consider the histology of the vagina (Chen et al., 2002; Goepel et al., 2003; Söderberg et al., 2004), most likely contributing to the variability of data in this area. Similarly, collagen III was found to be increased in the uterosacral ligament of women with prolapse (Gabriel et al., 2005). It is currently unclear whether these changes in collagen content and collagenase activity are the causes of prolapse or the result of remodeling to prolapse conditions.

Treatment using biomaterials: prolapse mesh

POP is a common disorder among women, as it is estimated to impact 50% of women over the age of 50 (Ellerkmann et al., 2001; Nygaard, 2012; Subak et al., 2001; Swift, 2000). While many women do not require surgical intervention, the lifetime risk for having a single repair procedure for POP is roughly 7% (Olsen et al., 1997). Unfortunately, up to 40% of women undergoing a repair of prolapse with her own tissues will fail by 2 years and up to one-third will undergo a repeat surgery within 5 years (Olsen et al., 1997; Barber et al., 2014). Because of these disappointingly high failure rates, surgeons and patients alike have turned to biomaterials to improve outcomes (Barber et al., 2014). The use of mesh in prolapse repairs has

(A)   (B)

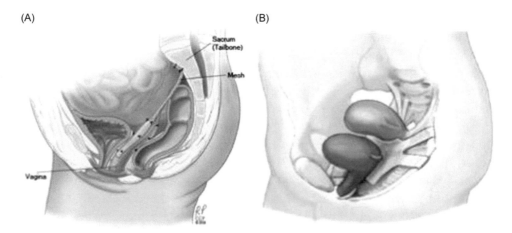

Figure 13.8 Two of the most common surgical procedures for prolapse repair that utilize mesh are abdominal sacrocolpopexy (A) and transvaginal (B) procedures. For sacrocolpopexy, mesh is introduced via an abdominal incision and attached to the anterior and/or posterior surface of the vagina. The mesh is then tensioned and anchored to the sacrum. Transvaginal procedures introduce mesh through a vaginal incision. Mesh is then attached to the anterior and/or posterior vagina and the arms of the vagina are anchored in various structures in the pelvic sidewall.

become widespread over the last decade, being used in 100,000 prolapse repair surgeries in 2010, roughly one-third of all POP surgeries (US FDA, 2011). In general, surgical treatment of POP using mesh provides mechanical support to the vagina by attaching the mesh to the vagina and anchoring the mesh into the pelvic sidewall or sacrum. This reapproximation of vaginal support attempts to restore patient anatomy, in theory returning the pelvic organs to their normal locations. Typically mesh reconstruction is performed transvaginally or via transabdominally via sacrocolpopexy, though procedure selection is surgeon and patient specific, depending on the site of prolapse and identified support defects (Figure 13.8). Transvaginal procedures are commonly used to repair anterior and posterior wall prolapse, known as a cystocele and rectocele respectively, while sacrocolpopexy is most often used to repair apical (vaginal vault) prolapse (Figure 13.7). Aside from the considerations of prolapse site, transvaginal mesh procedures are less invasive and technically easier for clinicians to perform.

For transvaginal procedures, an incision is made through a full thickness vaginal dissection and the underlying defect is exposed (Figure 13.9). To restore support, the body of the graft is placed underneath the bulging viscera, while the arms of the graft are then anchored to, or pulled through structures in the pelvic sidewall and placed on tension. Sidewall attachments include the ATFP and sacrospinous ligament. Given these attachments, a transvaginal mesh provides lateral support to the anterior and/or posterior vaginal wall as well as the vaginal apex to prevent bulging. As mentioned,

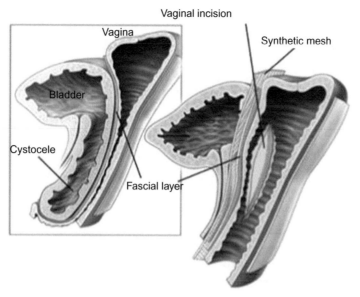

Figure 13.9 For a transvaginal mesh repair mesh, it introduced via a vaginal incision. Here an incision is made on the anterior vaginal wall and the graft is placed in the plane between the bladder and vagina.

many consider transvaginal mesh placement to be a technically easier procedure relative to an abdominal approach, with a quicker patient recovery. This is reflected in clinical practice as roughly 75% of all mesh procedures for POP repair are performed transvaginally (US FDA, 2011). Interestingly, many studies have shown that abdominal approaches yield twice as many "ideal" outcomes, citing better efficacy at the expense of a higher rate of serious complications (Nygaard et al., 2004). This disparity between outcome and the procedure selection highlights the need to consider the impact of both surgical technique and route of mesh implantation. During an abdominal sacrocolpopexy, a surgeon attaches a strap of mesh to the anterior and/or posterior surface of the vagina via an abdominal approach, often laparoscopic or robotic. Following attachment to the vagina, the graft is directed and anchored to the sacrum at the S1–S3 level. As such, an abdominal sacrocolpopexy provides support in a longitudinal direction. Procedures similar to an abdominal sacrocolpopexy repair date to the early 1900s when the vaginal apex was fixed to the abdominal wall with fascia (Nygaard et al., 2004). Over the next 50 years, fixation continually migrated posteriorly until the sacrum was determined to best mimic the normal vaginal angle. Moreover, this is the site of attachment of the uterosacral ligaments, the primary apical support to the vagina. Historically, graft materials have included both biological and synthetic materials, though recent studies have found failure rates as high as 43% after 1 year for autologous fascia repairs, while frozen allograft fascia has seen failure rates of 83% after

17 months (FitzGerald et al., 2000). Due to the poor quality of tissue and high fail-ure rates observed for native tissue repair, synthetic meshes have gained prominence for prolapse repair procedures (Boreham et al., 2002; Budatha et al., 2011; Feola et al., 2010; Moalli et al., 2005; Mosser and Edwards, 2008; Zong et al., 2010b).

Biological materials

Given the shortcomings of both autograft and allograft repairs, much focus has been turned to the use of xenografts for POP repair or tissue procured from a species other than the graft recipient. Xenografts often consist of extracellular matrix (ECM) derived from porcine dermis, small intestinal submucosa (SIS), or bladder (Chen et al., 2007). Additional sources for xenograft devices include bovine pericardium and dermis (Chen et al., 2007). All biological materials (autografts, allografts, and xenografts) can be further classified into non-cross-linked and chemically cross-linked materials.

In general, non-cross-linked biological grafts are subject to decellularization processes to improve biocompatibility. Decellularization treatments are designed to eliminate cellu-lar and genetic debris while preserving the 3D structure of the ECM proteins. Therefore, non-cross-linked devices permit cellular infiltration allowing the implanted matrix to readily undergo a rapid remodeling response (Hodde, 2006; Badylak et al., 2001; Badylak, 2002). To date, the emphasis on prolapse biological grafts has been on mechanical integ-rity rather than regeneration, with product designs consisting of multilayered and heav-ily chemically cross-linked materials. Consequently, multilayered materials (typically 6–8 ply) have been used in sacrocolpopexy. In general, these products have experienced low rates of erosion and infection, though objective recurrence rates are often increased rela-tive to synthetic meshes. For non-cross-linked grafts, erosion and infection rates are fairly low (1.2% and 1.3%, respectively) while recurrence rates for non-cross-linked grafts were found to be 14.5% (Dillion, 2011). Given that non-cross-linked grafts typically degrade over a relatively short time frame, much of the response to these materials, including complications, likely results from a rapid remodeling response.

Unlike non-cross-linked devices, cross-linked biologics are comprised of collagen fibrils that are chemically cross-linked, typically with carbodiimide, to slow the rate of degradation of the implanted matrix. Several studies have shown that chemical cross-linking does indeed decrease the amount of cellular infiltration into the implanted matrix (Badylak, 2002; Gandhi et al., 2005; Jarman-Smith et al., 2004; Kimuli et al., 2004). The increased number of cross-links, however, also increases the stiffness of the graft and is believed to affect the differentiation of infiltrating cells; thereby, altering the subsequent remodeling of the biological scaffold material (Buxboim et al., 2010). However, there appears to be a noticeable foreign body reaction to cross-linked materials as these grafts are often encapsulated following implantation (Gandhi et al., 2005). Clinically, cross-linked biologics for POP repair have experienced worse out-comes relative to their non-cross-linked counterparts. Most strikingly the incidence of

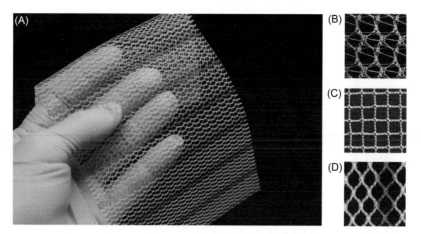

Figure 13.10 In recent decades, synthetic materials have become the gold standard for mesh repair for prolapse. Gynemesh PS, shown here (A,B), is a popular mesh product in todays urogynecological mesh market. Gynemesh PS (A,B), Restorelle (C), and UltraPro (D) are all examples of knitted, Type I, polypropylene, macroporous mesh, despite a wide range of pore architectures (B–D).

erosion, pain, and objective recurrence rates are noticeably increased relative to non-cross-linked products, occurring in 6.2%, 21.6%, and 24% of cases respectively (Dillion, 2011). Further, cross-linked grafts repairs are associated with a nontrivial incidence of seroma formation likely related to residual foreign material in the product. See Chapter 4 for additional information regarding the host response to biologic materials.

Synthetic

Similar to the trends for surgical SUI treatment, shortcomings of biological materials have led to the prominence of synthetic mesh for POP repair (Figure 13.10). The predominance of these synthetic devices was highlighted in a recent FDA release, stating that 100,000 of the approximately 300,000 annual surgical repairs for prolapse utilized mesh (US FDA, 2011). Throughout the last two decades, the materials and features of prolapse meshes have undergone significant changes. Ultimately, the introduction and success of TVT sling for SUI repair led to type I polypropylene mesh as the material of choice for prolapse meshes. Still, polypropylene devices were initially heavier in terms of mesh weight (g/m^3) relative to contemporary mesh products. The shift toward lower weight mesh was found through trial and error as surgeons noted lower rates of complication for such meshes. To date much of our knowledge of ideal mesh properties is derived from mesh studies in the abdominal wall though several recent studies have demonstrated factors that are necessary to consider for mesh design for use in the pelvic floor. These factors, including both those learned from abdominal and pelvic floor studies, will be discussed later in this chapter. Despite complications rates ranging from 5% to 30%, synthetic mesh has demonstrated noticeable efficacy over biological grafts, with objective anatomic cure rates consistently greater than 85% (Chen et al., 2007; Dillion, 2011). Moreover, type I polypropylene mesh is often reported to have cure rates greater than 90% in sacrocolpopexy, showing greater consistency and efficacy than other synthetic mesh materials and biologics (Chen et al., 2007; Dillion, 2011; Nygaard, 2012). Unfortunately the surgical successes of these products are hampered by relatively high rates of complications, many of which are severe and may impact a patient's quality of life more than prolapse.

BIOMATERIAL-RELATED COMPLICATIONS IN THE PELVIC FLOOR

Autologous grafts are rarely associated with complications postimplantation; however, donor site morbidity, increased surgical time required to harvest grafts, and prolonged recovery are primary concerns for these procedures (Moalli, 2006). Similarly, complications related to biological allograft or nonchemically cross-linked xenografts in most studies have been found to be low. However, high failure rates of 17–29% have provided a tremendous increase in the acceptance of synthetic mesh, striking a balance between the risk of complication and surgical efficacy (Clemons et al., 2013).

Following the introduction of the technically easier transvaginal application of prolapse mesh, along with an increase in the use of the midurethral sling to treat incontinence, synthetic mesh use in reconstructive pelvic surgeries escalated between 2005 and 2011. Unfortunately, as mesh use increased so did mesh-related complications, prompting the FDA to issue two public health notifications. The first issued in 2008 warned physicians and patients of potential complications associated with the transvaginal application of mesh, and a second issued in 2011 warned that these complications are not rare events (US FDA, 2008, 2011). Reports addressing the rise in complications associated with synthetic mesh and the observation that complications may take years to develop and may not completely resolve with removal of the mesh have stirred significant controversy over mesh use (Iglesia et al., 1997; Baessler et al., 2005). It is unclear if the act of introducing a device through the vaginal wall alone is a risk, or if the specificity of transvaginal mesh complications is simply due to the increased use of these procedures over the past decade, again bringing to question the role of implantation method and surgical technique. To date there has been virtually no consideration of the role of the host tissue response as a significant or causative variable in prolapse mesh outcomes, in spite of the host response having been shown to play a key role in patient outcomes in virtually every other field in which biomaterials are employed.

Complications most reported following mesh implantation include mesh erosion, mesh exposure, infection, dyspareunia, and pain. Mesh exposure is characterized by the visualization of the mesh through the vaginal epithelium (Figure 13.11). Mesh erosion is characterized by perforation of the mesh into adjacent structures. Other complications include infection, contraction, and bunching. Contraction, or shrinkage of the

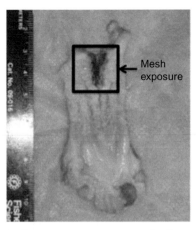

Figure 13.11 Mesh exposure is the most common complication associated with vaginal mesh implantation. Exposure is characterized by the visualization and palpation of the mesh through the vaginal epithelium. Shown here is a mesh exposure on the anterior wall of an explanted vagina from a rhesus macaque sacrocolpopexy model.

mesh implant area, may be caused by two potential mechanisms: mechanical loading and fibroblast-induced contraction as part of the foreign body response, which is an expected outcome though the amount is variable and patient specific. Both mechanisms are likely related to the geometry of the mesh and the loading environment in which the mesh is placed as well as mesh characteristics such as pore size. These factors will be discussed later in this chapter. Women with mesh complications may complain of vaginal discharge, pain, and dyspareunia. Often, management of mesh-related complications includes repeat surgery with removal of mesh (Mattox et al., 2004; Duckett and Jain, 2005; Baessler and Maher, 2006; Collinet et al., 2006). Moreover 20% of women who undergo mesh surgery require a repeat surgery for recurrent symptoms or complications (Baessler et al., 2005; Bako and Dhar, 2008; Patel et al., 2012a).

Early clinical findings for synthetic SUI slings found complication rates ranging from 0.3% to 23%, though these findings considered all types of sling products including woven and nonporous (Brophy et al., 2001). Interestingly, the complication rate for TVT was found to be markedly reduced in early reports as well as more contemporary studies, with erosion rates of 1% (Abouassaly et al., 2004). Meanwhile, no single prolapse mesh has had such success in terms of reducing complications, as mesh exposure occurs in up to 15% of transvaginal repairs and 10.5% of sacrocolpopexies (US FDA, 2008; Letouzey et al., 2010; Brubaker et al., 2008; Deffieux et al., 2007; Nygaard et al., 2008). In most cases, exposure requires the mesh to be removed surgically in order to manage symptoms pain, discharge, odor, and dyspareunia; however, there are many reports that symptoms may persist even after mesh has been removed (Abed et al., 2011; Collinet et al., 2006; US FDA, 2011; Araco et al., 2009).

While the exact cause of mesh-related complications is unclear, recent studies have enhanced our understanding of the impact of mesh on the morphology, composition, and biomechanical behavior of vaginal tissue. Liang et al. examined the impact of mesh stiffness on vaginal morphology and structural proteins utilizing a rhesus macaque model. Meshes were implanted via abdominal sacrocolpopexy and the vagina–mesh complex was explanted after 3 months. The goal of the study was to compare the prototype and most widely used prolapse mesh, Gynemesh PS, to newer lighter weight, higher porosity, and lower stiffness mesh. Notably, Gynemesh PS was the most detrimental to the vaginal tissue on which it was implanted. While all meshes examined noticeably disrupted the organization of vaginal tissue, the smooth muscle layer was most profoundly impacted as Gynemesh PS was found to decrease the thickness of this layer by 55% relative to sham controls (Liang et al., 2013). In addition, Gynemesh PS was the only mesh that dramatically increased the number of apoptotic cells in the subepithelium and adventitia layers, rising from 0.43% and 1.56% of cells to 7.22% and 22.34% respectively (Figure 13.12). A majority of these apoptotic cells were located around the individual mesh fibers. Gynemesh PS implantation also had a significant effect on structural proteins, decreasing collagen and elastin content by 20% and 43%, respectively. While no other synthetic meshes tested were as detrimental to collagen content, other mesh devices decreased elastin content by as much as 49%. Lastly, sulfated glycosaminoglycans (GAG) content was increased by 20% relative to sham samples, while collagenase activity rose by 135% following Gynemesh PS implantation. Combined, these results suggest that the vagina undergoes a maladaptive remodeling response following Gynemesh PS implantation, as the tissues were found to have high rates of collagen turnover and overall loss of structural proteins. While other meshes tested appeared to impact the tissues appearance and composition, Gynemesh PS, the stiffest of all the type I polypropylene meshes tested was

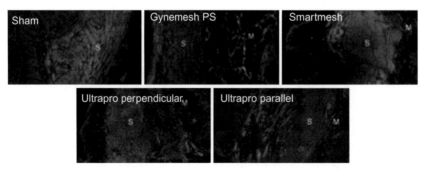

Figure 13.12 Liang et al. (2013) examined the impact of synthetic mesh implantation of vaginal tissue using a rhesus macaque model. Here, immunofluorescent labeling is used to highlight smooth muscle and *in situ* cell apoptosis, where the red signal is a positive stain for alpha smooth muscle actin, green represents apoptotic cells, and blue represents cell nuclei. In addition, S indicates the smooth muscle layer and M indicates individual mesh fibers.

found to elicit the most dramatic changes in vaginal tissue. These findings may be attributed to a phenomenon known as stress shielding, which will be discussed later in this chapter. In addition, increased sulfated GAG content is consistent with acute soft tissue injury and tissue turnover (Plaas et al., 2000). Independent of the mechanism, these results are consistent with a mechanistic process leading to the most common mesh complication—mesh exposure.

Mesh implantation has also been shown to induce a deterioration in both the active (smooth muscle contractility) and passive (stiffness) mechanical properties of the underlying and associated vagina (Feola et al., 2013). In a rhesus macaque 2acrocolpopexy model, Gynemesh PS virtually abolished smooth muscle contractility relative to sham samples with a concomitant decrease in the thickness of vaginal muscularis due to atrophy (Liang et al., 2013). While the impact of lighter weight, higher porosity meshes were not as significant, disruption in smooth muscle organization may explain the reductions in contractility that occurs after implantation of most polypropylene prolapse meshes. Passive properties, typically reflecting the mechanical integrity of the fibrillar ECM proteins, collagen and elastin, were evaluated via ball burst testing. When accounting for the combined stiffness of both mesh and tissue, it was determined that Gynemesh PS drastically reduced the mechanical integrity of the tissue, with the estimated vaginal tissue stiffness in Gynemesh PS implanted samples decreasing nearly 10-fold (Feola et al., 2013). Given that tissue stiffness values approached $0\,N/mm$, it can be concluded that Gynemesh PS implantation nearly abolished mechanical integrity of vaginal tissues. These findings are also in agreement with reports of reduced total collagen and elastin in the vagina (Liang et al., 2013) that occurs after implantation of this mesh. Overall, mesh implantation appears to be detrimental to the mechanical properties of the vagina, particularly when mesh stiffness is high. The degradation of smooth muscles is particularly concerning, as this integral component of vaginal tissue is believed to be already compromised in women with prolapse (Boreham et al., 2002). Thus, further damage via biomaterial implantation is not ideal. In addition, depletion of collagen and elastin content would further compromise the supportive capabilities of the vagina.

FACTORS INFLUENCING THE HOST RESPONSE TO SYNTHETIC MESH

Much of our current knowledge of urogynecological mesh products has been derived from the hernia mesh literature (Iglesia et al., 1997). This transfer of knowledge is especially true in regard to the impact of mesh design on the host response to these devices. Even current literature and marketing pamphlets distributed by urogynecological mesh manufacturers demonstrate biocompatibility of SUI and POP products via implantation studies in the abdominal wall. These studies are certainly necessary to initially demonstrate the ability for mesh designs to be implanted in a host without overt rejection, though the abdominal wall and pelvic floor are quite distinct in terms of both biological factors and the structural functions that a mesh device is intended to withstand. Therefore, current urogynecological mesh designs are more similar to a prototype solution rather than an optimal one. That said, much has been learned from these abdominal wall studies and the findings have greatly enhanced outcomes in the pelvic floor. Perhaps the most important concepts shown to impact the host response to synthetic meshes in the pelvic floor are filament type, pore size, and the effect of these variables upon the host response.

Structure

Filament type

In addition to the material, the filament structure of the mesh has been linked to the host response, specifically in relation to the presence of infection. Filamental structure can be classified as either mono- or multifilament, where multifilament fibers consist of braided or interwoven filaments. Multifilament meshes are linked to significantly higher bacterial presence (Engelsman et al., 2010). These findings are believed to be a result of the increased surface area of multifilament fibers, suggested to increase the surface area by a factor of at least 1.57 (Klinge et al., 2002a). The larger surface is thought to provide more space for bacteria adhesion and increased area for bacteria proliferation. Further, multifilament fibers are thought to have spaces within the fibers themselves, which are less than 10 μm in diameter. This opening would allow for the passage of bacteria, but prevent macrophage infiltration, providing a harbor for bacterial proliferation (Iglesia et al., 1997).

Fiber pattern

While individual fibers, whether monofilament or multifilament, provide the basic structural element of synthetic mesh implants, the behavior of the entire mesh is governed by the method in which the mesh is constructed. Two of the most common textile construction techniques used to create a mesh structure are knitting and weaving. Woven meshes are constructed using a simple interlacing technique, using of two sets of threads (fibers), running perpendicular to one another. There are several weave styles, including plain, twill, and satin weaves (Figure 13.13). Woven meshes have superior mechanical strength and shape memory; however, woven meshes are susceptible to fraying when cut and conform poorly to boundaries such as the organs of the pelvic floor (Cosson et al., 2003). Unlike woven mesh, knit mesh is constructed by successive looping of a single fiber. In addition, there are several types of knit structures including warp-lock, interlock, and circular knit, though the latter is uncommon for urogynecological meshes (Figure 13.13). Knit meshes are characterized by flexible behavior, allowing surgeons to easily manipulate the device. In addition, knit mesh provides high conformity to adjacent anatomical structures.

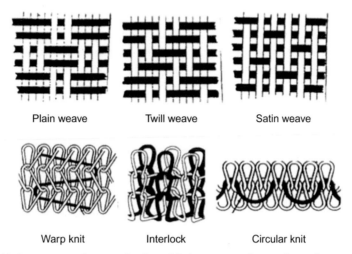

Plain weave   Twill weave   Satin weave

Warp knit   Interlock   Circular knit

Figure 13.13 Various types of weave (top) and knit patterns (bottom) can be used to construct synthetic mesh products. The construction technique has been found to greatly impact both the mechanical behavior of the device and the host response to the implant.

The mechanical behavior of mesh is directly dependent on the filament type and thread morphology (fiber pattern). Since multifilament fibers contain small gaps within the fiber, the fibers must undergo tightening, or come into contact with each other before the full stiffness of fiber is attained. This slight recruitment behavior is similar to that of a rope. The combined effect of such small recruitment across a mesh comprised of multifilament fibers contributes to its nonlinear load–elongation behavior, meaning that stiffness is a function of mesh elongation. Conversely, monofilament fibers exhibit their full stiffness values immediately upon loading, entering the linear region of the loading curve instantaneously, similar to a steel rod. However, it should be noted that individual fibers of mesh materials (nylon, polypropylene, etc.) have stiffness values much greater than that of an entire mesh.

The ability for a mesh to have a lower stiffness value than the components such as polypropylene, from which it is constructed, arises from the construction technique used to create the mesh. Mesh products utilize linkages (created via knitting or weaving) between fibers, allowing thin extrusions of stiff materials, such as polypropylene, to become a flexible structure. In addition, the fiber pattern impacts the orientation of individual fibers relative to axes of loading. For example, woven meshes orient fibers perpendicular to one another. Since all of the fibers in a woven mesh are only oriented in two orthogonal directions, the mesh is stiff along these two directions. Further, weaving techniques leave little room for fibers to rotate or reorient to off axis loads, creating stiff intersections between fibers and an overall rigid structure with a small toe region of the load–elongation curve. Unlike woven mesh, knitted mesh contains fibers that can be oriented in a number of directions. Additionally, linkages in knitted mesh contain gaps between the fibers allowing fibers to rotate freely relative to woven mesh. These characteristics allow fibers of knit mesh to rotate and reorient in the direction of applied force. This phenomenon is the primary mechanism responsible for the non-linear load-elongation behavior associated with contemporary mesh products (Moalli et al., 2008).

Since the method of construction has been shown to greatly affect the mechanical behavior of a mesh, it can be altered in order to obtain the desired mechanical and tactile properties a manufacturer desires. For this reason, a single filament material can be used to create meshes with a wide range of properties. This is overtly apparent in the current urogynecological mesh market, as nearly all SUI and POP meshes are comprised of polypropylene and classified as type I meshes, yet their mechanical behaviors (characterized by structural properties in mechanics literature) are markedly different (Jones et al., 2009; Moalli et al., 2008; Shepherd et al., 2012). In addition, it is not uncommon for materials of differing construction techniques to be marketed as distinct materials, given that their behavior is quite dissimilar. For instance, a polyester material, Dacron, is known as Mersilene when knitted and Ligatene when woven (Cosson et al., 2003).

Fiber pattern is not only a major factor in determining the biomechanical behavior of mesh, but it also appears to significantly impact the host response following implantation. Notably woven mesh has been found to greatly increase the number of mesh-related complication relative to knitted mesh. Comparison between construction methods is easily illustrated by comparing Marlex, a woven polypropylene mesh, and Prolene, a knitted polypropylene mesh. When first used to treat abdominal hernias, Marlex exposure rates were nearly 44%, while Prolene exposure rates were minimal (Cosson et al., 2003).

Porosity and pore size

From a design perspective, the pore size and porosity of a mesh appear to be the greatest factors that dictate the host response. The impact of pore size has been well characterized in hernia literature, specifically for polypropylene mesh, where larger pores have been shown to improve the mechanical integrity of the resulting mesh–tissue complex, increasing both strength and collagen deposition. Conversely, small pores restrict both vascular growth and the local tissue ingrowth, with resulting structures containing less mature collagen (Greca et al., 2001, 2008). In addition, the foreign body response to mesh is highly dependent on the pore size and has been shown to be greatly reduced with increasing pore size (Klinge et al., 2002c; Chvapil et al., 1969; Patel et al., 2012b). Pores with dimensions less than 10 μm provide beds for bacterial proliferation and persistent infection, as macrophages and neutrophils are unable to enter these pores (Amid, 1997). Further, it has been documented that the surface of each fiber becomes encased by a granulomatous inflammatory reaction as part of the foreign body response (Muhl et al., 2007; Otto et al., 2014; Junge et al., 2011). Reduction in pore size brings these peri-fiber inflammatory reactions closer together, and once sufficiently close the fibrous granulation tissue can form a bridge with neighboring fibrous granulations. This bridging, known as "bridging fibrosis," leads to the formation of a continuous scar plate and prevents tissue from growing into the mesh structure (Klinge et al., 2002b,c). Notably, it has been shown that effective tissue in-growth with polypropylene mesh, characterized by the quality of the tissue which forms around mesh fibers, only occurs in mesh pores with a diameter of 1000 μm or greater (Klinge and Klosterhalfen, 2011). Pore sizes less than 1000 μm have greatly enhanced inflammatory and fibrotic responses (Weyhe et al., 2006; Bellon et al., 2002). While a pore size of 1000 μm appears to be the threshold for polypropylene, the thickness of fibrous encapsulation is expected to vary depending on the polymer used as that the degree of fibrous connective tissue deposition is believed to be dependent on protein interaction with the fiber surface and related to hydrophobicity of the polymer (Klinge et al., 2002d). It is important to note that these findings on pore size were all determined using an abdominal wall model. Though the general foreign body response to mesh should consist of similar mechanisms in the vagina and adjacent supportive tissues, there are distinct differences in the biology of these sites, which likely impacts the host response to SUI, and POP meshes. Therefore, the critical pore diameter for urogynecological meshes to minimize scar plate formation may be distinct from that found in abdominal wall studies.

Interestingly the specific gravity of the mesh, which is referred to as the mesh weight, does not seem to play a significant role in dictating this response. This is contrary to those who have suggested that the POP mesh erosion rates are higher than SUI meshes due to the increased amount of mesh implanted (Bent et al., 2008). Rather than the total amount of material implanted, the relative density or spatial distribution of the implanted material drives this host response. Typically, heavyweight meshes (those with higher specific gravities, typically above $1\,\text{g/cm}^3$) are often constructed to have small pore sizes. Therefore, the observed effects of most heavyweight meshes may be due solely to the small pore design. Conversely, lower weight meshes ($< 1\,\text{g/cm}^3$) are often constructed with a large range of pore sizes. Studies by Weyhe et al. (2006) demonstrate that pore size, rather than mesh weight, is more predictive of the host response as lightweight, microporous mesh was found to provoke a more intense foreign body response with poor tissue integration relative to heavyweight meshes with larger pore sizes. Further, Junge et al. (2011) has suggested that weight classification be avoided.

Given the importance of pore size, it may be considered the primary characterization method for synthetic mesh products. Indeed such classification exists, though its origin in 1997 (Amid, 1997) reflects older generation of materials which are not necessarily used today. Moreover, the previous generations of materials, in general, were less porous than current materials. Nevertheless, this outdated system is helpful when conceptually dividing mesh types. Accordingly, type I meshes are macroporous, with primary pore sizes greater than 75 μm (Bent et al., 2008; Baessler and Maher, 2006). These meshes are associated with improved tissue integration, as their pores provide sufficient space for tissue ingrowth (Baessler and Maher, 2006). Clearly this diameter is much smaller than threshold pore size, which was found to minimize the foreign body reaction for polypropylene mesh, suggesting that not all type I meshes will elicit the same host response. Type II meshes are completely microporous meshes, with pore sizes less than 75 μm. Gore-Tex (expanded polytetrafluoroethylene) is the primary example of type II meshes. These meshes do not form adhesions with tissue and deter fibroblast and macrophage infiltration (Baessler and Maher, 2006). Therefore, tissue formation and treatment of infections is difficult with type II mesh, often requiring the mesh to be removed in the event of complications (Weinberger and Ostergard, 1995). Type III meshes are primarily macroporous with microporous components and include polyethylene terephthalate (Mersilene) and polytetrafluoroethylene (Teflon) meshes. Type II and III meshes have both been linked to high rates of complications, likely due to the effects of small interstices that develop between the fibers (Bent et al., 2008). Type IV meshes, which are coated meshes with submicroscopic pore size (< 1 μm), have also been utilized, though clinical results have been poor (Bent et al., 2008). It should be noted that this method of characterizing mesh does not consider the polymer, only the primary pore size of a mesh. As previously discussed, the polymer type may dictate the minimum pore size required to reduce the immune response and promote tissue integration. Further, this classification does not consider the spaces created due to the methods of construction. For example, knit construction creates small voids around the location at which filaments are joined. The size of these pores should be considered as they provide microporous elements even in large pore meshes. Clinically, type I meshes have been found to have the lowest incidence of infection and erosion, helping to decrease complication and erosion rates (Bent et al., 2008; Rodrigues Macield da Fonseca et al., 2013; Karlovsky et al., 2005). As of 2004, these rates were thought to have dropped below 2% and 1%, respectively; albeit, mesh complications have not been well studied. However, after introduction of transvaginal delivery of type I polypropylene prolapse meshes, complications have substantially increased with rates as high as 20%, prompting physicians and patients alike to reconsider their use in transvaginal prolapse repairs (US FDA, 2008, 2011; Manodoro et al., 2012).

Material type

Several materials have been used in the construction of prolapse and incontinence meshes with a wide range of results. These materials include polyethylene terephthalate (Mersilene), polypropylene (Marlex), polytetrafluoroethylene (Teflon), and expanded polytetrafluoroethylene (Gore-Tex) (Iglesia et al., 1997). Since meshes are a composite structure, comprised of an extruded material which is then assembled, the mechanical behavior of these devices is classified in terms of structural properties, rather than mechanical properties. Mechanical properties imply a homogenous, continuous composition, whose data can be normalized and presented as stress, strain, and tangent modulus. Conversely, structural properties characterize multimaterial constructs or discontinuous materials (such as porous mesh) and are described via parameters such as load, elongation, and stiffness. As such, direct comparison between many structural properties (other than stiffness or relative elongation) can only be made if test samples are of the same initial dimensions.

Ex vivo and *in vitro* comparisons of these materials have shown that all are non-toxic and have a high tensile strength. While many implants are not exposed to such high forces *in vivo*, tensile strength is considered as a safety factor to ensure the mesh is not likely to result in surgical failure. In this regard, the tensile strength of the material or composite should be considered though most meshes are overdesigned in terms of this requirement. As the tensile strength (the load at which failure occurs) of synthetic mesh is unlikely to be approached under the loading conditions of the pelvis, this parameter likely plays no role in the host response to mesh implants (Cobb et al., 2005; Noakes et al., 2008). Rather the relationship between the material elongation and applied load, known as stiffness, may be important in governing the host response based on previous findings that cells respond to the stiffness of materials (Liang et al., 2013; Feola et al., 2013). This concept has been demonstrated as the stiffness of a substrate has been found to elicit specific tissue and cellular responses (Discher et al., 2005; Yeung et al., 2005).

Two materials that have had poor results in the incontinence and prolapse surgeries are Teflon and Gore-Tex. Perhaps their most distinctive trait is that they did not integrate well into the tissues, which is thought to be related to the pore design and chemical makeup of these materials (Iglesia et al., 1997). Initially this lack of integration was thought to be beneficial as Gore-Tex mesh could easily be removed in the presence of an infection. In addition, it was reported that these devices initiated only a minimal inflammatory response. However, clinical use of Gore-Tex was plagued with numerous complications of alarming severity (Bent et al., 2008). Gore-Tex slings for SUI repair had a removal rate of at least 35%, with a significant number of sinus tract formations (10%) and infections in addition to reports of vaginal exposures (Weinberger and Ostergard, 1995). For sacrocolpopexy, Gore-Tex was found to be one of the primary risk factors for mesh exposure into the vagina (Nygaard et al., 2008; Cundiff et al., 2008). The primary concern for Gore-Tex POP meshes was the number of rejections, likely due to infection, again requiring mesh removal (Iglesia et al., 1997).

Woven multifilament materials such as polyethylene terephthalate, a member of the polyester polymer family manufactured as Mersilene, has also been associated with increased rates of exposure and infection. The mechanism is thought to be due to interstices between the fibers of woven materials that can be as small as 1 μm. As such the risk for infection is a concern, while tissue integration is poor.

Over time, knitted polypropylene has become the primary material for synthetic mesh used in incontinence and prolapse surgeries. Early studies found polypropylene to elicit a strong inflammatory response with formation of fibrotic tissue and multi-nucleated giant cells (i.e., foreign body response) (Elliott and Juler, 1979). Additionally, polypropylene mesh was found to be conducive to tissue ingrowth, providing a scaffold on which tissue could attach and penetrate. Clinically, polypropylene was found to have relatively low erosion rates for both SUI and POP procedures relative to other material types. Perhaps most influential in the rise of polypropylene as the dominant mesh material was the success of the TVT (Ulmsten et al., 1996). However, more recently, with the publication of large case series and other clinical trials (eCARE), there has been an increased awareness of complications associated with both the transvaginal and transabdominal insertion of polypropylene and the finding that complications after the purportedly safer transabdominal route increase in time (Nygaard et al., 2013) have led some to question the use of polypropylene in urogynecological procedures.

PELVIC FLOOR CONSIDERATIONS FOR MESH IMPLANTS

While many concepts regarding hernia repair mesh design are useful for pelvic floor meshes, these criteria may only serve as an initial design rather than an optimal one. As suggested by Junge et al. (2011), the structural requirements for mesh repair will vary from situation to situation, not just in regard to site of implantation but potentially from patient to patient. The environment of the pelvic floor is much more complicated from a biological and mechanical perspective, requiring consideration of the role of the implant in this anatomic location.

Biological environment

Unlike hernia repair meshes, which are in direct contact only with the abdominal fascia, urogynecological mesh is placed in an environment with a wide range of soft tissues, ranging from muscle (smooth and striated), various types of connective tissue, and specialized organs. Moreover, the vagina heavily colonized with bacteria is considered a clean-contaminated surgical field. In general, the soft tissues of the pelvic floor are metabolically active, with compositions that have been shown to change dramatically with normal aging and in response to hormone-driven events such as pregnancy, menstrual cycle, and menopause (Moalli et al., 2004, 2005). Several studies have compared the biological response to surgical mesh between abdominal hernia repair and prolapse repair models and have found markedly different host responses. Using a rabbit model, Pierce et al. (2009) implanted polypropylene and cross-linked porcine dermis grafts in the abdomen and posterior vagina for a period of 9 months. Interestingly, no mesh exposures were observed for abdominally implanted mesh, while exposure rates for polypropylene and chemically cross-linked porcine dermis (Pelvichol) were 27% and 15%, respectively, at the vaginal site. In addition, the authors state that the length of polypropylene graft was often decreased upon explanation and that such decreases in length were associated with mesh exposure. Histological analysis revealed that inflammation and fibroblast proliferation scores were significantly increased in the vagina for both implant materials studied, while the scores were decreased relative to the abdominal site. Further, the cross-linked porcine graft was degraded in 37% of abdominal implants, while 70% of these biological grafts degraded when implanted in the vagina. Porcine graft degradation was so drastic in the pelvic floor that in nearly half of vaginal implantations the graft was thought to be missing upon sample harvesting, though the sutures used for securing these products remained (Pierce et al., 2009). Manodoro et al. (2012) also noted that vaginal polypropylene mesh appeared more folded and found that the degree of mesh "contraction" was nearly twice that of abdominally implanted mesh. Again, mesh erosion was not observed in the abdomen, while 30% of vaginal implants resulted in erosion. These later findings are based on a relatively small sample size and in the sheep model, though they appear quite similar to the previous findings in the rabbit. It should be noted that both of these studies simply sutured the mesh to the vagina, rather than placing the mesh in tension as is done for many pelvic reconstruction procedures. Still, these studies provide evidence that the biological response to a material is vastly different in the vagina relative to the abdominal wall. The increased inflammation and foreign body response, along with the noticeable increase in degradation of porcine dermis, suggest that the vagina in particular is a much harsher and biologically active environment for mesh products. In addition to the postimplantation environment, surgical entry for transvaginal procedures may result in contamination of the surgical graft upon insertion due to vaginal microflora. As such, this potential contamination may result in subclinical infection adding to the intensity of the vaginal environment. While the biology of the vagina appears to play a large role in the complication rate of mesh, the impact of mechanical loads in this location must also be considered in order to determine the role biomaterials in this space.

Mechanical environment

Like most biological tissues, the structures comprising the pelvic floor respond to the presence or absence of mechanical loads. As the connective tissues which support the vagina are often compromised in women with SUI and POP, the primary objective of mesh is to restore support to the vagina and/or urethra. Therefore, the response of the vagina to mechanical stimuli is an important design consideration when selecting a suitable reconstruction method for pelvic floor disorders. Zong et al. (2010a) recently demonstrated the impact of mechanical loading on vaginal tissue. In this study, vaginal fibroblasts were obtained from a full thickness biopsy from the vaginal apex. Cells were cultured on media and were placed under repetitive stretch to either 8% or 16% and collagenase activity was measured. Relative to fibroblasts cultured without mechanical stimuli, MMP activity for 8% stretched cells was increased by 76%, while cells undergoing 16% stretch had an increase of 188%. Interestingly, addition of 17-β-estradiol and progesterone to the culture media returned collagenase activity to control levels, suggesting hormones may help to mediate the mechanosensitive response of the vagina (Zong et al., 2010a). While the *in vivo* stretch of vaginal tissue is unknown, there is likely some physiological stretch or force that is beneficial to maintain structure, likely applied by abdominal pressure and the interaction of the vagina with its supportive structures. Understanding of how these forces are transmitted to the vagina and the mechanosensitive behavior of the vagina may explain complications such as exposure and erosion and improve reconstructive techniques used in the pelvic floor.

Support to the vagina and hence the organs supported by it is a complex mechanical system in which many tissue interactions are combined to maintain static equilibrium and resist transient changes in abdominal pressure. As previously mentioned, this system is comprised of sheets of connective tissue and musculature, focused around the vagina. While understanding and recreating a nonpathological support system may seem implausible, there are several mechanical factors to consider when using synthetic mesh products in reconstructive pelvic surgeries.

One of the most significant mechanical considerations for mesh use in SUI and POP repair is that they are subjected to predominately uniaxial tensile loading conditions. This is quite different from the loading conditions a mesh experiences when used for abdominal hernia repair. During a hernia repair, the mesh is placed within the abdominal wall, fixed along its entire perimeter. Since the abdominal cavity can be thought of as a pressurized vessel, the mesh graft must function as the wall of a pressurized vessel. Under the pressure exerted within the abdominal cavity, the abdomen expands or is "inflated," and the abdominal wall resists and limits this expansion. Given this loading condition, hernia mesh is placed in tension along all axes simultaneously, much like the surface of a balloon upon inflation. This loading environment helps the mesh maintain its original geometry and pore sizes (Figure 13.14). However, incontinence meshes are used as suspension structures for slings in the retropubic or transobturator space. Similarly prolapse meshes act as suspension cables, attaching the vagina to the sacrum or pelvic sidewall. These configurations load the mesh, particularly the fixation arms of these devices, primarily in a tensile uniaxial fashion. Even while the name TVT suggests that the device does not experience tension, its intended function is to have the urethra compressed along the sling, which would place the mesh in tension. The tension-free component is thus more representative of the surgical technique rather than the long-term *in vivo* function of the device.

Hernia   Prolapse

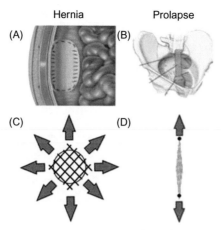

Figure 13.14 The site of implantation dictates the mechanical environment a mesh experiences. For hernia repair, mesh is implanted in the abdominal wall via sutures along the entire boundary (A and C). This loads the all axes of the mesh simultaneously. For prolapse repair, mesh is loaded in a predominately uniaxial fashion (B and D). Uniaxial loading is more likely to result in collapse of mesh pores.

This concept of mechanical loads becomes extremely relevant when considering the importance of mesh porosity on the host response. Studies performed in our lab in addition to work by Otto et al. have demonstrated that under uniaxial loads, the maximum pore size and porosity of nearly all synthetic meshes is dramatically reduced (Moalli et al., 2008; Shepherd et al., 2012; Otto et al., 2014). When loaded in a uniaxial fashion, the material extends in the direction of applied force as the fibers of the mesh rotate and reorganize to resist the applied force. This reorganization is largely governed by the geometry of a mesh. As the mesh extends along the direction of the applied force, it narrows in the direction perpendicular to the force (Figure 13.15). This phenomenon, known as Poisson's effect, is often accompanied by a reduction in pore size. Indeed, application of uniaxial tension to mesh dramatically reduces pore size and in many cases, all of the pores in a tensioned mesh are less than 1 mm in diameter, diminishing the potential for tissue ingrowth and promoting bridging of fibrous encapsulations such that long-term tissue incorporation is compromised (Muhl et al., 2007; Otto et al., 2014). Thus, mechanical behavior may provide an explanation or contribute to the clinical observation of mesh "shrinking" or "contraction" after implantation (Baessler and Maher, 2006; Manodoro et al., 2012). Moreover, dramatic reductions in pore size were found to occur at just 5 and 10 N of force, which are low levels of force relative to those anticipated to occur *in vivo* (Cobb et al., 2005; Noakes et al., 2008). While the actual cause of mesh shrinkage may involve active contraction of fibrotic tissue or other biological mechanisms, it appears plausible that application of these tensile forces have the potential to cause such mesh deformation alone or induce

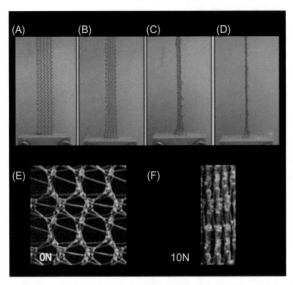

Figure 13.15 In response to uniaxial tensile testing, synthetic mesh contracts in the direction perpendicular to the axis of loading (A–D). In addition, the individual fibers of the mesh reorient to withstand mechanical forces and often lead to the collapse of pores (E and F).

significant fibrosis. Therefore the deformation of mesh under tensile forces must be considered when "tensioning" or placing a mesh surgically, as well as during *in vivo* loading conditions both before and after host tissue integration occurs.

In addition to the distribution of forces applied to the mesh (multiaxial vs. uniaxial), the porosity of a mesh during tensile loading is highly dependent on the orientation of the mesh pores to the direction of applied force. This concept is clearly demonstrated by mesh products whose pores initially have a square geometry (Figure 13.16). With application of a tensile force in the direction of the mesh fibers (either vertical or horizontal), the pores will maintain their shape effectively until the mesh is placed under relatively high loads. Conversely, loading the mesh at an angle 45° offset will result in a nearly immediate collapse of the pores, at forces below 1 N. More intricate product designs such as those found in transvaginal mesh devices are also subject to these effects, as various orientations within the same transvaginal mesh experience differing pore behavior under the same tensile force (Otto et al., 2014). This anisotropic behavior is exhibited by all synthetic meshes, though the degree of anisotropy varies depending on the method of construction, initial pore geometry, and mechanical boundary conditions.

Despite the tendency of mesh pores to collapse under *ex vivo* uniaxial testing procedures, it should be noted that mesh reorganization in most *ex vivo* mechanical studies consider only idealized deformations with an even distribution of force at the sample

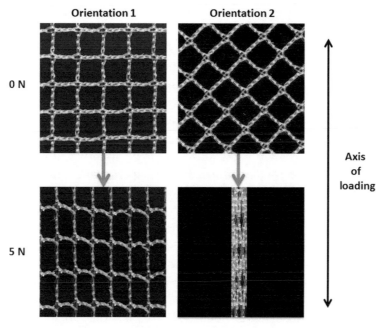

Figure 13.16 The deformation of mesh under uniaxial loading is highly dependent on the mesh orientation relative to the axis of loading. Consider the two orientations of Restorelle shown when pulled in tension along the vertical axis. In orientation 1, many mesh fibers are aligned with the vertical axis (top left). In orientation 2, we rotate the mesh by 45° (top right). Loading each orientation to 5 N (bottom row) results in dramatically different mesh appearances. Pores in orientation 1 remain open, allowing for potential tissue integration, while pores in orientation 2 are completely collapsed, appearing as a dense region of polypropylene.

midsubstance. The conditions of this test produce a predominately planar deformation, with a drastic collapse of pores and limited out-of-plane bending or curling of the mesh. These observations are consistent with the planar assumption used for uniaxial testing protocols, though they do not necessarily reflect those deformations noted upon implantation. Mesh deformations at the vaginal interface are largely determined by the method of fixation. Surgically, mesh products are fixed to the vagina using sutures, which apply discrete points of attachment to the vagina. Depending on the spatial arrangement and number of point loads applied, one would anticipate a variety of results. For instance, if one were to use a single suture to attach the mesh to the vagina and a single suture to anchor the mesh to the sacrum, it is expected that mesh pores along a line connecting the two suture locations would be responsible for resisting applied force and therefore are subject to the greatest risk for collapse. Meanwhile, pores not on this line would carry little, if any, force, and thus are not likely to experience a decrease in pore size. Still these pores may wrinkle or deform out of plane depending on the bending stiffness of the mesh. This wrinkling or buckling behavior is due to the nonhomogenous distribution of force throughout the mesh, again, since forces are only transferred between the points of attachment. Conversely, using many points of attachment (i.e., suture attachments) would help to distribute this force resulting in a more planar and homogenous alteration of pore geometry, similar to the deformations observed in standard uniaxial tensile test.

When considering the interface between two materials, such as the vagina and implanted mesh, one must consider how forces are transferred, in terms of both the distribution of force and the properties of the materials to which they are connected. As previously discussed, isolated point loads may result in localized increases in force, while sites further from the point of attachment experience no mechanical loading. In addition, when two materials are in contact, the locations at which they are joined are subject to stress concentrations or stress raisers. Stress raisers are localized increases in stress (force per unit area) found at a material interface. It should be noted that the greater the disparity between mechanical properties of the two materials, the greater the stress observed at this interface (Simon et al., 2003; Spalazzi et al., 2008). From a design perspective, this principal is evident when examining composition of tendons, specialized tissues that transfer force from muscle to bone. Tendons have properties between that of muscles and bone, and serve not only to transmit forces, but also to provide a buffer between two materials of vastly different stiffness. In order to accomplish this gradual load transfer, the composition of a tendon varies along its length ranging from a more compliant tissue at the site of muscle attachment to a stiffer, nearly cartilaginous tissue (fibrocartilage) at their bony insertion (Spalazzi et al., 2008; Thomopoulos et al., 2003). The gradual transition in composition serves to transmit forces from soft tissue to hard bone while minimizing stress concentrations.

Indeed, there is significant evidence demonstrating that the stiffness of implantable devices can alter tissue remodeling and response (Zong et al., 2010a; Huiskes et al., 1987; Goel et al., 1991). In general, increased implant stiffness is believed to induce a maladaptive remodeling response through a phenomenon known as stress shielding. Stress shielding occurs when a stiffer material resists applied loads and buffers or "shields" surrounding tissues from these forces. One of the most notable occurrences of stress shielding arose with implants for hip arthroplasty in the 1990s. Implantation of these devices resulted in bone loss around the implant, leading to hip fractures in this location (Jacobs et al., 1993; Rubash et al., 1998). Soft tissues have also been found to have increased breakdown of both collagen and elastin upon implantation of implants of increasing stiffness (Majima et al., 1996; Ozog et al., 2011). Additional studies have confirmed increases in collagen turnover and collagenase activity in the absence of mechanical loading (Liang et al., 2013).

The concepts of force distribution and stress shielding are extremely important to consider as the vagina has been shown to respond to mechanical stimuli (Zong et al., 2010a). Recently the relevance of these mechanical principles was demonstrated for current lightweight polypropylene prolapse meshes. Meshes of increased stiffness were most detrimental to functional behavior of vaginal tissue, dramatically decreasing thickness of the vaginal muscularis and reducing the total amount of collagen (Liang et al., 2013; Feola et al., 2013). While stiffer materials may seem ideal to maintain the anatomy of the pelvic floor, they appear to be less compatible with the properties of native tissues, and even more dissimilar if prolapsed tissues are already mechanically compromised (Moalli et al., 2005). Ideally, mesh would provide support to the vagina in a manner that promotes remodeling which maintains or restores the native mechanical integrity of the vagina.

In line with stress shielding, point loading induced by suture attachment can result in regions of high stress at the point of attachment. This discrete loading is a rather significant departure from the even distribution of force that would be provided by the broad contact area of normal musculature and connective tissue support. These local regions of high-force transmission may result in a host maladaptive remodeling response with localized increases in collagenase activity, potentially forming a site of erosion. Conversely, regions further away from suture attachments may experience reduced load as they receive little biomechanical stimuli and the effects of stress shielding may induce remodeling to form a mechanically inferior tissue.

While it is quite evident that mechanical loading alters mesh pore dimensions and potential impacting the host response to mesh, it provides only a 2D measure of the distance between mesh fibers. Given that interfiber distance is heavily implicated in bridging fibrosis, the 3D confirmation of the mesh should be considered. In this regard, folding or bunching of the mesh would increase the amount of mesh material per unit volume and bring mesh fibers closer in 3D space. Such an increase in density would have the same impact as reduction in porosity as mesh fibers become sufficiently close for bridging of fibrotic tissue, as well as an enhanced inflammatory response. Indeed there are reports of mesh bunching or palpable "edges" associated with sites of exposure, suggesting that meshes are subject to out-of-plane deformations which are not observed during a uniaxial test. Recent studies in our lab have confirmed that introduction of point loads via suture attachment increased the overall surface wrinkling by more than an order of magnitude (Figure 13.17) compared to standard uniaxial protocols. Again, this observed wrinkling of the mesh surface is largely due to the nonuniform loading imparted by point loads (i.e., suture points), resulting from transfer of force through the mesh fibers between anchoring points. As such, the locations and number of anchoring points should be considered in development of surgical procedures utilizing mesh.

Clearly it is a difficult task to mimic the natural support system of the vagina and urethra. Connective tissues offer a wide base of support with attachments along the entire vaginal length ensuring a relatively even distribution of force across the tissue. These forces are likely vital in promoting healthy tissue development with mechanisms for proper homeostasis. In addition to the presence of a foreign body, grafts used

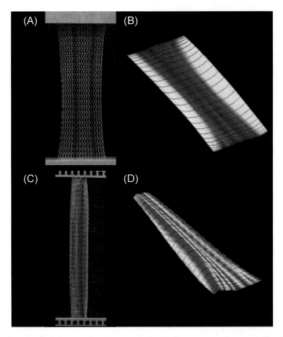

Figure 13.17 The mechanical deformation a mesh experiences varies greatly depending on boundary conditions applied. In response to standard uniaxial tensile testing, mesh contracts in the direction perpendicular to the axis of loading, though this deformation is planar (A). Analysis of the surface curvature upon loading confirms that the mesh indeed remains in plane (B), with cool colors representing 0 curvature and warm colors representing greater curvature. Introduction of point loads via suture attachment dramatically alters this deformation (C). Curvature analysis confirms increased surface wrinkling and out-of-plane deformation, evident by alternating warm and cool colors.

for pelvic floor reconstruction typically do not provide support to the same extent. While current procedures are quite effective in terms of reducing symptoms of pelvic floor dysfunction and restoring a desirable level of function, alleviation of complications such as exposure, erosion, and pain may not occur until surgical approaches more adeptly address the mechanical environment in which these devices are utilized.

LOOKING TO THE FUTURE

Without question there remains room for improvement in developing biomaterials and accompanying procedures for use in the pelvic floor. The current standards of synthetic mesh do indeed appear to achieve significantly higher efficacy rates, however, these treatments should not be weighed against such severe, and relatively frequent complications. Rather than adapting treatments from outside fields, we must strive to understand the environment and conditions of the vagina and its supportive tissues, along with anatomic site-specific factors that affect the host response to biomaterials. These ideals must be considered and approached in order to create devices that help restore normal function. Indeed, all factors as outlined in Chapter 1 should be considered in the design of devices for the repair of incontinence and prolapse.

Currently it is unclear whether the future of urogynecological biomaterials will consist of synthetics, biologics, or a combination of these two in order to fulfill the highly complex and poorly understood physiological requirements of the vagina. Moving forward, it is important to consider the history of previous biomaterials in this space, but not become constrained by the materials or procedures currently in use. Rather, we must reassess both the successes and shortcomings from this history and develop new products and techniques that are optimized for restoring pelvic organ support. As a community, more studies are required to examine native support under *in vivo* loads and to better understand the environment of the vagina in terms of the biological response to not simply the material which is implanted, but in response to the forces imparted by these materials. To date many of the considerations discussed have been neglected during device design for SUI and POP repairs. As such the ideal product, whether it is a mesh or tissue engineered construct, is still on the horizon and unlike previous generations of treatment, we must take the proper steps to successfully attain our goals.

REFERENCES

Abed, H., Rahn, D.D., Lowenstein, L., Balk, E.M., Clemons, J.L., Rogers, R.G., 2011. Incidence and management of graft erosion, wound granulation, and dyspareunia following vaginal prolapse repair with graft materials: a systematic review. Int. Urogynecol. J. 22 (7), 789–798. (Epub 2011/03/23).

Abouassaly, R., Steinberg, J.R., Lemieux, M., Marois, C., Gilchrist, L.I., Bourque, J., et al., 2004. Complications of tension-free vaginal tape surgery: a multi-institutional review. BJU Int. 94, 100–113.

Abramowitch, S.D., Feola, A., Jallah, Z., Moalli, P.A., 2009. Tissue mechanics, animal models, and pelvic organ prolapse: a review. Eur. J. Obstet. Gynecol. Reprod. Biol. 144S, S146–S158.

Albo, M.E., Steers, W., Diokno, A., Khandwala, S., Brubaker, L., FitzGerald, M.P., et al., 2008. The trial of mid-urethral slings (TOMUS): design and methodology. J. Appl. Res. 8 (1), 1–13.

Alperin, M., Moalli, P.A., 2006. Remodeling of vaginal connective tissue in patients with prolapse. Curr. Opin. Obstet. Gynecol. 18 (5), 544–550.

Amid, P.K., 1997. Classification of biomaterials and their related complications in abdominal wall hernia surgery. Hernia (1), 15–21.

Araco, F., Gravante, G., Sorge, R., Overton, J., De Vita, D., Primicerio, M., et al., 2009. The influence of BMI, smoking, and age on vaginal erosions after synthetic mesh repair of pelvic organ prolapses. A multicenter study. Acta Obstet. Gynecol. Scand. 88 (7), 772–780. (Epub 2009/05/20).

Badylak, S., 2002. The extracellular matrix as a scaffold for tissue reconstruction. Semin. Cell Dev. Biol. 13 (5), 377–383.

Badylak, S.F., Park, K., Peppas, N., McCabe, G., Yoder, M., 2001. Marrow-derived cells populate scaffolds composed of xenogeneic extracellular matrix. Exp. Hematol. 29 (11), 1310–1318.

Baessler, K., Maher, C.F., 2006. Mesh augmentation during pelvic-floor reconstructive surgery: risks and benefits. Curr. Opin. Obstet. Gynecol. 18, 560–566.

Baessler, K., Hewson, A.D., Schuessler, B., Maher, C.F., 2005. Severe mesh complications following intra-vaginal slingplasty. Obstet. Gynecol. 106 (4), 713–716. (Epub 2005/4/10).

Bako, A., Dhar, R., 2008. Review of synthetic mesh-related complication in pelvic floor reconstructive surgery. Int. Urogynecol. J. (20), 103–111. (Epub 2008/9/9).

Barber, M.D., Brubaker, L., Burgio, K.L., Richter, H.E., Nygaard, I., Weidner, A.C., et al., 2014. Comparison of 2 transvaginal surgical approaches and perioperative behavioral therapy for apical vaginal prolapse: the OPTIMAL randomized trial. JAMA 311 (10), 1023–1034.

Bellon, L.M., Jurado, F., Garcia-Honduvilla, N., Lopez, R., Carrera-San Martin, A., Bujan, J., 2002. The structure of a biomaterial rather than its chemical composition modulates the repair process at the peritoneal level. Am. J. Surg. 184 (2), 154–159.

Bent, A.E., Cundiff, G.W., Swift, S.E., 2008. Ostergard's Urogynecology and Pelvic Floor Dysfunction, sixth ed. Lippincott Williams & Wilkins, Philadelphia, PA.

Birk, D.E., Fitch, J.M., Babiarz, J.P., Doane, K.J., Linsenmayer, T.F., 1990. Collagen fibrillogenesis *in vitro*: interaction of types I and V collagen regulates fibril diameter. J. Cell Sci. 95, 649–657.

Boreham, M.K., Wai, C., Miller, R.T., Schaffer, J.I., Word, R.A., 2002. Morphometric analysis of smooth muscle in the anterior vaginal wall of women with pelvic organ prolapse. Am. J. Obstet. Gynecol. 187 (1), 56–63. (Epub 2002/07/13).

Brophy, M.M., Klutke, J.J., Klutke, C.G., 2001. A review of the tension-free vaginal tape procedure: outcomes complications and theories. Curr. Urol. Rep. 2, 364–369.

Brubaker, L., Nygaard, I., Richter, H.E., Visco, A., Weber, A.M., Cundiff, G.W., et al., 2008. Two-year outcomes after sacrocolpopexy with and without burch to prevent stress urinary incontinence. Obstet. Gynecol. 112 (1), 49–55. (Epub 2008/07/02).

Brubaker, L., Norton, P.A., Albo, M.E., Chai, T.C., Dandreo, K.J., Lloyd, K.L., et al., 2011. Adverse events over two years after retropubic or transobturator midurethral sling surgery: findings from the Trial of Midurethral Slings (TOMUS) study. Am. J. Obstet. Gynecol. 205 (5), 498. e1–498.e6.

Budatha, M., Roshanravan, S., Zheng, Q., Weislander, C., Chapman, S.L., Davis, E.C., et al., 2011. Extracellular matrix proteases contribute to progression of pelvic organ prolapse in mice and humans. J. Clin. Invest. 121 (5), 2048–2059. (Epub 2011/04/27).

Buxboim, A., Ivanovska, I.L., Discher, D.E., 2010. Matrix elasticity, cytoskeletal forces and physics of the nucleus: how deeply do cells "feel" outside and in? J. Cell Sci. 123, 297–308.

Chen, B.H., Wen, Y., Li, H., Polan, M.L., 2002. Collagen metabolism and turnover in women with stress urinary incontinence and pelvic prolapse. Int. Urogynecol. J. Pelvic Floor Dysfunct. 13 (2), 80–87.

Chen, C.C., Ridgeway, B., Paraiso, M.F., 2007. Biologic grafts and synthetic meshes in pelvic reconstructive surgery. Clin. Obstet. Gynecol. 50 (2), 382–441. (Epub 2007/05/22).

Chvapil, M., Holuša, R., Kliment, K., Štoll, M., 1969. Some chemical and biological characteristics of a new collagen–polymer compound material. J. Biomed. Mater. Res. Part A 3 (2), 315–332. (Epub 2004/9/13).

Clemons, J.L., Weinstein, M., Guess, M.K., Alperin, M., Moalli, P., Gregory, W.T., et al., 2013. Impact of the 2011 FDA transvaginal mesh safety update on AUGS members' use of synthetic mesh and biological grafts in pelvic reconstructive surgery. Female Pelvic Med. Reconstr. Surg. 19 (4), 191–198.

Cobb, W.S., Burns, J.M., Kercher, K.W., Matthews, B.D., Norton, H.J., Heniford, B.T., 2005. Normal intraabdominal pressure in healthy adults. J. Surg. Res. 129, 231–235.

Collinet, P., Belot, F., Debodinance, P., Ha Duc, E., Lucot, J.P., Cosson, M., 2006. Transvaginal mesh technique for pelvic organ prolapse repair: mesh exposure management and risk factors. Int. Urogynecol. J. Pelvic Floor Dysfunct. 17 (4), 315–320. (Epub 2005/10/18).

Cosson, M., Debodinance, P., Boukerrou, M., Chauvet, M.P., Lobry, P., Crépin, G., et al., 2003. Mechanical properties of synthetic implants used in the repair of prolapse and urinary incontinence in women: Which is the ideal material? Int. Urogynecol. J. Pelvic Floor Dysfunct. 14 (3), 169–178.

Cundiff, G.W., Varner, E., Visco, A.G., Zyczynski, H.M., Nager, C.W., Norton, P.A., et al., 2008. Risk factors for mesh/suture erosion following sacrocolpopexy. Am. J. Obstet. Gynecol. 199 (6), 688. e1–688.e5.

Deffieux, X., de Tayrac, R., Huel, C., Bottero, J., Gervaise, A., Bonnet, K., et al., 2007. Vaginal mesh erosion after transvaginal repair of cystocele using Gynemesh or Gynemesh-Soft in 138 women: a comparative study. Int. Urogynecol. J. Pelvic Floor Dysfunct. 18 (1), 73–79. (Epub 2006/01/05).

DeLancey, J.O.L., 1994. The anatomy of the pelvic floor. Curr. Opin. Obstet. Gynecol. 6 (4), 313–316.

DeLancey, J.O.L., 2002. Fascial and muscular abnormalities in women with urethral hypermobility and anterior vaginal wall prolapse. Am. J. Obstetr. Gynecol. 187 (1), 93–98.

Dillion D.J., 2011. Docket No FDA-2011-N-0002: Cook Medical; (cited 303.14). This is a succinct and updated review of graft-related complications and postoperative sequelae such as pain and dyspareunia after biologic, synthetic, and standard anterior compartment repairs. Available from: <http://www.fda.gov/downloads/AdvisoryCommittees/CommitteesMeetingMaterials/MedicalDevices/MedicalDevicesAdvisoryCommittee/ObstetricsandGynecologyDevices/UCM270781.pdf>.

Discher, D.E., Janmey, P., Wang, Y.-L., 2005. Tissue cells feel and respond to the stiffness of their substrate. Science 310 (5751), 1139–1143.

Duckett, J.R., Jain, S., 2005. Groin pain after a tension-free vaginal tape or similar suburethral sling: management strategies. BJU Int. 95, 95–97.

Ellerkmann, R.M., Cundiff, G.W., Melick, C.F., Nihira, M.A., Leffler, K., Bent, A.E., 2001. Correlation of symptoms with location and severity of pelvic organ prolapse. Am. J. Obstet. Gynecol. 185 (6), 1332–1337. discussion 7–8. (Epub 2001/12/18. http://dx.doi.org/10.1067/mob.2001.119078).

Elliott, M.P., Juler, G.L., 1979. Comparison of Marlex mesh and microporous Teflon sheets when used for hernia repair in the experimental animal. Am. J. Surg. 137, 342–344.

Engelsman, A.F., van Dam, G.M., van der Mei, H.C., Busscher, H.J., Ploeg, R.J., 2010. *In vivo* evaluation of bacterial infection involving morphologically different surgical meshes. Ann. Surg. 251, 133–137.

Feola, A., Abramowitch, S., Jones, K., Stein, S., Moalli, P., 2010. Parity negatively impacts vaginal mechanical properties and collagen structure in rhesus macaques. Am. J. Obstet. Gynecol. 203 (6), 595.e1–595.e8. (Epub 2010/08/10).

Feola, A., Abramowitch, S., Jallah, Z., Stein, S., Barone, W., Palcsey, S., et al., 2013. Deterioration in biomechanical properties of the vagina following implantation of a high-stiffness prolapse mesh. BJOG An Int. J. Obstet. Gynaecol. 120 (2), 224–232.

FitzGerald, M.P., Mollenhauer, J., Brubaker, L., 2000. The antigenicity of fascia lata allografts. BJU Int. 86 (7), 826–828.

Gabriel, B., Denschlag, D., Gobel, H., et al., 2005. Uterosacral ligament in postmenopausal women with or without pelvic organ prolapse. Int. Urogynecol. J. Pelvic Floor Dysfunct. 16, 475–479.

Gandhi, S., Kubba, L.M., Abramov, Y., Botros, S.M., Goldberg, R.P., Victor, T.A., et al., 2005. Histopathologic changes of porcine dermis xenografts for transvaginal suburethral slings. Am. J. Obstet. Gynecol. 192 (S5), 1643–1648.

Gillard, J., Reed, M.W.R., Buttle, D., Cross, S.S., Brown, N.J., 2004. Matrix metalloproteinase activity and immunohistochemical profile of matrix metalloproteinase-2 and -9 and tissue inhibitor of metalloproteinase-1 during human dermal wound healing. Wound Repair Regen. 12 (3), 295–304.

Goel, V.K., Lim, T.-H., Gwon, J., Chen, J.-Y., Winterbottom, J.M., Park, J.B., et al., 1991. Effects of rigidity of an internal fixation device: a comprehensive biomechanical investigation. Spine 16 (3 Suppl.), S155–S161.

Goepel, C., Hefler, L., Methfessel, H., Koelbl, H., 2003. Periurethral connective tissue status of postmenopausal women with genital prolapse with and without stress incontinence. Acta Obstet. Gynecol. Scand. 82 (7), 659–664.

Greca, F.H., De Paula, J.B., Biondo-Simões, M.L.P., Da Costa, F.D., Da Silva, A.P.G., Time, S., et al., 2001. The influence of differing pore sizes on the biocompatibility of two polypropylene meshes in the repair of abdominal defects: experimental study in dogs. Hernia 5 (2), 59–64.

Greca, F.H., Souza-Filho, Z.A., Giovanini, A., Rubin, M.R., Kuenzer, R.F., Reese, F.B., et al., 2008. The influence of porosity on the integration histology of two polypropylene meshes for the treatment of abdominal wall defects in dogs. Hernia 12 (1), 45–49.

Hendrix, S.I., Clark, A., Nygaard, I., 2002. Pelvic organ prolapse in the women's health initiative: gravity and gravidity. Am. J. Obstet. Gynecol. 186, 1160–1166.

Hinton, R., Jinnah, R.H., Johnson, C., Warden, K., Clarke, H.J., 1992. A biomechanical analysis of solvent-dehydrated and freeze-dried human fascia lata allografts. A preliminary report. Am. J. Sports Med. 20 (5), 607–612.

Hodde, J., 2006. Extracellular matrix as a bioactive material for soft tissue reconstruction. ANZ J. Surg. 76 (12), 1096–1100.

Huiskes, R., Weinans, H., Grootenboer, H.J., Dalstra, M., Fudala, B., Slooff, T.J., 1987. Adaptive bone-remodeling theory applied to prosthetic-design analysis. J. Biomech. 20 (11–12), 1135–1150.

Iglesia, C.B., Fenner, D.E., Brubaker, L., 1997. The use of mesh in gynecologic surgery. Int. Urogynecol. J. 8, 105–115.

Jacobs, J.J., Sumner, D.R., Galante, J.O., 1993. Mechanisms of bone loss associated with total hip replacement. Orthop. Clin. North Am. 24 (4), 583–590.

Jarman-Smith, M.L., Bodamyali, T., Stevens, C., Howell, J.A., Horrocks, M., Chaudhuri, J.B., 2004. Porcine collagen crosslinking, degradation and its capability for fibroblast adhesion and proliferation. J. Mater. Sci. Mater. Med. 15 (8), 925–932.

Jones, K.A., Moalli, P.A., 2010. Pathophysiology of pelvic organ prolapse. Female Pelvic Med. Reconstr. Surg. 16 (2), 79–87.

Jones, K.A., Feola, A., Meyn, L., Abramowitch, S.D., Moalli, P.A., 2009. Tensile properties of commonly used prolapse meshes. Int. Urogynecol. J. Pelvic Floor Dysfunct. 20 (7), 847–853.

Junge, K., Binnebosel, M., von Trotha, K.T., Rosch, R., Klinge, U., Neumann, U.P., et al., 2011. Mesh biocompatibility: effects of cellular inflammation and tissue remodeling. Langenbecks Arch. Surg. 397, 255–270.

Karlovsky, M., Thakre, A., Rastinehad, A., Kushner, L., Badlani, G.H., 2005. Biomaterial for pelvic floor reconstruction. Urology 66, 469.

Kimuli, M., Eardley, I., Southgate, J., 2004. *In vitro* assessment of decellularized porcine dermis as a matrix for urinary tract reconstruction. BJU Int. 94 (6), 859–866.

Kjaer, M., Langberg, H., Miller, B.F., Boushel, R., Crameri, R., Koskinen, S., et al., 2005. Metabolic activity and collagen turnover in human tendon in response to physical activity. J. Musculoskelet. Neuronal. Interact. 5 (1), 41–52.

Klinge, U., Klosterhalfen, B., 2011. Modified classification of surgical meshes for hernia repair based on the analysis of 1000 explanted meshes. Hernia 16, 251–258. (Epub 2012/5/5).

Klinge, U., Junge, K., Spellerberg, B., Piroth, C., Klosterhalfen, B., Schumpelick, V., 2002a. Do multifilament alloplastic meshes increase the infection rate? Analysis of the polymeric surface, the bacteria adherence, and the *in vivo* consequences in a rat model. J. Biomed. Mater. Res. 63, 765–771.

Klinge, U., Junge, K., Stumpf, M., Öttinger, A.P., Klosterhalfen, B., 2002b. Functional and morphological evaluation of a low-weight monofilament polypropylene mesh for hernia repair. J. Biomed. Mater. Res. 63, 129–136.

Klinge, U., Klosterhalfen, B., Birkenhauer, V., Junge, K., Conze, J., Schumpelick, V., 2002c. Impact of polymer pore size on the interface scar formation in a rat model. J. Surg. Res. 103, 208–214.

Klinge, U., Klosterhalfen, B., Öttinger, A.P., Junge, K., Schumpelick, V., 2002d. PVDF as a new polymer for the construction of surgical meshes. Biomaterials 23 (16), 3487–3493.

Kobashi, K.C., Dmochowski, R., 1999. Erosion of woven polyester pubovaginal sling. J. Urol. 162 (2), 2070–2072.

Langberg, H., Skovgaard, D., Petersen, L.J., Bulow, J., Kjaer, M., 1999. Type 1 collagen synthesis and degradation in peritendinous tissue after exercise determined by microdialysis in humans. J. Physiol. 521, 299–306.

Lanir, Y., 1979. A structural theory for the homogeneous biaxial stress–strain relationships in flat collagenous tissues. J. Biomech. 12, 423–436.

Larsen, W.I., Yavork, J., 2007. Pelvic organ prolapse and urinary incontinence in nulliparous college women in relation to paratrooper training. Int. Urogynecol. J. 18, 769–771.

Letouzey, V., Deffieux, X., Gervaise, A., Mercier, G., Fernandez, H., de Tayrac, R., 2010. Trans-vaginal cystocele repair using a tension-free polypropylene mesh: more than 5 years of follow-up. Eur. J. Obstet. Gynecol. Reprod. Biol. 151 (1), 101–105. (Epub 2010/04/27).

Liang, R., Abramowitch, S., Knight, K., Palcsey, S., Nolfi, A., Feola, A., et al., 2013. Vaginal degeneration following implantation of synthetic mesh with increased stiffness. BJOG 120 (2), 233–243. (Epub 2012/12/18).

Lowder, J.L., Park, A.J., Ellison, R., Ghetti, C., Moalli, P., Zyczynski, H., et al., 2008. The role of apical vaginal support in the appearance of anterior and posterior vaginal prolapse. Obstet. Gynecol. 111 (1), 152–157.

Lukacz, E.S., Lawrence, J.M., Contreras, R., Nager, C.W., Luber, K.M., 2006. Parity, mode of delivery, and pelvic floor disorders. Obstet. Gynecol. 107 (6), 1253–1260.

MacLennan, A.H., Taylor, A.W., Wilson, D.H., Wilson, D., 2000. The prevalence of pelvic floor disorders and their relationship to gender, age, parity and mode of delivery. Br. J. Obstet. Gynaecol. 107 (12), 1460–1470.

Majima, T., Yasuda, K., Fujii, T., Yamamoto, N., Hayashi, K., Kaneda, K., 1996. Biomechanical effects of stress shielding of the rabbit patellar tendon depend on the degree of stress reduction. J. Orthop. Res. 14 (3), 377–383.

Mangera, A., Bullock, A.J., Roman, S., Chapple, C.R., Macneil, S., 2013. Comparison of candidate scaffolds for tissue engineering for stress urinary incontinence and pelvic organ prolapse repair. BJU Int. 112 (5), 674–685.

Manodoro, S., Endo, M., Uvin, P., Ablersen, M., Vlacil, J., Engels, A., et al., 2012. Graft-related complications and biaxial tensiometry following experimental vaginal implantation of flat mesh of variable dimensions. BJOG 120 (2), 244–250.

Mant, J., Painter, R., Vessey, M., 1997. Epidemiology of genital prolapse: observations from the oxford family planning association study. Br. J. Obstet. Gynaecol. 104 (5), 579–585.

Mattox, T.F., Stanford, E.J., Varner, E., 2004. Infected abdominal sacrocolpopexies: diagnosis and treatment. Int. Urogynecol. J. Pelvic Floor Dysfunct. 15, 319–323.

Moalli, P.A., 2006. Cadaveric fascia lata. Int. Urogynecol. J. Pelvic Floor Dysfunct. 17 (Suppl. 7), S48–S50.

Moalli, P.A., Talarico, L.C., Sung, V.W., Klingensmith, W.L., Shand, S.H., Meyn, L.A., et al., 2004. Impact of menopause on collagen subtypes in the arcus tendineous fasciae pelvis. Am. J. Obstet. Gynecol. 190 (3), 620–627.

Moalli, P.A., Shand, S.H., Zyczynski, H.M., Gordy, S.C., Meyn, L.A., 2005. Remodeling of vaginal connective tissue in patients with prolapse. Obstet. Gynecol. 106 (5 Pt 1), 953–963. (Epub 2005/11/02).

Moalli, P.A., Papas, N., Menefee, S., Albo, M., Meyn, L., Abramowitch, S.D., 2008. Tensile properties of five commonly used mid-urethral slings relative to the TVT. Int. Urogynecol. J. Pelvic Floor Dysfunct. 19 (5), 655–663.

Mosser, D.M., Edwards, J.P., 2008. Exploring the full spectrum of macrophage activation. Nat. Rev. Immunol. 8 (12), 958–969. (Epub 2008/11/26).

Muhl, T., Binnebosel, M., Klinge, U., Goedderz, T., 2007. New objective measurement to characterize the porosity of textile implants. J. Biomed. Mater. Res. Part B Appl. Biomater., 176–183.

Muir, T.W., Aspera, A.M., Rackley, R.R., et al., 2004. Recurrent pelvic organ prolapse in a women with bladder exstrophy: a case report of surgical management and review of the literature. Int. Urogynecol. J. Pelvic Floor Dysfunct. 15, 436–438.

Noakes, N.F., Pullan, A.J., Bissett, I.P., Cheng, L.K., 2008. Subject specific finite elasticity simulations of the pelvic floor. J. Biomech. 41, 3060–3065.

Nolfi A.L., Brown B., Palcsey S.L., Turner L.C., Moalli P. (Eds.), 2014. An M1 Pro-inflammatory Profile Persists in Tissue Excised from Women with Mesh Complications Years After Mesh Insertion. AUGS/IUGA Scientific Meeting, Washington, DC.

Nygaard I. (Ed.), 2012. A 7-Year Follow Up Study of Abdominal Sacrocolpopexy with and Without BURCH Urethropexy: The Extended Colpopexy and Urinary Reduction Efforts Study. 33rd Annual American Urogynecologic Society Meeting, Chicago, IL.

Nygaard, I., McCreery, R., Brubaker, L., Connolly, A., Cundiff, G., Weber, A.M., et al., 2004. Abdominal sacrocolpopexy: a comprehensive review. Am. Coll. Obstet. Gynecol. 104 (4), 805–823.

Nygaard, I., Barber, M.D., Burgio, K.L., Kenton, K., Meikle, S., Schaffer, J., et al., 2008. Prevalence of symptomatic pelvic floor disorders in US women. JAMA 200 (11), 1311–1316. (Epub 2008/09/19).

Nygaard, I., Brubaker, L., Zyczynski, H.M., Cundiff, G., Richter, H., Gantz, M., et al., 2013. Long-term outcomes following abdominal sacrocolpopexy for pelvic organ prolapse. JAMA 309 (19), 2016–2024. Available from: http://dx.doi.org/10.1001/jama.2013.4919.

Olsen, A.L., Smith, V.J., Bergstrom, J.O., Colling, J.C., Clark, A.L., 1997. Epidemiology of surgically managed pelvic organ prolapse and urinary incontinence. Obstet. Gynecol. 89 (4), 501–506. (Epub 1997/04/01).

Orringer, J.S., Kang, S., Johnson, T.M., Karimipour, D.J., Hamilton, T., Hammerberg, C., et al., 2004. Connective tissue remodeling induced by carbon dioxide laser resurfacing of photodamaged human skin. Arch. Dermatol. 140 (11), 1326–1332.

Otto, J., Kaldenhoff, E., Kirschner-Harmanns, R., Muhl, T., Klinge, U., 2014. Elongation of textile pelvic floor implants under load is related to complete loss of effective porosity, thereby favoring incorporation in scar plates. J. Biomed. Mater. Res. Part A 102 (4), 1079–1084. http://dx.doi.org/10.1002/jbm.a.34767. (Epub 2013 Jun 11).

Ozog, Y., Konstantinovic, M.L., Werbrouck, E., De Ridder, D., Mazza, E., Deprest, J., 2011. Persistence of polypropylene mesh anisotropy after implantation: an experimental study. BJOG An Int. J. Obstet. Gynaecol. 118 (10), 1180–1185.

Patel, B.N., Lucioni, A., Kobashi, K.C., 2012a. Anterior pelvic organ prolapse repair using synthetic mesh. Curr. Urol. Rep. (13), 211–215. (Epub 2012/5/6).

Patel, H., Ostergard, D., Sternschuss, G., 2012b. Polypropylene mesh and the host response. Int. Urogynecol. J. Pelvic Floor Dysfunct. 23 (6), 669–679.

Petros, P.E., Ulmsten, U., 1997. Role of the pelvic floor in bladder neck opening and closure I: muscle forces. Int. Urogynecol. J. Pelvic Floor Dysfunct. 8 (2), 74–80.

Petros, P.E.P., Woodman, P.J., 2008. The integral theory of continence. Int. Urogynecol. J. Pelvic Floor Dysfunct. 19 (1), 35–40.

Pierce, L.M., Rao, A., Baumann, S.S., Glassberg, J.E., Kuehl, T.J., Muir, T.W., 2009. Long-term histologic response to synthetic and biologic graft materials implanted in the vagina and abdomen of a rabbit model. Am. J. Obstet. Gynecol. 200 (5), 546.e1–546.e8 (Epub 2009/03/17).

Plaas, A.H.K., Wong-Palms, S., Koob, T., Hernandez, D., Marchuk, L., Frank, C.B., 2000. Proteoglycan metabolism during repair of the ruptured medial collateral ligament in skeletally mature rabbits. Arch. Biochem. Biophys. 374 (1), 35–41.

Rodrigues Macield da Fonseca, A.M., Vale de Castro Monteiro, M., Mello de Figueiredo, E., Cardoso, F.A., Lopes da Silva Filho, A., 2013. Factors influencing the incidence of mesh erosion after transobturator sling placement for stress urinary incontinence. J. Gynecol. Surg. 29 (5), 231–234.

Rubash, H.E., Sinha, R., Shanbhag, A.S., Kim, S.-Y., 1998. Pathogenesis of bone loss after total hip arthroplasty. Orthop. Clin. North Am. 29 (2), 173–186.

Shepherd, J.P., Feola, A.J., Abramowitch, S.D., Moalli, P.A., 2012. Uniaxial biomechanical properties of seven different vaginally implanted meshes for pelvic organ prolapse. Int. Urogynecol. J. Pelvic Floor Dysfunct. 23 (5), 613–620.

Simon, U., Augat, P., Ignatius, A., Claes, L., 2003. Influence of the stiffness of bone defect implants on the mechanical conditions at the interface—a finite element analysis with contact. J. Biomech. 36 (8), 1079–1086.

Söderberg, M.W., Falconer, C., Bystrom, B., Malmström, A., Ekman, G., 2004. Young women with genital prolapse have a low collagen concentration. Acta Obstet. Gynecol. Scand. 83 (12), 1193–1198.

Soergel, T.M., Shott, S., Heit, M., 2001. Poor surgical outcomes after fascia lata allograft slings. Int. Urogynecol. J. Pelvic Floor Dysfunct. 12 (4), 247–253.

Spalazzi, J.P., Dagher, E., Doty, S.B., Guo, X.E., Rodeo, S.A., Lu, H.H., 2008. In vivo evaluation of a multiphased scaffold designed for orthopaedic interface tissue engineering and soft tissue-to-bone integration. J. Biomed. Mater. Res. Part A 86 (1), 1–12.

Subak, L.L., Waetjen, L.E., van den Eeden, S., Thom, D.H., Vittinghoff, E., Brown, J.S., 2001. Cost of pelvic organ prolapse surgery in the United States. Obstet. Gynecol. 98 (4), 646–651. (Epub 2001/09/29).

Swift, S.E., 2000. The distribution of pelvic organ support in a population of female subjects seen for routine gynecologic health care. Am. J. Obstet. Gynecol. 183 (2), 277–285. (Epub 2000/08/15).

Sze, E.H.M., Meranus, J., Kohli, N., Miklos, J.R., Karram, M.M., 2001. Vaginal configuration on MRI after abdominal sacrocolpopexy and sacrospinous ligament suspension. Int. Urogynecol. J. Pelvic Floor Dysfunct. 12 (6), 375–380.

Sze, E.H.M., Sherard III, G.B., Dolezal, J.M., 2002. Pregnancy, labor, delivery, and pelvic organ prolapse. Obstet. Gynecol. 100 (5), 981–986.

Thomopoulos, S., Williams, G.R., Gimbel, J.A., Favata, M., Soslowsky, L.J., 2003. Variation of biomechanical, structural, and compositional properties along the tendon to bone insertion site. J. Orthop. Res. 21 (3), 413–419.

Ulmsten, U., Henriksson, I., Johnson, P., Varhos, G., 1996. An ambulatory surgical procedure under local anesthesia for treatment of female urinary incontinence. Int. Urogynecol. J. Pelvic Floor Dysfunct. 7 (2), 81–86.

U.S. Food and Drug Administration. 2008, October 20. Serious complications associated with transvaginal placement of surgical mesh in repair of pelvic organ prolapse and stress urinary incontinence. Retrieved from: <http://www.fda.gov/MedicalDevices/Safety/AlertsandNotices/PublicHealthNotifications/ucm061976.htm>.

U.S. Food and Drug Administration. 2011, July 13. Surgical placement of mesh to repair pelvic organ prolapse poses risks. Retrieved from: <http://www.fda.gov/NewsEvents/Newsroom/PressAnnouncements/ucm262752.htm>.

Walters, M.D., Karram, M.M., 1993. Clinical Urogynecology. Mosby- Year Book Inc., St. Louis, MO.

Weinberger, M.W., Ostergard, D.R., 1995. Long-term clinical and urodynamic evaluation of polytetrafluoroethylene sling for treatment of genuine stress incontinence. Obstet. Gynecol. 86, 92–96.

Weyhe, D., Schmitz, I., Belyaev, O., Garbs, R., Muller, K.M., Uhl, W., et al., 2006. Experimental comparison of monofile light and heavy polypropylene meshes: less weight does not mean less biological response. World J. Surg. 30 (8), 1586–1591.

Yeung, T., Georges, P.C., Flanagan, L.A., Marg, B., Ortiz, M., Funaki, M., et al., 2005. Effects of substrate stiffness on cell morphology, cytoskeletal structure, and adhesion. Cell Motil. Cytoskeleton 60 (1), 24–34.

Zong, W., Jallah, Z.C., Stein, S.E., Abramowitch, S.D., Moalli, P.A., 2010a. Repetitive mechanical stretch increases extracellular collagenase activity in vaginal fibroblasts. Female Pelvic Med. Reconstr. Surg. 16 (5), 257–262. (Epub 2011/05/24).

Zong, W., Stein, S.E., Starcher, B., Meyn, L.A., Moalli, P.A., 2010b. Alteration of vaginal elastin metabolism in women with pelvic organ prolapse. Obstet. Gynecol. 115 (5), 953–961. (Epub 2010/04/23).

CHAPTER 14

Methods Used to Evaluate the Host Responses to Medical Implants *In Vivo*

David W. Baker, Jun Zhou and Liping Tang
Bioengineering Department, University of Texas at Arlington, Arlington, TX, USA

Contents

INTRODUCTION

All medical implants prompt varying degrees of inflammatory tissue reactions and fibrosis which may, in chronic conditions, lead to the failure of the implant or device (Tang and Eaton, 1995). While the events surrounding implant failure are complex and convoluted, it is generally agreed that such processes begin with implant-mediated fibrin clot formation followed by acute inflammatory responses (Tang and Eaton, 1995, 1999). Cellular-mediated signals from neutrophils and mast cells propagate this preliminary response. Neutrophils release a large amount of granular enzymes and reactive oxygen species (ROS) including hydrogen peroxide and superoxide anions (Kasahara et al., 1997; Okusa, 2002). Mast cells are known granulocytic cells which release a multitude of factors, most importantly histamine (Eming et al., 2007). Histamine functions as a vasoactive mediator increasing capillary permeability leading to further translocation of plasma constituents,

Host Response to Biomaterials.
DOI: http://dx.doi.org/10.1016/B978-0-12-800196-7.00014-1

such as fibrinogen, and cellular migration to the tissue sites. The inflammatory response may then become exacerbated through continuous cytokine and chemokine release from adherent immune cells triggering further migration signals of macrophages (MΦs) and fibroblasts. This hyperactivity may also lead to tissue acidosis of the surrounding inflamed tissue (Mainnemare et al., 2004). MΦs then dominate the response driving many interwoven reactions leading to chronic inflammation, extracellular matrix (ECM) production, fibrosis, and eventual implant failure.

The events surrounding the successful integration of biomaterials and host tissue remains largely elusive due mainly to the complexity of the host tissue response. While substantial progress has been made on the production of a wide variety of bioactive materials, significant efforts have been placed in recent years on the development of methods to evaluate and monitor the host response. While the traditional methods of histological, analytical, and immunohistochemical analysis remain the "gold standards," there is a compelling need to develop faster, more cost-effective, noninvasive, and real-time strategies to analyze biomaterial-mediated tissue reactions. Several noninvasive imaging techniques including computed tomography, magnetic resonance imaging (MRI) (McAteer et al., 2007), positron emission tomography (PET) (Zhuang and Alavi, 2002), and ultrasonography (Lindner et al., 2000) have been developed to visualize and quantify inflammatory responses and infection *in vivo*; however, these technologies rely primarily on structural changes (Tsai et al., 2014a), making them inept at monitoring acute, nontraumatic, and localized host inflammatory reactions. In order to determine specific inflammatory cellular responses, more cost-effective optical imaging approaches utilizing fluorescence, chemiluminescence, or ratiometric techniques to investigate the cellular, protein-mediated, and biochemical cues of the host tissue response are being investigated. In this chapter, we summarize both traditional and emerging techniques used to evaluate the host response to biomaterial implants.

EX VIVO METHODS TO EVALUATE THE HOST RESPONSE

The histological approach

Histological stains such as Hematoxylin and Eosin (H&E), Masson trichrome, Wright's stain, and countless others are by far the most common and well-accepted "gold standards" in evaluation of the host response. These methods provide us with the tools to analyze almost any part of the tissue response at a single time point and a single tissue location at a time. Tissue sections are fixed, embedded, sectioned, stained, coversliped and finally analyzed under an optical microscope. The data must then be collected in replicates for each test subject or sample, repeated at each time point in the study, images from the microscope collected, and lastly the data can be compiled and analyzed. The entire process is then often repeated, as many times as necessary, with alternate stains to determine alternate factors. The process continues to be time-consuming, cumbersome, and repetitive, despite the assistance (when available) of automated tissue sectioning and staining processes. General histological stains like H&E are the most common, providing an overall picture of the host response from which data such as the capsule thickness or a cellular count of the foreign body response (FBR) may be determined (Baker et al., 2011). More specific stains can be used to identify cell types or certain characteristics of the response, such as staining with toluidine blue for mast cells (Tang et al., 1998; Thevenot et al., 2011) or proteins such as collagens with Masson trichrome (Baker et al., 2011). While histology often provides clear visual delineation and qualitative assessment, quantitative results are often difficult to achieve.

Analytical techniques and immunohistochemistry

Alternatives to traditional histology include numerous analytical techniques that can provide more quantitative analysis of specific molecular, cellular, and tissue characteristics. For instance, specific assays such as Sircol or hydroxyproline can determine collagen content in tissues or production by cells. Other techniques such as immunohistochemistry (IHC) can be used to detect the specific types of cells and cellular products in tissue at different time points. However, the same pitfalls as in histological staining occur. The use of fluorescently tagged antibodies has become a vital methodology for identifying cells, biomarkers, and proteins and is further enhanced by the use of techniques such as flow cytometry. As a method to evaluate the host response however, sample biopsies are continually needed to provide a kinetic analysis, significantly limiting the approach. Finally, enzyme-linked immunosorbent assays (ELISA) may be used to detect various components in the solubilized tissues as body fluids. The downside of these techniques however is that they do not offer real-time delineation of processes and are often tedious, requiring additional steps such as tissue digestion or continuous and multiple biopsies. Beyond these individual methods, a combinational approach may also be taken.

Combinational approaches

The main reason the above mentioned *ex vivo* methods remain the gold standards despite their tediousness is that they provide validation for the *in vivo* studies. For instance, the degree of implant-associated neutrophil responses may be quantified by either myeloperoxidase enzyme measurement (Tang and Eaton, 1993; Tang et al., 1993), histological staining for neutrophils (Lefer et al., 1998; Josefsson et al., 1992), or through IHC. As in most cases with histological analysis, there are multiple ways to determine a single aspect thereby validating one method or another. The histological techniques may be combined to gain insight regarding a relationship or correlation such as that presented in Figure 14.1. In this example, histological techniques are combined with immunolabeling of cell types to determine a correlation between a specific cell type and an associated histological response.

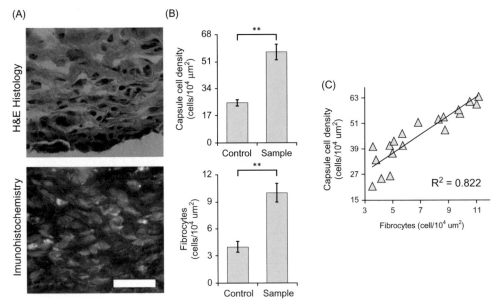

Figure 14.1 The histological approach. (A) H&E and IHC images of the FBR and fibrocyte accumulation surrounding a PDMS implant, respectively. The scale bar shows 50 μm. (B) Resultant average counts for the total capsule cell density and the specifically stained fibrocytes for a control and test sample, $**P < 0.01$. (C) Correlation between fibrocytes and the cell density across all the samples in the study based on IHC and H&E staining, respectively. (*Adapted from Baker et al., 2011*).

Emerging methodologies

While *ex vivo* methods are vital to the analysis of the host response, several inherent limitations exist. Kinetics-based approaches require numerous animals to obtain sufficient tissue samples and statistically significant results at various time points, which in turn increases the amount of labor, time, and cost for large-scale investigations of material properties and mechanisms. To reduce extraneous costs, smaller studies may be performed; however, with an insufficient number of animals, misleading conclusions may be drawn. The need therefore exists for rapid, accurate, and cost-effective strategies to enable the assessment of the host response to biomaterials. Several promising strategies have recently emerged as a means to detect and monitor various aspects of the host response such as protein deposition, pH change, ROS imaging, and cell-specific monitoring. Of these strategies, several particle-based sensors have been developed for a wide range of applications in biological research and clinical diagnosis (McNamara et al., 2001; Xu et al., 2001; Tan et al., 2004; Wang et al., 2005). Herein, we present an introduction to a few methods which offer an evaluation strategy in a continuous, noninvasive, real-time manner.

EARLY DETECTION OF MOLECULAR CUES AND EVENTS

Host protein deposition and the resultant immune responses

Fibrinogen/fibrin accumulation is known to be an instigating step in triggering host responses such as coagulation, inflammation, and infection (Hu et al., 2001; Tang and Eaton, 1993, 1999; Smiley et al., 2001). The localized fibrin deposition is generally accepted to be responsible for localized immune cell recruitment through expression of adhesion-promoting receptors (Languino et al., 1993; Altieri et al., 1988; Loike et al., 1991). Several studies have investigated methods to detect fibrin deposition at localized sites of inflammation using short fibrin-specific peptides and agents such as gadolinium for MRI-based imaging (Pan et al., 2008; Botnar et al., 2004; Overoye-Chan et al., 2008). Others have gone further combining an MRI with fluorescently tagged peptide functionalized particles for dual monitoring modalities (McCarthy et al., 2009). A recent study investigated a more novel approach to fibrin deposition as a means to determine the degree of implant-associated mast cell activation (Tsai et al., 2014b). In this study, a near infrared (NIR) peptide-specific fibrin-affinity probe was used to detect the extent of implant-associated fibrin deposition. This technique was accomplished around various particle implants, as well as under direct mast cell stimulation with chemical agent compound 48/80, and in mast cell deficient mice (Figure 14.2). This study determined that real-time evaluation of fibrin deposition may serve as an indicator for mast cell activation as well as rapid assessment of a biomaterials' tissue compatibility (Tsai et al., 2014b).

Detecting ROS

The accumulation of phagocytic cells such as neutrophils, MΦs, mast cells, dendritic cells, and others is a hallmark of inflammation and inflammatory process. As this cell accumulation occurs, ROS are produced most notably by polymorphonuclear neutrophils (PMNs) (Zhou et al., 2012a). PMNs activate a respiratory burst releasing superoxide, hydrogen peroxide, and hyperchlorous acid, resulting in oxidative killing of microorganisms and cells alike (Greenhalgh, 1998). Due to the extent of ROS production, ROS offers a distinctive method to monitor inflammatory reactions for prognosis and implant assessment. Several methods have targeted ROS production including electron paramagnetic resonance, fluorescence, and chemiluminescence detection (Hirayama et al., 2005; Panizzi et al., 2009; Kielland et al., 2009). Chemiluminescence is uniquely suited for detection of ROS generation as emitted light is produced upon the biological reactions with minimal background interference and emission quantification at the single-photon level (Zhou et al., 2012a). A recent study designed such a probe using L-012 (Zhou et al., 2012a), a luminal derivative with improved sensitivity toward ROS compared to other ROS probes such as luminal and lucigenin (Daiber et al., 2004a,b). This study found that the L-012 probe had an

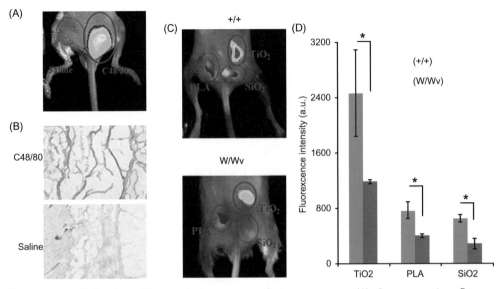

Figure 14.2 Fibrin deposition and immune mediate responses. (A) Representative fluorescence imaging of the enhanced fibrin signal from mast cell stimulation by compound 48/80. (B) Immunohistological staining verifies the enhanced fibrin deposition by compound 48/80. (C) Imaging of PLA, titanium oxide (TiO$_2$), and silicone oxide (SiO$_2$) particles implanted in wild type (+/+) or mast cell deficient mice (W/Wv). (D) Corresponding fluorescence intensities showing the reduced accumulation of fibrin probes in mast cell deficient mice. *$P < 0.05$. *(Adapted from Tsai et al., 2014b)*.

improved reliable signal for noninvasive detection of ROS *in vivo* (Zhou et al., 2012a). By using various models, the investigators determined that the chemiluminescence signal may be used to monitor and assess the kinetics of inflammatory reactions over time. Additionally, investigation into several types of inflammatory reactions including allergy-mediated inflammatory responses, device-associated FBRs, and infection studies, they demonstrate that chemiluminescence of ROS production is a valuable method for evaluating the host response.

Measuring changes in pH

Left unchecked, inflammatory reactions often lead to tissue acidosis and cell death within the localized host tissue response. Inflamed tissue and malignant tumors are often found with a high hydrogen ion concentration resulting in a very low pH, down to approximately pH 5.4 in inflammation, and even a pH of 4.7 in fracture-related hematomas (Steen et al., 1995; Reeh and Steen, 1996). Several studies suggest that acidification of diseased tissues is tied to inflammatory products such as ROS, hypochloric acid, and hydrogen peroxide (Mainnemare et al., 2004; Conus and Simon, 2008; Whiteman and Spencer, 2008). Therefore, the ability to monitor the pH shift

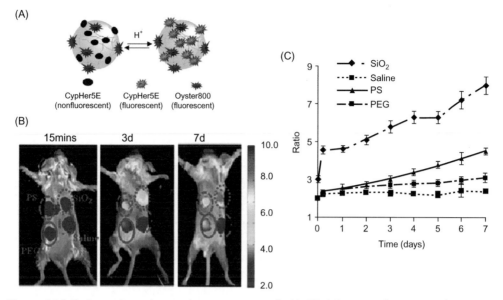

Figure 14.3 Ratiometric probes and measurement of pH. (A) Schematic illustration of PNIPAM–CypHer5E–Oyster800 pH sensors. (B) Ratiometric imaging of mice implanted with different nanosphere made of silicone oxide (SiO_2), polystyrene (PS), PEG, or saline at various time points (15 min, 3 days, and 7 days after implantation). (C) The observed ratiometric change at the implantation site over time. *(Adapted from Tsai et al., 2014a).*

within the host tissue response could be invaluable for determining the progression of an inflammatory state. With this goal in mind, several pH-sensitive dyes have been developed (Andreev et al., 2007; Carmo et al., 2008). However, the dyes have limited capabilities for use *in vivo* due to high diffusion in and out of cells and tissues at various rates. To overcome these limitations, an imaging probe has recently been developed which combines a pH-sensitive dye (CypHer5E) with a pH-insensitive dye (Oyster800) to monitor the ratio of fluorescent intensities at the respective wavelengths of the dyes (Tsai et al., 2014a) (Figure 14.3A). This approach allows for continuous *in vivo* monitoring of pH changes with minimal disruption from sensor concentration (ratio of the two wavelengths will remain the same with a change in concentration). In this study, both dyes were covalently linked to poly(*N*-isopropylacrylamide) (PNIPAM) nanospheres to prolong diffusion and retention within the tissue (Tsai et al., 2014a). The study found that not only were the ratiometric probes suitable for *in situ* use, but they can be used to monitor changes due to anti-inflammatory agents and biomaterial implants *in vivo* (Tsai et al., 2014a). Part of this study is described in Figure 14.3 whereby the pH change is monitored around several different particle implants with associated various degrees of inflammation. The extent of the histological change was also shown to correlate with histological results.

METHODS TO EVALUATE INNATE IMMUNE RESPONSES LEADING TO INFLAMMATION AND FIBROSIS

Evaluation of cell-specific responses, neutrophils

It has long been suggested that accumulation of activated neutrophils around biomaterial implants may lead to increased fibrotic reactions and tissue damage (Freeman et al., 2009; Hoemann et al., 2010). Additionally, the impaired bactericidal activities of implant-associated neutrophils are thought to be involved in the pathogenesis of device-centered infection (Kaplan et al., 1999). Neutrophil activity, as an integral part of the host response, is commonly monitored by enzyme measurements and histological evaluation. However, these methods cannot accurately depict dynamic cellular responses. Several imaging methods have therefore been investigated to monitor neutrophil migration. For instance, two-photon microscopy and time-lapse imaging haven shown neutrophil migration in the lungs of mechanically ventilated mice (Kreisel et al., 2010). A leukotriene LTB4 receptor antagonist was shown to exhibit neutrophil targeting and was developed for imaging acute myocardium inflammation (Riou et al., 2002). Additionally, chemotactic peptide receptor agonists were found useful for imaging infection and associated inflammatory cell accumulation *in vivo* (Babich et al., 1997; van der Laken et al., 1997). Finally, several optical imaging systems using various peptides such as cinnamoyl-Phe-(D)Leu-Phe-(D)Leu-Phe (cFLFLF), or formyl-methionyl-leucylphenylalanine (FMLF) peptide have been utilized to target the formyl peptide receptor of neutrophils (Locke et al., 2009; Xiao et al., 2010). Careful selection of peptides is necessary to avoid unwanted side effects such as inducing neutropenia (Xiao et al., 2010; Locke et al., 2009). The peptides may additionally be coupled to NIR dyes and polyethylene glycol (PEG) polymers to improve the hydrophilicity of the probe providing enhanced efficacy. These methods have been used to detect severe neutrophil-associated lung inflammation and infection (Xiao et al., 2010; Zhang et al., 2010), as well as the degree of neutrophil recruitment to medical-device-associated FBRs and infection (Figure 14.4) (Zhou et al., 2012b). The use of PEG polymers as carriers may not only enhance nanoprobe hydrophilicity, but also reduce nonspecific binding, improve bioavailability and clearance *in vivo* (Suzuki et al., 1984; Healy et al., 2004). While optical imaging enables quick, noninvasive real-time imaging, it is still plagued by low tissue penetration depth, thus limiting the clinical application. Conjugation with radionucleotides and PET or MRI may therefore be needed to enhance clinical application.

MΦs and the alteration of phenotype

MΦs are critical to host defense. MΦs are phagocytic cells which seek out and destroy potential pathogens. Therefore, it is not all that surprising that when MΦs encounter a "foreign" implant, they treat it as a pathogen and, arguably, prompt the most essential

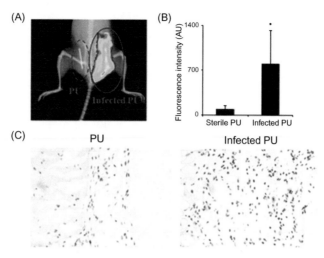

Figure 14.4 In an infected polyurethane (PU) catheter inflammation model, PU catheters were colonized with luciferase transgene *Staphylococcus aureus* and then transplanted subcutaneously on the back of mice. After 1 day, the mice were injected by tail vein with formyl peptide receptor-targeting probes. Fluorescence images were taken 3 h postinjection. (A) Representative fluorescence image reveals formyl peptide receptor-targeting probe accumulation at the surrounding area of infected PU catheters. (B) Quantification analysis of fluorescence intensity shows that 8.8 times higher fluorescence intensity from the infected catheters versus the controls ($P < 0.05$). (C) Immunohistochemical staining of neutrophils (400×) reveals that significantly higher numbers of neutrophils accumulated around the infected PU catheters compared to sterile catheters.

and dominating reactions in the host response. When the pathogen is a nondegradable implant which cannot be destroyed, the result is chronic inflammation and regenerative capabilities. Quantifying the degree of MΦ activation may therefore be a vital strategy to assess the extent of inflammation in disease models as well as around biomaterial implants. Some studies have investigated via fluorescently tagging MΦ antibodies to image MΦ recruitment at implant sites (Bratlie et al., 2010). Another investigation sought to monitor inflammatory responses by developing a folate-targeting NIR nanoprobe (Zhou et al., 2011), as the folate receptor is known to be overexpressed on activated MΦ (Low et al., 2008; Hilgenbrink and Low, 2005). These studies, and others, have indicated that targeting MΦs with indicator probes is a viable method for quantifying degree of inflammatory reactions.

In normal tissue repair, as opposed to chronic stimulation, MΦs are observed to shift along a spectrum of activation from one functional phenotype to another termed MΦ polarization (Stout and Suttles, 2004). Chapter 6 provides an in-depth discussion of MΦ phenotypes. At the opposing ends of this spectrum, MΦs have typically been classified as M1 (classical activation) or M2 (alternative activation) and tend to act (in a general sense) as pro-inflammatory or regulation, respectively, influencing both tissue destruction and regeneration (Martinez et al., 2008; Stout and Suttles, 2004). Therefore as a means to evaluate the normal host response, a method which could quantify not only the classically activated inflammatory MΦ response but the regulatory MΦ response as well would significantly aid in determining the biocompatibility or regenerative capabilities of an implant, device, or disease state. A recent study examining the role of MΦs in the remodeling response of surgical mesh used histological methods to investigate an M2/M1 ratio for various implants (Brown et al., 2012). The investigators determined that an increased M2/M1 ratio was associated with more positive remodeling outcomes, providing support to the MΦ polarization paradigm. Presently, a dual imaging probe modality was developed to monitor MΦ polarization *in vivo*.

As previously discussed, M1 inflammatory MΦs are known to have an increased expression of folate receptor. Similarly, M2 MΦs express high levels of the mannose receptor which is up-regulated by regulatory cytokines such as interleukin-4 (IL-4), IL-10, and IL-13 (Martinez-Pomares et al., 2003; Gordon, 2003; Stein et al., 1992). To further investigate the process of MΦ polarization and determine if an M2/M1 ratio could be utilized *in vivo* to monitor biocompatibility, analogous imaging probes were developed coupling NIR indicators to target MΦ folate and mannose receptors (Baker et al., 2014). This study identifies the shifting patterns of polarized MΦs *in vitro*, as well as *in vivo* around both prominent changes in an infection model and very subtle changes such as various biomaterial implants. Figure 14.5 presents an imaging analysis performed on two biocompatible polymeric particle implants Poly-L-lactic acid (PLA) and PNIPAM. Both materials are commonly employed biocompatible microparticles for tissue engineering. PLA microparticles are known to elicit an inflammatory response (Jiang et al., 2007) where PNIPAM has shown milder tissue reactivity (Weng et al., 2004). This study demonstrates that subtle changes in the MΦ response, such as the shifting of polarized phenotypes, may be determined *in vivo* in real time. The noninvasive characterization of such processes may provide a critical step forward as a method to determine the host response.

MATHEMATICAL MODELING AND PREDICTION METHODS

Despite intensive research efforts in wound healing, few methods are currently able to systematically predict the dynamic behavior of immunological and inflammatory reactions. With the goal of forecasting outcomes of tissue responses to biomaterials, mathematical modeling may offer unique insight through a kinetics-based approach to analyze the outcome of complex reactions of cells/proteins and biochemical processes (Dale et al., 1996; Dallon et al., 2001; Lemon et al., 2009). For instance, surface-mediated and acute inflammatory responses are known to propagate a gradient release of growth factors into the surrounding tissue. This reaction, which results in

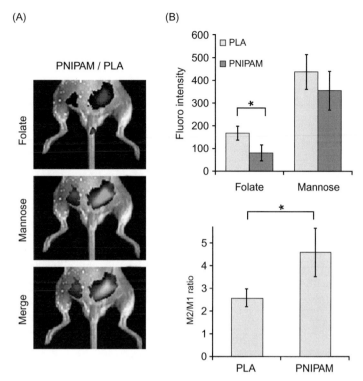

Figure 14.5 MΦ polarization paradigm showing M1 and M2 imaging probe assessment in a biomaterial response. (A) Imaging analysis of PNIPAM (left side of mouse) and PLA (right side of mouse) implants at 4 days showing the separate and merged NIR fluorescence channels. (B) Bar graphs of relative fluorescence intensity and M2/M1 ratio. Statistics were performed with the student's *t*-test and show *$P < 0.05$. *(Adapted from Baker et al., 2014).*

the migration of various cell types toward the implant, may be captured in essence by either mathematical chemotactic equations in a continuum model or cell motion equations of discrete cells in multiscale models (Su et al., 2011). The initial cell recruitment results in greater and more diverse cell recruitment which may be further modeled by chemotactic equations (Mantzaris et al., 2004). Such predictive models based on biochemical and biophysical mechanisms have previously been developed for analysis of treatments (Schugart et al., 2008). In the same way, modeling the host inflammatory and fibrotic response is possible. A recent study investigated expanding previous mathematical models to "forecast" the process of foreign body reactions by considering several features of MΦs, treating MΦ as either a continuum or as discrete cells. They found that discrete cell modeling of MΦ is capable of showing very interesting development patterns of the healing process, while continuum modeling provides good estimation of average cell behaviors (Su et al., 2011). For this reason, a multiscale model approach was conducted combining the continuous modeling for the cellular and chemical fields along with discrete modeling for limited cell numbers (Su et al., 2011). By using this multivariate approach, the model can predict the trends of MΦ migration, collagen production, and enzyme regulation in FBRs. The advantage of such models lies in the systematic approach to evaluating multiple variables and complex interactions. Furthermore, such models may be used to evaluate multiscale kinetic responses to identify critical time points for treatment applications to alter the fibrotic outcomes of the host response.

CONCLUSION AND SUMMARY

The immunological and inflammatory reactions of the host response have long been known to be critical determinants of medical device success or failure. The methods used to interpret these reactions are therefore critical to the future development of implants, treatments, and regenerative strategies in tissue engineering. The histologic methods used to identify trends in the host response provide a solid foundation upon which to grow. Although limited and time-consuming, histology will continue to provide the verification required to develop more rapid, noninvasive, and cost-efficient technologies. By identifying specific characteristics of the host response and targeting our methods at the clear delineation of chemical-, biological-, and cellular-mediated processes, large-scale studies become more rapid, and materials and treatments become easier to develop. Many of the mechanisms driving the host response are well known. The continued development of methods which push the envelope and shorten the gap of evaluation and analysis of medical devices will continue to improve.

REFERENCES

Altieri, D.C., Bader, R., Mannucci, P.M., Edgington, T.S., 1988. Oligospecificity of the cellular adhesion receptor Mac-1 encompasses an inducible recognition specificity for fibrinogen. J. Cell. Biol. 107 (5), 1893–1900.

Andreev, O.A., Dupuy, A.D., Segala, M., Sandugu, S., Serra, D.A., Chichester, C.O., et al., 2007. Mechanism and uses of a membrane peptide that targets tumors and other acidic tissues *in vivo*. Proc. Natl. Acad. Sci. USA 104 (19), 7893–7898.

Babich, J.W., Tompkins, R.G., Graham, W., Barrow, S.A., Fischman, A.J., 1997. Localization of radiolabeled chemotactic peptide at focal sites of *Escherichia coli* infection in rabbits: evidence for a receptor-specific mechanism. J. Nucl. Med. 38 (8), 1316–1322.

Baker, D.W., Liu, X., Weng, H., Luo, C., Tang, L., 2011. Fibroblast/fibrocyte: surface interaction dictates tissue reactions to micropillar implants. Biomacromolecules 12 (4), 997–1005.

Baker, D.W., Zhou, J., Tsai, Y.T., Patty, K.M., Weng, H., Tang, E.N., et al., 2014. Development of optical probes for *in vivo* imaging of polarized macrophages during foreign body reactions. Acta. Biomater 10 (7), 2945–2955. PMCID: 4041819.

Botnar, R.M., Perez, A.S., Witte, S., Wiethoff, A.J., Laredo, J., Hamilton, J., et al., 2004. *In vivo* molecular imaging of acute and subacute thrombosis using a fibrin-binding magnetic resonance imaging contrast agent. Circulation 109 (16), 2023–2029.

Bratlie, K.M., Dang, T.T., Lyle, S., Nahrendorf, M., Weissleder, R., Langer, R., et al., 2010. Rapid biocompatibility analysis of materials via *in vivo* fluorescence imaging of mouse models. PLoS. One. 5 (4), e10032.

Brown, B.N., Londono, R., Tottey, S., Zhang, L., Kukla, K.A., Wolf, M.T., et al., 2012. Macrophage phenotype as a predictor of constructive remodeling following the implantation of biologically derived surgical mesh materials. Acta. Biomater. 8 (3), 978–987.

Carmo, V.A., Ferrari, C.S., Reis, E.C., Ramaldes, G.A., Pereira, M.A., De Oliveira, M.C., et al., 2008. Biodistribution study and identification of inflammation sites using 99mTc-labelled stealth pH-sensitive liposomes. Nucl. Med. Commun. 29 (1), 33–38.

Conus, S., Simon, H.U., 2008. Cathepsins: key modulators of cell death and inflammatory responses. Biochem. Pharmacol. 76 (11), 1374–1382.

Daiber, A., August, M., Baldus, S., Wendt, M., Oelze, M., Sydow, K., et al., 2004a. Measurement of NAD(P)H oxidase-derived superoxide with the luminol analogue L-012. Free Radic. Biol. Med. 36 (1), 101–111.

Daiber, A., Oelze, M., August, M., Wendt, M., Sydow, K., Wieboldt, H., et al., 2004b. Detection of superoxide and peroxynitrite in model systems and mitochondria by the luminol analogue L-012. Free Radic. Res. 38 (3), 259–269.

Dale, P.D., Sherratt, J.A., Maini, P.K., 1996. A mathematical model for collagen fibre formation during foetal and adult dermal wound healing. Proc. Biol. Sci. 263 (1370), 653–660.

Dallon, J.C., Sherratt, J.A., Maini, P.K., 2001. Modeling the effects of transforming growth factor-beta on extracellular matrix alignment in dermal wound repair. Wound. Repair. Regen. 9 (4), 278–286.

Eming, S.A., Krieg, T., Davidson, J.M., 2007. Inflammation in wound repair: molecular and cellular mechanisms. J. Invest. Dermatol. 127 (3), 514–525.

Freeman, T.A., Parvizi, J., Della Valle, C.J., Steinbeck, M.J., 2009. Reactive oxygen and nitrogen species induce protein and DNA modifications driving arthrofibrosis following total knee arthroplasty. Fibrogenesis Tissue Repair 2 (1), 5.

Gordon, S., 2003. Alternative activation of macrophages. Nat. Rev. Immunol. 3 (1), 23–35.

Greenhalgh, D.G., 1998. The role of apoptosis in wound healing. Int. J. Biochem. Cell. Biol. 30 (9), 1019–1030.

Healy, J.M., Lewis, S.D., Kurz, M., Boomer, R.M., Thompson, K.M., Wilson, C., et al., 2004. Pharmacokinetics and biodistribution of novel aptamer compositions. Pharm. Res. 21 (12), 2234–2246.

Hilgenbrink, A.R., Low, P.S., 2005. Folate receptor-mediated drug targeting: from therapeutics to diagnostics. J. Pharm. Sci. 94 (10), 2135–2146.

Hirayama, A., Nagase, S., Ueda, A., Oteki, T., Takada, K., Obara, M., et al., 2005. *In vivo* imaging of oxidative stress in ischemia–reperfusion renal injury using electron paramagnetic resonance. Am. J. Physiol. Renal. Physiol. 288 (3), F597–F603.

Hoemann, C.D., Chen, G., Marchand, C., Tran-Khanh, N., Thibault, M., Chevrier, A., et al., 2010. Scaffold-guided subchondral bone repair: implication of neutrophils and alternatively activated arginase-1+ macrophages. Am. J. Sports. Med. 38 (9), 1845–1856.

Hu, W.J., Eaton, J.W., Ugarova, T.P., Tang, L., 2001. Molecular basis of biomaterial-mediated foreign body reactions. Blood 98 (4), 1231–1238.

Jiang, W.W., Su, S.H., Eberhart, R.C., Tang, L., 2007. Phagocyte responses to degradable polymers. J. Biomed. Mater. Res. A. 82 (2), 492–497.

Josefsson, E., Tarkowski, A., Carlsten, H., 1992. Anti-inflammatory properties of estrogen. I. *In vivo* suppression of leukocyte production in bone marrow and redistribution of peripheral blood neutrophils. Cell. Immunol. 142 (1), 67–78.

Kaplan, S.S., Heine, R.P., Simmons, R.L., 1999. Defensins impair phagocytic killing by neutrophils in biomaterial-related infection. Infect. Immun. 67 (4), 1640–1645.

Kasahara, Y., Iwai, K., Yachie, A., Ohta, K., Konno, A., Seki, H., et al., 1997. Involvement of reactive oxygen intermediates in spontaneous and CD95 (Fas/APO-1)-mediated apoptosis of neutrophils. Blood 89 (5), 1748–1753.

Kielland, A., Blom, T., Nandakumar, K.S., Holmdahl, R., Blomhoff, R., Carlsen, H., 2009. *In vivo* imaging of reactive oxygen and nitrogen species in inflammation using the luminescent probe L-012. Free Radic. Biol. Med. 47 (6), 760–766.

Kreisel, D., Nava, R.G., Li, W., Zinselmeyer, B.H., Wang, B., Lai, J., et al., 2010. *In vivo* two-photon imaging reveals monocyte-dependent neutrophil extravasation during pulmonary inflammation. Proc. Natl. Acad. Sci. U.S.A. 107 (42), 18073–18078.

Languino, L.R., Plescia, J., Duperray, A., Brian, A.A., Plow, E.F., Geltosky, J.E., et al., 1993. Fibrinogen mediates leukocyte adhesion to vascular endothelium through an ICAM-1-dependent pathway. Cell 73 (7), 1423–1434.

Lefer, A.M., Campbell, B., Scalia, R., Lefer, D.J., 1998. Synergism between platelets and neutrophils in provoking cardiac dysfunction after ischemia and reperfusion: role of selectins. Circulation 98 (13), 1322–1328.

Lemon, G., Howard, D., Tomlinson, M.J., Buttery, L.D., Rose, F.R., Waters, S.L., et al., 2009. Mathematical modelling of tissue-engineered angiogenesis. Math. Biosci. 221 (2), 101–120.

Lindner, J.R., Song, J., Xu, F., Klibanov, A.L., Singbartl, K., Ley, K., et al., 2000. Noninvasive ultrasound imaging of inflammation using microbubbles targeted to activated leukocytes. Circulation 102 (22), 2745–2750.

Locke, L.W., Chordia, M.D., Zhang, Y., Kundu, B., Kennedy, D., Landseadel, J., et al., 2009. A novel neutrophil-specific PET imaging agent: cFLFLFK-PEG-64Cu. J. Nucl. Med. 50 (5), 790–797.

Loike, J.D., Sodeik, B., Cao, L., Leucona, S., Weitz, J.I., Detmers, P.A., et al., 1991. CD11c/CD18 on neutrophils recognizes a domain at the N terminus of the A alpha chain of fibrinogen. Proc. Natl. Acad. Sci. USA 88 (3), 1044–1048.

Low, P.S., Henne, W.A., Doorneweerd, D.D., 2008. Discovery and development of folic-acid-based receptor targeting for imaging and therapy of cancer and inflammatory diseases. Acc. Chem. Res. 41 (1), 120–129.

Mainnemare, A., Megarbane, B., Soueidan, A., Daniel, A., Chapple, I.L., 2004. Hypochlorous acid and taurine-*N*-monochloramine in periodontal diseases. J. Dent. Res. 83 (11), 823–831.

Mantzaris, N.V., Webb, S., Othmer, H.G., 2004. Mathematical modeling of tumor-induced angiogenesis. J. Math. Biol. 49 (2), 111–187.

Martinez-Pomares, L., Reid, D.M., Brown, G.D., Taylor, P.R., Stillion, R.J., Linehan, S.A., et al., 2003. Analysis of mannose receptor regulation by IL-4, IL-10, and proteolytic processing using novel monoclonal antibodies. J. Leukoc. Biol. 73 (5), 604–613.

Martinez, F.O., Sica, A., Mantovani, A., Locati, M., 2008. Macrophage activation and polarization. Front. Biosci. 13, 453–461.

McAteer, M.A., Sibson, N.R., von Zur Muhlen, C., Schneider, J.E., Lowe, A.S., Warrick, N., et al., 2007. *In vivo* magnetic resonance imaging of acute brain inflammation using microparticles of iron oxide. Nat. Med. 13 (10), 1253–1258.

McCarthy, J.R., Patel, P., Botnaru, I., Haghayeghi, P., Weissleder, R., Jaffer, F.A., 2009. Multimodal nanoagents for the detection of intravascular thrombi. Bioconjug. Chem. 20 (6), 1251–1255.

McNamara, K.P., Nguyen, T., Dumitrascu, G., Ji, J., Rosenzweig, N., Rosenzweig, Z., 2001. Synthesis, characterization, and application of fluorescence sensing lipobeads for intracellular pH measurements. Anal. Chem. 73 (14), 3240–3246.

Okusa, M.D., 2002. The inflammatory cascade in acute ischemic renal failure. Nephron 90 (2), 133–138.

Overoye-Chan, K., Koerner, S., Looby, R.J., Kolodziej, A.F., Zech, S.G., Deng, Q., et al., 2008. EP-2104R: a fibrin-specific gadolinium-based MRI contrast agent for detection of thrombus. J. Am. Chem. Soc. 130 (18), 6025–6039.

Pan, D., Caruthers, S.D., Hu, G., Senpan, A., Scott, M.J., Gaffney, P.J., et al., 2008. Ligand-directed nanobialys as theranostic agent for drug delivery and manganese-based magnetic resonance imaging of vascular targets. J. Am. Chem. Soc. 130 (29), 9186–9187.

Panizzi, P., Nahrendorf, M., Wildgruber, M., Waterman, P., Figueiredo, J.L., Aikawa, E., et al., 2009. Oxazine conjugated nanoparticle detects *in vivo* hypochlorous acid and peroxynitrite generation. J. Am. Chem. Soc. 131 (43), 15739–15744.

Reeh, P.W., Steen, K.H., 1996. Tissue acidosis in nociception and pain. Prog. Brain. Res. 113, 143–151.

Riou, L.M., Ruiz, M., Sullivan, G.W., Linden, J., Leong-Poi, H., Lindner, J.R., et al., 2002. Assessment of myocardial inflammation produced by experimental coronary occlusion and reperfusion with 99mTc-RP517, a new leukotriene B4 receptor antagonist that preferentially labels neutrophils *in vivo*. Circulation 106 (5), 592–598.

Schugart, R.C., Friedman, A., Zhao, R., Sen, C.K., 2008. Wound angiogenesis as a function of tissue oxygen tension: a mathematical model. Proc. Natl. Acad. Sci. USA 105 (7), 2628–2633.

Smiley, S.T., King, J.A., Hancock, W.W., 2001. Fibrinogen stimulates macrophage chemokine secretion through toll-like receptor 4. J. Immunol. 167 (5), 2887–2894.

Steen, K.H., Steen, A.E., Reeh, P.W., 1995. A dominant role of acid pH in inflammatory excitation and sensitization of nociceptors in rat skin, *in vitro*. J. Neurosci. 15 (5 Pt 2), 3982–3989.

Stein, M., Keshav, S., Harris, N., Gordon, S., 1992. Interleukin 4 potently enhances murine macrophage mannose receptor activity: a marker of alternative immunologic macrophage activation. J. Exp. Med. 176 (1), 287–292.

Stout, R.D., Suttles, J., 2004. Functional plasticity of macrophages: reversible adaptation to changing micro-environments. J. Leukoc. Biol. 76 (3), 509–513.

Su, J., Todorov, M., Gonzales, H.P., Perkins, L., Kojouharov, H., Weng, H., et al., 2011. A predictive tool for foreign body fibrotic reactions using 2-dimensional computational model. Open Access Bioinformatics 2011 (3), 19–35.

Suzuki, T., Kanbara, N., Tomono, T., Hayashi, N., Shinohara, I., 1984. Physicochemical and biological properties of poly(ethylene glycol)-coupled immunoglobulin G. Biochim. Biophys. Acta. 788 (2), 248–255.

Tan, M.Q., Wang, G.L., Hai, X.D., Ye, Z.Q., Yuan, J.L., 2004. Development of functionalized fluorescent europium nanoparticles for biolabeling and time-resolved fluorometric applications. J. Mater. Chem. 14 (19), 2896–2901.

Tang, L.P., Eaton, J.W., 1993. Fibrin(ogen) mediates acute inflammatory responses to biomaterials. J. Exp. Med. 178 (6), 2147–2156.

Tang, L., Eaton, J.W., 1995. Inflammatory responses to biomaterials. Am. J. Clin. Pathol. 103 (4), 466–471.

Tang, L., Eaton, J.W., 1999. Natural responses to unnatural materials: a molecular mechanism for foreign body reactions. Mol. Med. 5 (6), 351–358.

Tang, L., Lucas, A.H., Eaton, J.W., 1993. Inflammatory responses to implanted polymeric biomaterials: role of surface-adsorbed immunoglobulin G. J. Lab. Clin. Med. 122 (3), 292–300.

Tang, L., Jennings, T.A., Eaton, J.W., 1998. Mast cells mediate acute inflammatory responses to implanted biomaterials. Proc. Natl. Acad. Sci. USA 95 (15), 8841–8846.

Thevenot, P.T., Baker, D.W., Weng, H., Sun, M.W., Tang, L., 2011. The pivotal role of fibrocytes and mast cells in mediating fibrotic reactions to biomaterials. Biomaterials 32 (33), 8394–8403.

Tsai, Y.T., Zhou, J., Weng, H., Shen, J., Tang, L., Hu, W.J., 2014a. Real-time noninvasive monitoring of *in vivo* inflammatory responses using a pH ratiometric fluorescence imaging probe. Adv. Healthc Mater. 3 (2), 221–229.

Tsai, Y.T., Zhou, J., Weng, H., Tang, E.N., Baker, D.W., Tang, L., 2014b. Optical imaging of fibrin deposition to elucidate participation of mast cells in foreign body responses. Biomaterials 35 (7), 2089–2096.

van der Laken, C.J., Boerman, O.C., Oyen, W.J., van de Ven, M.T., Edwards, D.S., Barrett, J.A., et al., 1997. Technetium-99m-labeled chemotactic peptides in acute infection and sterile inflammation. J. Nucl. Med. 38 (8), 1310–1315.

Wang, L., Yang, C., Tan, W., 2005. Dual-luminophore-doped silica nanoparticles for multiplexed signaling. Nano. Lett. 5 (1), 37–43.

Weng, H., Zhou, J., Tang, L., Hu, Z., 2004. Tissue responses to thermally-responsive hydrogel nanoparticles. J. Biomater. Sci. Polym. Ed. 15 (9), 1167–1180.

Whiteman, M., Spencer, J.P., 2008. Loss of 3-chlorotyrosine by inflammatory oxidants: implications for the use of 3-chlorotyrosine as a bio-marker *in vivo*. Biochem. Biophys. Res. Commun. 371 (1), 50–53.

Xiao, L., Zhang, Y., Liu, Z., Yang, M., Pu, L., Pan, D., 2010. Synthesis of the Cyanine 7 labeled neutrophil-specific agents for noninvasive near infrared fluorescence imaging. Bioorg. Med. Chem. Lett. 20 (12), 3515–3517.

Xu, H., Aylott, J.W., Kopelman, R., Miller, T.J., Philbert, M.A., 2001. A real-time ratiometric method for the determination of molecular oxygen inside living cells using sol-gel-based spherical optical nanosensors with applications to rat C6 glioma. Anal. Chem. 73 (17), 4124–4133.

Zhang, Y., Xiao, L., Chordia, M.D., Locke, L.W., Williams, M.B., Berr, S.S., et al., 2010. Neutrophil targeting heterobivalent SPECT imaging probe: cFLFLF-PEG-TKPPR-99mTc. Bioconjug. Chem. 21 (10), 1788–1793.

Zhou, J., Tsai, Y.T., Weng, H., Baker, D.W., Tang, L., 2011. Real time monitoring of biomaterial-mediated inflammatory responses via macrophage-targeting NIR nanoprobes. Biomaterials 32 (35), 9383–9390.

Zhou, J., Tsai, Y.T., Weng, H., Tang, L., 2012a. Noninvasive assessment of localized inflammatory responses. Free Radic. Biol. Med. 52 (1), 218–226. PMCID: 3249500.

Zhou, J., Tsai, Y.T., Weng, H., Tang, E.N., Nair, A., Dave, D.P., et al., 2012b. Real-time detection of implant-associated neutrophil responses using a formyl peptide receptor-targeting NIR nanoprobe. Int. J. Nanomedicine. 7, 2057–2068.

Zhuang, H., Alavi, A., 2002. 18-fluorodeoxyglucose positron emission tomographic imaging in the detection and monitoring of infection and inflammation. Semin. Nucl. Med. 32 (1), 47–59.

INDEX

Note: Page numbers followed by "*f*" and "*t*" refer to figures and tables, respectively.

Printed in the United States
By Bookmasters